Etched in Hope

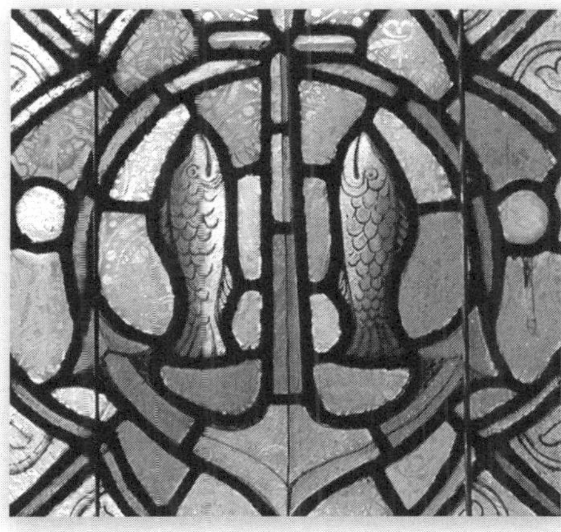

In the service of love, only the wounded soldier can serve.

Thorton Wilder

Etched in Hope

A weekly journal
for those living with or affected by
HIV/AIDS

Paul J. Ashton

acta
PUBLICATIONS

Dedicated in honor of my grandmother Ruth and mother Nancy,
whose examples anchored my heart to the ministry of love's service.

Etched in Hope
A weekly journal for those living with or affected by HIV/AIDS
by Paul J. Ashton

Edited by Gregory F. Augustine Pierce
Cover Design by Tom A. Wright
Text design and typesetting by Patricia Lynch

Published by ACTA Publications, 5559 W. Howard Street, Skokie, IL 60077-2621, (800) 397-2282, www.actapublications.com

ISBN: 978-0-87946-344-1

Printed in the United States of America by Versa Press

Year 15 14 13 12 11 10 09 08 07
Printing 15 14 13 12 11 10 9 8 7 6 5 4 3 2 First

Contents

Introduction
Week 1: Go Gently
Week 2: Our Bodies Are True Temples
Week 3: Reframing Your Life
Week 4: Finding Peace and Meaning in Suffering
Week 5: Courage and Bravery
Week 6: All Are Welcome Here
Week 7: Humility
Week 8: Knowing Our Limitations
Week 9: Streams in the Desert
Week 10: Do What You Love
Week 11: Discernment
Week 12: The Most Powerful Beginning Is Choice
Week 13: Determination
Week 14: Searching to Know God
Weel 15: Getting Involved
Week 16: Respecting the Choices of Others
Week 17: Unity in Diversity
Week 18: Interdependence
Week 19: Hanging by a Thread
Week 20: Christ Has No Hands but Ours
Week 21: Seeing and Believing
Week 22: Fear
Week 23: Confronting Skills
Week 24: Recognizing and Using Our Talents
Week 25: Remembering
Week 26: Simplify
Week 27: Excuses
Week 28: Beginning Anew
Week 29: Cookies and Milk
Week 30: An Attitude of Gratitude
Week 31: Full Disclosure
Week 32: Confronting Stigmas
Week 33: Saying No
Week 34: Flight/Fight/Community
Week 35: Love as a Verb
Week 36: Sanctuary
Week 37: Victim Solidarity
Week 38: Survivor Solidarity
Week 39: Thriving
Week 40: Faith through Others
Week 41: Spirituality
Week 42: Religion
Week 43: Replaying Tapes
Week 44: Loneliness/Aloneness
Week 45: Negative Self-Talk
Week 46: Just as I Am
Week 47: Challenging Friendship
Week 48: Prayer
Week 49: Forgiveness and Peace
Week 50: Kidding Ourselves
Week 51: Confidentiality
Week 52: Rejoice in Hope
Acknowledgments
About the Author

Introduction

Etched in ten-inch frosted print on a twelve-foot-high mirror were four letters forming the simple word HOPE. If you looked too quickly, you would miss it. Hundreds of people walked by it, but few stopped to admire it, except to steal a glance at their outfit in the mirror. The mirror sat on the wall of the dance floor of a huge auditorium and reflected the gyrating bodies of the motliest crowd ever gathered. There were infants dancing in their parents' arms and elderly couples gliding across the dance floor using canes and walkers. There were people dancing in wheelchairs and with crutches. There were beautiful people and not so beautiful people of every age, creed, color and background imaginable. All these people were there for one reason: to raise money to help eliminate AIDS.

This dance-a-thon fundraiser was the first of many I have attended since the mid-eighties, and it remains one of the most memorable. The word HOPE etched in that mirror has forever haunted my mind. That mirror reflected the dreams of the many people there suffering with HIV/AIDS: the need to be accepted, loved and freed from the stigma of their illness. It also reflected the pain and the sorrow of mothers, fathers, sisters, brothers, aunts, uncles, cousins, husbands, wives, lovers, and friends of those with HIV/AIDS.

I watched the mirror reflect joy, excitement and intense happiness as songs like Sister Sledge's "We Are Family" echoed throughout the room and witnessed tears and hugs being mirrored in waltzing embraces to Dionne Warwick's "That's What Friends Are For." What I thought then is what I think now: "These men and women are saints. Nothing stops them from serving their brothers and sisters. Thank God for them. They are HOPE for the hopeless."

This fifty-two-week journal is designed to help those living with HIV/AIDS and those who love them in two ways. The first is to offer readers a source of inspiration and reflection. The second is to offer a simple way to work on various issues.

I know from personal experience how difficult it is for people to stick with things, so this little workbook is written so you may pick it up at any point in your life, put it down, and then pick it up again when you need the boost of HOPE. You can journey through it alone, with a friend or loved one, or as part of a group. You can use it for your own needs, whether your are living with HIV/AIDS yourself or care for and about someone who is. It is intended to be a blessing, not a burden to your life.

Each weekly entry contains five parts:

- A reflection meant to enlighten and stir things up. The reflections are to remind us of the issues we all face and the gifts and talents we already possess.
- A mini-biography of a saint or holy person whose life mirrors God's love in practical, concrete ways. Although there are thousands of such people, I chose these diverse fifty-two with the hope that they would speak to a wide audience.

- An inspiring passage from Scripture for you to ponder.
- A challenging quote of the week from someone who understands life in a mighty way.
- An activity that gently nudges us to action. Pages of this workbook are perforated so that the activity pages can be easily removed.

My prayer is that this workbook will prove helpful to some people struggling to live with HIV/AIDS. If it does, the glory belongs to God, who has etched HOPE into each of our hearts:

> God of all hope, you call us to be one with you, yet we fear that we are never worthy enough. Fill us with the grace we need to discover nourishing streams in the people, places and things you send into our lives. Allow us to be aware of our worthiness and give us the courage to thrive. Help us transform the darkness of our pain into blinding and healing light, and continue to fill us with the ability to laugh and rejoice in the face of every anxiety that causes us fear. Remind us that we do not journey alone but with you, who transforms our doubts and fears into trust and acceptance. We rejoice in the deep and certain hope of eternal life, while clinging fast to the anchors that bind us to you in the here and now. Amen.

Paul J. Ashton
Boston, Massachusetts

WEEK 1

Go Gently

Taking a page from an imaginary book called *The Loving Care Manual for Mothers*, a book most mothers seem to read and follow, we choose to start this first week of reflections and activities gently. We put aside the expectations and desires others have for us and concentrate on our own. Without protest, we approach the newness of the endeavor by gingerly placing ourselves under the guidance of Mary, Mother of Good Counsel. We know that we control only what we can control, and we ask her to do the rest. We deserve her help. We need it. We operate better when we accept it.

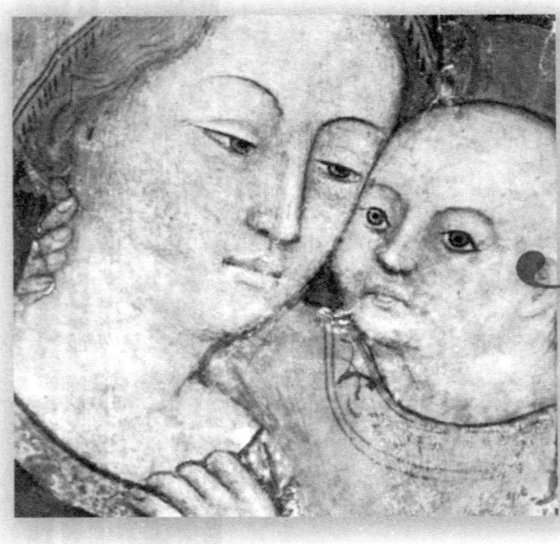

When this year of journaling gets tough, we can turn back to this page and remind ourselves, "Go gently, as Mother Mary would have us do."

Mary, Mother of Good Counsel

There is nothing like a mother's love, care and concern. Through Mary, as the "Mother of Good Counsel," we can find the love we need to live our lives with fullness and joy, even in the face of AIDS/HIV, for with her love comes guidance. Few of us like to be told what to do, but sooner or later we must admit that we need help. Devotion to Mary as the Mother of Good Counsel is centuries old and has been a comfort for many who have sought her wisdom. Turning to her is a comfort like no other. Mother is always right.

Isaiah 30:15

In quietness and in trust shall be your strength.

Quote for the Week

When people care for you and cry for you,
they can straighten out your soul.

Langston Hughes

Activity

Find fifteen minutes to half an hour and do nothing and say nothing. Just think about your mother. If you have had a good relationship with her, think about what she might advise you now. If not, ask Jesus to share his mother with you and listen to her. Write below things your hear mother saying to you. This week think about your mother at least a few minutes each day.

What Mother Is Telling Me

1.

2.

3.

4.

5.

6.

7.

WEEK 2

Our Bodies Are True Temples

We need to take care of our bodies, for they are true temples of God. To tend a garden means to find the right proportion of water, sunshine and nutrients so that full growth potential is maximized. If our own bodies are like a garden that needs tending, what are we overlooking and what needs our attention this week? Sometimes when we are immersed in the work of dealing with AIDS/HIV, we can forget to eat and to nourish ourselves. If we take a natural break to sit and eat with others, we allow them to help bandage the wounds that are hard for us to reach. We may even find that the answer to our most pressing concerns is right at our fingertips. Saint Basil understood this truth.

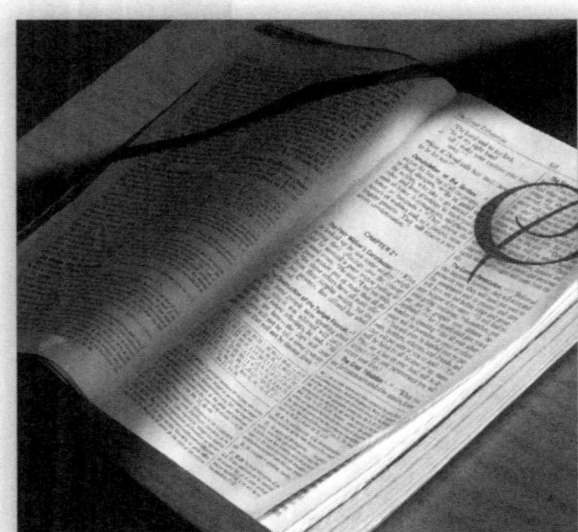

Saint Basil

An extremely intelligent man who came from a family of saints and nobility, Basil gave up his wealth to attend to the needs of the poor. His scholarly works are many and his theological contribution to the church is exemplary; however, he is best known for preaching that we can never bring people to God until they are no longer hungry, tired or wounded. Basil teaches us much about attending to our physical bodies first.

Psalm 147:3

He heals the broken-hearted and binds up their wounds.

Quote for the Week

Everyone who is born holds dual citizenship
in the kingdom of the well
and in the kingdom of the sick.

Susan Sontag

Activity

Fill in the schedule below for a typical day. Look at it. Did you allot time each day for food, fun, rest, relaxation, spiritual re-energizing, physical exercise, and interaction with those you love? Fix your schedule below to allow time for these things this week.

6:00 a.m.	
7:00 a.m.	
8:00 a.m.	
9:00 a.m.	
10:00 a.m.	
11:00 a.m.	
noon	
1:00 p.m.	
2:00 p.m.	
3:00 p.m.	
4:00 p.m.	
5:00 p.m.	
6:00 p.m.	
7:00 p.m.	
8:00 p.m.	
9:00 p.m.	
10:00 p.m.	
11:00 p.m.	
midnight	

WEEK 3

Reframing Your Life

Reframing our life situation is at the same time both simple and profound. You may stand in awe when you view a beautifully finished watercolor, but what you do not see are the artist's hours of frustration and the determination to get the hues of light and sand just right. It is hard work, requiring practice and perseverance and often starting over. Let us look at our lives as we deal with AIDS/HIV as an opportunity to reframe our entire lives—taking what we have and beginning anew, looking at our lives in new, different and fulfilling ways. Saint Elizabeth Ann Seton certainly had this ability.

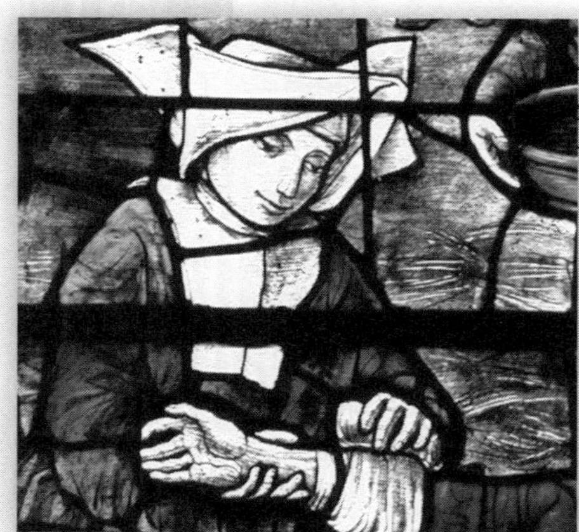

Saint Elizabeth Ann Seton

Elizabeth Ann Seton is a model for every American woman. This strong, determined pioneer woman experienced many changes in her life and accepted them with a zest like few others have demonstrated. A wife and mother of five children, she had a special interest in helping children, especially poor children. She recognized needs in her community and worked to fulfill them. After being widowed, she founded the Sisters of Charity, a religious community whose mission is to educate poor children. Her good works live on through these Sisters and many other women who have taken up her cause. She certainly reframed her life several times.

Hebrews 12:12

Therefore lift your drooping hands and strengthen your weak knees, and make straight paths for your feet, so that what is lame may not be put out of joint, but rather be healed.

Quote for the Week

Life is a process where people mix and match,
fall apart and come together.

Nikki Giovanni

Activity

Make a list of five things you can no longer do because of changes in your life brought about by dealing with AIDS/HIV. Now try to reframe them, to approach them from a different angle. This week, apply one of these new approaches and see how it works. (For example, you may no longer be able to run 10 miles a day, but perhaps you can walk with a friend or a pet around the block or through a park each day.)

What I Can't Do Anymore	What I Could Do If I Tried
1.	
2.	
3.	
4.	
5.	

WEEK 4

Finding Peace and Meaning in Suffering

Finding peace and meaning in suffering is a challenge that confronts all of us, as it did Saint John Neumann. It is often difficult to see how we can draw strength from suffering, but it always seems to be the case. We endure one more injection, take one more medication, survive one more uncomfortable medical test, embrace one more x-ray, and we gain strength from the very act of doing so. Our trials and pains can somehow allow us to find peace and meaning if we look to the cross to gain just one more moment of courage and endurance. The prayer we share at the Good Friday service states it best: "We worship you Lord; we venerate your cross; we praise your resurrection. Through the cross you brought joy to the world."

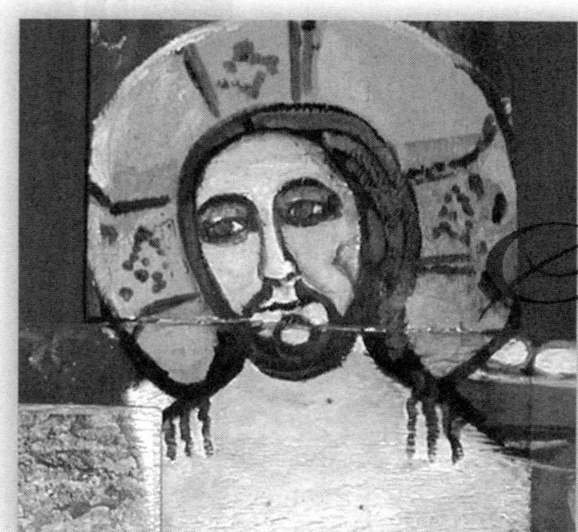

Saint John Neumann

John Neumann was born in Germany. He immigrated to the United States and began serving other immigrants in remote regions of New York State. In 1842, he took vows as a Redemptorist father and continued his work among immigrants in Baltimore. In 1852, he was consecrated Bishop of Philadelphia, where he continued his prodigious and exhausting ministry to poor and immigrant people. *Passio Christi, conforta me!* ("Passion of Christ, strengthen me!") was John Neumann's personal motto. He found that his own lack of physical health helped him to more fully appreciate the passion and suffering that Jesus experienced. In turn, this gave him a greater insight into the sufferings of others and propelled him to teach and minister through his own experience.

1 Peter 2:24

He himself bore our sins in his body on the cross....
By his wounds you have been healed.

Quote for the Week

Hearts live by being wounded.

Oscar Wilde

Activity

Make a list of the things in your life that overwhelm you right now. Rework the list by placing them in the three columns below. How can you make changes to accept what can't be changed, work on changing the things that can be changed, and forget the rest? Now circle one item in column one and work on changing it this week.

What Can Be Changed	What Cannot Be Changed	Who Cares, Really?

WEEK 5

Courage and Bravery

Courage and bravery come to us when we face the demons of our lives as Martin Luther King, Jr., certainly did. At those times, when we close our eyes, we see a glimmer of light somewhere, somehow, and hold fast to that pinpoint of light. Courage comes from within, but it is reinforced by those people who surround us. Don't worry if you cannot see them; they are there. They come in familiar uniforms or odd disguises. You will recognize them in a kind word, warm gesture, or thoughtful look when you least expect but most appreciate it. They give us courage to stand up for who we are and what we believe.

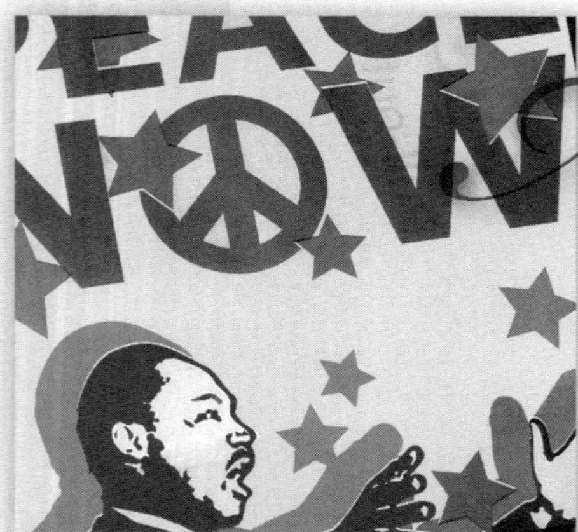

Martin Luther King, Jr.

Many have worked for a cause, but few have effected the range of change that Dr. Martin Luther King, Jr. brought upon the world. The price he paid for standing up and preaching an end to racism was his death. Yet his mission continues to be fought today by thousands if not millions of unnamed and unsung heroes who have found new meaning in the courage and bravery of his example. Martin Luther King, Jr., preached an unpopular message in a way few others could, and he left a legacy that changed the world. For this reason, we can include him in the pantheon of our saints.

John 16:33

I have said this to you, so that in me you may have peace. In the world you face persecution. But take courage; I have conquered the world!

Quote for the Week

Sometimes even to live is an act of courage.

Seneca

Activity

What is the one legacy that you would like to be remembered for? Write it down below in big, bold letters. Underneath it, write the names of five people who are already working on this same concern—either friends or those in public life. This week do one thing to further deepen and develop this mission in your life.

My Legacy

Who Is Working on This Goal as Well?

1.
2.
3.
4.
5.

WEEK 6

All Are Welcome Here

One of the saddest moments in my ministry with the HIV/AIDS community occurred in the mid-1980s, when an IV drug user came to one of our support group meetings. After she explained who she was and the challenges she faced in her life, many in the group were uncomfortable. One person said, "Don't you think you would be better off in a meeting with other drug users?" As a facilitator, I was shocked and speechless. I felt very bad for our newest member. Finally, it was the the voice of another group member, a mother who had recently lost her son, that broke the dreadful silence. She proclaimed, "The mission statement we read each week says, *All are welcome here.*" Saint John Bosco welcomed everyone into his ministry.

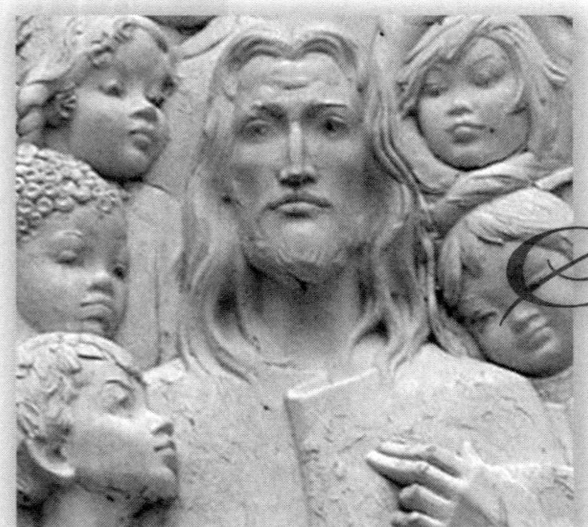

Saint John Bosco

John Bosco devoted his life to the care and education of children. The schools he established worldwide used a threefold approach — "reason, religion and kindness" — to educate the young. In his memoirs, he tells of a dream he had as a youngster that greatly influenced his life. In his dream, he saw a group of young boys arguing and fighting. John Bosco tried to stop the fighting but ended up being drawn into the melee. A man appeared nearby and said, *"Bonta!"* — Italian for "kindness!" John Bosco realized that only through kindness would he be able to bring peace and change to the lives of homeless children. His good works are continued today through the two religious communities he founded, the Salesians and the Daughters of Mary, Help of Christians.

Matthew 18:5

Whoever welcomes one such child in my name welcomes me.

Quote for the Week

Jesus began to do before he began to preach.

Saint John Bosco

Activity

Write down the names of people in your life you have ignored or even mistreated lately. This week, go out of your way to give each of them some sign of kindness—a note, a smile, a phone call, a nod, a simple "hello."

People I Have Ignored or Mistreated

1. ____________________

2. ____________________

3. ____________________

4. ____________________

5. ____________________

6. ____________________

7. ____________________

8. ____________________

9. ____________________

10. ____________________

WEEK 7 Humility

Reaching out to others is not only the privilege of the spiritual, gifted and famous. Extending outside our own zone of comfort, reaching beyond our perceived limits, and forgetting our own inadequacies are the hallmarks of a person who lives with humility. Those with humility offer themselves just as they are, no matter what. We can learn much from people like Saint Bridget. Acceptance of who we are should not limit how we treat others. We can actually save the world if we learn to act out of our own self-awareness and through our own humility.

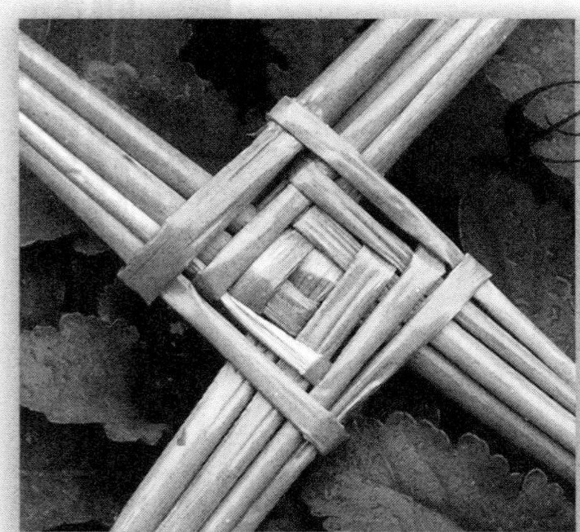

Saint Bridget

According to legend, Bridget, a friend of Saint Patrick, became a nun at an early age. She devoted her life to charitable works and to developing and sharing her spirituality. Bridget founded a school whose artists produced the famous illuminated manuscript *The Book of Kildare*. Many miracles are attributed to the intercession of Saint Bridget, but it is her humility that has led many to the God she loved and served so well throughout her whole life.

Colossians 3:12

As God's chosen ones, holy and beloved, clothe yourselves with compassion, kindness, humility, meekness, and patience.

Quote for the Week

Everyone must row with the oars he or she has.

English Proverb

Activity

Name and describe three gifts or talents that others have recognized in you but you have been hesitant to claim. This week, make a conscious effort to share one of these gifts with someone who will benefit from it, but do so with self-awareness and humility.

Gift One

Gift Two

Gift Three

WEEK 8

Knowing Our Limitations

Knowing our limitations is an on-going journey of discovery. Some days we can climb mountains; other days we can take just a couple of steps. Accepting the uncertainty of our limitations is hard, depressing, bothersome, and often disappointing. But it is something we must accept, live with, and get to know all too well. Yet we can't let our limitations become the center of our life. We must accomplish what we can and leave what we cannot to another day, spending our energy doing the things that last, as Saint Valentine did so well.

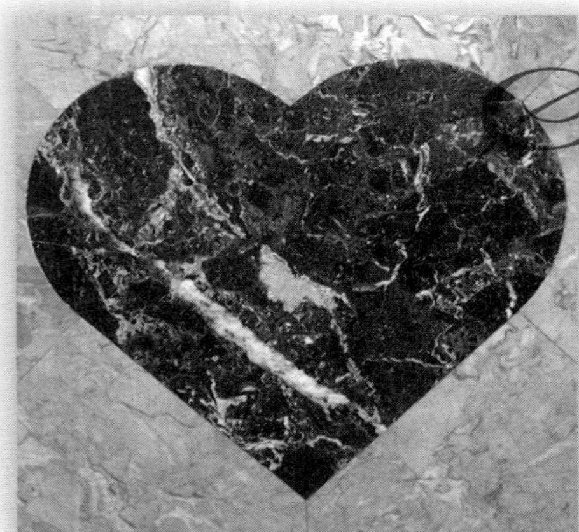

Saint Valentine

Valentine lived in the third century in Rome, a time when Christians were considered traitors to the empire because they refused to worship the gods of Rome, including the emperor. It was not easy to be a Christian back then. Valentine was both a priest and a bishop, and he preached the word of God whenever and however he could. Finally, he was arrested for secretly officiating at marriages, which is why he is the patron saint of lovers. The emperor was at first fascinated by this gentle man of faith and made him his guest, but when Valentine tried to convert the emperor he was martyred.

Psalm 121:1-2

I lift up my eyes to the hills,
from where will my help come?
My help comes from the Lord,
who made heaven and earth.

Quote for the Week

God will not look you over for medals, degrees or diplomas, but for scars!

Elbert Hubbard

Activity In the first column below, write a list of things you think you must do. In the second column, write a list of things you want to do. Compare the lists. What do they teach you? Pick one thing from each list this week and try to accomplish it.

Must Do	Want to Do

WEEK 9 Streams in the Desert

When we are in a dry spell and find ourselves thirsting, nothing quenches that longing like a cool, glass of water. "Streams in the desert" is the promise that God gives all who are in the midst of arid and lifeless days and nights. Where can we find the life-giving springs of water? If we look closely at our everyday relationships, we find glimpses of these pools. We might need to rethink our relationships, but the life-giving water is there. Sometimes we mistrust ourselves and others and think these streams of water are mirages in a hopeless situation, sent to fool us and make us even thirstier. But they are real, if we but stop and drink. Soon we will realize that we are a stream for others as well, as Saint Katherine Drexel was.

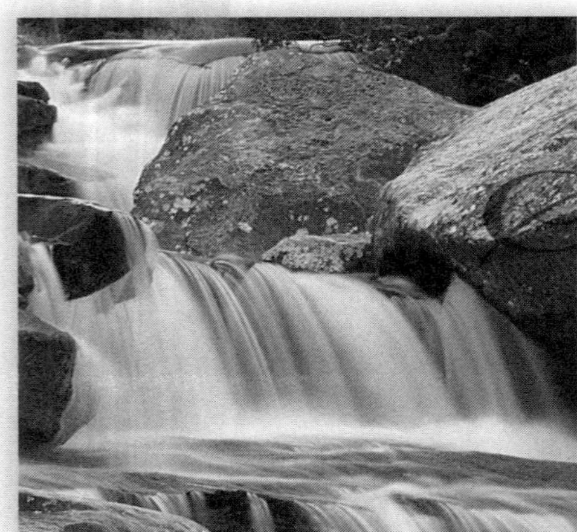

Saint Katherine Drexel

Katherine Drexel, raised in a prominent Baltimore family, could not help but notice the needs of others around her, especially Africans and Native Americans. She initially donated money to improve their well-being, but soon she realized that she should do more. Katherine dedicated her life to the benefit of the needy. She founded the Sisters of the Blessed Sacrament to help her accomplish this critical work. At her death in 1955, 63 schools were staffed by over 500 sisters whose mission was to minister to African-American and Native American children throughout the United States.

Isaiah 35:6

Then the lame shall leap like a deer, and the tongue of the speechless sing for joy. For waters shall break forth in the wilderness, and streams in the desert.

Quote for the Week

There is no hope of joy except in human relations.

Antoine Saint-Exupery

Activity

List your favorite comfort foods and drinks below. Treat yourself to at least one of them this week. Find a friend to share your treat with you.

My Favorite Comfort Foods/Drinks

1. ____________________
2. ____________________
3. ____________________
4. ____________________
5. ____________________
6. ____________________
7. ____________________
8. ____________________
9. ____________________
10. ____________________

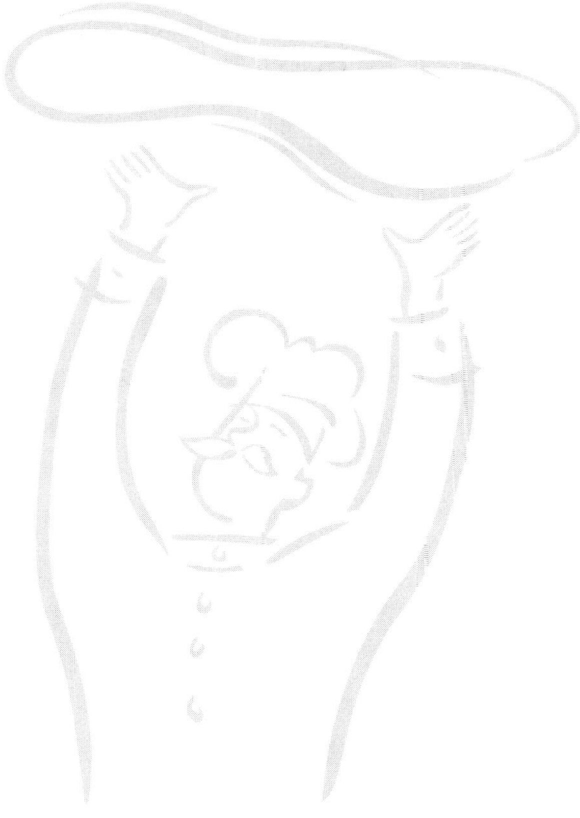

Friend I Will Share with This Week

____

Name

WEEK 10

Do What You Love

We must know what we love. This is hard for some people because society does not always support our talents and our desires to do the things that give us life and energy. Affirmation of gifts and talents is scarce in a world where material success is valued most. So it takes courage and determination to seek out and stick to the "loves" we have in our life — courage like Saint Casimir exhibited with his own family. If our passion is writing poetry, painting, playing a musical instrument, woodworking, computer programming, cooking, athletics, trivia, or something else, we need to reacquaint ourselves with that activity. We need to do what we love, even if it means giving up something others see as more important.

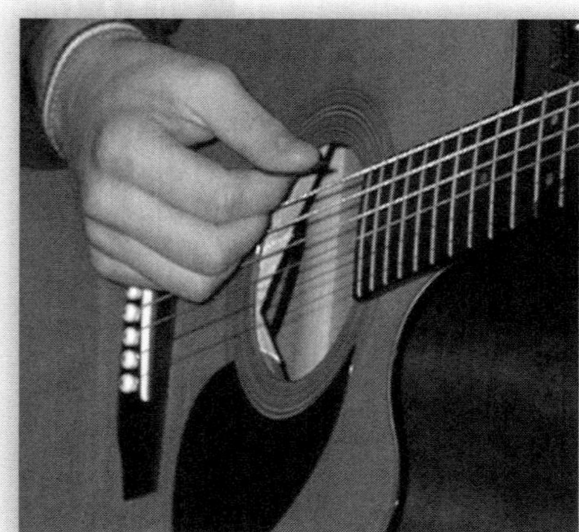

Saint Casimir

Casimir, son of King Casimir IV of Poland, was the third child of thirteen. His predetermined role was to support and cement his father's political position throughout central Europe in the fifteenth century. Along with royal position and wealth, however, Casimir was also filled with a strong faith. He placed his first loyalties with God, despite threats and punishment from his father, and he worked with the poor and needy in his country. Casimir was eventually exiled by his father and died at age 24 of a lung disease he acquired while in exile. He died without wealth or the trappings of fortune, but he experienced the peace that cannot be replaced by anything else: He died being faithful to what he believed and doing what he loved.

Proverbs 15:15

All the days of the poor are hard, but a cheerful heart has a continual feast.

Quote for the Week

It is neither wealth nor splendor,
but tranquility and occupation,
which gives happiness.
Thomas Jefferson

Activity

List things you love doing below. Put a check by any of them that someone has discouraged you from doing, because of an illness or some other reason. During this week, pick one of those and just do it!

	Things I Love to Do	Been Discouraged from Doing It? (check)
1.	______________________	☐
2.	______________________	☐
3.	______________________	☐
4.	______________________	☐
5.	______________________	☐
6.	______________________	☐
7.	______________________	☐
8.	______________________	☐
9.	______________________	☐
10.	______________________	☐

WEEK 11 Discernment

It is a difficult process to discern the path or direction that our life should take. There are many roads to choose and many paths to follow. Often, we seem to be on a path that was laid before us and keep going along without thought or question. When we ask, "Is this the right path for me?" we feel overwhelmed with the thought of starting over again and finding another way. Sometimes, the journey is interrupted by illness or hurt or a broken relationship. Life often seems like a journey with no road map. Saint John of God certainly experienced a life that followed many roads and paths. Then he discovered the road that was right for him and made the decision to follow it. We can do the same, although the new road may take us to places we might never have traveled or places we fear or avoid.

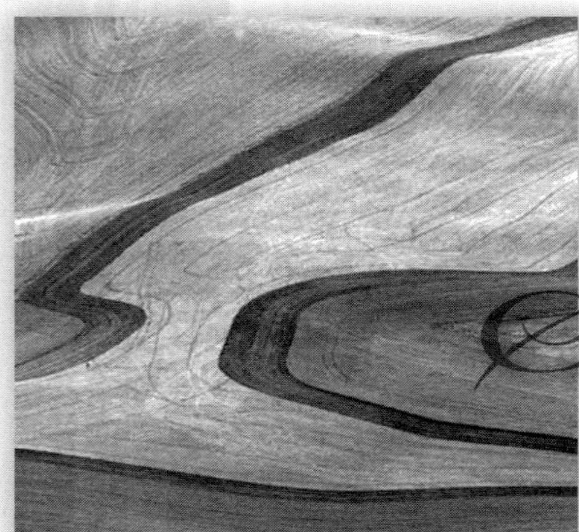

Saint John of God

The life journey of John of God was interesting and dramatic. He spent his youth as a shepherd, and he lived a wild life. Later, he became a soldier who traveled the countryside as a mercenary. He was briefly hospitalized in an insane asylum before he became a servant to a noble family that had been exiled to Africa. Because of his experiences, he had great compassion for those in difficult situations. In his forties, John changed his life and began helping the sick, the poor, and the homeless. The two religious communities he founded, the Order of Charity and the Order of Hospitallers of Saint John of God, continue his work to this day.

Jeremiah 29:13-14

When you search for me, you will find me; if you seek me with all your heart, I will let you find me, says the Lord, and I will restore your fortunes and gather you from all the nations and all the places where I have driven you, says the Lord, and I will bring you back to the place from which I sent you into exile.

Quote for the Week

Until the deer tried to clear the fence,
he thought himself a donkey.

Gregory Pierce,
with acknowledgment to Arthur Guterman

Activity

At the fork in the road below, write two options in your life right now. Spend the week thinking about which is the best for you, perhaps discussing it with a friend or loved one. At the end of the week, make your decision.

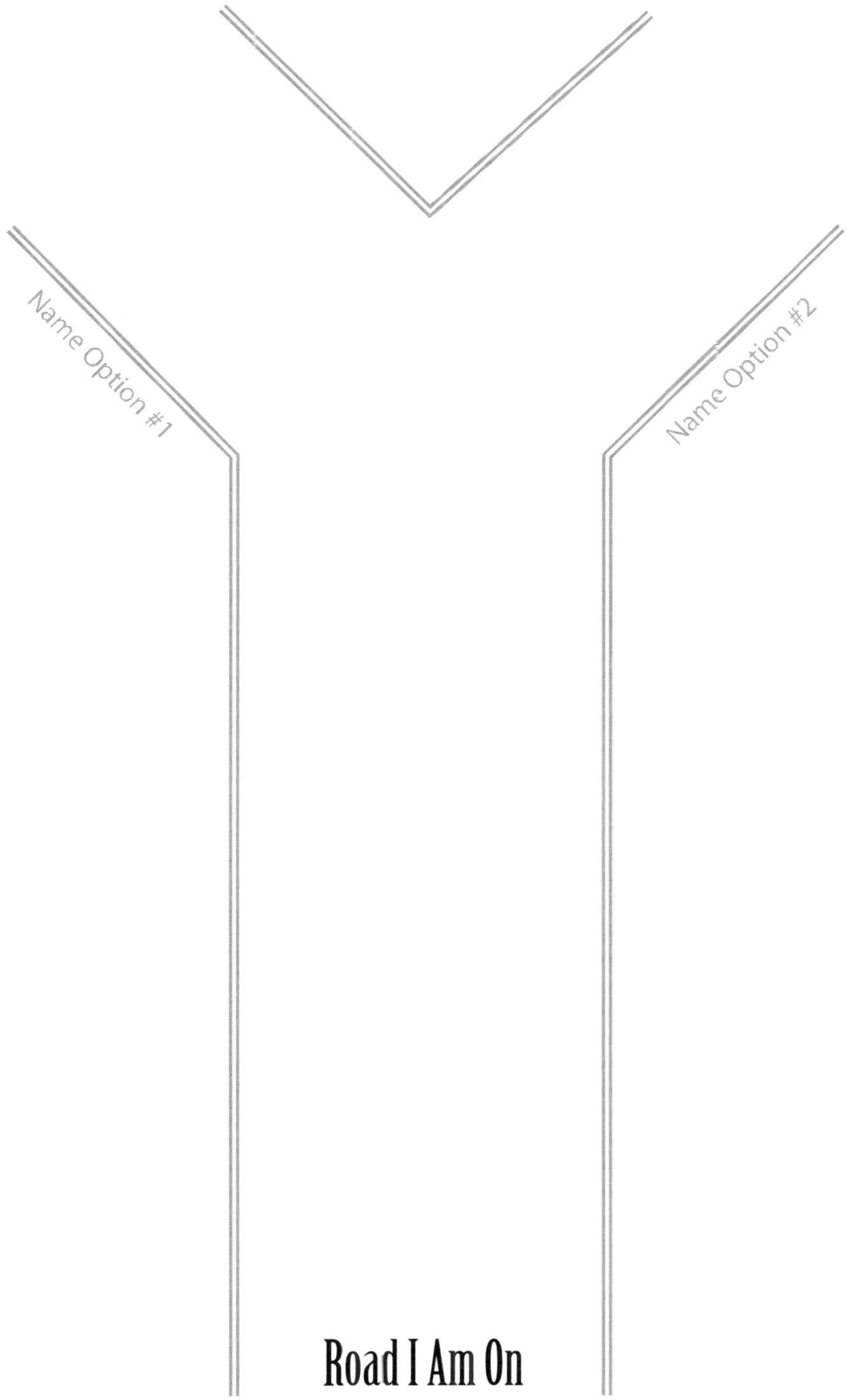

WEEK 12 The Most Powerful Beginning Is Choice

It has been said that "the most powerful beginning is choice." It is a powerful experience to choose from the options before us, to choose from the changes that confront us, before the ability to choose is taken away. To be in control over our own life, body, health and spirituality is the goal of every person. Sometimes fighting change is necessary, because it helps us to accept or own the change when it happens. One person with HIV/AIDS says his doctor wants him to take his medication every day at noon, but he says, "I take it at 3:00 pm. It works better for me at that time. What does the doctor know anyway?" As with Saint Joseph, many changes in our life are largely out of our hands, but we can at least control the little choices that make the bigger ones tolerable.

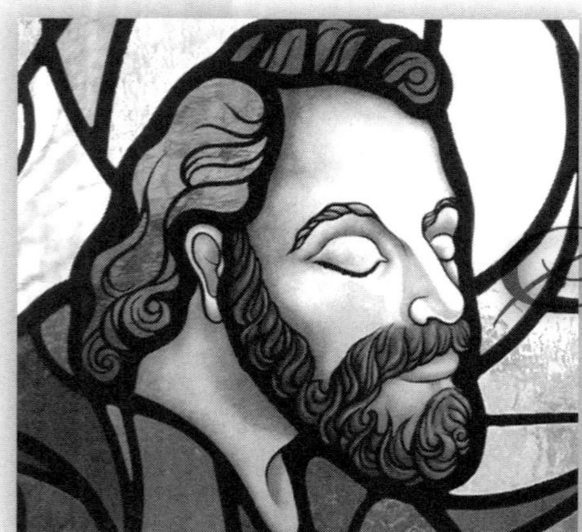

Saint Joseph

We know very little about Joseph, the husband of Mary and foster father of Jesus. We do know that he was a man of simple yet profound faith, a man who listened to God and tried to do God's will. He chose to respond to the news of Mary's pregnancy by bringing her into his home rather than having her sent away in disgrace. Joseph put the needs of others ahead of his own—obeying the emperor's order to go to Bethlehem to register for the census, even though his wife was pregnant; taking his family to Egypt when they were in danger, and bringing them home when things were safe; bringing his child to Jerusalem to pray, and finding the boy when he was lost. He was not always in control of his circumstances, but he was always in control of his response.

Job 34:4

Let us choose what is right;
let us determine among ourselves what is good.

Quote for the Week

AIDS may take my body,
but I refuse to give it my spirit.
Chelsie

Activity

In the columns below, list words that describe you as you are and that describe you as you'd like to be. Circle the words that are in both columns. During the week, try to work on ways to build on those aspects of yourself.

	The Way I Am	The Way I'd Like to Be
1.		
2.		
3.		
4.		
5.		
6.		
7.		
8.		
9.		
10.		

WEEK 13 Determination

Determination is the thing that gets us through difficult times. Finishing a task, completing a medical trial, reading a good book, writing a long overdue letter, or making a promised visit to someone can give us great gratification. When we are determined to get something completed, regardless of obstacles, we focus on the end and not the beginning. Sometimes the end seems too far away, and we become discouraged and give up. Like Bishop Oscar Romero, however, we cannot be discouraged by those who hate our efforts, mock us, or try to keep us down. Like him, we need to move toward our goal. Even when we are discouraged, we must have faith in our determination.

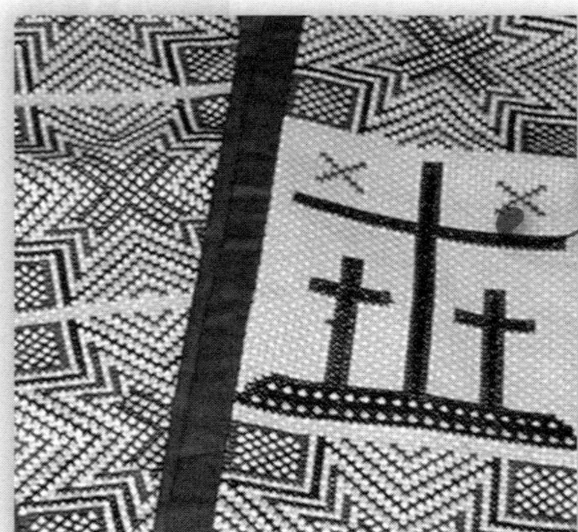

Archbishop Oscar Romero

"We must not love ourselves so much as to avoid getting involved in the risks of life that history demands of us." Oscar Romero, Archbishop of El Salvador, spoke these words moments before he was assassinated while he was celebrating the Eucharist. Archbishop Romero's life was not the stuff of most saints and martyrs. He was hated by the El Salvadoran government because he would not back down on his criticism of those in power. Yet El Salvadoran rebels opposed him because he steadfastly preached his support for the right of peasants to organize co-operatives rather than participate in violent revolution. He was determined never to turn his back on the poor, and it cost him his life. It was this determination that makes him a "saint of the people."

Hebrews 2:18

Because he himself was tested by what he suffered,
he is able to help those who are being tested.

Quote for the Week

I am only one but I am one.
I cannot do everything, but I can do something;
and what I can do, that I ought to do;
and what I ought to do, by the grace of God I shall do.

Edward Everett Hale

Activity

Recall below something you tried to accomplish recently that was successful and something that was not. Under each, write what happened and how you felt. This week, think about the determination in you that made the difference.

Successful	Unsuccessful
What it was:	
______________________	______________________
What happened:	
______________________	______________________
How I felt:	
______________________	______________________

WEEK 14 Searching to Know God

Your relationship with God is personal, but sharing with others who God is for you can be a wonderful experience. God can be found in the ordinary persons, places and things of our everyday lives. The search is not so much a theological quest as it is a day-to-day journey of discovery. High-powered conversations with your family, friends and neighbors about religion and theology are not necessary. Rather, simply sharing with others the cycle of life events that draw you together is what is important. Saint Julie Billiart's search for God was not hindered by the horrors of revolution or the challenges she faced as a paralyzed woman. She sought God through very difficult times—sometimes the perfect situation in which to start a search.

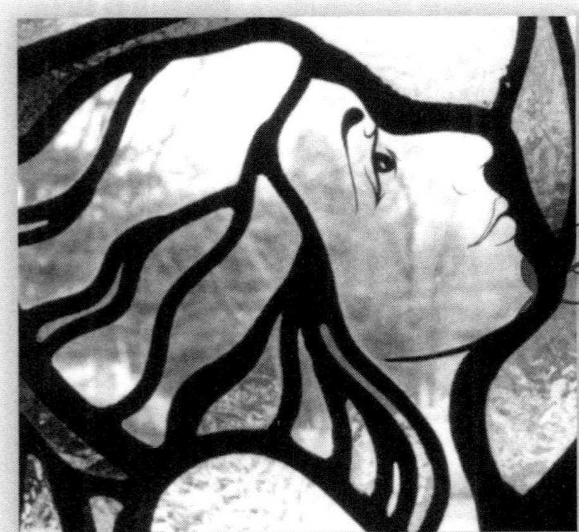

Saint Julie Billiart

Saint Julie Billiart founded the Sisters of Notre Dame de Namur, a congregation of teachers in France. She struggled twenty-two years with the pain of paralysis and endured assassination attempts on the life of her father. Julie offered her home as a safe haven to priests during the French Revolution and managed to escape capture and execution by the revolutionaries. She cared for the needy children she saw around her. Her search for God in a time of war, poverty and oppression included all those in her circle and beyond it. She found inspiration in her motto, "How good is the good God!" Many continue to live by that motto today.

Psalm 95:6-7

O come, let us worship and bow down, let us kneel before the Lord, our Maker!
For he is our God, and we are the people of his pasture, and the sheep of his hand.
O that today you would listen to his voice!

Quote for the Week

Wherever we go, whatever we do,
self is the sole subject we study and learn.
Ralph Waldo Emerson

Activity

Write a letter to yourself from God, asking all the questions you want answered. If you feel comfortable, share your letter with a minister, friend or loved one this week.

Dear God,

I believe. Help my unbelief. Here are some questions I have for you:

1. ______________________________
____

2. ______________________________
____

3. ______________________________
____

4. ______________________________
____

5. ______________________________
____

6. ______________________________
____

7. ______________________________
____

8. ______________________________
____

9. ______________________________
____

10. ______________________________
____

Your Wanting-to-Be-Faithful Servant,

____

WEEK 15 Getting Involved

Living with a life threatening illness often causes people to pull back, to shrink from the light, to avoid any kind of attention. It is frightening to face a world of healthy people when you fear their rejection. Society praises health and wholeness. Those who are ill are considered weak, in need of assistance, pitiable. Sometimes those who are ill are even ostracized. Often those who are ill are placed in nursing homes, health care facilities, hospices, assisted living homes or rehabilitation centers so that they can be "looked after." People of health feel that they have much to offer those who are unwell, but they fail to recognize that those living with HIV/AIDS could possibly teach them wonderful things. How can we change this attitude? By getting involved ourselves, no matter what our own level of health, in the spirit of Blessed Damien Molokai.

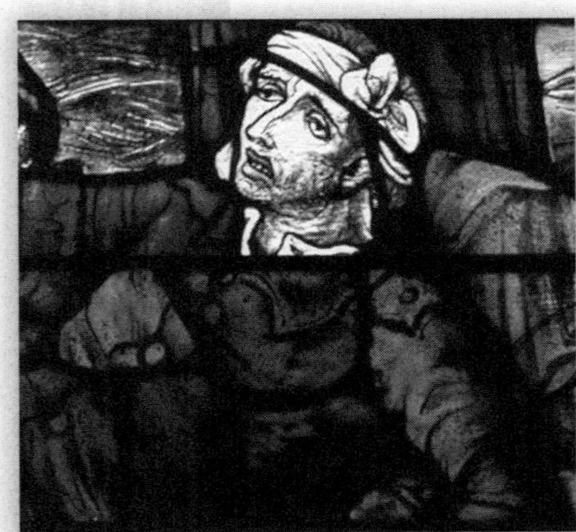

Blessed Damien of Molokai

Joseph de Veuster of Belgium entered the Congregation of the Sacred Hearts of Jesus and Mary at the age of nineteen. He took the religious name of Damien, a fourth century physician and martyr. He volunteered to take his ailing brother's place in an assignment to the Hawaiian Islands. Father Damien answered the request of the Hawaiian government to work on the remote island of Molokai, an island given over to those with Hansen's disease, then popularly known as leprosy. Damien loved the people there. He built homes, schools, clinics and hospitals for their benefit. When his own health failed and he was encouraged to leave the island, he insisted on remaining. Eventually, Father Damien contracted leprosy. He died of its complications in 1889, surrounded by the people he loved and ministered to so well.

Matthew 5:14-16

You are the light of the world. A city built on a hill cannot be hidden. No one after lighting a lamp puts it under the bushel basket, but on the lampstand, and it gives light to all in the house. In the same way, let your light shine before others, so that they may see your good works and give glory to your Father in heaven.

Quote for the Week

The challenge is to cleanse our wounds, attitudes and deeds of stigma — even toward those who hide behind stigma and refuse to respect and reach out to those we care about and care for with HIV/AIDS.

Rev. Rodney J. DeMartini

Activity

Do something this week to help someone in need. Write the name under the stick person below of someone who seems to be ostracized or left out in your community. On the arms and legs write some ways you might reach out to him or her in some small way.

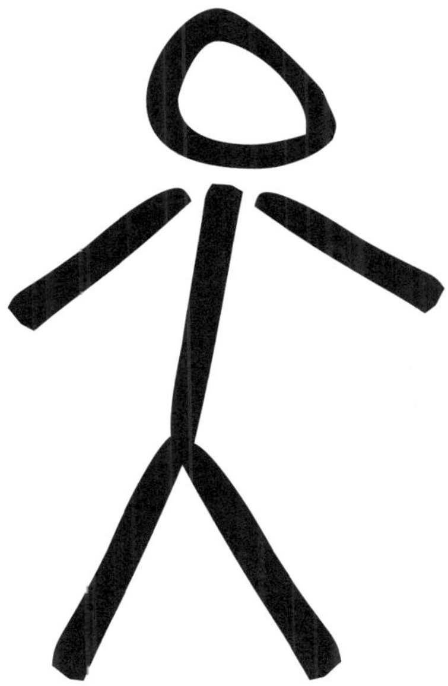

____

Name

WEEK 16 Respecting the Choices of Others

Many people in our lives think they know what is best for us. They find it easy to tell us what to do, how to do it, when to do it, and what not to fear. Perhaps their enthusiasm comes from a wealth of experience and a deep-rooted love for us. But people need to understand that the individual is the best expert in his or her own life. Otherwise, like Saint Anselm, we might do what others want us to do and never feel comfortable in our own lives. There are different ways to share our own experiences, but we must allow individuals the privilege to make their own choices. Many support groups fail to see this important point. Walking with people and journeying with them, being empathetic, is the key to helping them understand the way to respond to their own life's choices. We all have the right to make mistakes.

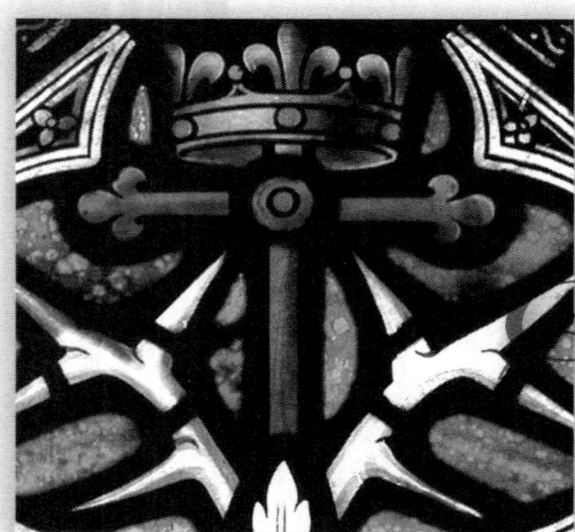

Saint Anselm

The great struggles Saint Anselm experienced in his life constantly pulled him in the wrong direction. He wanted to spend his life as a religious monk, living a life of solitude and prayer, but his father objected. Anselm caved in to his father's wishes. Eventually, however, his desire for a religious vocation won out and he entered a monastery in Normandy. At that time, the monarchy had much political influence in the Church, and King William Rufus used his influence to pull Anselm from the cloister and make him Archbishop of Canterbury, England. Anselm never gave in to political influences and remained faithful to the teaching of the Church under the care and guidance of the Virgin Mary. His profound writings continue to give witness to his fidelity to the gospels to this day.

Hebrews 13:1-2

Let mutual love continue. Do not neglect to show hospitality to strangers,
for by doing that some have entertained angels without knowing it.

Quote for the Week

Grace is given or offered to all, but in odd ways. We cannot judge.
Fortunately, it is not our business just now.
Our business is, on the contrary, not to judge,
and we shall not be judged.

Dom John Chapman

Activity

List examples of advice you've received and examples of advice you've given. What do they share in common? This week, be more aware of how advice is being dished out by yourself and others.

Advice I've Received

Advice I've Given

1. ______________________________ ______________________________

2. ______________________________ ______________________________

3. ______________________________ ______________________________

What They Share in Common

____

WEEK 17 Unity in Diversity

In many support groups, one question rears its ugly head again and again. It is a question that causes separation, not unity. That question is "How did you get it?" The best reply is, "The usual way." The answer doesn't really matter. No one is to blame for the infection, and it is no one else's business how the virus was contracted. We have heard this before, yet we are intrigued about the people we encounter who say they are infected. Ask yourself, "Will knowing how this person was infected change the way I treat him or her or the way that I feel about him or her?" In the early days of church ministry with the HIV/AIDS community a simple yet profound slogan arose — "The Body of Christ has AIDS." Like Saint Zita, we should look beyond what we possess and where we live and concentrate more on who we are. That is, we are all the same and, though we differ in appearance, we must remain united as brothers and sisters on a journey.

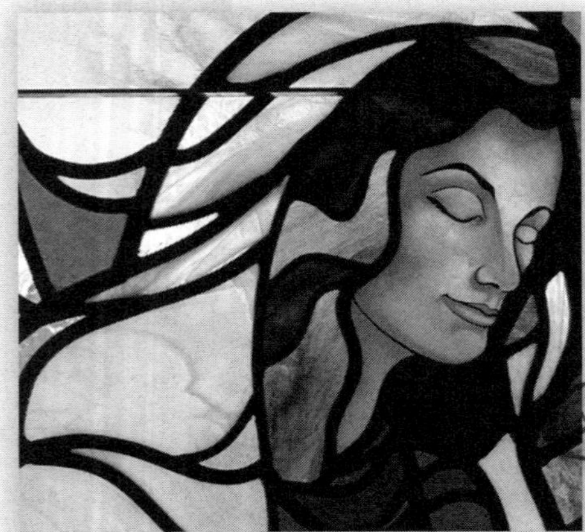

Saint Zita

Saint Zita lived in the early thirteenth century in Lucca, Italy. She was from a poor family, so she helped support them by working for property owners in the area. She was a kind of Robin Hood of her time. She took food and clothing from her employers and gave it to the poor and homeless. Zita's employers were not always happy with her practices, but they were convinced that she was special when the things she took were miraculously replaced. These miracles occurred so often that her employers began to understand the origin of Zita's zeal to heal those who needed her, even though she was also needy.

Romans 12:4-5

For, as in one body we have many members, and not all the members have the same function, so we, who are many, are one body in Christ, and individually we are members one of another.

Quote for the Week

It is simply a matter of the way of the cultural tradition in which the faith is presented. If we cling to the past, we simply become irrelevant. If we have the courage to change, then the message comes through in a way that is meaningful to people. That is the hope.

Bede Griffith, OSB

Activity

Fill in the following blanks about your own prejudices and stereotypes. You can put in more than one answer. Use a pencil with an eraser if you want. Be honest. No one else will ever read this. Then the rest of the week, pray about your answers.

All ______________________________ are alike.

All ______________________________ do (or are) ______________________________.

______________________________ bring it on themselves.

______________________________ make me uncomfortable.

I just don't want to be around ______________________________.

I like ______________________________ people, but I wouldn't want my sibling or child to marry one.

WEEK 18 Interdependence

When we are sick or feel down or depressed, we often long to be left alone. Sometimes privacy allows us to be comfortable in our own misery. While this can be good for a short time, too much isolation leads to increased and deeper pain. To want to be "left alone" is unhealthy. We humans were not created to be alone. We need the assistance of others in many ways—listening ears, helping hands, and compassionate hearts. Accepting these gestures of concern from others can turn our world around in moments. A wise saying enlightens this truth: "It is a gift to be able to receive a gift." Being open to take what others have to offer allows us to be transformed and encourages us to give to others whatever we have to share. Sharing ourselves is a sure and certain remedy to despair and loneliness. Saint Peter Celestine's yearning for a life of prayer and solitude was based on the support of the community to which he belonged. He knew that his brothers and sisters in religious life shared and supported him through their own prayerful lives of good works.

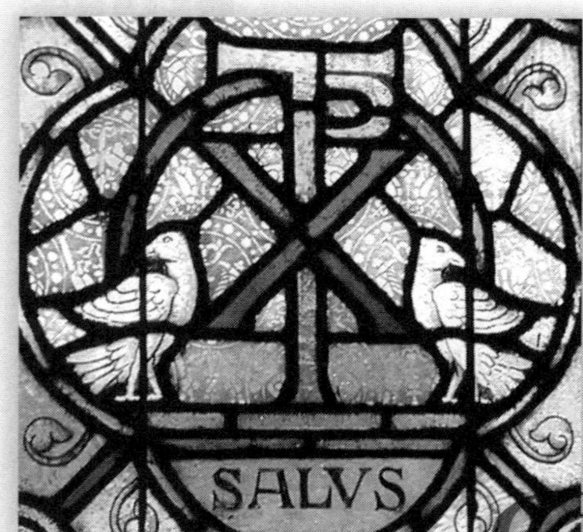

Saint Peter Celestine

From an early age, Saint Peter Celestine longed for nothing more than living the life of a monk in prayer and devotion to God. Coming from a large family of twelve children made it attractive to him to live a life of solitude and prayer in the mountains around his home. In time, word circulated about the holiness of his life, and Peter was unable to shake those who wanted to learn from him. In response, Peter prepared a rule for others to follow. He established the Celestines, who would follow his way of living in the tradition of the Benedictines. So holy was Peter's life that he was elected Pope, which was far from his early desire to live a life of solitude.

1 Corinthians 12:21-23

The eye cannot say to the hand, "I have no need of you" nor again the head to the feet, "I have no need of you." On the contrary, the members of the body that seem to be weaker are indispensable, and those members of the body that we think less honorable we clothe with greater honor, and our less respectable members are treated with greater respect.

Quote for the Week

Community is like a large mosaic...a fellowship of little people
who together make God visible in the world.

Henri Nouwen

Activity

Take a few moments to reflect on the times you most need solitude and the times it is important to have people around you. List them below. Add to the lists during the week as you recognize additional times for each.

Times I Need to Be Alone	Times I Need to Be with Others

WEEK 19

Hanging by a Thread

It seems we often find ourselves hanging by a thread, but we don't always know whether anyone is holding the other end. But we hang there, hoping that the person will not let go. We hold on for dear life and, in the holding, we become numb—unable to feel anything but the pain of the moment. The times we are hanging by a thread can be filled with grace, although we may not realize it at the time. Grace is an invisible booster shot of courage that infuses us with strength and determination we never thought we had. God sends grace to us through people, places and things that reveal who we are and who God is for us. Saint Rita knew pain throughout her life, and she hung on through prayer and accepted what came her way. When we pray to Saint Rita, however, we should beware. The saying goes that Saint Rita sends the roses, but she also sends the thorns: Our prayers will be answered (the roses), but the answer may not always be what we expected (the thorns).

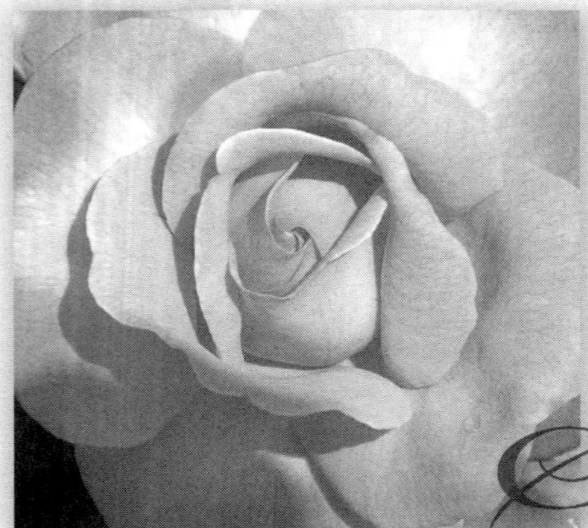

Saint Rita of Cascia

Saint Rita of Cascia, Italy, lived in the Middle Ages when it was common for a young girl to be married to an older man to assure the girl's security. Rita spent eighteen unhappy years married to a man who treated her badly. Even so, she was a devoted mother to her two sons. Eventually, when Rita's husband died, she attempted to enter the Augustinian convent but was refused because she was a widow and not a virgin. Her dream of acceptance to the order persisted, and she pursued the superiors until they relented and allowed her to enter. Rita was known for her deeply prayerful life and a bleeding mark of a crown of thorns on her forehead, something she received in the midst of a chronic ailment. This mark exemplified her union with the suffering of Jesus' own passion on earth.

1 Corinthians 15:10

But by the grace of God I am what I am, and his grace towards me has not been in vain. On the contrary, I worked harder than any of them though it was not I, but the grace of God that is with me.

Quote for the Week

We reject the idea that HIV/AIDS is a direct punishment from God….
Nothing in the Bible or in Catholic teaching can be used to justify
prejudicial or discriminatory attitudes and behaviors.

United States Conference of Catholic Bishops

Activity

Name three people in the past few years who have held tightly to the other end of your thread when you were in crisis. This week, call each person and say "thank you." If one of them has died, visit his or her grave or recall the person during your prayers.

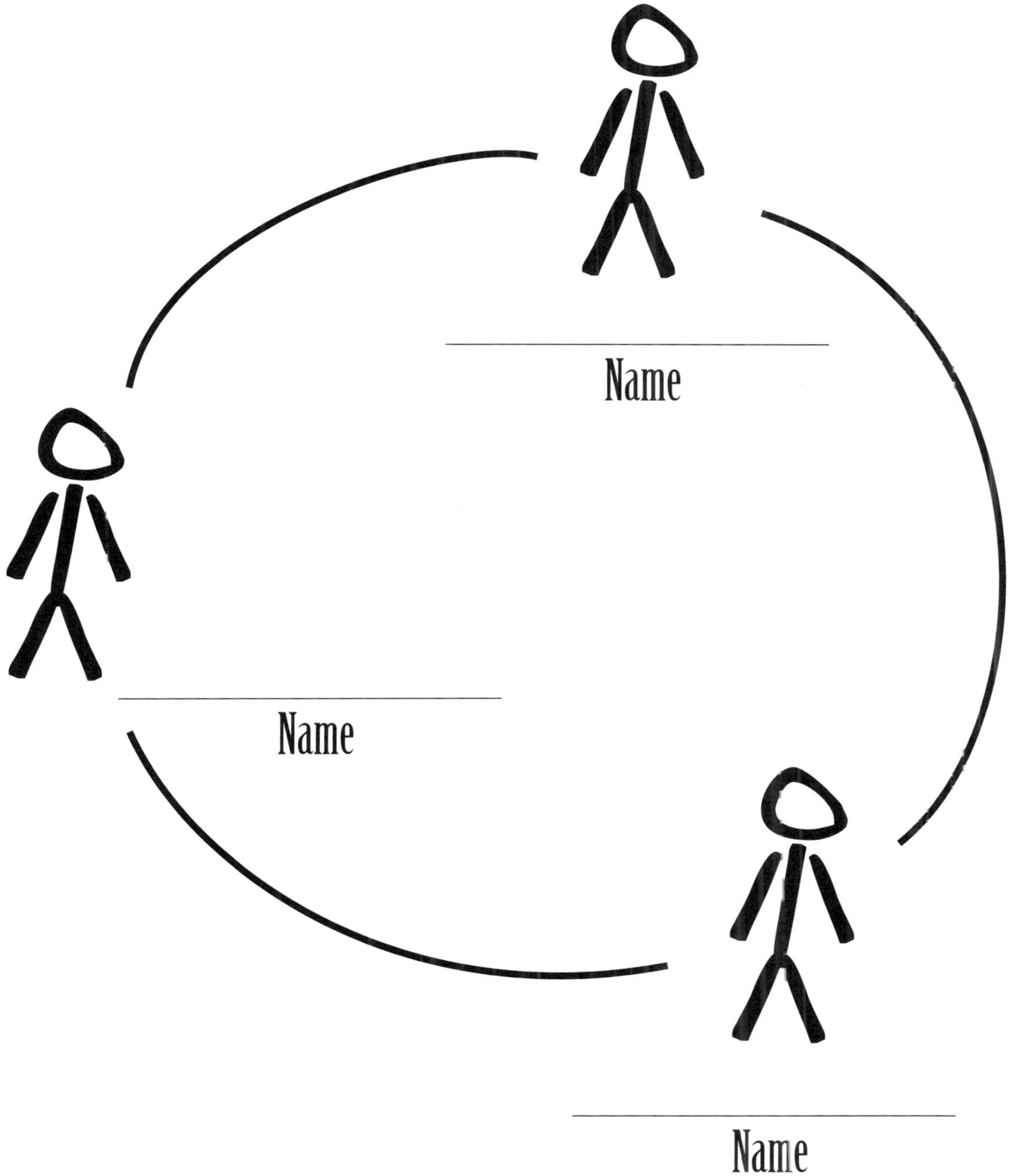

WEEK 20 Christ Has No Hands but Ours

World War II destroyed a German boarding school, leaving the buildings in shambles. The students and faculty of the school worked hard for many months to rebuild the school, its chapel, and the dormitories. When it was almost completed, they wondered what would replace the six-foot marble statue of Jesus that had greeted all visitors at the entrance of the building. The statue had been toppled over and the hands of Jesus, which had been outstretched, were broken off. The art teachers and their students were summoned to see if the statue could be repaired. They succeeded in mending its many wounds—all except the hands. These they could not restore. The faculty and students decided to place the statue of Jesus back in its original home—without the hands. This time, however, the caption they engraved under the base of the statue was changed to read: "Christ has no hands but yours." Saint Joan of Arc became the hands of Christ in a vivid way, even in the face of her own suffering and death. In her compelling story we see a simple yet profound message: no matter how difficult our circumstance, we can be the hands of Christ for others and make their lives more bearable.

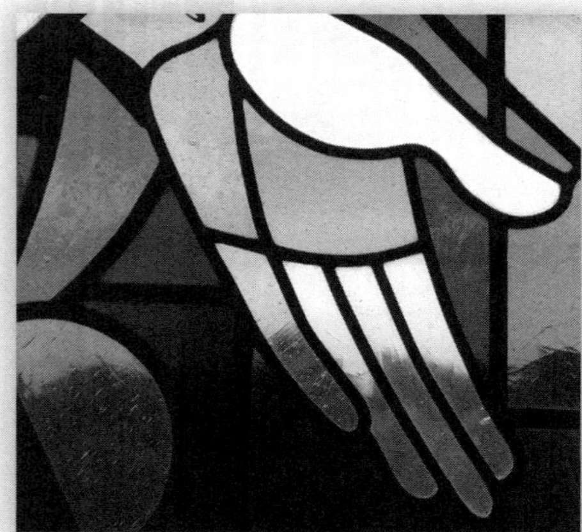

Saint Joan of Arc

Saint Joan of Arc, the "Maid of Orleans," was a brave young woman who followed God's will literally—in a way few others have. Her fervent zeal to serve God and assist King Charles VII of France caused many to doubt her. She was an ordinary girl who lacked formal education and was, perhaps, even naïve. But Saint Joan answered God's call and fought bravely for her country. Eventually, she was tried by the English as a heretic and—confused, frightened and abandoned by the Church and the people she had served so well—burned at the stake in 1431.

Micah 6:8

He has told you, O mortal, what is good; and what does the Lord require of you
but to do justice, and to love kindness, and to walk humbly with your God?

Quote for the Week

In the service of love, only the wounded soldier can serve.

Thorton Wilder

Activity

Write a paragraph or a poem below about what it feels like to be the hands of Christ. Then find one hour this week and visit someone in the hospital or nursing home, or at least call a sick friend or do an errand for a person in need.

The Hands of Christ

WEEK 21

Seeing and Believing

Amidst claims of new and improved miracle products, we have become consumers who live by the adage "seeing is believing." We think we are too sophisticated to believe in things that cannot be proved, but sometimes it is important that we believe in what we cannot see. For example, our own resourcefulness is a difficult thing for some of us to see, but it should not be the last place we look for surety of talent, knowledge and ability. Likewise, we must believe in others, because they will come through for us and help us do what we must do, even if we do not always see how they do it. Pope John XXIII is a great model for those seeking to believe what they cannot yet see. His love for people and his great respect for their gifts and talents teach us about faith and belief in ourselves and in others.

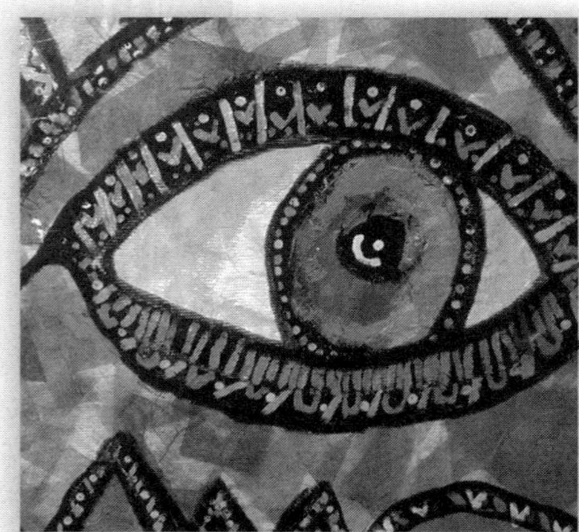

Blessed Pope John XXIII

In 1960, Angelo Cardinal Roncalli, the seventy-seven year old Patriarch of Venice and former diplomat of the Vatican to Bulgaria, Turkey, Greece and France, was thought too old to do much of anything if elected Pope. Yet Pope John XXIII, as he was called, changed the Church in ways that hadn't been done in hundreds of years. His vision led the Church to rediscover herself and the riches she possessed in her membership. He prepared the Catholic Church to move into the twenty-first century and created a whole new mindset, one that would forever change the roles of lay men and women in the Church. Pope John XXIII was a man of great humility, wit and charm. He was the perfect person to undertake such an awesome task, and his keen vision left a great legacy.

John 20:29

Jesus said to him, "Have you believed because you have seen me? Blessed are those who have not seen and yet have come to believe."

Quote for the Week

See everything; overlook much; correct little.

Blessed Pope John XXIII

Activity On a clear night this week, go outside and look up at the stars. How often do you walk under them and forget that they are there? Put the name of something or someone you want to believe in on each star below.

I Want to Believe In

☆ ______________________________

☆ ______________________________

☆ ______________________________

☆ ______________________________

☆ ______________________________

☆ ______________________________

☆ ______________________________

☆ ______________________________

☆ ______________________________

☆ ______________________________

WEEK 22 Fear

We fear rejection, ridicule and failure. Yet fear can overwhelm us, like a tidal wave out of control, keeping us from succeeding and growing. Try taking the word "FEAR" apart, piece by piece: **F**ace what bothers you; name it; recognize it; make friends with it. **E**nergize yourself with positive images; put yourself in a peaceful place where you are in control. **A**ssess the situation; decide what is the best and the worst that can happen if you take action. **R**espond as best you can; if you are able to accept the challenge of your fear, go for it; if not, buy some time and make a promise to try again soon. Saint Marcellin Champagnat worked hard to overcome the obstacles in his path from his youngest days. Learn from him.

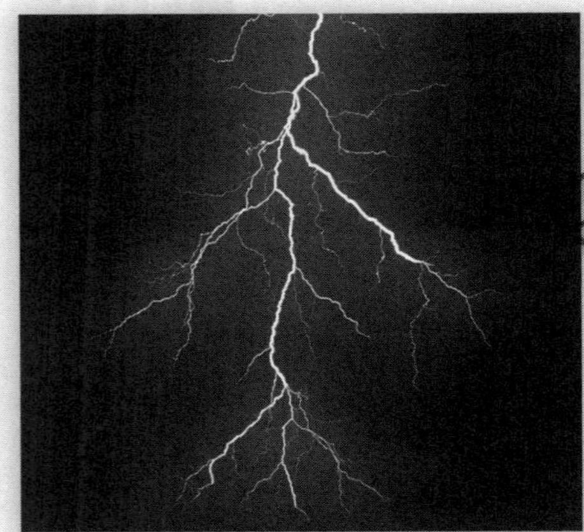

Saint Marcellin Champagnat

Joseph Benedict Marcellin Champagnat was born the year the French Revolution began. Reared in a religious family, he wanted to become a priest but lacked the education to do so. Marcellin had to work much harder than anyone else just to meet the standards for the schools he needed to attend. But this concerted effort established a work ethic that served him well for the rest of his life. Because of the shortage of schools, Marcellin and several friends banded together and formed the Marist Brothers and dedicated their lives to the education of youth. Despite personal obstacles and insufficiencies, as well as a negative social environment, Saint Marcellin Champagnat faced his fears and overcame them.

Mark 5:36

But overhearing what they said, Jesus said to the leader of the synagogue, "Do not fear, only believe."

Quote for the Week

The only way I get rid of my fears
is to make films about them.

Alfred Hitchcock

Activity

Name a fear in your life that you would like to overcome. Now name a larger fear that underlies the original one. Keep doing so until you have reached your deepest fear. Now use the model on the previous page of **F**ace, **E**nergize, **A**ssess, **R**espond to plot out a plan to address that fear during this week.

Fear name ______________________________

____

Fear name ______________________________

____

Fear name ______________________________

____

Fear name ______________________________

____

What I will do to **face** my deepest fear:

What I will do to **energize** myself to face this fear:

What I will do to **assess** this fear:

What I will do to **respond** to this fear:

WEEK 23 Confronting Skills

Confronting those we love is not an easy task. People can make us crazy by the things they say or do. As a result, we often find ourselves frustrated when we cannot find the courage to confront them with our version of the truth. Even when naming our truths, however, we often confront other persons with something they do not know, hoping that they will come to understand what we have risked to tell our truth. Try this technique the next time you confront someone: Say "When you (state what the other person does), I feel (state your feelings) because (give the reason behind your feeling.) For example: "When you call me names, I feel inadequate and helpless because that is what mean kids did to me when I was young." Using an "I Message" communicates your truth gently and invites the listener to engage in conversation. With hope, the conversation will lead to understanding, forgiveness and reconciliation. Saint Anthony of Padua taught us that sincerity and simplicity in speech ensure that the truth—sometimes hard to express and accept—is revealed in a gentle manner.

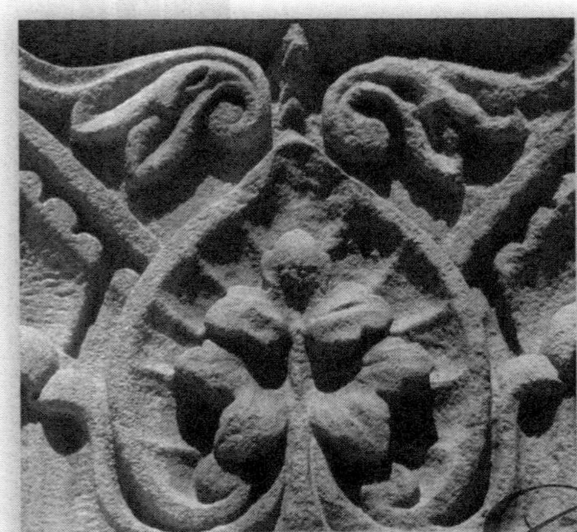

Saint Anthony of Padua

Saint Anthony of Padua began his religious life as an Augustinian. After he saw the beheaded and beaten bodies of Franciscan martyrs being returned from Morocco, he became a Franciscan in hope of dying as a martyr as well. Even though he was intent on going to North Africa, Anthony was diverted to Italy. There he was discovered to have a great facility for preaching and explaining the faith with profound simplicity. Hundreds of people would come to him to learn and to hear him speak. He was said to possess a "golden tongue."

Isaiah 7:4

And say to him, "Take heed, be quiet, do not fear, and do not let your heart be faint."

Quote for the Week

We should make it a point never to do anything when we are "hot and bothered," but strive first of all to calm down, to hand ourselves over to the will of God and of the Immaculate Mary, and then to act with serenity so that we may not commit blunders.

Saint Maximillian Mary Kolbe

Activity

Fill in the "I message" below on something important you need to say to someone. Then practice it in front of a mirror. Finally, deliver it sometime this week to the person you need to confront. Be sure to do it in person or at least in a note (not on the telephone or in an e-mail if it can be avoided, because these are more impersonal and open to misinterpretation). Say what you have to say with kindness, love and confidence, and do not be defensive or overreact to the other person's response.

When You...

____

____

____

____

____

____

I Feel...

____

____

____

____

____

____

Because...

____

____

____

____

____

____

WEEK 24 Recognizing and Using Our Talents

Tom gave 100% of himself to everyone and everything he got involved with. He would make you feel like a movie star when you were with him, his full attention on your words and your concerns. Physical and spiritual fitness was extremely important for Tom. When he went to speak to high school students about being HIV positive, they could not believe he was infected. He was 6'3" tall and was 190 pounds of muscle. He appeared more healthy than most and was mentally sound. He loved the feedback from the students and was proud he could share his knowledge of HIV/AIDS prevention and put a face on the disease for them. Tom was a "manna personality": Like the manna (bread) God sent from heaven to feed the starving Israelites in the desert, Tom was food for the soul. If he could not help you emotionally by listening to your concerns and problems, he would help physically, by silently attending to your needs. Like the bread from heaven, Tom fed, nurtured, and cared for many. Like Saints Peter and Paul, Tom used his own humanity and weaknesses to build up others.

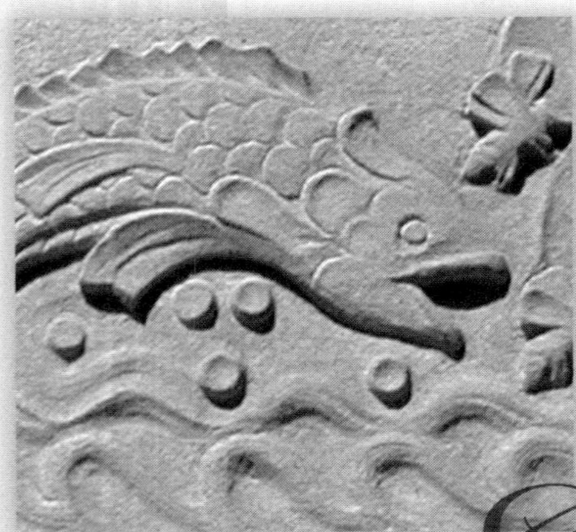

Saints Peter and Saint Paul

God uses our gifts, our talents, and our inadequacies to benefit ourselves and those around us. Saint Peter and Saint Paul are perfect examples of God's desire to use ordinary human beings to do extraordinary work. Scripture presents Peter as wishy-washy, having denied the Lord when He needed him the most. Paul was a feared persecutor of Christians. But God worked wonders in their lives. Peter became the "rock" on which the Church was built, and Paul led many to the faith through his missionary activities and prolific writings on love.

Isaiah 42:16

I will lead the blind by a road they do not know, by paths they have not known I will guide them. I will turn the darkness before them into light, the rough places into level ground. These are the things I will do, and I will not forsake them.

Quote for the Week

The human passions transform us from a mere thing into a hero, into a being that, in spite of tremendous handicaps, tries to make sense of life.

Erich Fromm

Activity

Think about good things others have seen in you that you did not see in yourself. List what they see in the first column on the left. Next, list good things you see in yourself that others don't necessarily recognize. List them in the column on the right. This week, try to practice at least one of your talents from each list.

Good Things Others See In Me	Good Things I See In Myself

WEEK 25 Remembering

Remembering can be painful, but it can also be healing and life-giving. To recall a time when we were young and carefree—when the world was an easier place to conquer—brings us to a time when our imaginations ran wild and our ideals were high and invincible. Through the tears of our memories, we may see our long-ago selves as champions of the world. We see ourselves without fear, without knowledge of a world that brings hurt, and without the pain of illness. We see ourselves as different from what we are now. Franciscan Father Junipero Serra used the memories of the Native American peoples to gather them closer to God and to build new communities. Like him, we should bring the past with us to new places. It is an important tool to build up, remodel and renew.

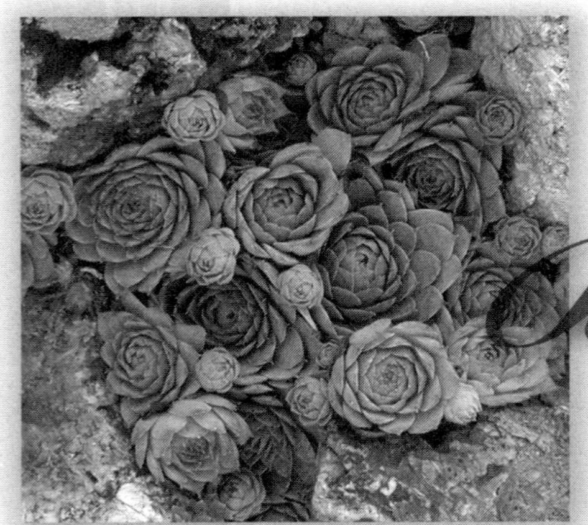

Blessed Junipero Serra

In the 1700s, Miguel José Serra was a Franciscan priest who became known as Father Junipero Serra. He established twenty-two Spanish missions along six hundred miles of the California coast. It was neither a doctorate in theology nor educational prowess that gave him his enormous energy. Instead, his passion for the gospel message and his love for the native peoples he met moved him to build communities wherever he found a need. A painful leg injury never stopped Father Junipero from making many visits to the missions he founded. His memory lives on in the hearts of many and is memorialized in bronze statues throughout California.

1 Corinthians 11:2

I commend you because you remember me in everything and maintain the traditions just as I handed them on to you.

Quote for the Week

Now I am laughing. I see it like this, a perfect sphere. I travel on the inside of that sphere as infinity of paths with a multiplicity of experience. AIDS is one of these experiences, but one that persistently taps, then throbs, then taps inside me. I am necessarily strengthened by it.

Maya Sue

Activity

Populate the table below with people and things from times you were happy. (Don't worry about the artwork, just put everyone and everything you can around or on the table, either by picture or word.) During the week, use this image as a focus for prayer and meditation.

Times I Was Happy

⇩

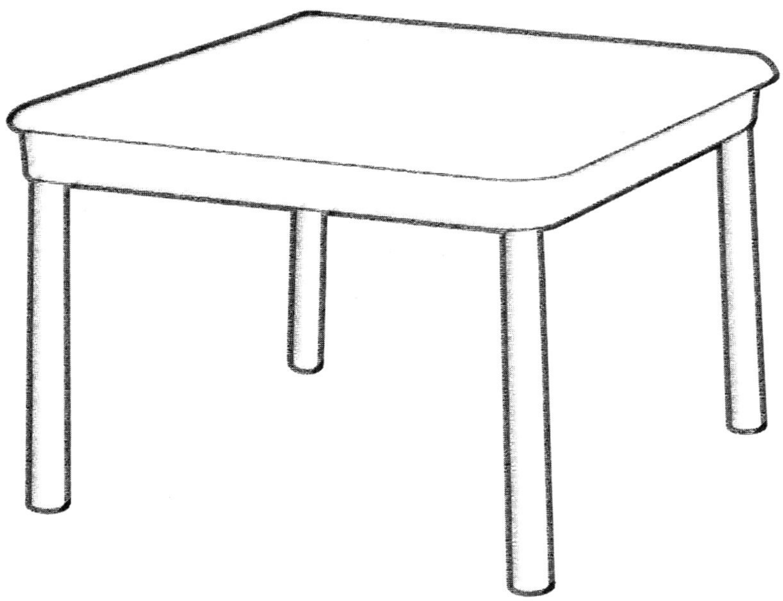

WEEK 26

Simplify

To simplify our lives is not just to get rid of things. To simplify, we must examine our things and decide which are helpful to our inner peace and which are a hindrance. One item may be a special gift from a loved one or something that gives us comfort, such as a favorite pillow or photo. Such material possessions can hold all the love in the world. Other things are just junk, like that treadmill we now use as a clothes rack or that surround-sound television system that keeps us at home alone most nights. God saw that the material world is good, but only when it is used with moderation and common sense. Saint Benedict's search for simplicity resulted in a balanced life of work, rest, recreation, and prayer. He discovered holistic practices way ahead of his time.

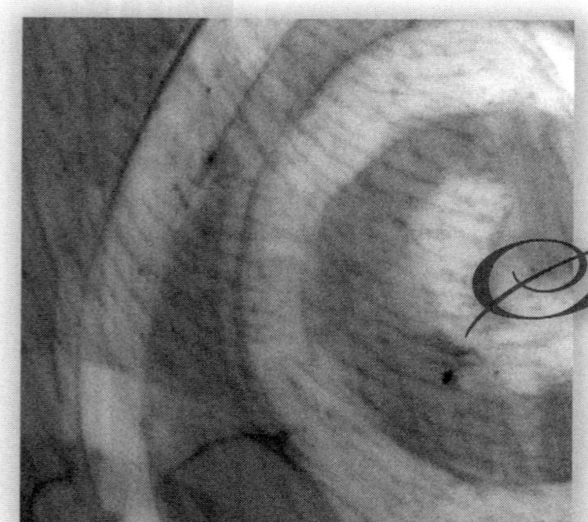

Saint Benedict

Benedict was born in the town of Nursia in the Umbrian region of Italy around the year 480 AD. As was customary for people of his upper class, he traveled to Rome to complete his education in rhetoric and law. During his time, much chaos surrounded the Churches of both the East and the West. Heresies erupted in Rome; people who held opposing views were often threatened physically by one another. Determined to simplify his life, Benedict withdrew in solitude. He immersed himself in prayer, study and hard labor. These practices lead him to establish a guide for those who desired a monastic life. "The Rule of Saint Benedict" remains the source of inspiration for a majority of monastic communities worldwide and for thousands of laypeople who find fuller meaning in their lives by following his simple dictum: *Ora et Labora*, "Prayer and Work."

Luke12:34

For where your treasure is, there your heart will be also.

Quote for the Week

We are fed or damaged spiritually by what we attend to.

Alan Helms

Activity

This week, find the messiest set of drawers in your house. Empty the contents drawer by drawer onto a flat surface and name them below. Now sort, clean, throw out and save. Cross out below all the things you discarded. This is a simple act of simplifying that will remind you to do so in other areas of your life.

What I Found

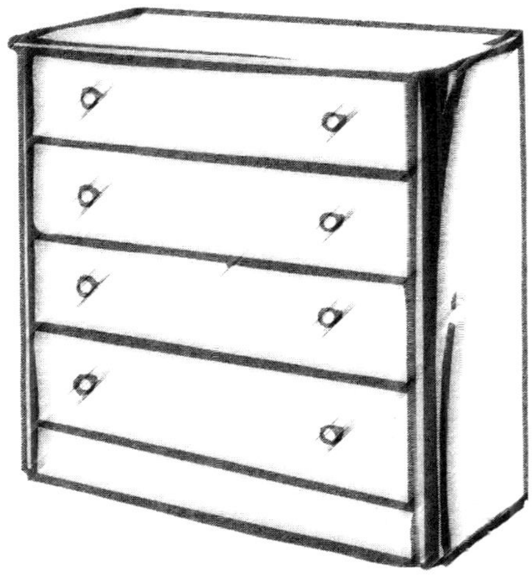

WEEK 27 Excuses

We often dance around what bothers us, haunts us, and torments us. In this dance, we make clever moves and side steps. These dance moves often keep us from fully seeing what is hidden and what issues are being skirted. People begin to know us by the dance. They begin to expect certain things and responses because we use the same dance so often. For example, when we are faced with tough decisions and need to think through all of the possibilities—everything that can or will occur as a result of our choices—it is sometimes easier to avoid the whole process. Instead of going to a support group, keeping a lunch date with a friend, or interacting with supportive family members, we use the excuse of being overworked or overextended. Anything can become an excuse for us to avoid the real issues because we fear the demons that lurk behind them. The Native American woman Kateri Tekakwitha is a model for those of us who seek to become our best selves by facing whatever holds us back from God.

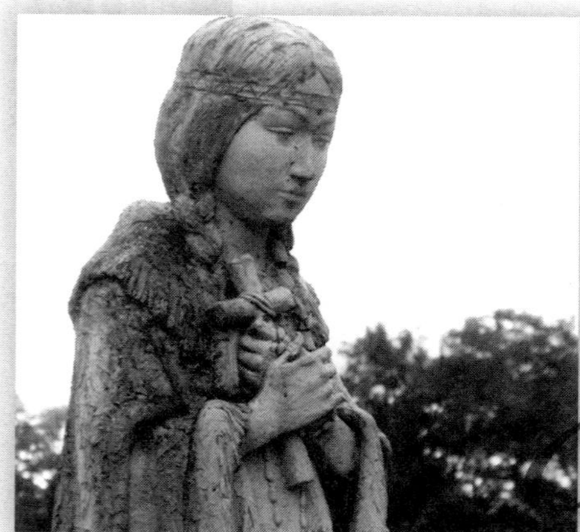

Blessed Kateri Tekakwitha

Kateri Tekakwitha, born in 1656, was the daughter of a Mohawk warrior. She was orphaned at a very young age when she lost her family in a smallpox epidemic. She converted to Catholicism in her teens and was baptized at twenty years old. Blessed Kateri spent her life tending to the sick and the aged. This earned her the title "Lily of the Mohawks." She died at an early age herself. Devotion to her is credited with establishing Native American ministries throughout the United States and Canada. Her simple life has been the inspiration for many to turn toward the good and change their lives.

James 5:12

Above all, my beloved, do not swear either by heaven or by earth or by any other oath, but let your "Yes" be yes and your "No" be no, so that you may not fall under condemnation.

Quote for the Week

All acts of courage communicate the same message: This is me!

Robert J. Furey

Activity

List below your favorite excuses for not dealing with things in your life that bind you, chain you down, or keep you from being the person you want to be. During the week, put an asterisk next to any of the excuses you use. At the end of the week, cross out any excuse you have not used.

Excuse #1

Excuse #2

Excuse # 3

Excuse #4

Excuse #5

WEEK 28 Beginning Anew

Painful memories can torture us and lead us to dark places where the only way to survive is to close ourselves off and hide. Sometimes even a holiday or anniversary or season of the year will bring back memories of a painful or abusive situation. We need to reclaim and rename our past. It can be done. We have the power within ourselves to begin again, to rename a bad holiday and make new memories. Mary of Magdala is perhaps the patron saint of beginning anew. Possessed by demons, she was cured by Jesus and became a key follower and financial supporter of his ministry. After the passion and death of Jesus, she was the first one to experience him as risen from the dead. She became the "Apostle to the Apostles."

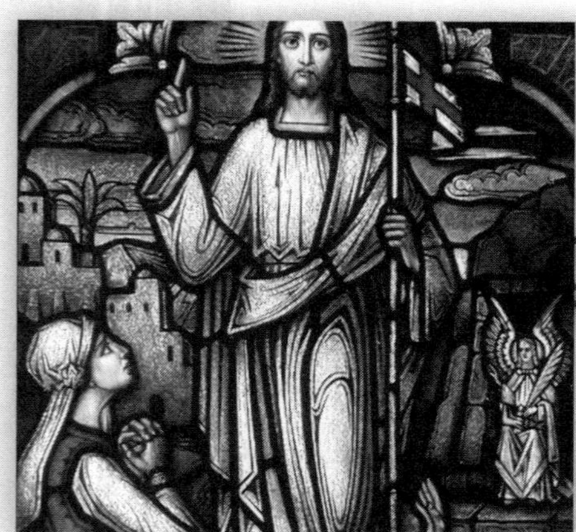

Saint Mary Magdalene

In the eighth chapter of Luke, we meet Mary of Magdala, also called Mary Magdalene, when Jesus heals her of her possession by seven demons. Mary then joined the other women who accompanied Jesus as he went about healing and teaching. She was at the foot of the cross with John and with Mary, the Mother of Jesus. Mary Magdalene was the first person to see the risen Lord, and Jesus sent her to tell the other disciples. Over the centuries, popes and others somehow confused Mary Magdalene with the woman caught in adultery or the woman who bathed Jesus' feet with her hair. This is not the case. Mary Magdalene was a faithful, powerful, dedicated and devout follower of Jesus. She is the model for us to let go of past pains and commit ourselves fully to the present and the future.

Hebrews 10:32

But recall those earlier days when, after you had been enlightened, you endured a hard struggle with sufferings.

Quote for the Week

I've worked with AIDS patients in the past. The key is to gently touch their pain at the very point where it hurts the most; then healing begins at this very point where they feel most unloved.

Cheryl

Activity

Write below about a terrible event, great tragedy, or real regret in your life. Now write how you might put it behind you and transform it into a new, more positive memory—or at least one that has no power over you. During the week, try to put your plan into action, even in small ways.

What I Remember

What I Will Do to Get Past It

WEEK 29 Cookies and Milk

The most beautiful greeting card can be one made on a computer or a heartfelt note scribbled on the back of a paper bag. The most delicious meal can be eating cookies with milk. Saint Martha placed thoughtfulness and hospitality above all else and knew how to serve everything with love and care. We often wait too long to invite our friends over for dinner or too long to visit them. Sometimes we wait so long to find the perfect card that we miss the actual birthday or holiday or event or anniversary. No matter what we make, buy, burn in the oven, or prepare, it should be a gift that our friend or loved one can treasure: a gift from the heart. One single cookie, one simple written word can lift the spirits of another for a week! Think of your own wonderful memories with loved ones and friends. They are probably the times when nothing was planned but everything was perfect.

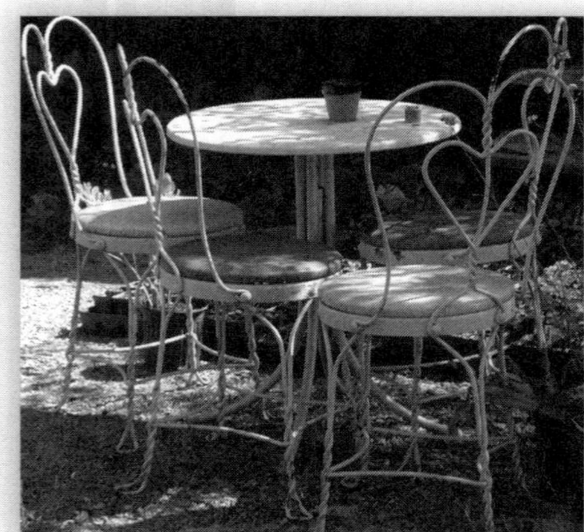

Saint Martha

Martha, Mary, and their brother Lazarus were good friends to Jesus. The hospitality they showed him in their home at Bethany was a blessed comfort. The gospel story shows that one day Martha had enough and complained to Jesus that Mary sat at his feet and listened to his stories while Martha cooked, cleaned and served. Jesus told her that Mary had chosen the better part—to listen to God's word—but what would Jesus' ministry have been like without Martha? She was faithful, warm, loving, and so hospitable that Jesus came back to her home again and again. It was Martha, not Mary, who finally realized that Jesus was "the Messiah, the Son of the Living God" (Matthew 27:54).

1 Timothy 6:18

They are to do good, to be rich in good works, generous, and ready to share.

Quote for the Week

O God, when I have food, help me to remember the hungry; when I have to work, help me to remember the jobless; when I have a home, help me to remember those who have no home at all; when I am without pain, help me to remember those who suffer; and remembering, help me to destroy my complacency, bestir my compassion, and be concerned enough to help, by word and deed, those who cry out for what we take for granted. Amen.

Samuel F. Pugh

Activity

Make some cookies this week, even if you have to buy the ready-to-bake kind. Then share some with a friend and bring the rest to someone you think might need them. Write below how you can become like Saint Martha in your life.

How I Can Be Like Saint Martha

WEEK 30 An Attitude of Gratitude

Many people see the glass as half empty instead of half full. Pessimism seems to be in their blood. There are others, however, who make everyone around them happier with their positive attitude. How can we learn from this second group? First, we can seek out the company of those who smile often, don't complain when they are completing an unpleasant task, and use words of praise and gratitude often. Next, we can copy what they do and keep copying until it becomes a part of how we operate. Third, we can notice that when we are positive, we receive a different response from people. Finally, we can put our own twist on this "Attitude of Gratitude." We don't have to be Pollyanna all the time. We don't have to deny that there are bad things in the world. We can be positive in our own way, even if we are curmudgeons! Like Edith Stein, we just have to persevere in our faith that God is good.

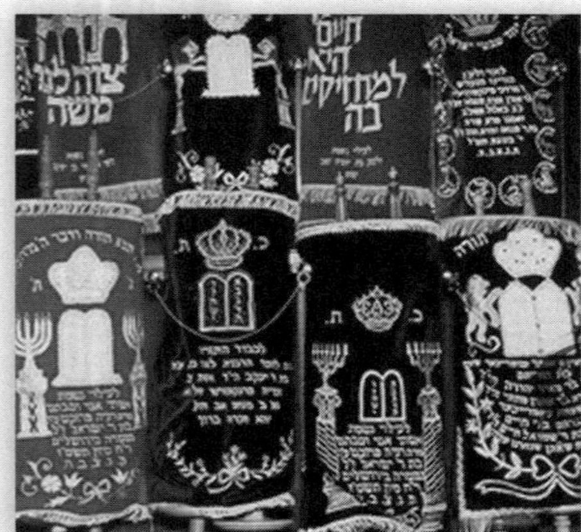

Saint Theresa Benedicta (Edith Stein)

Born to a Jewish family, Edith Stein did not have any particular feelings about God. She was an extremely intelligent girl who studied philosophy and phenomenology under Max Scheler, a Jew who converted to Catholicism. Edith, inspired by the deep love of a Catholic widow who suffered greatly during World War I, converted to Catholicism. She became a Carmelite nun and took the religious name Sister Theresa Benedicta. During the Nazi persecution she was arrested and sent to Auschwitz, where she was subjected to the tortures of the Nazi concentration camps. Her deep faith sustained her, and her gratitude to God was unfailing, even in the most difficult of situations. She died at Auschwitz on August 9, 1942, and her writings continue to be an inspiration to many.

Colossians 3:15

And let the peace of Christ rule in your hearts, to which indeed you were called in the one body. And be thankful.

Quote for the Week

If there is one thing all this has given me it is a love of life. To me, living every moment with happiness and optimism is paramount. I no longer take anything or anyone for granted. I have learned that I am my own best friend. I know where I stand with myself, and I trust myself completely.

Pearl

Activity

Try to recall someone who has inspired and affirmed you. Below, write that person a letter of gratitude and describe what he or she did for you. If you can, locate this person and mail a copy of the letter this week.

Dear ______________________________,

I just want to tell you what you have done for me and how much I appreciate it:

Sincerely,

____

WEEK 31 Full Disclosure

Full disclosure is not for everyone, especially when it comes to HIV/AIDS. This single topic has been the cause of more heated discussions in HIV/AIDS workshops, public health meetings, support groups, therapy sessions, and gatherings than any other. Whom should we tell that we are HIV-positive or have AIDS? When should we tell them? How do we tell them? Do we tell them before we go out on a date with them? Before we engage in sexual activity? Do we tell our children? Do we tell our church community, our extended families, our employers? Do we disclose our status to former husbands, wives, lovers? There is no single answer that fits every situation. In the early days of the AIDS epidemic, many infected people lost their jobs, their relationships with family members, and their health insurance coverage because they disclosed their HIV/AIDS status. Now, laws prohibit this kind of prejudice in the workplace, but not in relationships and in families. How does Saint Clare enlighten us about disclosure? She lived in silence most of her life, but her life was the lesson she wanted to preach and teach to others. Her message is simple: respect others, do the best you can, and remain faithful.

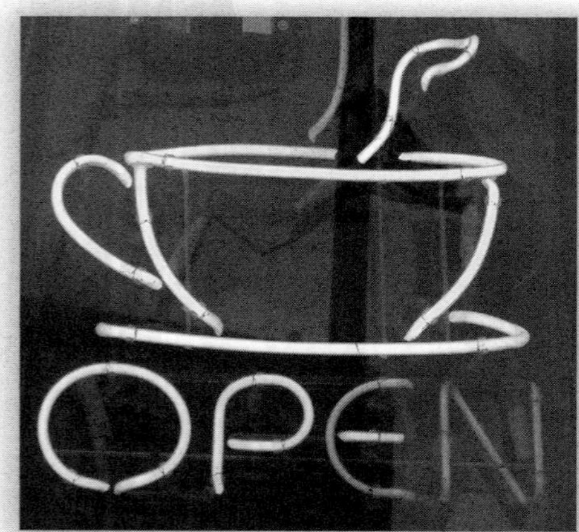

Saint Clare of Assisi

"Behind every great man is a great woman" rings true in the life of Saint Francis of Assisi, whose "great woman" was Clare, a beautiful, Italian noblewoman who gave up everything to embrace voluntary poverty. She founded the Poor Clare community of women, who imitate her lifestyle to this day. Saint Clare worked tirelessly to promote the life of prayer and simplicity that Francis had begun. She lived by example and won the hearts of many through her faithful silence and determination.

Hebrews 11:1

Now faith is the assurance of things hoped for, the conviction of things not seen.

Quote for the Week

The fruit of Silence is Prayer.
The fruit of Prayer is Faith.
The fruit of Faith is Love.
The fruit of Love is Service.
And the fruit of Service is Peace.
Blessed Mother Teresa of Calcutta

Activity

Write down very specific things you want to tell in the first column below and very specifically to whom you want to tell them. Then this week set up very specific times and places to do so with each person. If you know other people who are struggling with HIV/AIDS, share your experiences of doing this exercise with them.

	What I Want to Tell	To Whom I Want to Tell It
1.	____________________	____________________
	____________________	____________________
	____________________	____________________
	____________________	____________________
2.	____________________	____________________
	____________________	____________________
	____________________	____________________
	____________________	____________________
3.	____________________	____________________
	____________________	____________________
	____________________	____________________
	____________________	____________________
4.	____________________	____________________
	____________________	____________________
	____________________	____________________
	____________________	____________________
5.	____________________	____________________
	____________________	____________________
	____________________	____________________
	____________________	____________________

WEEK 32 Confronting Stigmas

Society often views and treats poorly those living with HIV/AIDS—or even sometimes those working with or caring for those infected. Everyone is lumped into a category of shame and guilt. But this terrible disease does not belong to the homosexual community, nor the IV-drug using community, nor to the poor, nor the uneducated, nor the African-American or any other ethnic group. It belongs to no one and to everyone. No one deserves this disease; no one is exempt from its effects. One HIV support group facilitator says it best: "It is what it is." We make of it whatever we wish. We can turn it around and find the courage to face ignorance and educate people that the victims are not the disease. This is what matters most. Saint Maximilian Mary Kolbe exhibited this kind of understanding and courage in the face of Nazi persecution.

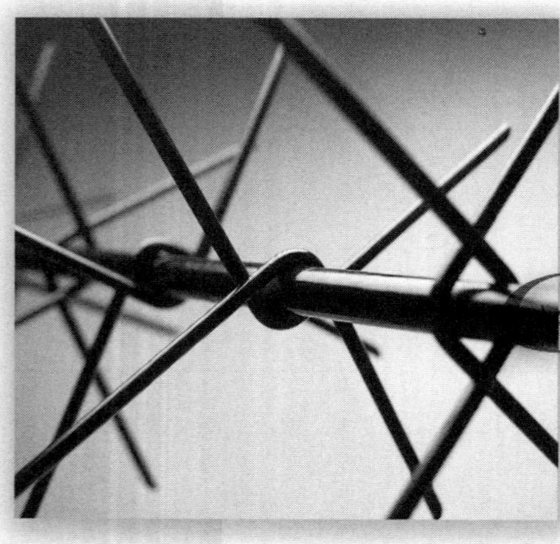

Saint Maximilian Mary Kolbe

Maximilian Kolbe was a Conventual Franciscan Friar with a very strong devotion to the Blessed Mother, whose name he took as a priest. He was no model child, but whatever energy he had in his wild youth was channeled into studies for the priesthood. As a priest, he used that childhood energy to influence the Polish people about their faith and against the tyranny of Nazi oppressors. He was arrested and sent to Auschwitz. Records tell us that when someone escaped from the prison, the camp protocol was to randomly select ten other people to be executed. One time, a married man with several children was one of those selected. He begged for mercy, and Father Kolbe stepped up to take the man's place. The priest was killed by a lethal injection of carbonic acid on August 14, 1941.

1 Corinthians 1:27

But God chose what is foolish in the world to shame the wise; God chose what is weak in the world to shame the strong.

Quote for the Week

I found out I was HIV positive when I was 23 years old.... I don't want people to know that I have HIV because they make you feel like you're no good; you're contaminated.... Not telling anyone that I have HIV makes me feel normal. I can't even tell my kids because I don't want people hurting them by saying bad things about me.

Starr

Activity

Below are five statements connected with HIV/AIDS. On a scale of 0-10, with 0 being "not at all prevalent" and 10 being "almost universally prevalent," estimate how widespread you feel this belief is today. During the week, try to talk with at least one person who has expressed a negative comment about people with HIV/AIDS and try to convince him or her of the truth.

"People with HIV/AIDS brought it upon themselves."

How prevalent a belief today:

0 — 1 — 2 — 3 — 4 — 5 — 6 — 7 — 8 — 9 — 10

"People with HIV/AIDS only care about themselves, not others."

How prevalent a belief today:

0 — 1 — 2 — 3 — 4 — 5 — 6 — 7 — 8 — 9 — 10

"If people know you have HIV/AIDS, they treat you differently."

How prevalent a belief today:

0 — 1 — 2 — 3 — 4 — 5 — 6 — 7 — 8 — 9 — 10

"Research and treatment of HIV/AIDS receives an inordinate amount of funding."

How prevalent a belief today:

0 — 1 — 2 — 3 — 4 — 5 — 6 — 7 — 8 — 9 — 10

"I can catch HIV/AIDS from casual, non-sexual contact with people who are infected."

How prevalent a belief today:

0 — 1 — 2 — 3 — 4 — 5 — 6 — 7 — 8 — 9 — 10

WEEK 33 Saying No

In our fast-paced, stressed-out, crazy world, it seems that everyone wants a piece of us. Everyone wants something, and they usually want it right away. Why is it difficult for us to say "No, I can't do this for you"? Why do we add stress to our lives when we know that we shouldn't make one more addition to our "to do" list? We torment ourselves by saying yes to people when we know the answer should be a firm "no." The next time you should say "no" but you don't, think about the reason. Do you want everyone to think you are wonderful? Do you want to be a superhero? Do you fear hurting others like you have been hurt when a "no" you received stung and lingered with pain? You have the right to say "no!" Practice. And don't say "yes" when you mean "no." Trying is what is most important. As Saint Augustine reminds us, "God bestows more consideration on the purity of the intention with which our actions are performed than on the actions themselves."

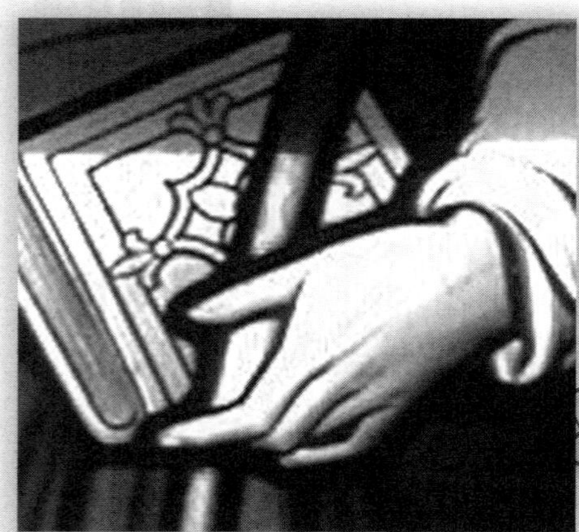

Saint Augustine of Hippo

Saint Augustine, a bishop in North Africa in the late fourth and early fifth centuries, left a legacy of teachings that has spanned the centuries and caused many to experience conversion and a deeper understanding of their faith. Important lessons he taught us by his example, however, are what not to do and when we should say "no." For example, he tried every popular philosophy and lifestyle of his era. But the prayers of his mother, Saint Monica, worked the miracle of his conversion at age thirty when he was baptized at the Easter Vigil in 387 AD. We remember Augustine not for the struggles of his humanity but for the profound way he changed his life and sought God with his whole heart. He learned through tribulation to finally say "no" to what was blocking him from a full knowledge of himself, others and God.

2 Timothy 1:7

For God did not give us a spirit of cowardice, but rather a spirit of power and of love and of self-discipline.

Quote for the Week

To be a witness does not consist in engaging in propaganda nor even in stirring people up, but in being a living mystery. It means to live in such a way that one's life would not make sense if God did not exist.

Emmanuel Célestin Cardinal Suhard

Activity

Make a list of things you should (or want to) say "no" to this week. Then this week mark with a star anytime you say "no" when you are being pressured to say "yes" to that request. If you say "no" to any one thing three times, draw a circle around it!

Things I Should (or Want to) Say "No" to This Week (*When I Do So)

1. ____________________ ________
____

2. ____________________ ________
____

3. ____________________ ________
____

4. ____________________ ________
____

5. ____________________ ________
____

6. ____________________ ________
____

7. ____________________ ________
____

8. ____________________ ________
____

9. ____________________ ________
____

10. ____________________ ________
____

WEEK 34 Flight/Fight/Community

Some people say that they can't bear to hear or say the term "HIV/AIDS" one more time or they will scream. It is a common response to want to run away. This "flight syndrome" happens when we feel overwhelmed and unable to handle anything added to our plate. We walk away or close down because we do not want to address the matter at hand. Flight syndrome is running away from an issue or problem. The opposite is the "fight syndrome." In this, we address the situation head on and "fight" through to the end. When we feel like running away it is, instead, the time we most need community. Being together lifts our spirits, lightens our burdens, and allows us to fully be who we are. A person living with HIV/AIDS said, "There is nothing better than coming to a support group and just being accepted and not having to say that I am HIV-positive because everyone knows and no one cares." "Flight" or "fight" are not the only choices. To be in a group of people who accept you as you are can help tremendously. Hildegard of Bingen knew both the flight/fight syndrome and the healing power of community.

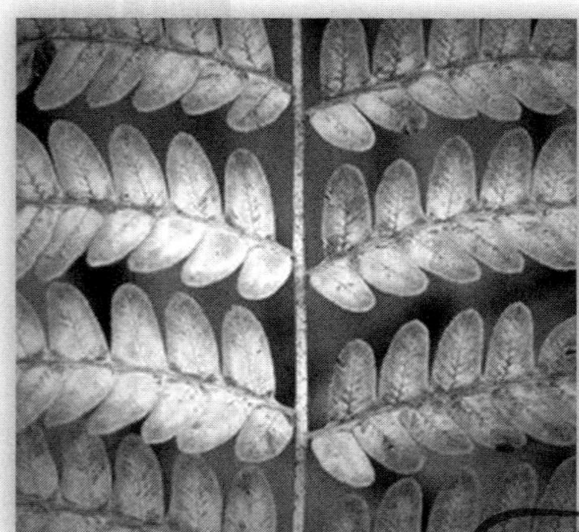

Hildegard of Bingen

Hildegard of Bingen was born in Bockelheim, Germany. From an early age she is reported to have had mystical visions. Around 1147, she founded Rupertsberg Convent near Bingen. Hildegard chose a life of total dedication to God and directed that she be bricked into her cell. Only through a window was she able to receive food and water and whatever simple needs she had. Her prayer and solitude, however, allowed her to create exceptional mystical writings, poems, music and treatises refuting the heresies and schisms of her day. She eventually became the superior of her congregation and an advisor to kings and Church leaders alike. Though never formally canonized by the Church, Hildergard is regarded as a saint by many.

Philemon 1:6

I pray that the sharing of your faith may become effective when you perceive all the good that we may do for Christ.

Quote for the Week

Experiences don't take up space like microwave ovens, but they can cook from the inside just as easily. You can store experiences in your brain and heart, even bad experiences. Don't throw them away. Bad experiences teach lessons you never forget. They temper you and give you strength. They provide contrast to make good experiences better.

Everett White

Activity

Name a problem you are facing right now. List how you might handle the problem by flight, by fight, and through community. During the week, try the method that seems best to you. If it doesn't work by the end of the week, try another method.

My Problem

How to Handle It through Flight

How to Handle It through Fight

How to Handle It through Community

WEEK 35 Love as a Verb

It is beautiful to feel loved, to be desired and cared for by another person. It makes the bad in our lives float away. Love renews and refreshes and energizes us to take on any task. Love gives us purpose and lifts our self esteem. What happens, though, when love just isn't present? What happens when we feel that no one loves us? Love is less a noun and more a verb. Love is something we need to do. Loves means understanding, forgiveness, compassion, respect, loyalty, devotion, care, concern, empathy, sympathy, mercy, joy, hope and faith. When we fall out of love or feel unloved, we need to try love as a verb instead of a noun by showing love to someone else. Love lives in the day to day of loving, not just in the happy feelings that are its byproduct. Saint Thomas of Villanova knew love as a verb, not just a noun.

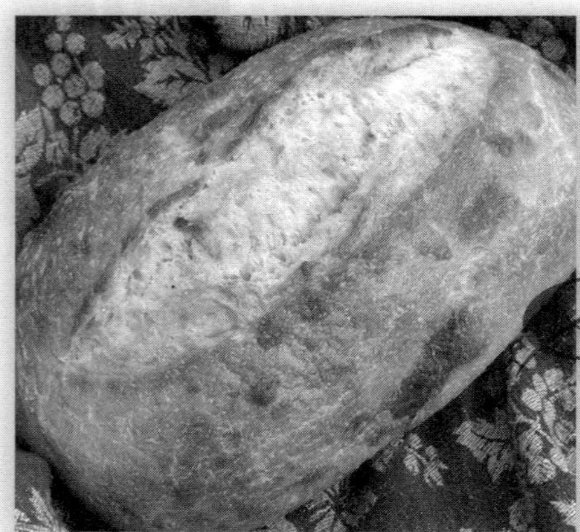

Saint Thomas of Villanova

Thomas of Villanova was an Augustinian Friar in the 1500s in Spain. He taught art, logic and philosophy. Thomas was totally devoted to the poor, and his love for them did not go unnoticed. The emperor proposed Thomas as archbishop of Granada, and the pope confirmed his suggestion. As bishop, Thomas constantly rejected the trappings of his position. Instead, he chose to wear the same habit he had received as a novice, mending it himself. He constantly fed the hungry and gave money to the poor. When given money to furnish his cathedral residence, Thomas gave it all away to the least fortunate of his flock.

1 Corinthians 13:4-7

Love is patient; love is kind; love is not envious or boastful or arrogant or rude. It does not insist on its own way; it is not irritable or resentful; it does not rejoice in wrongdoing, but rejoices in the truth. It bears all things, believes all things, hopes all things, endures all things.

Quote for the Week

Then there are those of us who have accepted the guilt of not being good enough, for whatever reason. Perhaps we feel guilty because of our sex or our sexuality. We may have tremendous guilt for having AIDS. Whatever our guilt feelings may be about, it is time to let them go. Then let us take our energy and use it to find out how we can help ourselves heal.

Louise L. Hay

Activity Think of people who would benefit from your practicing love as a verb—including yourself. Circle each of the verbs you will practice this week, and fill in how you plan to do so. For the rest of the week, try to carry each verb out.

Verb	How I Plan to Practice It This Week
To Believe	
To Understand	
To Empathize	
To Forgive	
To Hope	
To Support	
To Encourage	
To Help	
To Envision	
To Respect	

WEEK 36

Sanctuary

Peter had been living and struggling with HIV for a couple of years, but he was doing well living with other HIV-positive roommates and working on his sobriety. The small quarters the men shared featured loud music, a noisy dog and cat, and a distracting parrot. It was pure bedlam. In a corner of the main room, however, Peter had created a tent-like structure furnished with two comfortable chairs, plants, flowers, a lava light, and a small bubbling fountain. When he and I entered this sanctuary, all other outside noise seemed to go away. This is how Peter survived the chaos. Creating sanctuaries like this in our own lives is not difficult, but we often make it so. We think we don't have the time or the right materials, but a sanctuary is a just a safe place created by us for our own safety, nourishment and enjoyment. It is our "world within our world." It is a place where we draw strength and inner peace, or perhaps just a few stolen quiet moments. Peter's namesake, Saint Peter Claver, knew how to create a sanctuary for those who needed one.

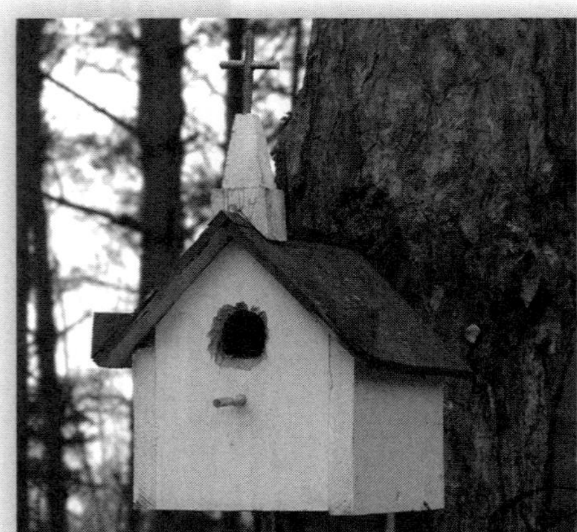

Saint Peter Claver

Saint Peter Claver was a Jesuit missionary from Spain who came to the New World. Once here, he was faced with the horrors of slavery and dedicated the remainder of his years to ministry with slaves. Because of his love for the slaves, Peter offered them sanctuary from the pain and torments of their lives. He cared for their physical and medical needs as well as many of their other material needs. Peter said, "We must speak to them with our hands by giving, before we try to speak to them with our lips." He offered these men, women and children a sense of peace and tranquility, despite his inabilty to stop the horrors brought on by slavery.

1 Chronicles 28:10

Take heed now, for the Lord has chosen you to build a house as the sanctuary; be strong, and act.

Quote for the Week

A Temple is a landscape of the soul.

Joseph Campbell

Activity

In the space below, sketch out your own holy place, your own sanctuary. Keep it simple and realistic. This week, set it up, and then keep it as your own place of comfort.

My Sanctuary

⇩

WEEK 37 Victim Solidarity

The "victim" label is applied to a person who struggles with a terrible thing that has happened to them: some trauma, abuse, loss, crime, unjust illness, or disease that has invaded life like a tsunami and crushed everything in its path. Victims feel trapped, caught, frozen, unable to move. They think they are out of place, dirty, unclean and unloved. They lack joy and happiness and feel constant sorrow and mistrust. The fact is that we are all victims in one way or another at different times in our lives. What is important is that we all recognize this and act in solidarity with one another. We all need affirmation and solid ground to stand on when that time comes. "Rejoice in Hope," says Romans 12:12, because God loves us no matter what, and we are bigger than what the world has labeled us. Saint Vincent de Paul knew that each person who needed him was a child of God, regardless of the label society had placed on them.

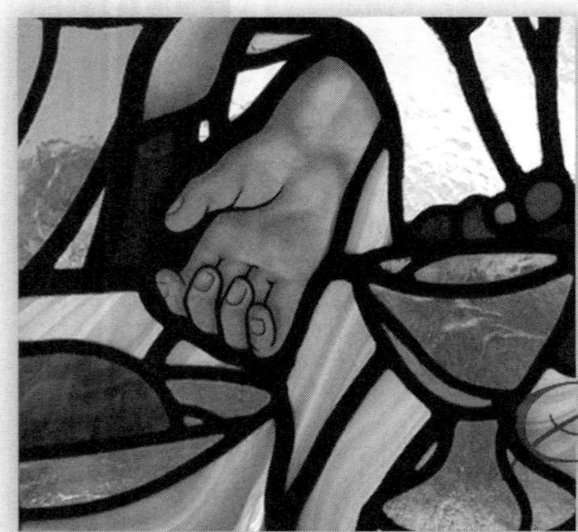

Saint Vincent de Paul

The name of Vincent de Paul is synomous with charity and good works. Thousands of thrift stores and organizations throughout the world are aptly named for Saint Vincent, who dedicated his life to helping the poor, homeless, underprivileged, forgotten and abandoned. Saint Vincent was so well known throughout his native France that nobility would readily open their coffers and donate funds to help support his many causes. Though his work with the poor was highly successful, greater still was Vincent's humility. He never felt he was above the people he served. Rather he was in solidarity with them.

2 Thessalonians 2:16-17

Now may our Lord Jesus Christ himself and God our Father, who loved us and through grace gave us eternal comfort and good hope, comfort your hearts and strengthen them in every good work and word.

Quote for the Week

Heaven shall not wait for the poor to lose their patience, the scorned to smile, the despised to find a friend. Jesus is Lord; he has championed the unwanted; in him injustice confronts its timely end.

John L. Bell

Activity

Read about someone in the newspaper who was a victim this week. Write that person a note below, showing your solidarity. If you can find an address, send him or her a copy, even if it is anonymous. If not, send a letter to the editor of the paper.

Dear ______________________________,

I am a victim, just as you are. Let me explain.

____

____

____

____

____

____

____

____

____

____

____

____

____

____

____

____

____

____

____

____

____

____

Sincerely,

____

Your name or anonymous

WEEK 38 Survivor Solidarity

We all go through periods where we merely survive. We only recognize these times when we look back on them after they are over. Once we have accepted and understood, even if only slightly, that we are victims, we begin to operate in the "survivor" mode. We begin to go on with our lives—making choices, performing tasks, holding down jobs, and being in relationships and marriages. Many of us are highly successful and extremely productive in society's terms. What we lack is a fuller sense of joy, happiness and freedom with which God has blessed us. We behave in the ways that protected us during the time of our victimization. We act, but never question why. Society and loved ones do not notice our terrible, secret feelings of shame, guilt and inferiority. Sometimes, it is hard to recognize that we are survivors. We appear perfect, organized, in control and capable. On the inside, however, we suffer. Saint Thérèse of Lisieux models for us the way we can survive each day and each moment through the simplest of ways.

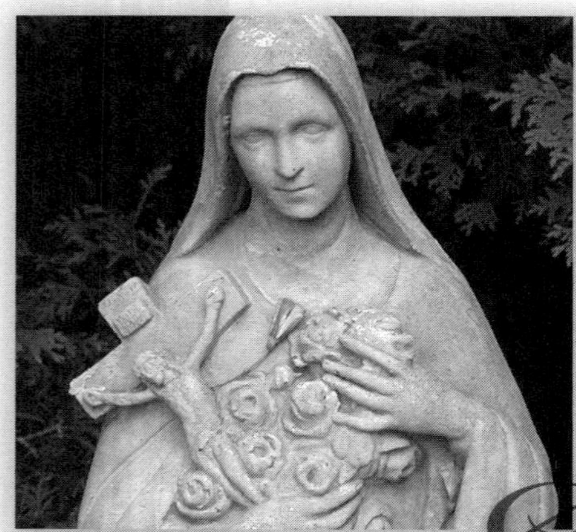

Saint Thérèse of Lisieux

Known to many as the "Little Flower," Thérèse Martin is also known as Saint Thérèse of Lisieux. Born to a middle class French family, Therese was miraculously cured from an illness at age eight. At fifteen, she entered the Carmelite community where she developed a deep spirituality. Her path to God is famously known as "The Little Way" and has been an inspiration for many to come to know God through simplicity and trust. The Little Flower's autobiography, *Story of a Soul*, tells of the peace she obtained through the simplicity of the search for God. All this she accomplished before her death at the age of 24.

Psalm 28:7

The Lord is my strength and my shield; in him my heart trusts; so I am helped, and my heart exults, and with my song I give thanks to him.

Quote for the Week

Jesus did not come to explain away suffering or remove it.
He came to fill it with his presence.

Paul Claudel

Activity

Write a prayer to God below. Ask for the things you need. Be specific.
Pray this prayer for the next week.

Dear God,

Thank you for helping me to survive, but I need the following things to continue:

1. ____
____
____

2. ____
____
____

3. ____
____
____

4. ____
____
____

5. ____
____
____

Your beloved child,

____

WEEK 39 Thriving

Some people are more than survivors. They are "thrivers." Thrivers will take anything—a smile, an experience, a piece of bread—and share it with another, finding in this simple act of gratitude an opportunity to spread joy. What we in the HIV/AIDS community need more than anything else are more thrivers, people who call out the gifts of others and affirm them for who they are. We might, however, need special glasses to help us identify who these people are in our lives. Sometimes they are hard to spot. Sometimes, truth be known, they are even hard to take. Saint Francis of Assisi, for example, could draw from people's pain the love that they held deep inside. But sometimes Francis was difficult for others to tolerate, with his constant joy and his total commitment. People like Saint Francis come into our lives. Sometimes we become unsettled or put off when they ask us to do something we do not have the energy or desire to do, or invite us to share our story when we wish to be silent. They may encourage us to go out in the sunshine when we want to close the draperies and pull up the covers. Moving from victim to survivor to thriver is no easy task, but people do it every day. We must be willing to reach our hand into the darkness and grasp the hand of a person we barely recognize.

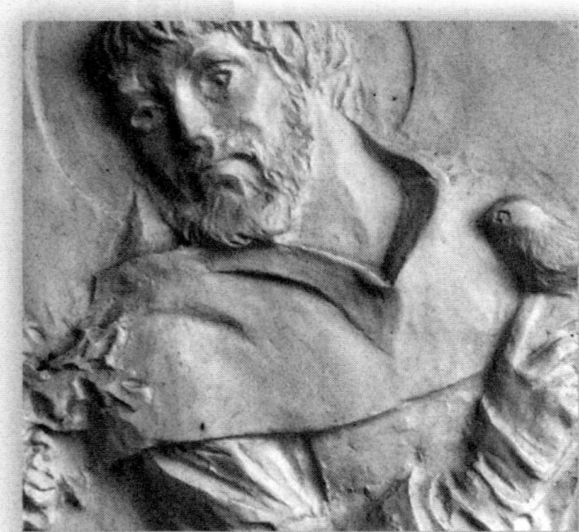

Saint Francis of Assisi

Saint Francis of Assisi is one of the most famous saints known in the world. The familiar brown habit worn today by the Franciscan community he founded is the same one he took when he stripped off his wealthy garments and began his ministry with the poor. Francis died in October 1225 at the age of 45. During the short years of his life, he forever changed the way we look at poverty. He saw the world and nature as the brothers and sisters of all mankind, and he raised poverty to holiness. In giving up his wealth and material possessions, he found that he gained far more in return. We are fortunate to live with his legacy.

Jeremiah 20:13

Sing to the Lord; praise the Lord! For he has delivered the life of the needy from the hands of evildoers.

Quote for the Week

To rid the world of the shame and hatred that make people more vulnerable to HIV infection is to bear the light of God.

Dan Lunney

Activity	List "thrivers" you know, either personally or in the media. Next to each name, jot down one quality each exhibits. During the week, put a star by each quality you practice.

Name of Thriver	Quality Exhibited	(*I Practiced This Week)
1.		
2.		
3.		
4.		
5.		

WEEK 40 Faith through Others

Faith is believing without seeing. It is a leap into the darkness and an act of courage that draws us closer to ourselves, to others, and to God. How do we manage to make this leap? As babies, we depended solely upon our parents and other close relatives to feed, shelter and clothe us. We especially depended on them to protect us and show us love. They represented the first faces of God for us. We found faith through them. Alas, for some of us, our families failed us in this basic task, and so we have had to find God through others in our lives: a kind minister or teacher, a wise counselor or therapist, a true friend or lover. The point is that we learn to recognize the holy, the sacred, the transcendent, the divine, the ultimately meaningful through others. Good relationships with others mirror who God is and allow us to understand and develop our faith. It is never too late to appreciate this wonderful gift from God, but we may need to take a closer look at our relationships, discovering who helps us in our faith and who is holding us back. Saint Callistus is an example of someone who never held anyone back.

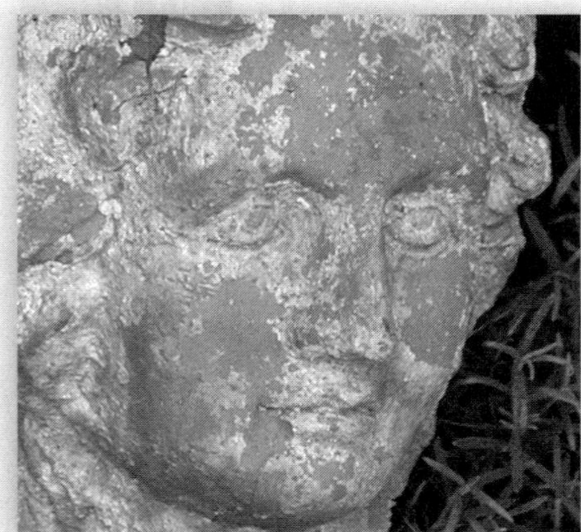

Saint Callistus

Callistus was born a Roman slave. He was imprisoned for being a Christian, but he was later released because he was a favorite of the emperor. Callistus also served Pope Victor, who was impressed by the slave's faithfulness in the face of adversity. Callistus became a deacon and later served as secretary to Pope Zephyrinus. In 217, by popular acclaim of clergy and people of Rome, Callistus was elected Pope. He devoted his papacy to the importance of the need for forgiveness of sin and the right for those forgiven to receive the sacraments. He gave great attention to the burial of the martyrs who filled the tombs on the Appian Way. Despite the trials of his life, Saint Callistus never lost sight of his faith.

Matthew 17:20

If you have faith the size of a mustard seed, you will say to this mountain, "Move from here to there," and it will move; and nothing will be impossible for you.

Quote for the Week

Faith is a living and unshakable confidence, a belief in the grace of God
so assured that a man would die a thousand deaths for its sake.

Martin Luther

Activity

Name below the people who have helped you have faith in God, yourself, and others. Say a prayer each day this week to God for having sent these people into your life.

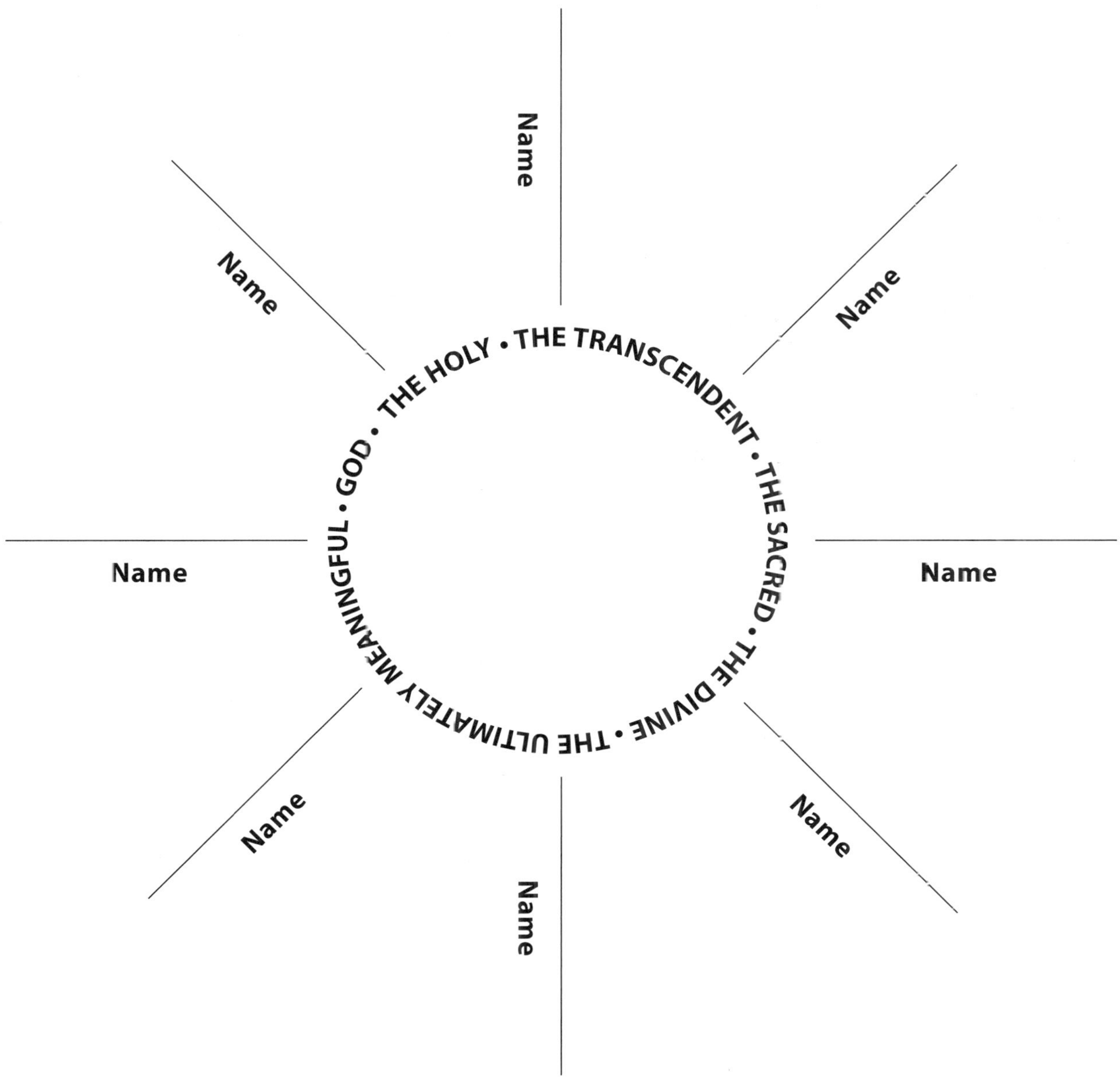

WEEK 41

Spirituality

Spiritual people make time for themselves every day. They attend to their physical, mental and emotional well-being. They seek out places, people and opportunities to feed their spirit. For some, a walk on the beach or on a wooded trail, a jog, or sitting in quiet meditation will lead to spirituality. For others, it can be more formalized and traditional practices, like saying the rosary or novenas or prayers that comfort. Others find spirituality in the midst of their daily work or social justice activity. Spirituality is simply awareness: a decision to get in touch with ourselves and with God by looking at who we are and what we do, then improving those behaviors and applying them to become the best person we can be. Spirituality is drawing deeply from the personal well buried deep inside. It is an awareness of faith in self, others and God that allows us to understand and to forgive and accept. It is the calm in the storms of life that everyone seeks. Spirituality is a way of living that brings us fullness. It is what we yearn for but often give up on because of lack of time and energy. Saint Teresa of Avila was an expert in spirituality and has much to teach us today.

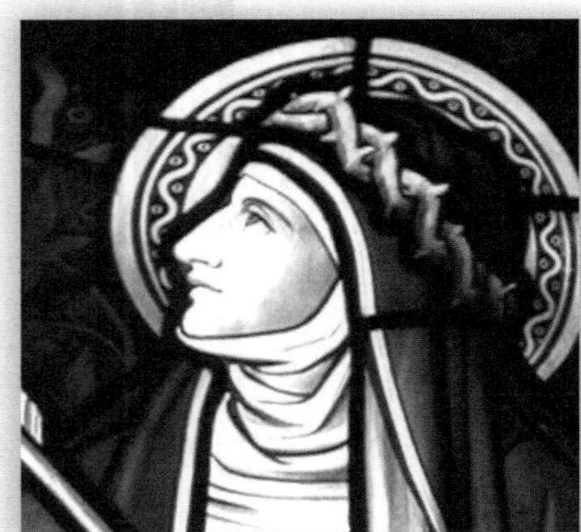

Saint Teresa of Avila

As a child, Teresa of Avila, whose human side was very much a part of who she was, loved clothes and loved to flirt with boys. As an adult, Teresa surprised her family by entering a Carmelite monastery. Religious life in the mid 1500s was often chosen by women as an escape from the world, not for anything to do with the pursuit of holiness. Teresa, however, recognized the Lord's call to her heart and soul, and it guided her on the way to holiness. Through a deeper understanding of her own prayer and spitiruality, Teresa pursued the reformation of the Carmelite Order to restore it to its original intention. We recognize Teresa not only for the holiness of her life but also the holy way she overcame great obstacles to draw herself and others nearer to God. Along with Saint Catherine of Siena, she is one of only two women Doctors of the Church.

Philippians 1:9

And this is my prayer, that your love may overflow more and more with knowledge and full insight.

Quote for the Week

Our spirituality is our opening to another as whole human beings,
each different and precious, and our exploring how we can truly love.

Jean Grasso-Fitzpatrick

Activity Name some of your spiritual practices in the balloons below. Carry out each one this week at least once. If you don't have any spiritual disciplines, start at least one. As you try others, draw and fill in more balloons.

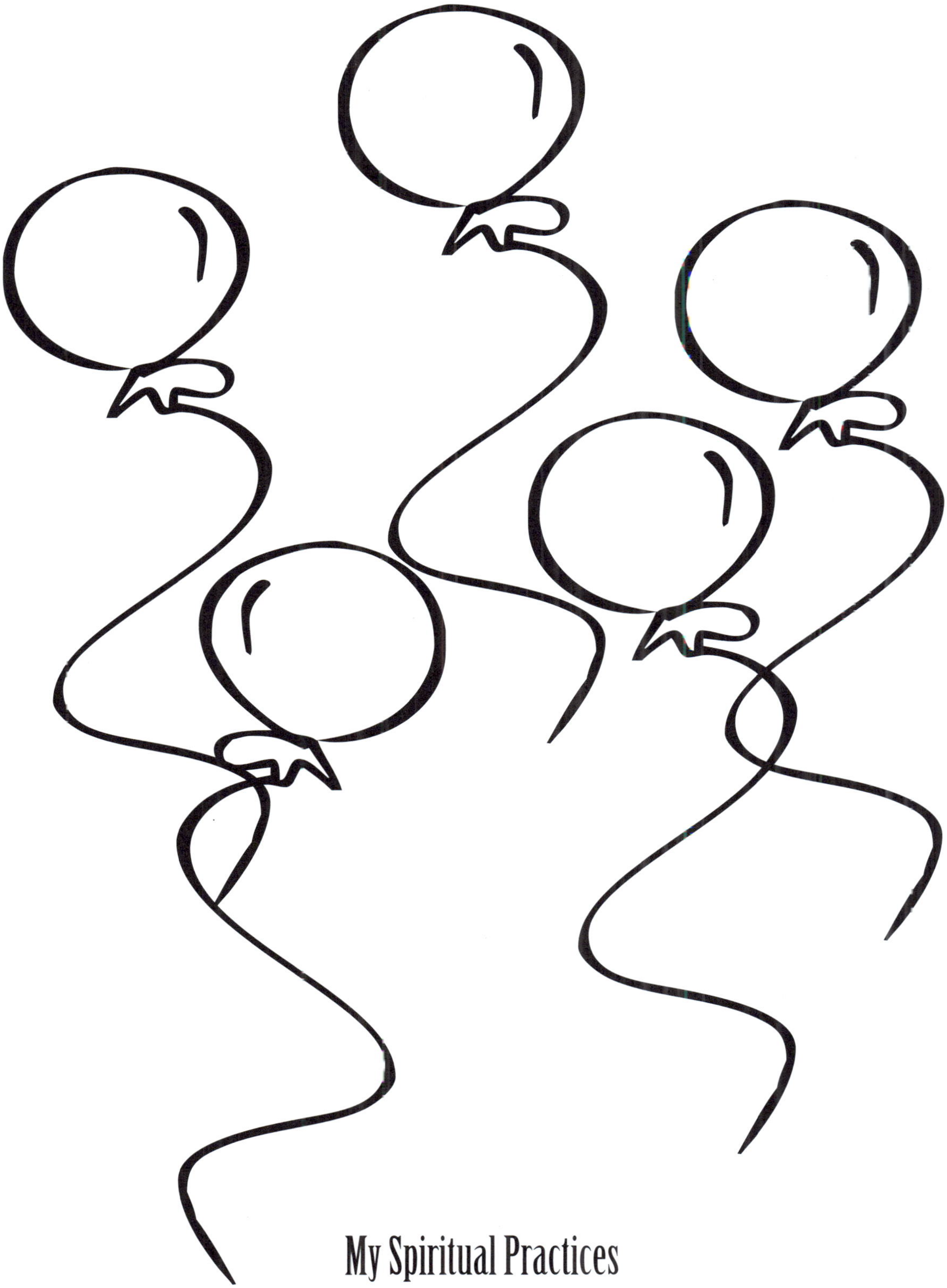

My Spiritual Practices

WEEK 42 Religion

Religion is about hospitality and belonging. Religion uses rites, rules, and regulations to help us encounter God and live moral lives. Religious doctrines and beliefs give us ways to deal with the complexities of life. Religion is hard for some people because it places responsibilities upon us. We can't practice religion alone; we need to be in community. Religion allows us many opportunities to come together to celebrate birth, life, commitments, death, and rites of passage. It allows us to put words and song to our deepest feelings. Religion is meant to keep us together and to invite others in. It is not closed or exclusive. It is not just for the rich, the healthy, and those without struggle. Saint Martin de Porres did not let his modest origins prohibit him from finding a home in religion and from using his religious faith to draw and heal those who needed it most. He knew, as we should, that without faith and spirituality, religion is nothing but a shell.

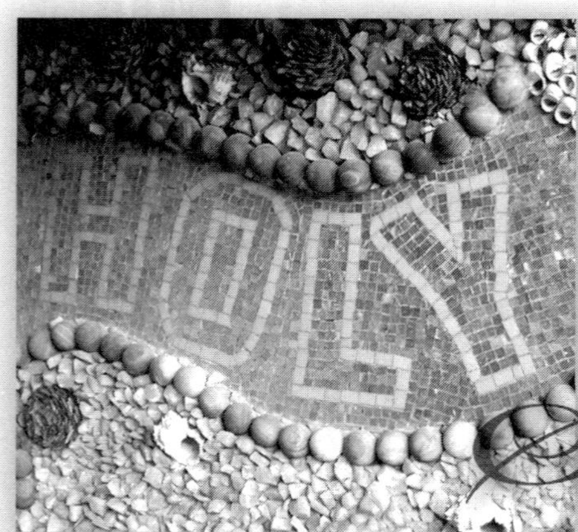

Saint Martin de Porres

Martin, born in Lima, Peru, was the illegitimate son of a Spanish nobleman and a young Indian woman. Martin's mother struggled to care for his sister and him, but she eventually had no choice but to place Martin in the care of a barber/surgeon to learn a trade. He later joined the Dominican brothers, where he used his skills to care for the sick and poor. Martin loved his life and his work with the poor, sick and marginalized. He prayed hard, worked harder, and sacrificed all for the love of God and his people. Many cures are attributed to Saint Martin de Porres, who is reported to have appeared in Africa, China, Algeria and Japan, yet he never left his home town in Peru.

Luke 4:18

The Spirit of the Lord is upon me, because he has anointed me to bring good news to the poor. He has sent me to proclaim release to the captives and recovery of sight to the blind, to let the oppressed go free.

Quote for the Week

Religion is something infinitely simple, ingenuous. It is not knowledge, not content of feeling, it is not duty and not renunciation, it is not restriction: but in the infinite extent of the universe it is a direction of the heart.

Rainer Maria Rilke

Activity

Take any formal prayer from the list below or another one you might have learned from your religious upbringing. Try to write it from memory below. If you have trouble, look it up on the Internet and then write it out. During the next week, say this prayer for all those who feel isolated and lost or need it the most.

Some Formal Prayers

- The Our Father
- The Hail Mary
- The Glory Be to the Father
- Hail, Holy Queen
- The Memorare
- The Prayer of Saint Francis
- The Serenity Prayer
- Prayer to Your Guardian Angel
- The Magnificat
- The Apostles Creed

Write One Prayer Here

WEEK 43

Replaying Tapes

Sometimes we become trapped into playing and replaying negative tapes over and over in our minds, then playing out these tapes in our lives. Facing HIV/AIDS head-on means facing these negative stories from our past and changing them into positive experiences. In her work, *The AIDS Book: Creating a Positive Approach*, Louise Hay states that if we have negative thinking patterns now is a good time to change them. She encourages us to replace: resentment with understanding; fear with peace; depression with forgiveness; rage with love; jealousy with rejoicing; despair with hope; self-pity with self-responsibility; rejection with acceptance; self-hatred with self-love. Saint Elizabeth of Hungary gave away her wealth and found peace and contentment in being poor. It is the mark of a great person who is able to turn around their life situations in such remarkable ways.

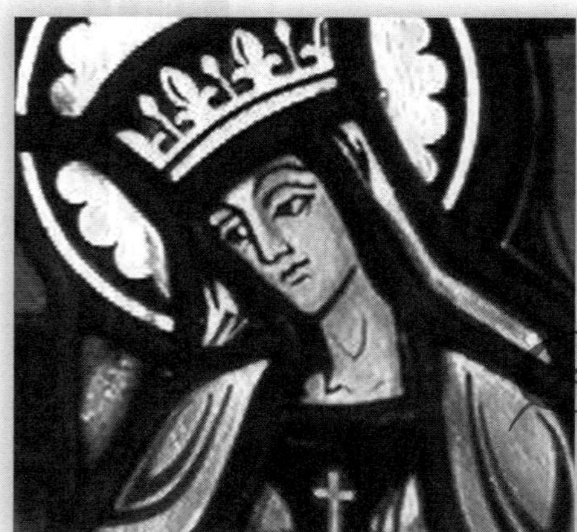

Saint Elizabeth of Hungary

Saints are often thought to come from poor families. Their struggles in poverty put them in touch with what is really important in life. This is not true of Saint Elizabeth of Hungary, who was born of royalty as a medieval princess. Greatly influenced by her saintly father, Louis of Thuringia, she refused all the trappings of her position. Instead, she used her resources to feed and clothe the poor. When her own funds were gone, she begged on behalf of the poor and gave them everything she earned. Praying, fasting and serving others was not the life Elizabeth was born to, but it was the life she chose. She lived only twenty-four years, but her people adored her. It was no wonder that she was canonized a saint only four years after her death.

Psalm 51:12

Restore to me the joy of your salvation, and sustain in me a willing spirit.

Quote for the Week

We keep a problem a problem
when we indulge it by obsessing over it.

Bob

Activity Take a long, hard look at the negative and positive thinking patterns below. Write instances in your life where you can replace negative ones with a positive response.

Negative	Positive	Instance Where I Can Change
Resentment	Understanding	
Fear	Peace	
Depression	Forgiveness	
Rage	Love	
Jealousy	Rejoicing	
Despair	Hope	
Self-Pity	Self-Responsibility	
Rejection	Acceptance	
Self-Hatred	Self-Love	

WEEK 44 Loneliness/Aloneness

Sometimes, it is difficult to see the difference between being lonely and being alone. We can be in a crowded room but feel very alone or be in a room by ourselves yet feel very connected and content. Loneliness is difficult to bear. It is the feeling that we face life with all its troubles, hardships, joys and happiness—entirely by ourselves. It is a place in life where no one is around to care or—just the opposite—many people are around but they are too busy to show that they care. "Aloneness," on the other hand, can often be a good thing. It is a place we go to get in touch with who we are and to clear our minds. Aloneness is the place that affords us the time to figure things out, to face our fears, to plan, to dream, to vision, to sing little songs of happiness to ourselves. Sometimes it is also a place where we cry our eyes out. It is a place where we renew ourselves, where we ready ourselves to join the rest of the world and deal with people who are perhaps crazier than we are. Saint Cecilia understood loneliness, because she was estranged from her family and her society, but she stood alone with great courage.

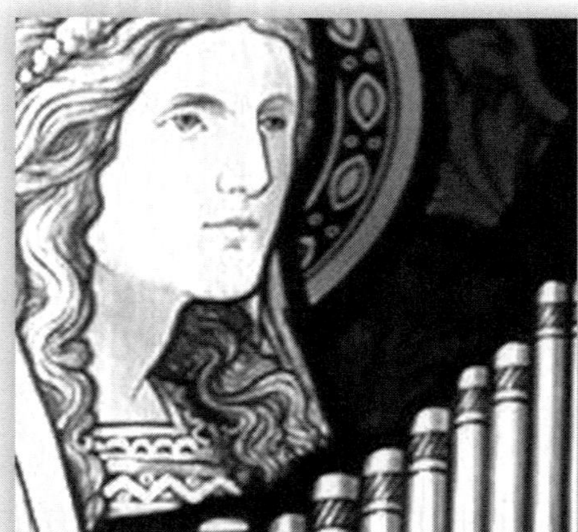

Saint Cecilia

Cecilia was born into a noble family of wealth. Although her other family members were non-Christian, Cecilia yearned to follow the teachings of Christ. Alone in her love for God and very lonely as she struggled to live in a family and society that spurned Christianity, Cecilia was forced to marry a pagan nobleman. Through her love, however, her husband was converted and baptized. Cecilia dedicated her life to helping other Christians who were tortured and persecuted. She attended those who were brutalized in the Christian persecutions at the Coliseum and helped give the Christian dead a proper burial. Cecilia was killed after she refused to deny her belief in God. A beautiful marble statue of Saint Cecilia lies in the catacombs of Christian martyrs. She is portrayed at her death with three fingers extended, telling the world that nothing would separate her from the love of her triune God: Father, Son and Holy Spirit.

Ecclesiastes 4:10

For if they fall, one will lift up the other; but woe to one who is alone and falls and does not have another to help.

Quote for the Week

Only in solitude do we find ourselves; and in finding ourselves,
we find in ourselves all our brothers in solitude.

Miguel DeUnamuno

Activity

Copy and then cut out the hearts below and tape them at random around your house where you will see them. Whenever you encounter one of them over the next week, spend a few minutes alone, rejoicing in your privacy and independence.

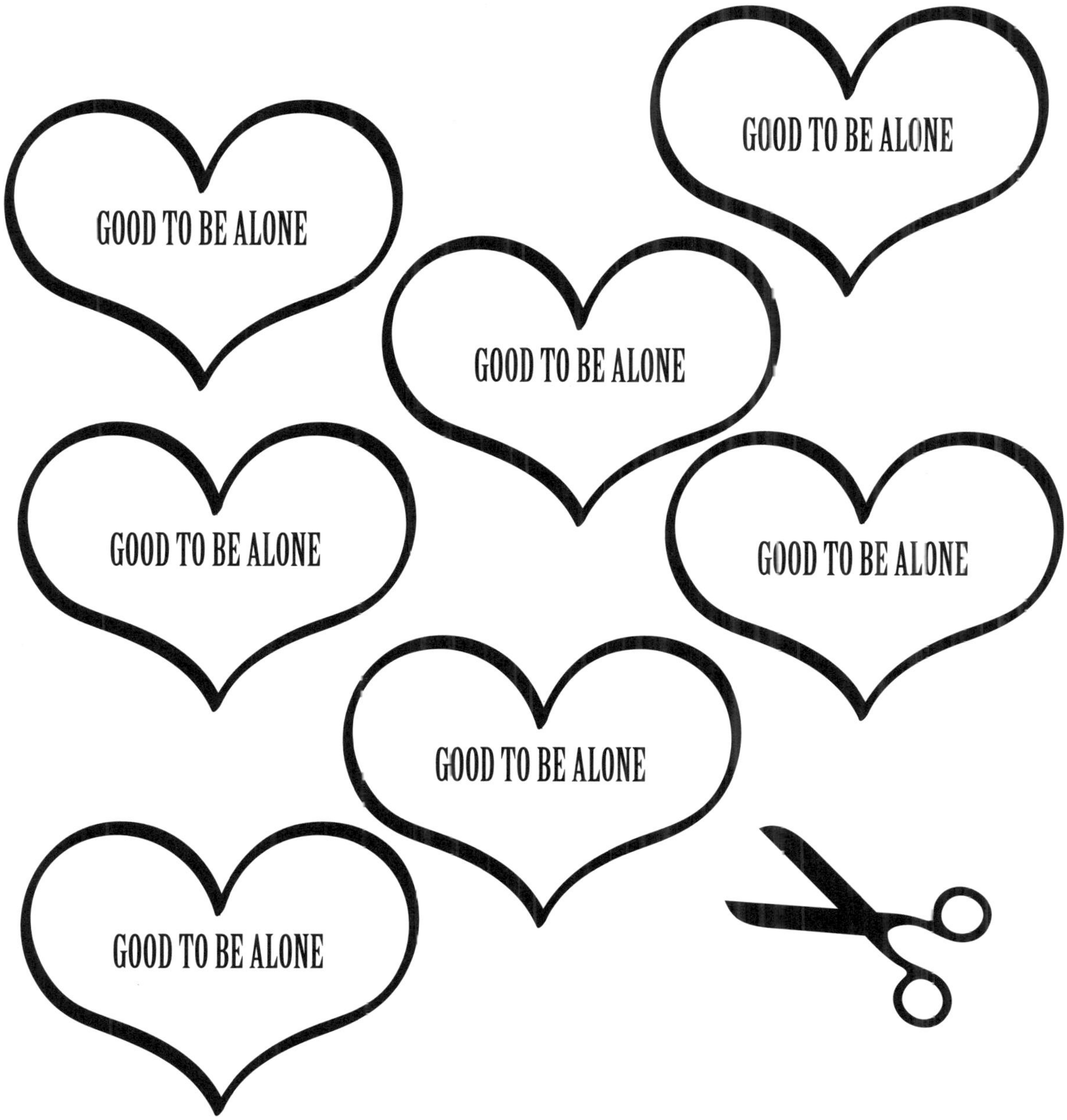

WEEK 45 Negative Self-Talk

Negative self-talk is what we say to ourselves in the present that chains us to past events and circumstances. Sometimes one particular person is responsible for the negative feelings we have about ourselves. Perhaps a parent, guardian, family member, or teacher did not give us the affirmation that we needed to be nurtured. Unfortunately, some people think that to put us down, scold or berate is the way to teach us or challenge us. More often, this technique convinces us that "I am no good. I can't do anything right." We need to realize that this negative thinking is wrong, and the behavior that caused it is destructive. We need to change negative self-talk into positive self-talk. We need to replace every "I can't" with "I can." We need to do our very best, even if we fail. We need to break away from the self-fulfilling prophecy phenomenon and stop causing ourselves to fail by talking ourselves into it. We doom ourselves to failure even before we tackle a challenge if we let the negative overcome the positive. Dorothy Day saw the positive in each and every person she met on her journey.

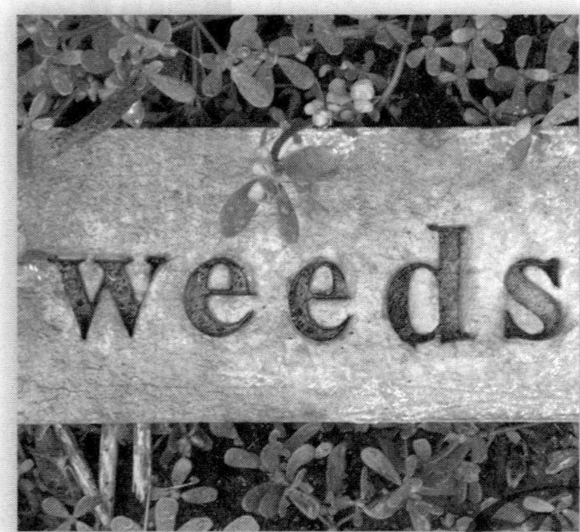

Dorothy Day

Dorothy Day was not only a bold advocate for the poor and marginalized, she was also a herald of peace and justice for our time. She was a self-made woman who embraced the social teachings of the gospel and promoted the "Catholic Worker Movement." Through her work, everyday Catholics embraced love of the poor and were moved to action. *Praxis*, a Greek word for "faith in action," was the underlying theme to all that Dorothy did. She raised up the lowly in a mighty way by teaching, feeding, and clothing them and by modeling the deep love that God posessed for each and every one of them.

Philippians 1:6

I am confident of this, that the one who began a good work among you will bring it to completion by the day of Jesus Christ.

Quote for the Week

What is this self inside us, this silent observer, severe and speechless critic, who can terrorize us, and urge us on to futile activity, and in the end, judge us still more severely, for the errors into which his own reproaches drove us?

T. S. Elliot

Activity

List three of your favorite songs of all time. Now, write down a favorite word or phrase from each song. Do these words or phrases challenge or inspire you? Do they make you happy or sad? Take one of the lines and make them your motto for the next week.

Song Title	Line or Phrase

WEEK 46 Just as I Am

For years, each time Billy Graham held a prayer service, the song "Just as I Am" would be sung when the people from the audience came forth to accept Jesus. The simplicity of the song sends forth a powerful message to each person who hears it. One verse of "Just as I Am" is a beautiful testimony to the trials of a person's life: "Just as I am, though tossed about, with many a conflict, many a doubt, fighting and fear from within, without, O Lamb of God, I come, I come!" We are all special, all valuable and pleasing to God and to many others. No matter how small, short, tall, fat, or thin we may be, we have a right to our space in this world. Like Jean Donovan, let us make sure we take all of our space—nothing more and nothing less—and only give some of it up when we choose to. We deserve to love ourselves just as we are, no matter how unfinished we think we might be.

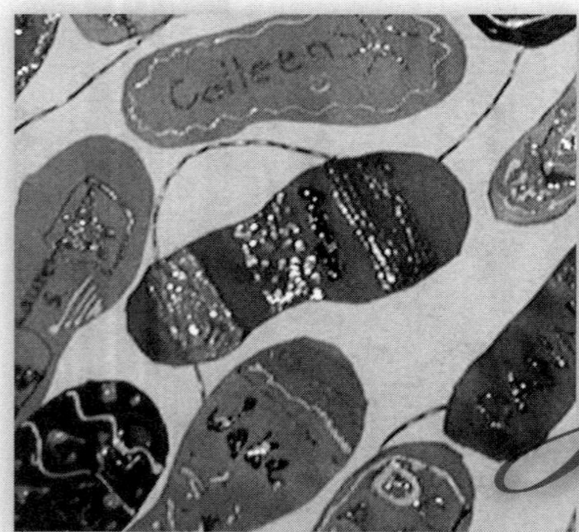

Jean Donovan

Jean Donovan was a young woman who accepted herself for who she was. After graduating from college with a Masters in Business Administration, she chose to follow her heart. She yearned to fill a void in her life and felt called to something more. Despite a promising future in the business world, she answered the call to be a lay missionary in El Salvador. She worked with the poor and those oppressed by the military, distributing food and clothing to them. Her reward for this simple gesture of love came on the night of December 2, 1980. Jean and three vowed religious women were assassinated and buried in shallow graves. Before she died, Jean wrote to a friend. She said that she would have left El Salvador when the bloodbath began if it were not for the children. "Who would care for them? Who could turn away from their eyes and their tears?"

Deuteronomy 14:2

For you are a people holy to the Lord your God; it is you the Lord has chosen out of all the peoples on earth to be his people, his treasured possession.

Quote for the Week

What does matter is a place where one who lives with HIV/AIDS, or one who is affected by HIV/AIDS, can be and feel safe. A place where someone will listen and give undivided attention, a place where there are no judgments, no hoops to jump through for entitlements like a food voucher or a blanket, a place where plain old acceptance "just as I am" is the order of the day.

Krysten Winter-Green

Activity Make a list below of things that make you "just as you are." Celebrate each one of them this week in some way.

Things that Make Me Just as I Am

1. ______________________________
____
2. ______________________________
____
3. ______________________________
____
4. ______________________________
____
5. ______________________________
____
6. ______________________________
____
7. ______________________________
____
8. ______________________________
____
9. ______________________________
____
10. ______________________________
____

WEEK 47 Challenging Friendship

Picking good friends is an art. Being a friend is a gift. It is knowing what to say or not to say and when. Surrounding ourselves with people who love us and care for us is the greatest gift we can give ourselves. Celebrating the joys and sorrows of life with a friend or confiding in a good friend is immensely comforting. Sometimes we find ourselves surrounded by friends who are kind and generous but do not offer us the challenges we truly need. Of great importance is the type of friend who can say, "What's wrong with you?" when we need to hear it. We need our friends to be straightforward and candid, to challenge us to live healthy, happy lives. They need to say things like, "Eat more" or "Eat less" or "Get out in the sunshine and go for a walk" or "Stay inside and get some rest." Saint Francis Xavier knew how to challenge his friends.

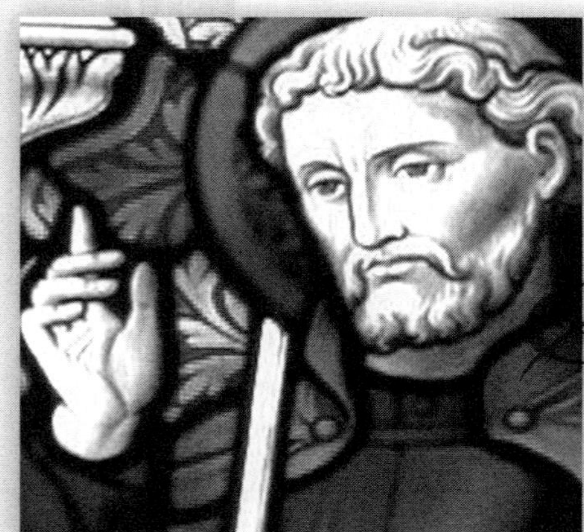

Saint Francis Xavier

Francis Xavier was an intelligent man trained by Saint Ignatius of Loyola. He spent his life working in India and other parts of Asia and brought many converts to God. Legend tells us that Francis had the "gift of tongues" and related extremely well to the different people and cultures he encountered. People were drawn to him, and he lived what he preached. He refused the conveniences offered to him and instead sought the poor and sick to minister to them with genuine love. Saint Francis gave up everything that was comfortable, including his home, so he could share the love of God he carried in his heart with many people.

1 John 4:7

Beloved, let us love one another, because love is from God; everyone who loves is born of God and knows God.

Quote for the Week

Friendship makes prosperity more brilliant,
and lightens adversity by dividing and sharing it.

Cicero

Activity

Call up one of your good friends and make an appointment to meet this week. Go to the local convenience store and buy your favorite soft drinks and snacks. Bring these to the meeting, and just enjoy each other's company. Discuss whether and how you challenge one another on issues of personal development. Write below what you learn.

What I Learned at Our Meeting

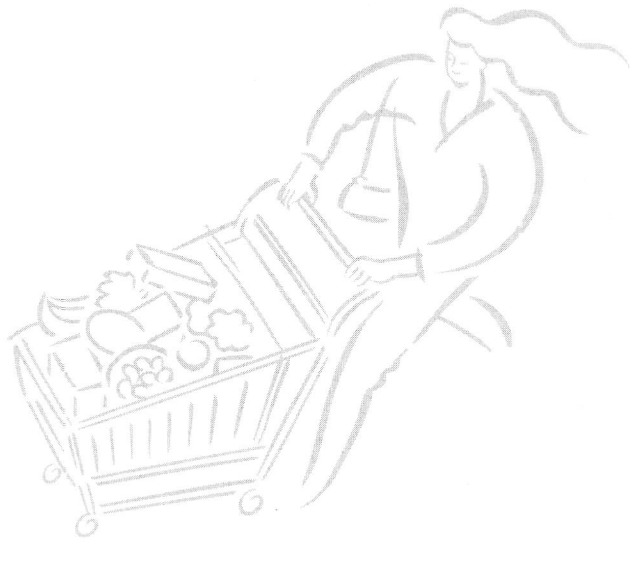

WEEK 48 Prayer

Prayer centers us on what matters most in our lives, no matter how painful or joyful. It calls us again and again to conversation with the most powerful witness in life—the One who loves us regardless of what we say or do. In difficult times, prayer can lift us up and help us focus on what is important. In times of great happiness, prayer can call us to share and to continue our journey with peace. Certainly, not everyone is called to devote their whole life to prayer as Thomas Merton was, but making prayer a part of our everyday actions is possible. Prayer can be formal or informal. It can be the recitation of comfortable and familiar devotions, favorite prayers, scripture passages, or the liturgies the Church offers. Prayer can be impromptu conversation with God. "God, please be with me today in a mighty way. I think it's going to be a rough one," is powerful in its spontaneity. Most importantly, prayer is heartfelt and straightforward.

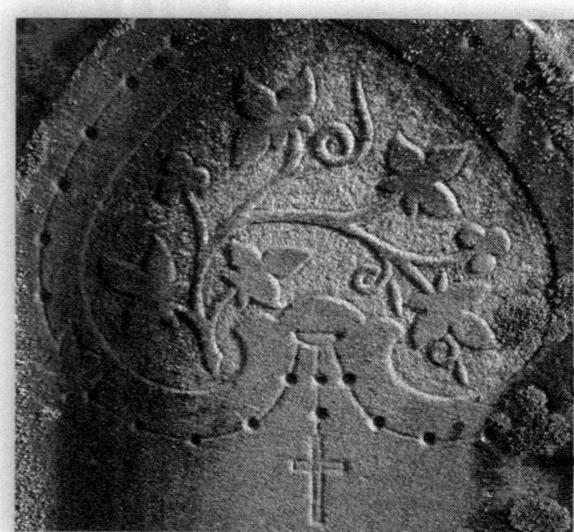

Thomas Merton

It is amazing how a cloistered, Trappist monk who spent his life in solitude and prayer has affected thousands of people. Thomas Merton began his journey as a vibrant, intelligent, capable and inquisitive young man. He was driven by a search for personal meaning, but his journey was transformed into a search for the love of God. His autobiographical memoire, *The Seven Storey Mountain*, describes his search for God through traditional Christian mysticism and the sacred gifts that ancient cultures offered his prayer life. The intensity of Merton's prayer life led him to profound writings. Those writings have moved people of later generations to address the political and social ills of their own time—civil rights, peace, justice, war, and nuclear disarmament. His prayerful life of contemplation brought inspiration to many.

1 Kings 8:28

Have regard to your servant's prayer and his plea, O Lord my God, heeding the cry and the prayer that your servant prays to you today.

Quote for the Week

To seek God is not difficult for the earnest soul, for He has left us countless clues to His presence—within us in conscience, behind us in history, around us in the best people we know, in our hands, in His word, before us in the heart's resilient hopefulness, and plainest of all in the ever-accessible Christ. God may not always be obvious, but He is there discernable, knowable, reachable, dependable, and ever welcoming.

Author Unknown

Activity

Write a short, one-sentence prayer for each of the forms of prayer below. Share your feelings, doubts and concerns with God. Set aside five minutes each day this week to have a conversation with God, using one of your prayers.

Prayer of Praise

Prayer of Contrition

Prayer of Thanks

Prayer of Petition

WEEK 49

Forgiveness and Peace

Seeking peace through forgiveness requires a lot of hard work, compassion and empathy. Many times we ask to be forgiven for something we have done, but we do not forgive ourselves. We do not let go but continue to punish ourselves over and over again. Forgiveness comes from deep within, from a desire to be at peace with who we are, what we did, and what we can do in the future to affect peace. We need to forgive ourselves for what we have done in the past, so that we can live fully in the present. Otherwise, we are wasting precious time. So, too, we are wasting beautiful time if we allow others who have harmed us to dominate our feelings and thoughts. We must not allow those who may not be remorseful to have power over us. We must let them go. Forgiveness frees us in many ways, allowing us to be positive individuals focused on health of body, mind and soul. For saints like Lucy, pardon and forgiveness seemed to come readily, even for those who betrayed and tortured them. It seems impossible to us, but her life was built on a strong faith that sustained her throughout terrible times.

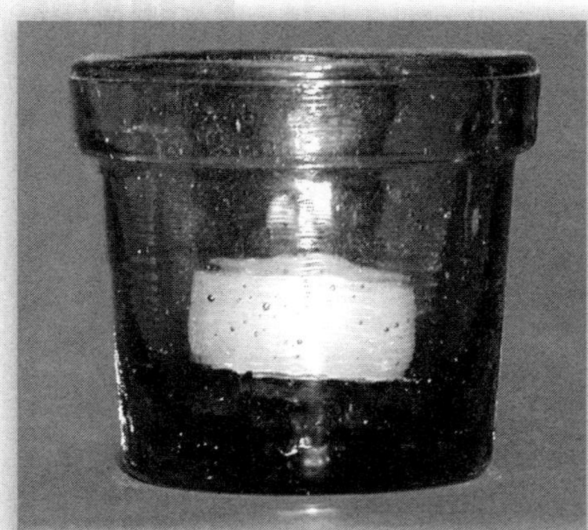

Saint Lucy

Lucy lived in the fourth century and was martyred during the persecution of the early Church. Legend tells us that Lucy spurned a pagan lover who betrayed her after she refused to participate in pagan rituals. She was brutally tortured. Her eyes were gouged out before she was stabbed to death. Lucy's great faith spawned many stories about her heroism. She was canonized in the sixth century. Lucy's name is derived from the Latin word *lux*, meaning "light," and she is the patron of all those who have troubles with their eyes. When Lucy lived, being a Christian often meant dying for your beliefs. This brave, courageous woman did just that.

Matthew 18:21-22

Then Peter came and said to him, "Lord, if another member of the church sins against me, how often should I forgive? As many as seven times?" Jesus said to him, "Not seven times, but, I tell you, seventy-seven times."

Quote for the Week

Forgiveness is the answer to the child's dream of a miracle by which
what is broken is made whole again, what is soiled is again made clean.

Dag Hammarskjold

Activity

Write below the name of someone you should forgive. Write the reason you need to forgive him or her. Then write down what blocks you from offering forgiveness. If it is possible and appropriate, seek to offer that person forgiveness this week. If not, write down one other action you could take this week to achieve a measure of inner peace.

Whom I Should Forgive

Why I Should Forgive That Person

What Is Blocking Me from Forgiving

One Action I Can Take This Week to Achieve Inner Peace

WEEK 50 Kidding Ourselves

We all kid ourselves. It is part of our system of self-preservation. We might say, "I have to lose twenty pounds" when it is really forty or more we have to trim. Our problems go up and down according to our self-perception. Kidding ourselves is a way of proving to ourselves that we aren't all that bad. We can stop kidding ourselves if we work on it. If we slip, fall or fail, we can start over, again and again and again. Knowing what we are struggling with, naming it, and admitting to it are the first and biggest steps on the road to acknowledgment, self-awareness and recovery. Like Saint John of the Cross, we need to look closely at our lives and then make the changes necessary to put ourselves on the track to truth and holiness.

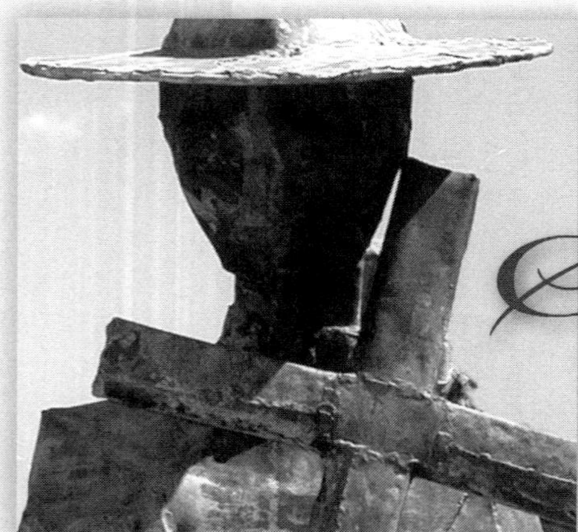

Saint John of the Cross

John, after an extraordinarily difficult youth, joined the Carmelites. Saint Teresa of Avila, also a Carmelite, asked him to join her in bringing reform to the Order, to restore its tradition of contemplative prayer. John is aptly associated with the Cross, as his life's journey bore many crosses. Many other Carmelites wanted nothing to do with the reform, and they felt threatened by the changes that John presented. In fact, some monks felt so threatened by the reform that they locked him into a tiny room where they would go to beat him three times a week. Instead of turning to anger and hatred, John turned to God, who filled him with joy and love. In his book *The Dark Night of the Soul*, Saint John of the Cross reflects on the suffering he experienced to bring about change and reform to his religious community.

1 Peter 3:6

Do what is good and never let fear alarm you.

Quote for the Week

When the record of any human life is set down,
there are three pairs of eyes who see it in a different light:
a. As I see it; b. As others see it; c. As God sees it.

Archbishop Fulton J. Sheen

Activity

In the blocks below, name a few of these obstacles in your life. Count them up and see what you are really facing. Are there more or fewer than you thought? This week, pick one obstacle and work on it. (You might find out the entire pile will begin to crumble.)

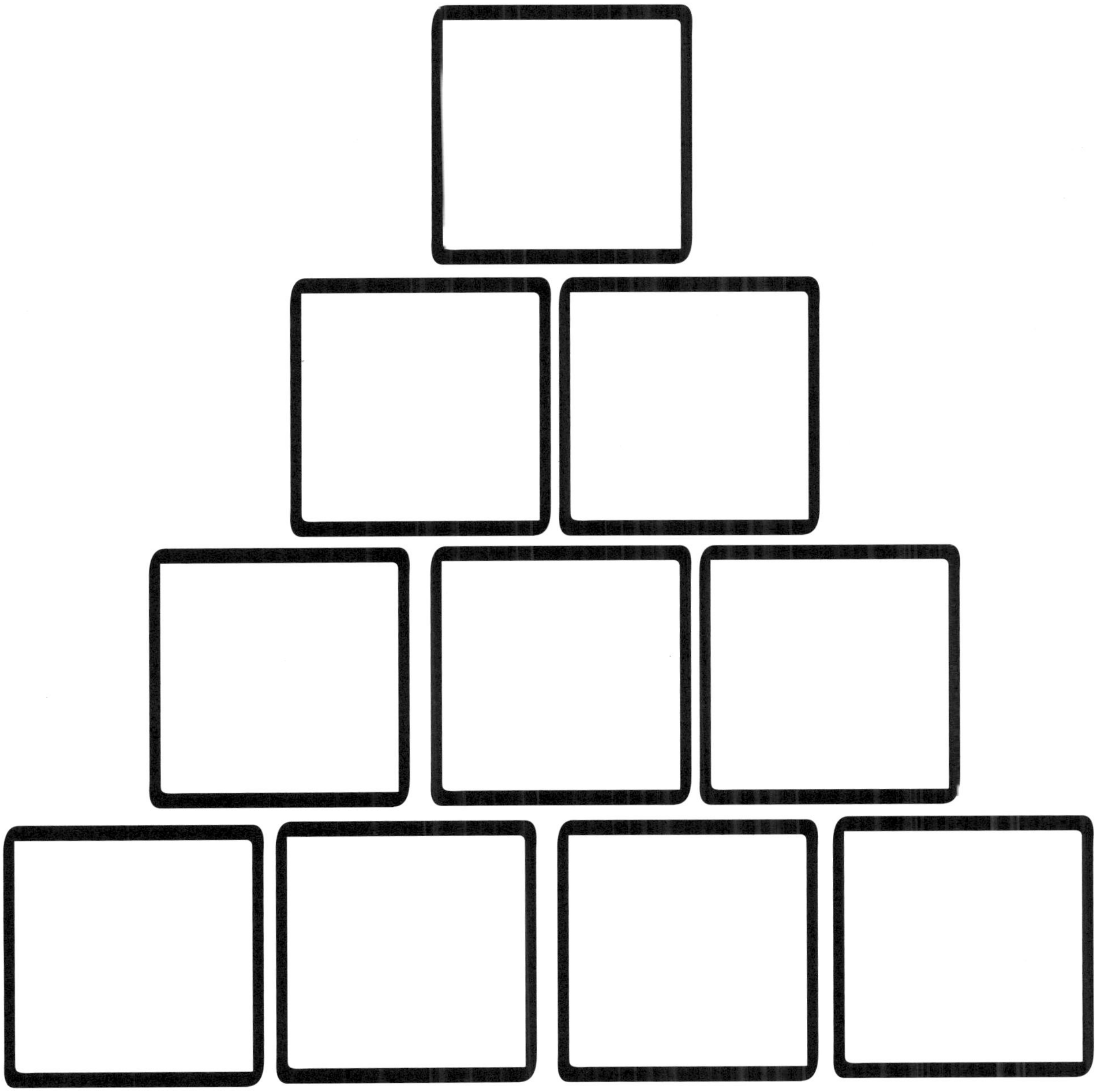

Obstacles I Face

WEEK 51

Confidentiality

In the world of HIV/AIDS, confidentiality is of the utmost importance. Many people who need services do not get them because they are afraid certain people will find out their status. People suffer more from the stigmas of the disease than from the symptoms of the syndrome itself. Mother Cabrini's life is a great model for those of us struggling to keep confidences. She treated the poor, the ill, and the homeless with great care and respect. She always put their need for dignity ahead of her own. We need to keep confidences to ourselves. We must respect others as we would want our own privacy respected. We must think before we speak. Sometimes an innocent comment can cause severe damage to a person's life. Not everyone is as open and understanding about the virus as we are. We need to respect all people, all the time.

Saint Frances Xavier Cabrini

Frances Xavier Cabrini, an Italian immigrant to the United States, was small in stature and often frail with ill health. But she was as tough as nails when it came to providing for poor immigrants, the sick, and the hungry. This naturalized American traveled throughout the United States, Europe, and Central and South America. She established 67 institutes for the poor—hospitals, orphanages, schools, and low income housing. Mother Cabrini attracted many women to follow in her footsteps in the religious order she founded, the Missionary Sisters of the Sacred Heart. She let nothing get in her way of serving those on the margins of society, yet she never broke a confidence.

Luke 16:10

Whoever is faithful in a very little is faithful also in much; and whoever is dishonest in a very little is dishonest also in much.

Quote for the Week

I dreamed in a dream, I saw a city invincible to the attacks of the whole of the rest of the earth, I dreamed that was the new City of Friends, nothing was greater there than the quality of robust love—it led the rest. It was seen every hour in the actions of the men of that city, and in all their looks and words.

Walt Whitman

Activity

List below in your past when you or someone else broke a confidence and how it made you feel. What resulted from each breach of confidence? This week, be more aware of confidences you hold.

A Confidence of Mine Someone Broke

How I Felt

What Was the Result

A Confidence of Someone That I Broke

How I Felt

What Was the Result

WEEK 52 Rejoice in Hope

Saint Paul wrote "Rejoice in hope, be patient in suffering, persevere in prayer" (Romans 12:12). At times, there is nothing else we can do but rejoice in hope. There is so much death, suffering, persecution, hatred, violence and prejudice around HIV/AIDS that hope is sometimes all we have. There are still no answers in the medical field and no money to do what needs to be done worldwide. Saint Charbel, in his humble yet profound way, offered hope to others through the simple way he lived his life. Those of us who journey together rejoice in the hope of our brothers and sisters who have gone before us, and we stand on their shoulders. We hope and pray that this suffering will end, that God will send the cure and stop the virus from spreading, that hatred towards those who are infected because of their lifestyle will cease. We have watched our brothers and sisters endure in affliction. We have cried out to God in prayer and continue to rejoice in hope. God is always near us in the persons, places, and things that we meet and dream of meeting every day.

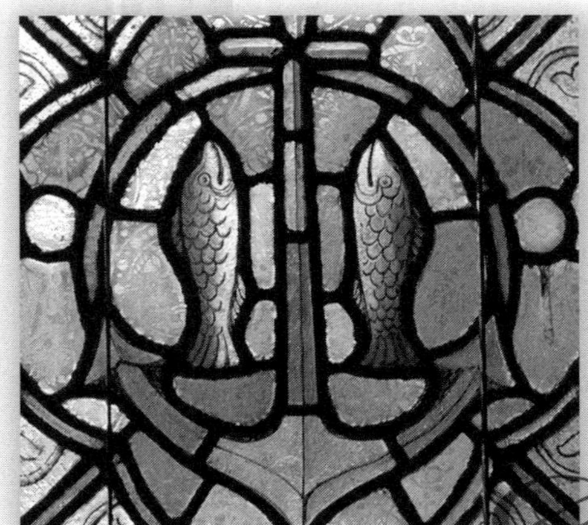

Saint Charbel

Youssef Makhlouf was born in 1828 in Lebanon, the son of devout Maronite parents. At a very early age, Youssef entered a Maronite monastery. There he took the name Charbel in honor of an early martyr from Antioch. He remained in the monastery for his entire life. For sixteen years after his ordination as a priest, he lived a life of simplicity and service in the monastery. For the last twenty-three years, he lived in prayer and solitude in its hermitage. Saint Charbel's life of penance, fasting and prayer was marked by complete serenity. He desired only to bear witness to God, and his life has been an inspiration to many. In life, he exuded God's love and rejoiced in God's hope. Now, in death, his incorrupt body exudes an oily liquid that has worked countless miracles and brought about much hope.

Romans 12:12

Rejoice in hope, be patient in suffering, persevere in prayer.

Quote for the Week

God turns our darkness into brightness, our ignorance into wisdom, and our despair into hope, through ordinary gestures, places, occasions, and people or stories. Since creation is in God and God is present in all creation, God can use anything or anybody to speak to us. Open your hearts and welcome God's voice.

Alexander Busch

Activity

Draw a picture of yourself below, rejoicing in hope. (Don't worry about the artistic quality; just try to capture the feeling.) For the rest of the week, and the rest of your life, try to be as hopeful as you have drawn yourself here.

Me Hopeful

⇩

Acknowledgments

I extend my heartfelt gratitude to these special people who have blessed my life with support, affirmation, loyalty, and good counsel:

> Rev. Edward J. Arsenault; Mark Belleau; Sr. Claudia Blanchette, SNDdeN; David W. Bonanno; Joseph Carney; Ruth M. Denault; Claire Detora; Betty Esposito; Kevin Heffernan; Atty. Michael F. Hogan; Dr. Merle R. Jordan; Sr. Agnes Kalinauskas, CJC; David Maher; Sr. Cecile Marcoux, SUSC; Most Rev. John B. McCormack; Dr. John H. Morgan; Mary H. Nedder; Rev. James D. Paradis, OSA; Very Rev. Donald F. Reilly, OSA; Rev. Dr. Eleftheria Sidiropoulou; Sr. Celestine Stakutis, CJC; Br. Robert M. Thornton, OSA; Sr. Mary Valliere, CJC; Dr. Krysten Winter-Green; Dr. Gerald Wyrwas; Sr. Julia Yucas, CJC.

Much gratitude to the members of Open Hearts HIV/AIDS Support Group, living and deceased, who taught and gave me so much.

Special thanks to Gregory Pierce whose tremendous hard work, faith and hope in this project made it a reality, and to Patricia Lynch, whose design, photography, and typesetting made it sing.

About the Author

Paul J. Ashton, Psy.D., D.Min., is a clinical psychologist who has worked with support and bereavement groups and buddy training programs and in direct care for those living with HIV/AIDS since 1987. He is the founder of Open Hearts, a support service group for those living with HIV/AIDS, which began in 1992. As a consultant to various dioceses and religious communities, Ashton offers retreats, workshops, seminars, and training programs and facilitates convocations around the country. He has written many articles and has trained people nationally and abroad in the area of sex abuse prevention. He lives and has his practice in Boston.

Recent Advances in Drug Delivery Technology

Raj K. Keservani
Rajiv Gandhi Proudyogiki Vishwavidyalaya, India

Anil K. Sharma
Delhi Institute of Pharmaceutical Sciences and Research, India

Rajesh Kumar Kesharwani
National Institute of Technology, Warangal, India

A volume in the Advances in Medical Technologies and Clinical Practice (AMTCP) Book Series

IGI GLOBAL
DISSEMINATOR OF KNOWLEDGE

www.igi-global.com

Published in the United States of America by
IGI Global
Medical Information Science Reference (an imprint of IGI Global)
701 E. Chocolate Avenue
Hershey PA, USA 17033
Tel: 717-533-8845
Fax: 717-533-8661
E-mail: cust@igi-global.com
Web site: http://www.igi-global.com

Library of Congress Cataloging-in-Publication Data

Names: Keservani, Raj K., 1981- editor. | Sharma, Anil K., 1980- editor. | Kesharwani, Rajesh Kumar, 1978- editor.
Title: Recent advances in drug delivery technology / Raj K. Keservani, Anil K. Sharma, and Rajesh Kumar Kesharwani, editors.
Description: Hershey PA : Medical Information Science Reference, [2017] | Includes bibliographical references and index.
Identifiers: LCCN 2016042234| ISBN 9781522507543 (hardcover) | ISBN 9781522507550 (ebook)
Subjects: | MESH: Drug Delivery Systems | Precision Medicine | Molecular Targeted Therapy | Functional Food | Cosmeceuticals | Phytotherapy
Classification: LCC RS199.5 | NLM QV 785 | DDC 615/.6--dc23 LC record available at https://lccn.loc.gov/2016042234

This book is published in the IGI Global book series Advances in Medical Technologies and Clinical Practice (AMTCP) (ISSN: 2327-9354; eISSN: 2327-9370)

British Cataloguing in Publication Data
A Cataloguing in Publication record for this book is available from the British Library.

All work contributed to this book is new, previously-unpublished material. The views expressed in this book are those of the authors, but not necessarily of the publisher.

For electronic access to this publication, please contact: eresources@igi-global.com.

Advances in Medical Technologies and Clinical Practice (AMTCP) Book Series

Srikanta Patnaik
SOA University, India
Priti Das
S.C.B. Medical College, India

ISSN: 2327-9354
EISSN: 2327-9370

Mission

Medical technological innovation continues to provide avenues of research for faster and safer diagnosis and treatments for patients. Practitioners must stay up to date with these latest advancements to provide the best care for nursing and clinical practices.

The **Advances in Medical Technologies and Clinical Practice (AMTCP) Book Series** brings together the most recent research on the latest technology used in areas of nursing informatics, clinical technology, biomedicine, diagnostic technologies, and more. Researchers, students, and practitioners in this field will benefit from this fundamental coverage on the use of technology in clinical practices.

Coverage

- Nutrition
- Clinical Data Mining
- Medical Informatics
- Biomedical Applications
- Telemedicine
- Clinical High-Performance Computing
- Diagnostic Technologies
- Biomechanics
- Nursing Informatics
- Patient-Centered Care

IGI Global is currently accepting manuscripts for publication within this series. To submit a proposal for a volume in this series, please contact our Acquisition Editors at Acquisitions@igi-global.com or visit: http://www.igi-global.com/publish/.

The Advances in Medical Technologies and Clinical Practice (AMTCP) Book Series (ISSN 2327-9354) is published by IGI Global, 701 E. Chocolate Avenue, Hershey, PA 17033-1240, USA, www.igi-global.com. This series is composed of titles available for purchase individually; each title is edited to be contextually exclusive from any other title within the series. For pricing and ordering information please visit http://www.igi-global.com/book-series/advances-medical-technologies-clinical-practice/73682. Postmaster: Send all address changes to above address.

Titles in this Series

For a list of additional titles in this series, please visit: www.igi-global.com

Emerging Research in the Analysis and Modeling of Gene Regulatory Networks
Ivan V. Ivanov (Texas A&M University, USA) Xiaoning Qian (Texas A&M University, USA) and Ranadip Pal (Texas Tech University, USA)
Medical Information Science Reference • copyright 2016 • 418pp • H/C (ISBN: 9781522503538) • US $195.00 (our price)

Applied Case Studies and Solutions in Molecular Docking-Based Drug Design
Siavoush Dastmalchi (Tabriz University of Medical Sciences, Iran) Maryam Hamzeh-Mivehroud (Tabriz University of Medical Sciences, Iran) and Babak Sokouti (Tabriz University of Medical Sciences, Iran)
Medical Information Science Reference • copyright 2016 • 367pp • H/C (ISBN: 9781522503620) • US $225.00 (our price)

Methods and Algorithms for Molecular Docking-Based Drug Design and Discovery
Siavoush Dastmalchi (Tabriz University of Medical Sciences, Iran) Maryam Hamzeh-Mivehroud (Tabriz University of Medical Sciences, Iran) and Babak Sokouti (Tabriz University of Medical Sciences, Iran)
Medical Information Science Reference • copyright 2016 • 456pp • H/C (ISBN: 9781522501152) • US $235.00 (our price)

Advancing Pharmaceutical Processes and Tools for Improved Health Outcomes
Tagelsir Mohamed Gasmelseid (International University of Africa, Sudan)
Medical Information Science Reference • copyright 2016 • 388pp • H/C (ISBN: 9781522502487) • US $185.00 (our price)

Classification and Clustering in Biomedical Signal Processing
Nilanjan Dey (Techno India College of Technology, India) and Amira Ashour (Tanta University, Egypt)
Medical Information Science Reference • copyright 2016 • 463pp • H/C (ISBN: 9781522501404) • US $225.00 (our price)

Virtual Reality Enhanced Robotic Systems for Disability Rehabilitation
Fei Hu (University of Alabama, USA) Jiang Lu (University of Houston -Clear Lake, USA) and Ting Zhang (University of Alabama, USA)
Medical Information Science Reference • copyright 2016 • 383pp • H/C (ISBN: 9781466697409) • US $210.00 (our price)

Editorial Advisory Board

Table of Contents

Preface xv

Section 1
Nanomedicine

Chapter 1
Personalized Approach in Nanomedicine: Understanding Adverse Effects and Their Risk Assessment 1
Maria Vlasova, University of Eastern Finland, Finland
Boris V. Smirin, University of Eastern Finland, Finland

Section 2
Pharmacogenetics

Chapter 2
Drug Delivery Strategies for Tolerogenic Therapy for Autoimmune Diseases in an Antigen-Specific Manner 23
Kevin J. Peine, The University of North Carolina at Chapel Hill, USA
Naihan Chen, The University of North Carolina at Chapel Hill, USA
Eric M. Bachelder, The University of North Carolina at Chapel Hill, USA
Kristy M. Ainslie, The University of North Carolina at Chapel Hill, USA

Chapter 3
Cancer Drug Delivery: Pharmacogenetics, Biomarkers, and Targeted Therapies 52
Jai N. Patel, Levine Cancer Institute, USA
Jeryl Villadolid, Levine Cancer Institute, USA

Section 3
Proteomics and Genomics

Chapter 4
Genomics and Proteomic Approach in the Treatment of Various Human Diseases: Applications of Genomics and Proteomics 97
Urmila Jarouliya, Jiwaji University, India
Raj K. Keservani, Rajiv Gandhi Proudyogiki Vishwavidyalaya, India

Section 4
Bioinformatics

Chapter 5
Bioinformatics and Its Therapeutic Applications 125
Sarvesh Kumar Gupta, IIIT Allahabad, India
Kamal Kumar Chaudhary, IIIT Allahabad, India
Nidhi Mishra, IIIT Allahabad, India

Section 5
Nutraceuticals and Phytopharmaceuticals

Chapter 6
An Overview and Therapeutic Applications of Nutraceutical and Functional Foods 160
Raj K. Keservani, Rajiv Gandhi Proudyogiki Vishwavidhyalaya, India
Anil K. Sharma, Delhi Institute of Pharmaceutical Sciences and Research, India
Rajesh K. Kesharwani, National Institute of Technology Warangal, India

Chapter 7
Phytoparmaceuticals and Its Applications in Therapy 202
Alejandra Hernández-Ceruelos, Cuerpo Académico de Salud Pública, Área Académica de Medicina, Universidad Autónoma del Estado de Hidalgo, Mexico
Sergio Muñoz-Juarez, Cuerpo Académico de Salud Pública, Área Académica de Medicina, Universidad Autónoma del Estado de Hidalgo, Mexico
Patricia Vázquez-Alvarado, Cuerpo Académico de Salud Pública, Área Académica de Odontología, Universidad Autónoma del Estado de Hidalgo, Mexico

Chapter 8
A Perspective on the Phytopharmaceuticals Responsible for the Therapeutic Applications 229
Rajesh K. Joshi, Regional Medical Research Centre (Indian Council of Medical Research), India

Chapter 9
Phytopharmaceutical Applications of Nutraceutical and Functional Foods 263
Dhan Prakash, Amity University, India
Charu Gupta, Amity University, India

Section 6
Cosmeceuticals

Chapter 10
Cosmeceuticals: Safety, Efficacy and Potential Benefits 287
Long Chiau Ming, University of Tasmania, Australia
Wei Chern Ang, University of Bath, UK
Quan Yang, University of Bath, UK
Premrutai Thitilertdecha, Mahidol University, Thailand
Tin Wui Wong, Universiti Teknologi MARA, Malaysia
Tahir Mehmood Khan, Monash University Malaysia, Malaysia

Chapter 11
Cosmeceuticals: Camel and Other Milk – Natural Skin Maintenance 309
Reuven Yagil, Ben-Gurion University, Israel & Beauty Treat Organic Cosmetics Ltd., Israel

Section 7
Red Blood Cells

Chapter 12
Resealed Erythrocytes as Drug Carriers and Its Therapeutic Applications 340
Prabhakar Singh, University of Allahabad, India
Sudhakar Singh, Kolkata Medical College, India
Rajesh Kumar Kesharwani, NIMS University, India

Section 8
Herbals

Chapter 13
New Herbal Approaches for the Treatment of Diabetic Kidney Diseases and Its Therapeutic Implications 368
Durgavati Yadav, Institute of Medical Sciences, India
Vivek Pandey, Institute of Medical Science, India
Shivani Srivastava, Institute of Medical Sciences, India
Yamini Bhusan Tripathi, Institute of Medical Science, India

Compilation of References 407

About the Contributors 503

Index 507

Detailed Table of Contents

Preface xv

Section 1
Nanomedicine

Chapter 1
Personalized Approach in Nanomedicine: Understanding Adverse Effects and Their Risk Assessment 1
Maria Vlasova, University of Eastern Finland, Finland
Boris V. Smirin, University of Eastern Finland, Finland

This chapter characterizes need for new patient-specific approaches in medicine. The authors here illustrate role of nanomedicine and particularly nanotheranostics, combining diagnostic and therapeutic functions, in the paradigm of personalized disease treatment. This chapter discusses current insights regarding the mechanisms of nano-bio interactions and the origin of adverse effects of nanoformulations. Furthermore, this chapter illustrates possible reasons behind an individual physiological response to a given nanomedicine, such as type and stage of disease, physiological conditions and lifestyle of a patient. Finally, a review of possible approaches for the initial choice of nanoformulation, suitable for a given patient is provided at the end of the chapter.

Section 2
Pharmacogenetics

Chapter 2
Drug Delivery Strategies for Tolerogenic Therapy for Autoimmune Diseases in an Antigen-Specific Manner 23
Kevin J. Peine, The University of North Carolina at Chapel Hill, USA
Naihan Chen, The University of North Carolina at Chapel Hill, USA
Eric M. Bachelder, The University of North Carolina at Chapel Hill, USA
Kristy M. Ainslie, The University of North Carolina at Chapel Hill, USA

Autoimmune diseases are the result of an improper immune response towards a self-antigen. Predominantly, autoimmune diseases have been treated using therapies that suppress systemic immune responses, which can result in significant side-effects like increased risk of infection and cancer. Alternatively, induction of immune tolerance through antigen-specific therapies can inhibit disease-associated responses without systemic suppression. Previously, immune tolerance has been accomplished by soluble antigen delivery through oral, nasal or sublingual routes. However, these therapies have shown minimal success in clinical settings. In an attempt to increase the efficacy of these therapies, recent work has utilized microparticulate delivery vehicles for the induction of immune tolerance. Microparticles are capable of increasing the solubility and circulation of cargo. In addition, their ability to passively target macrophages and dendritic cells increases their capacity for modulating the immune response. Recent work has shown microparticles fabricated with disease-associated antigens have limited disease progression and severity in animal models of Multiple Sclerosis, Type 1 Diabetes and Rheumatoid Arthritis. Inhibition of disease progression has corresponded with an antigen-specific decrease in inflammatory responses. The emerging field of inducing tolerance through microparticle-based therapies can limit therapeutic side-effects and increase patient quality of life by providing for long-term suppression of autoimmune disorders without compromising systemic immune function.

Chapter 3
Cancer Drug Delivery: Pharmacogenetics, Biomarkers, and Targeted Therapies 52
Jai N. Patel, Levine Cancer Institute, USA
Jeryl Villadolid, Levine Cancer Institute, USA

Advancements in cancer drug delivery have led to the development of personalized oncology care through molecularly-driven targeted therapies. Understanding molecular and cellular mechanisms which drive tumor progression and resistance is critical in managing new treatment strategies which have shifted from empiric to biomarker-directed therapy selection. Biomarker-directed therapies have improved clinical outcomes in multiple malignancies as monotherapy and in combination with other treatment modalities, however the changing scope of treatment options presents new opportunities and challenges for research. Furthermore, pharmacogenetics may provide a rationale method of personalizing anticancer drug dosing and supportive care management for oncology patients. This chapter reviews biomarker classifications and pharmacogenetics in anticancer therapy and supportive care. Examples of biomarker-directed therapies and clinical assays, in addition to future directions of molecular profiling in oncology therapy management are discussed.

Section 3
Proteomics and Genomics

Chapter 4
Genomics and Proteomic Approach in the Treatment of Various Human Diseases: Applications of Genomics and Proteomics 97
Urmila Jarouliya, Jiwaji University, India
Raj K. Keservani, Rajiv Gandhi Proudyogiki Vishwavidyalaya, India

World wise genomic analysis is beginning to move from the laboratories of basic investigators to large-scale clinical trials. The potential of this technology is to improve diagnosis and tailored treatment of various human diseases. In addition, new data from the emerging proteomics platforms add another layer of molecular information to the study of human disease, as scientists attempt to catalogue a complete list of the proteins encoded by the genome and to establish a 'bio-signature' profile of human health and disease. In the medical sciences identification of human genome sequence is a significant milestone for all the genes and their regulatory regions which provides the required framework for the genetic blueprint of humankind and that will make possible to recognize the molecular premise of disease. It is accepted that, together, these technologies genomic and proteomic will make easier to study all aspects of genes, gene products and signaling pathways so that the objective of personalised molecular medicine can be achieved.

Section 4
Bioinformatics

Chapter 5
Bioinformatics and Its Therapeutic Applications 125
Sarvesh Kumar Gupta, IIIT Allahabad, India
Kamal Kumar Chaudhary, IIIT Allahabad, India
Nidhi Mishra, IIIT Allahabad, India

Bioinformatics has emerged as a major element in contemporary biomedical and pharmaceutical region. Bioinformatics deals with growth in biological data and has led to development of many databases. Bioinformatics deals with collection of data that is relevant clinically and these days separate term clinical information has come up. Data mimics are another field which is gaining importance. This chapter shall deal with introduction of bioinformatics and its applications in medicine and health care.

Section 5
Nutraceuticals and Phytopharmaceuticals

Chapter 6
An Overview and Therapeutic Applications of Nutraceutical and Functional Foods 160
Raj K. Keservani, Rajiv Gandhi Proudyogiki Vishwavidhyalaya, India
Anil K. Sharma, Delhi Institute of Pharmaceutical Sciences and Research, India
Rajesh K. Kesharwani, National Institute of Technology Warangal, India

Healthy nutrition is important for human beings for good health provided by global industry. Nutraceutical and functional food provide a prospect to reduce health care costs and improve the human health. Researchers carried out plenty of work for the preparation of nutraceutical and functional food product. This article also focused on recent advances on the nutraceutical and functional foods product on health benefits and their application in prevention of disease. Here we discussed about the health benefit of recently introduced nutraceutical and functional food products. With the modernised, competitive lifestyle and ever increasing stressful conditions this product is the need of the day.

Chapter 7
Phytoparmaceuticals and Its Applications in Therapy.. 202
Alejandra Hernández-Ceruelos, Cuerpo Académico de Salud Pública, Área Académica de Medicina, Universidad Autónoma del Estado de Hidalgo, Mexico
Sergio Muñoz-Juarez, Cuerpo Académico de Salud Pública, Área Académica de Medicina, Universidad Autónoma del Estado de Hidalgo, Mexico
Patricia Vázquez-Alvarado, Cuerpo Académico de Salud Pública, Área Académica de Odontología, Universidad Autónoma del Estado de Hidalgo, Mexico

Medicinal plants have been used to treat illnesses since medicine began. Nowadays, 80% of the population in the planet uses drugs directly or indirectly derived from plants. In the past, natural products were used empirically; people experimented with them as helpful for their well-being and learned to treat ailments with specific plants. Henri Leclerc introduced the terminology of phytotherapy into medical science and this concept refers to study of the use of extracts of natural origin as medicines or health-promoting agents. Usually pharmacology isolates an active compound from a given plant, phytotherapy aims to reserve the complexity of constituents from a plant with moderately less processing. Phytopharmaceuticals (PP) are composed by one plant species or by complex mixtures of plants, presented in a natural or in a pharmaceutical form. The tendency is to use standardized plant extracts in the formulation, obtained by a patented extraction process. PP need to fulfill the same requirements as other medical products: safety, efficacy and consistent quality.

Chapter 8
A Perspective on the Phytopharmaceuticals Responsible for the Therapeutic Applications.............. 229
Rajesh K. Joshi, Regional Medical Research Centre (Indian Council of Medical Research), India

The word phytopharmaceutical deals with a complex mixture of compounds derived from the plant source that is used as a medicine or drug. Primitive human societies have been depending on plants and plant products for various remedies. Several plants in the different forms have been reported in traditional medicine and to find a rational for the treatment of various diseases than to isolated single compounds. Many of the single compounds isolated from the plant origin are effectively used in the medicine. The search of natural products in drug discovery has been greatly enhanced in the last few years. The impetus to use phytopharmaceutical agents for the treatment of disease, most of the plant based drugs are quite safe and have lesser adverse effects and are claimed that it works as synergistic effects.

Chapter 9
Phytopharmaceutical Applications of Nutraceutical and Functional Foods...................................... 263
Dhan Prakash, Amity University, India
Charu Gupta, Amity University, India

Nutraceuticals are actually "Bioactive herbal formulations" that contains selective combinations of specific bioactive constituents of plants and/or their parts that possess health-promotive, disease preventing and medicinal properties. The important phytochemical constituents commonly found in plants are polyphenols, flavonoids, isoflavonoids, anthocyanidins, carotenoids, fibers, limonoids, glucosinolates, phytoestrogens, phytosterols and terpenoids. They play positive pharmacological activities in human health such as antioxidant activity, anti-microbial activity, anti-inflammatory, anti-allergic, anti-spasmodic, chemo-preventive, hepato-protective, neuro-protective, hypolipidemic, hypotensive, anti-aging, diabetes, osteoporosis, repair DNA damage, heart diseases, diuretic, Central Nervous System (CNS) stimulant, immuno-modulator, carminative, Thus the present chapter summarizes the phyto-pharmaceutical applications of nutraceuticals and functional foods and would lay emphasis on its importance for future generations for their well-being.

Section 6
Cosmeceuticals

Chapter 10
Cosmeceuticals: Safety, Efficacy and Potential Benefits 287
Long Chiau Ming, University of Tasmania, Australia
Wei Chern Ang, University of Bath, UK
Quan Yang, University of Bath, UK
Premrutai Thitilertdecha, Mahidol University, Thailand
Tin Wui Wong, Universiti Teknologi MARA, Malaysia
Tahir Mehmood Khan, Monash University Malaysia, Malaysia

Cosmeceuticals are topical cosmetic-pharmaceutical hybrids used to maintain and improve appearance and beauty of the skin. The strong demand from the consumers to constantly look youthful and flawless has driven the research and development as well as sale volume of cosmeceuticals. Present studies show that many cosmetic products, which were assumed to be inert in the past, may modulate dermatological structure or function. The key players of cosmeceuticals are anti-aging therapy along with bleaching agent, sunscreen, and hair cosmeceuticals. This book chapter aims to explore the safety, toxicity and efficacy of these cosmeceuticals. Challenges and possible advancement potentials would be discussed. As patients are increasingly seeking advice from physicians and pharmacists regarding cosmeceuticals, the authors hope to provide health care professional and pharmaceutical scientists a resource that would aid to educate patients in using evidence-based cosmeceuticals to enhance their appearance and alleviate dermatological problems.

Chapter 11
Cosmeceuticals: Camel and Other Milk – Natural Skin Maintenance 309
Reuven Yagil, Ben-Gurion University, Israel & Beauty Treat Organic Cosmetics Ltd., Israel

This chapter will deal with delivering of a substance in a natural product, milk, via the skin – cosmeceuticals, from a variety of sources, camels, equine, ruminant and breast milk. The large quantities of bacteria on the normal skin, both friendly and "bad" bacteria provide skin and body health. The activity of cosmeceuticals of camel milk is due to the specific milk components, whose efficacy is retained in skin preparations which have not been destroyed in their preparation. By using camel milk which is pathogen-free the preparations are probiotic by definition and rapidly penetrate the outer skin layers to be active in the deeper layers. Massage therapy has been shown to improve flexibility and range of motion and strengthen the immune system. A list of the organic substances used for making the cosmeceuticals is provided.

Section 7
Red Blood Cells

Chapter 12
Resealed Erythrocytes as Drug Carriers and Its Therapeutic Applications.. 340
Prabhakar Singh, University of Allahabad, India
Sudhakar Singh, Kolkata Medical College, India
Rajesh Kumar Kesharwani, NIMS University, India

In this pharma innovative world, there are more than 30 drug delivery systems. Today's due to lacking the target specificity, the present scenario about drug delivery is emphasizing towards targeted drug delivery systems. Erythrocytes are the most common type of blood cells travel thousands of miles from wide to narrow pathways to deliver oxygen, drugs and nutrient during their lifetime. Red blood cells have strong and targeted potential carrier capabilities for varieties of drugs. Drug-loaded carrier erythrocytes or resealed erythrocytes are promising for various passive and active targeting. Resealed erythrocyte have advantage over several drug carrier models like biocompatibility, biodegradability without toxic products, inert intracellular environment, entrapping potential for a variety of chemicals, protection of the organism against toxic effects of the drug, able to circulate throughout the body, ideal zero-order drug-release kinetics, no undesired immune response against encapsulated drug etc. Resealed erythrocytes are rapidly taken up by macrophages of the Reticuloendothelial System (RES) of the liver, lung, and spleen of the body and hence drugs also. Resealed erythrocytes method of drugs delivery is secure and effective for drugs targeting specially for a longer period of time. This chapter will explain the different method of drug loading for resealed erythrocytes, their characterization, and applications in various therapies and associated health benefits.

Section 8
Herbals

Chapter 13
New Herbal Approaches for the Treatment of Diabetic Kidney Diseases and Its Therapeutic Implications 368
Durgavati Yadav, Institute of Medical Sciences, India
Vivek Pandey, Institute of Medical Science, India
Shivani Srivastava, Institute of Medical Sciences, India
Yamini Bhusan Tripathi, Institute of Medical Science, India

Diabetic Kidney Diseases (DKD) is a very serious complication of diabetes. There is recent steep rise in the prevalence of metabolic syndrome and DKD worldwide. Factors responsible for intraglomerular hypertension include activation of various vasoactive systems, polyol pathway, oxidative stress, inflammation and protein kinase C. Sodium-Dependent Glucose Co-Transporter (SGLT-2) inhibitors, DPP-IV (Dipeptidyl peptidase-4) inhibitors are being develop to manage the hyperglycemia and oxidative stress induced inflammatory cascade. Herbal drugs have gained increasing popularity; are complex mixtures of polyphenols and phytochemicals from any raw or processed part of a plant, including leaves. Herbal drugs in this modern era are preferred due to its lesser side effects. Various preparations are presently used for ameliorating the effect of DKD. Since, medicinal plants have been reported to affect various metabolic receptors, enzymes and signaling cascade. Above book chapter explains the involvement of different phytochemicals in biological pathway associated with the kidney damage.

Compilation of References 407

About the Contributors 503

Index 507

Preface

The efficient delivery of a drug is function of numerous biopharmaceutical as well as physiochemical characteristics. This has posed obstacles to the development of diverse drug delivery systems by researchers from academia and industry. There is need to customize the dosage forms according to biological and physical variables. The science of drug delivery technology is ever evolving with introduction of new systems with progress in time. We are witnessing the journey of techniques from conventional to novel ones. Several of such novel drug delivery systems have been found to overcome the pit falls associated with their customary counterparts. Novel drug delivery systems is an approach of delivering a drug, can have a significant effect on its efficacy. Some drugs have an optimum concentration range within which maximum benefit is derived, and concentrations above or below this range can be toxic or produce no therapeutic benefit at all. On the other hand, the very slow progress in the efficacy of the treatment of severe diseases, has suggested a growing need for a multidisciplinary approach to the delivery of therapeutics to targets in tissues. From this, new ideas on controlling the pharmacokinetics, pharmacodynamics, non-specific toxicity, immunogenicity, biorecognition, and efficacy of drugs were generated. Nevertheless, it would be appropriate to comment that novel drug delivery systems are also not devoid of limitations like cost, intricacies involved in development, bio-toxicity profile of materials employed etc. Therefore, the exercise of caution while using novel drug carriers is desired. The natural as well as synthetic carriers are reported to be explored as drug carriers.

The current book project was driven by the ever going quest to have an updated pool of research information scattered over diverse facets of science. It has attempted to cover the innovations being introduced while keeping the merits offered by the traditional dosage forms. This book offers an overview of the therapeutic application of drug delivery strategies, polymeric systems, nanotechnology, nanomedicine, biosimilar, pharmacogenetics, proteomics and genomics, bioinformatics, nutraceuticals and phytopharmaceuticals, cosmeceuticals and herbals with special emphasis on their pharmaceutical applications in different disease which really helps authors and readers.

The content of these chapters is written by highly skilled, experienced and renowned scientists, researchers across all over the world with updated knowledge to provide drug delivery information to readers, researchers, academician, scientists and industrialists around the globe.

CHAPTER COMPOSITION

This book has 13 chapters and divided into 8 sections.

Section 1 has Chapter 1, "Personalized Approach in Nanomedicine: Understanding Adverse Effects and Their Risk Assessment," written by Maria Vlasova and Boris V. Smirin from Finland illustrates possible reasons behind an individual physiological response to a given nanomedicine, such as type and stage of disease, physiological conditions and lifestyle of a patient. This chapter illustrates possible reasons behind an individual physiological response to a given nanomedicine, such as type and stage of disease, physiological conditions and lifestyle of a patient. The different approaches of nanoformulations have been summarized at the end of the chapter.

Section 2 has two chapters. Chapter 2, "Drug Delivery Strategies for Tolerogenic Therapy for Autoimmune Diseases in an Antigen-Specific Manner," is written by Kevin J Peine, Naihan Chen, Eric Bachelder and Kristy Ainslie from USA, demonstrates the emerging field of inducing tolerance through microparticle-based therapies can limit therapeutic side-effects and increase patient quality of life by providing for long-term suppression of autoimmune disorders without compromising systemic immune function. The chapter describes an attempt to increase the efficacy of these therapies, recent work has utilized microparticulate delivery vehicles for the induction of immune tolerance. Microparticles are capable of increasing the solubility and circulation of cargo. In addition, their ability to passively target macrophages and dendritic cells increases their capacity for modulating the immune response. Recent work has shown microparticles fabricated with disease-associated antigens have limited disease progression and severity in animal models of Multiple Sclerosis, Type 1 Diabetes and Rheumatoid Arthritis. Chapter 3, "Cancer Drug Delivery: Pharmacogenetics, Biomarkers, and Targeted Therapies," by Jai N. Patel and Jeryl Villadolid from USA, reviews biomarker classifications and pharmacogenetics in anticancer therapy and supportive care. Advancements in cancer drug delivery have led to the development of personalized oncology care through molecularly-driven targeted therapies. Understanding molecular and cellular mechanisms which drive tumor progression and resistance is critical in managing new treatment strategies which have shifted from empiric to biomarker-directed therapy selection. Examples of biomarker-directed therapies and clinical assays, in addition to future directions of molecular profiling in oncology therapy management are discussed.

Section 3 has Chapter 4, "Genomics and Proteomic Approach in the Treatment of Various Human Diseases: Application of Genomics and Proteomics," written by Urmila Jarouliya and Raj K. Keservani from India, has dealt in genomics and proteomic approach will make easier to study all aspects of genes, gene products and signaling pathways so that the objective of personalized molecular medicine can be achieved. World wise genomic analysis is beginning to move from the laboratories of basic investigators to large-scale clinical trials. The potential of this technology is to improve diagnosis and tailored treatment of various human diseases.

Section 4 has Chapter 5, "Bioinformatics and Its Therapeutic Applications," written by Sarvesh Kumar Gupta, Kamal Kumar Chaudhary and Nidhi Mishra from India, describes introduction of bioinformatics and its applications in medicine and health care. Bioinformatics has emerged as a major element in contemporary biomedical and pharmaceutical region. Bioinformatics deals with growth in biological data and has led to development of many databases. A number of applications could be customized to help the ailing mankind by exploring the principles of bioinformatics in drug delivery. This may prove beneficial to the patients by offering an alternative to existing synthetic analogues.

Section 5 has four chapters. Chapter 6, "An Overview and Therapeutic Applications of Nutraceutical and Functional Foods," written by Raj K. Keservani, Anil K. Sharma and Rajesh K. Kesharwani from India, discussed about the health benefit of recently introduced nutraceutical and functional food products. With the modernised, competitive lifestyle and ever increasing stressful conditions this product is the need of the day. The chapter entails the therapeutic benefits of food beyond its basic roles. The fundamentals of nutrition and pharmaceuticals are clubbed together to impart cure to the human beings. There are nowadays various concerns over the safety of synthetic drugs used, the nutraceuticals majority of them are considered to be safe, could substitute a few drug applications. There is need to explore the clinical evaluation of nutraceutical products in order to ascertain their innocuousness in biological milieu. Chapter 7, "Phytoparmaceuticals and Its Applications in Therapy," written by Alejandra Hernández-Ceruelos, Sergio Muñoz-Juarez and Patricia Vázquez-Alvarado from Mexico demonstrates phytoparmaceuticals and its applications in therapy. Henri Leclerc introduced the terminology of phytotherapy into medical science and this concept refers to study of the use of extracts of natural origin as medicines or health-promoting agents. The use of herbs for treatment has been in parlance from the beginning of civilizations. A wide number of plants products may be used to treat diverse diseases/disorders. Chapter 8, "A Perspective on the Phytopharmaceuticals Responsible for the Therapeutic Applications," by Rajesh K. Joshi from India, has summarized use of phytopharmaceutical agents for the treatment of disease, most of the plant based drugs are quite safe and have lesser adverse effects and are claimed that it works as synergistic effects. Several plants in the different forms have been reported in traditional medicine and to find a rational for the treatment of various diseases than to isolated single compounds. Chapter 9, "Phytopharmaceutical Applications of Nutraceutical and Functional Foods," written by Charu Gupta and Dhan Prakash from India, concluded phyto-pharmaceutical applications of nutraceuticals and functional foods and would lay emphasis on its importance for future generations for their well-being. The applications of nutraceuticals derived from plants are enumerated in the present chapter. Further, the future prospects are also discussed.

Section 6 has two chapters. Chapter 10, "Cosmeceuticals: Safety, Efficacy, and Potentials Benefits," is written by Long Chiau Ming, Wei Chern Ang, Quan Yang, Premrutai Thitilertdecha, Tin Wui Wong and Tahir Mehmood Khan from Malaysia discussed about health care professional and pharmaceutical scientists a resource that would aid to educate patients in using evidence-based cosmeceuticals to enhance their appearance and alleviate dermatological problems. The chapter has described several products used to beautify human skin employing principles of pharmaceutics to make a viable formulation. The present chapter would provide information to the manufactures to exploit the advantages associated with cosmetic formulations. As we all are aware that good looks have been in fresh demand irrespective of gender, ethnicity or country specific limitations. Chapter 11, "Camel and Other Milk for External Drug Delivery," written by Reuven Yagil from Israel, discussed cosmeceuticals prepared from camel and other milk for natural skin maintenance and massage therapy has been shown to improve flexibility and range of motion and strengthen the immune system. The chapter has quoted interesting case studies by which camel milk has been found to heal lesions associated with the skin. The readers may find this fascinating as it provides clinical evidences for each of the use of camel milk. The chapter has beautifully described the utility of ship of the desert's milk.

Section 7 has Chapter 12, "Resealed Erythrocytes as Drug Carriers and Its Therapeutic Application," by Prabahkar Singh, Sudhakar Singh and Rajesh K. Kesharwani from India has described about application potential of the resealed erythrocytes and explained the different method of drug loading for resealed erythrocytes, their characterization, and applications in various therapies and associated health benefits. The use of such biocompatible drug carrier appears fascinating for the researchers worldwide. The limitations linked with various synthetic and natural carriers may be overcome by employing RBCs as drug carriers. However, the cost and immunogenicity in certain cases should be taken into account while going for manufacturing RBC products.

Section 8 has one chapter. Chapter 13, "New Herbal Approaches for the Treatment of Diabetic Kidney Diseases and Its Therapeutics Implications," is written by Durgavati Yadav, Vivek Pandey, Shivani Srivastava and Yamini Bhusan Tripathi from India, explains the involvement of different phytochemicals in biological pathway associated with the kidney damage. The kidney damage is manifested as secondary complications while progression of diabetes. Herbal drugs in this modern era are preferred due to its lesser side effects. As the diabetes type 2 being associated with modern day lifestyle is usually worsen upon progression. The alternate therapy approaches originated from nature could prove as a boon to the patients.

The present book will be helpful to add the set of specific research updates to the existing ocean of science. This could be assumed as collection of few drops collected from the contributors spread over the earth to the repository of the knowledge. We all are aware that honing of the skills, knowledge is warranted in order to keep pace with the advancing world. This all comes through variety of sources which enables its end user with ability to withstand the challenges whatsoever they are. The editors humbly submit here that this is not all about the developments taking place in modern world, it is merely a beginning. We are quite hopeful that this particular compilation would receive the interest of its target audience. This book presents recent technology and future prospective and different drug delivery in addition highlighted its pharmaceutical and medical application. In last section book contains compilation of references, list of contributors and subject index. This should be taken as primary move similar to early steps taken by the toddlers. The editors are an email away to accept any suggestion, comment or critics.

Raj K. Keservani
Rajiv Gandhi Proudyogiki Vishwavidyalaya, India

Anil K. Sharma
Delhi Institute of Pharmaceutical Sciences and Research, India

Rajesh K. Kesharwani
National Institute of Technology, Warangal, India

Section 1
Nanomedicine

Chapter 1
Personalized Approach in Nanomedicine:
Understanding Adverse Effects and Their Risk Assessment

Maria Vlasova
University of Eastern Finland, Finland

Boris V. Smirin
University of Eastern Finland, Finland

ABSTRACT

This chapter characterizes need for new patient-specific approaches in medicine. The authors here illustrate role of nanomedicine and particularly nanotheranostics, combining diagnostic and therapeutic functions, in the paradigm of personalized disease treatment. This chapter discusses current insights regarding the mechanisms of nano-bio interactions and the origin of adverse effects of nanoformulations. Furthermore, this chapter illustrates possible reasons behind an individual physiological response to a given nanomedicine, such as type and stage of disease, physiological conditions and lifestyle of a patient. Finally, a review of possible approaches for the initial choice of nanoformulation, suitable for a given patient is provided at the end of the chapter.

INTRODUCTION

The current approaches to diagnostics and therapy, where the type of therapy and drug doses are selected according to the data obtained from a large cohort of patients, is accompanied by a number of severe adverse effects as well as cases of ineffective treatments. A need to individualize diagnostics and therapy according to the health status of an individual patient has become obvious and urgent. With the use of individualized medicine, clinical trials are likely to become more efficient by lowering the cost incurred due to drug's side effects or prescription of ineffective or potentially life-threatening drugs to the patients of certain genotype and in a certain physiological condition. Recent developments in nanomedicine offer

DOI: 10.4018/978-1-5225-0754-3.ch001

a great number of tools to achieve the target of personalized medicine. The most advanced creations of nanotechnology –nanotheranostics combine several functions and can be used for individual diagnostics, therapy and monitoring of the therapeutic response. However, due to the structural complexity, administration of nanoformulations can result in unexpected physiological effects. This chapter aims to discuss the current view on the interactions between nanoformulations and human body and to consider the determinants of these interactions. The importance of "personalized protein corona" formation and factors governing this process are reviewed in order to formulate the procedure of nanomedicine risk assessment for an individual patient.

BACKGROUND

Individual variability in disease course as well as in efficacy and safety of therapeutics is one of the main challenges in current clinical practice. Predisposition, progression, severity and recovery from diseases vary from patient to patient. Simultaneously, response of the patients to the same therapeutic agent can also vary significantly although diagnosed with the same disease.

A balance between drug efficacy and adverse drug effects determines clinical outcome of a medication. This balance can be calculated based on the concept of "therapeutic window". The therapeutic window is as a range of medication dosages that lie between a dosage with highest therapeutic effect and a dosage, which shows apparent adverse reactions (Figure 1 A). Smaller dosage gives sub-optimal therapeutic effect with almost no side effects while the higher doses enhance therapeutic effect, but at the same time evoke new or stronger side effects. In other words, within the therapeutic window, patients experience maximal therapeutic effect with minimum side effects.

As a rule, therapeutic window is determined for a large patient population. In current clinical practice, this *averaged therapeutic window* is a base for the choice of therapy. However, for most of medications, there are groups of patients, who have atypical dose-response curves for either therapeutic or adverse effect of the drug, or both. Application of a drug within averaged therapeutic window in these subgroups may result either in non-efficient treatment or in unexpected, undesirable and possibly life-threatening outcomes in these patients (Figure 1B and 1C). It is noteworthy that the probability of successful clinical outcome in current medical approach dramatically decreases in case of application of several drugs simultaneously. The lower probability for a patient to be within average therapeutic window for each of applied drugs can explain this.

Thus, there is a need to change the approach for the disease management from traditional "one treatment fits all" concept towards a more personalized medicine, where the individual health status of the patients defines a choice of the medical treatments. The concept of individual diagnostics and therapeutic strategy can already be found in Hippocrates' works: "Endogenously determined difference of human beings from each other together with age, physique, the season of the year" (Hippocrates, 1931) affect both the progression of the disease and how it responds to the treatment. In modern terms, diagnosis and therapy planning should take into account a combination of genetic, as well as physiological and environmental factors. Patient-specific approach in medicine would significantly increase the efficacy as well as safety of therapies and ensure that the medication is given only to patients who are more likely to respond to this treatment. This approach of personalized medicine can take health care to a higher standard with ultimate goal being "to help *and* do no harm".

Figure 1. Application of the drugs in current medicine and advantages of forming patient subgroups. A. Therapeutic window of a drug: the range of drug dosages, which can effectively treat disease while staying within the safety range. B. Risk of a drug application in a dose ranges, close to the borders of a drug therapeutic window. C. Subdivision of patients into subgroups by their drug sensitivity

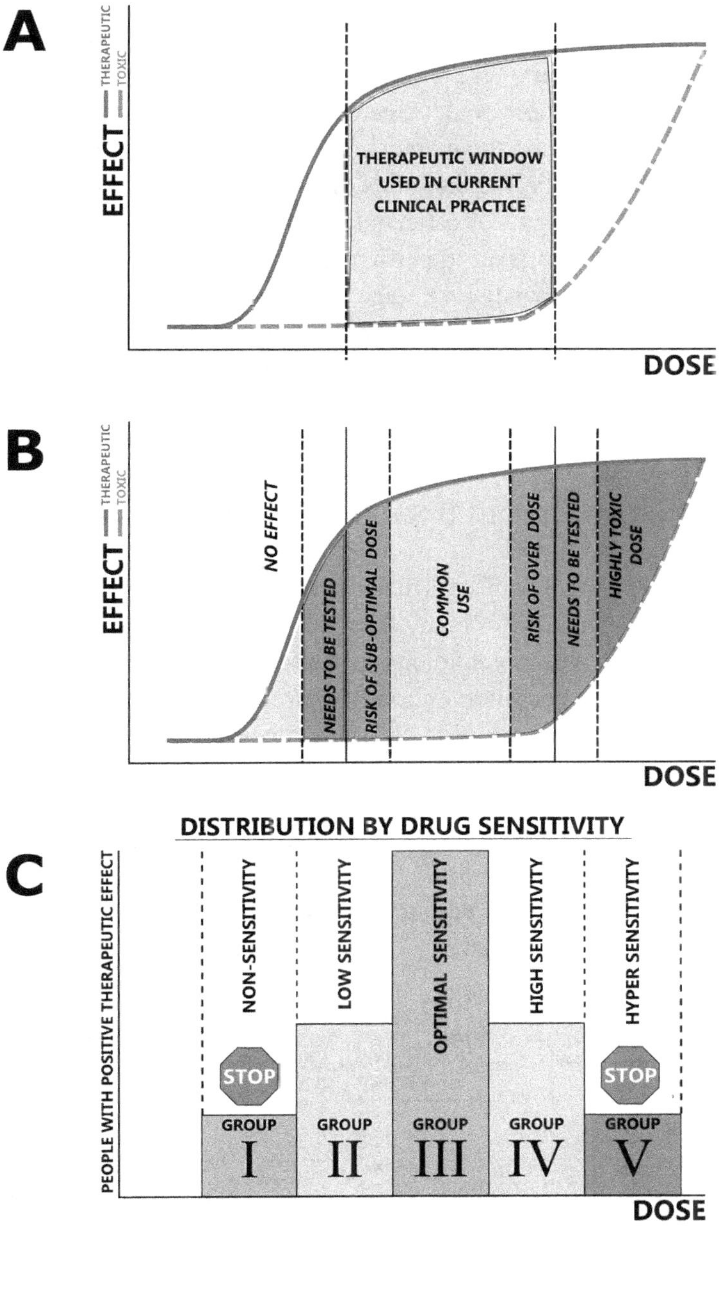

In practice, developing individual treatment approach for each patient is economically untenable. Rather, a large patient population can be divided into subgroups by efficacy and toxicity to certain medications (Figure 1) as well as by the disease stage and prognosis (Sadee & Dai, 2005). In fact, division of the patients into smaller sub-groups would expand the therapeutic window of the applied therapeutics. The most important problem here would be to define criteria for this sub-division.

Genetic polymorphisms of drug targeting and metabolizing proteins is likely to have a major contribution to variable drug response. Therefore, pharmacogenomics became one of the important approaches in personalized medicine. For example, to date, genetic tests are effective and used for a list of drugs to define the group of patients for whom the medication is not applicable, i.e. causes severe side effects.

In diagnostics, identification of type and number of biomarkers in individuals has been shown to have a high correlation with different forms of cancers (Liotta & Petricoin, 2000). However, the predictive power of tests, based on single biomarker identification is limited. In most of the cases, an interplay of several biomarkers describes a certain disease stage, and their identification requires techniques that are more sophisticated. Besides this, a variety of factors strongly influence disease progression and drug response, therefore only the integration of patient's genotyping with analysis of his physiological status and environmental factors can result in reliable therapeutic planning, suited at the time of treatment for an individual patient (Ma & Lu, 2011; Sadee & Dai, 2005).

Role of Nanomedicine in Patient Specific Medical Approach

Field of nanomedicine offers a number of significant advantages to improve clinical outcomes of medication and to extend therapeutic window for many drugs, i.e. to improve the balance between their efficacy and toxicity. Here we summarize nanotechnology-based tools, which are involved in an increased safety and enhanced efficacy of therapeutic interventions (Figure 2). Due to high medical need and extremely narrow therapeutic window of routinely used chemotherapeutic drugs (i.e. their high toxicity and low

Figure 2. Nanotechnology-based tools for extension of drug's therapeutic window

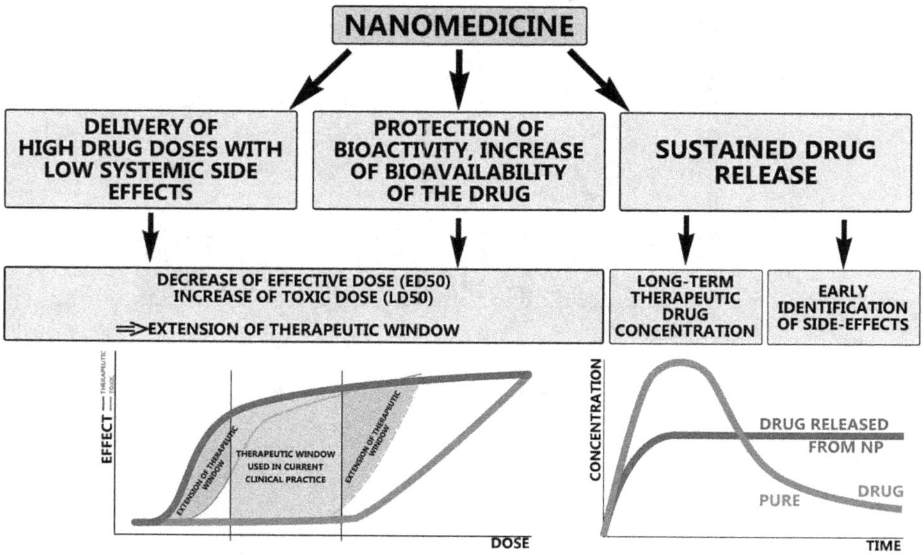

efficacy) majority of these efforts in nanomedicine are concentrated on cancer. Controlled release of the drug delivered in nanoparticulate formulations aim to maintain the long-term therapeutic concentrations of the drug and to avoid peaks of high drug concentration. Besides optimizing the therapeutic effect, it also improves drug safety since the probability of adverse effect is decreased (Kim et al., 2013) (Figure 2). It could be of great interest to have a nanoparticle-based drug delivery system in future, which can be switched on/off based on how a patient responds to a drug.

- Nanoparticles enable delivery of poorly soluble and/or easily degradable drugs, protect biological activity and increase bioavailability of the drug in the diseased organ. For example, they expand clinical application of a large class of peptide drugs (Carmona-Ribeiro & de Melo Carrasco, 2014; do Carmo et al., 2014), and allow the use of smaller drug concentrations.
- Passive targeting and accumulation at the disease site is possible for the drugs, entrapped or conjugated with nanoparticles, due to small size of nanoformulations and their increased circulation time (enabled by nanoparticle's surface modification). These properties increase the chances of nanoparticles to extravagate from leaky tumor vasculature and stay in tumor interstitial space due to compromised lymphatic filtration in the tumor (enhanced permeation and retention effect).
- Systemic delivery of highly toxic drugs to the target site prevent them from accumulating in healthy tissues and simultaneously enhance effectiveness of the drug by concentrating near the target site, thus extending the therapeutic window for a given drug. Therefore, the clinical use of several nanoformulations, containing highly toxic chemotherapeutics, was approved, namely non-PEGylated liposomal doxorubicin Myocet, PEGylated liposomal doxorubicin Doxil, and albumin-based paclitaxel Abraxane. The main advantage of these nanoformulations compared to pure drugs is their significantly reduced systemic toxicity. However, only moderate effectiveness of these nanoformulations is recognized (Jain & Stylianopoulos, 2010; Lammers et al., 2012).
- Furthermore, many nanoparticle types (metallic and magnetic nanoparticles) offer the advantage of non-invasive molecular imaging.
- At the same time, nanoparticles have high surface area to volume ratio; therefore, they possess high loading capacity for imaging probes, targeting moieties and therapeutic molecules.

Nanotheranostics

Due to all the above-mentioned properties, nanoparticles can be a perfect base for a single multifunctional system, widely referred to as nanotheranostics and combining diagnostic and therapeutic functions (Figure 3).Such advanced systems and greatly increase the quality and possibilities of personalized medicine. Nanotheranostics can offer a number of advantages as compared to existing imaging techniques, used in clinics.

Routinely, positron emission tomography (PET), magnetic resonance imaging (MRI), computed tomography (CT) and ultrasound are the methods to analyze the type and the course of a given pathology. Diagnostic information obtained with these methods is a base for stratifying the treatments for relatively large cohorts of patients. To date, none of the approved contrast agents is suitable for specific visualization of native gene and/or protein expression (molecular imaging). A number of studies show relative usefulness of radiolabeled antibodies for tumor identification (Lammers et al., 2012). However, most of them accumulate in tumor due to their physicochemical and pharmacokinetic properties and not by receptor expression levels. Therefore, non-invasive imaging with radiolabeled antibodies can be

Figure 3. Key properties of nanotheranostics: combination of functions

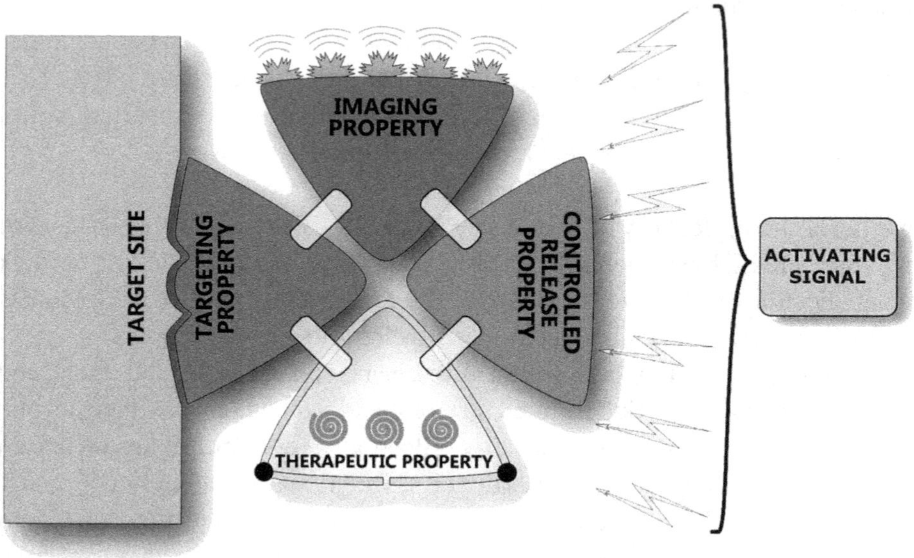

considered as a sub-optimal diagnostic method that has a limited potential to improve personalization of medicine(Lammers et al., 2012). Thus, there is a high medical need for the methods holding a better potential for target site recognition and possibility of non-invasive imaging.

Nanotechnology based theranostic systems can target, non-invasively image and follow biomarkers, characterizing the disease stage and progression (Figure 4).This information is more precise than only identifying genetic status, since it enables clinicians to identify the degree to which a certain biomarker is present in the body at a given time. Visualization of nanotheranostics by the above listed MRI, CT and PET makes these methods quantitative and thus folds more informative.

A more sophisticated system, which follows the complex protease signaling mechanism, can image several enzymes at the same time. A single nanoparticle that entrappers multiple quenchers is a base for this platform. The presence of multiple proteases produce multiple fluorescence signals.

Targeting the molecular events, such as hypoxia, apoptosis, angiogenesis, inflammation, proliferation and metastasis is another real-time diagnostic approach for personalized medicine. Here, nanotheranostics can go beyond *in vitro* identification of these biomarkers and diagnose significant disease stages *in vivo*. For this application, nanoparticles can be functionalized with probes which can be activated, which would increase their fluorescence in the presence of certain enzymes (Kim et al., 2013).

Personalization of therapy methods include use of therapeutic that activates upon a certain stimulus. In this case, nanoplatforms deliver to the target site a pro-drug, which becomes therapeutically active only upon transformation *via* specific stimulus. Environmental or chemical stimuli, like heat, light, magnetic field, sound, pH or presence of particular biomolecules transform the pro-drug into drug (Kim et al., 2013).Recently, a nanocomposite, which combine therapy with the treatment monitoring was developed and tested in a mouse tumor model. Reduced graphene oxide-iron oxide nanoparticle- PEG nanocomposite was used for phototermal therapy, image- guided by MRI (Yang et al., 2012).

Figure 4. Role of nanotheranostics (NT) in personalized medicine. PET-positron emission tomography, MRI-magnetic resonance imaging, CT–computed tomography, SA–sample analyzing, RA–radiolabeled antibodies

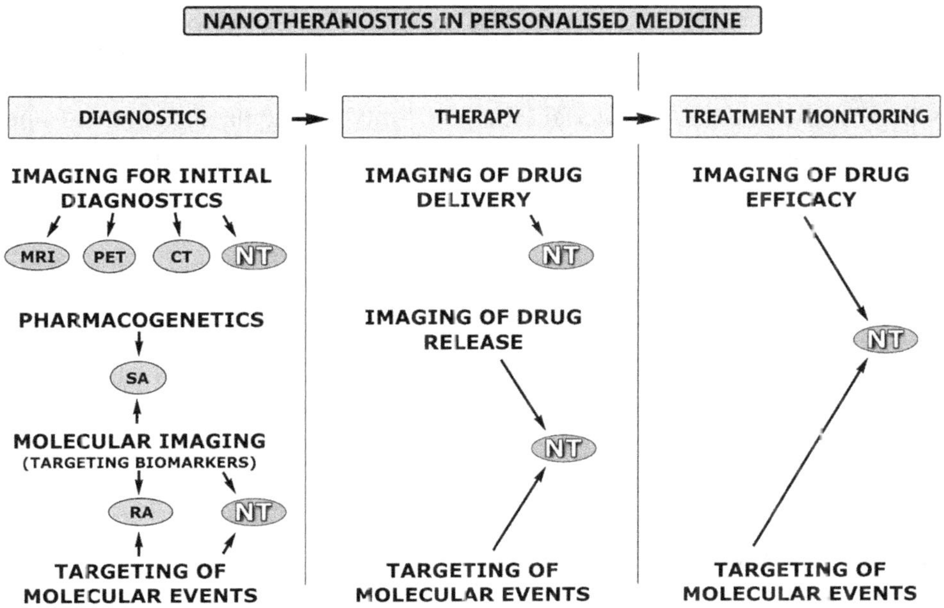

Due to only temporal presence of some biomarkers characterizing a specific disease state, targeted therapy, delayed even for a few days, may be ineffective. Here, an important advantage of theranostics is that both, detection of biomarker expression and targeted treatment, based on biomarker's presence, are possible *in vivo* and at the same time.

Moreover, nanoparticle based imaging systems can also be used to monitor treatment (Figure 4), which would be particularly valuable in early determination of the therapeutic success. Imaging of the tumor vasculature after an anticancer vasculature-disrupting treatment with the platform based on iron oxide nanoparticles (IONP) can serve as an example (Zhang et al., 2012). Another possibility is to mix trace amounts of radiolabeled nanomedicines with drug treatment (for example, in 2nd or 3^{d} cycle of therapy). Then the next step would be continuous anatomical CT-imaging of a patient in conjunction with 3D-PET to visualize the intervention efficacy in real time. This information would importantly assist the decision to adjust the drug dose or continue/discontinue the therapy.

This is the way to tune the use of theranostic nanomedicines for individual patient's therapy. Together with analysis of genetic polymorphism and biomarkers, the prescription of further therapy to a given patient would rely on imaged prediction and measurement of the therapeutic response.

In general, application of nanomedicine is similar to application of a combination of several drugs to one patient. Personalized approach suggests that before the therapy is prescribed, it is utmost important to test the suitability and safety of the nanocarrier. This topic deserves special attention and is the focus of the present chapter.

ADVERSE EFFECTS AND RISK ASSESSMENT OF NANOFORMULATIONS

Adverse Effects of Nanoformulation for Medical Use

Application of nanoparticles in medicine is increasing much faster than the knowledge on potential side effects they may have on human health. The use of nano-formulations in medicine results in direct exposure of body tissue to the nanomaterial. The possibility to tune the nanoparticle's physicochemical properties (primarily surface characteristics) offers unique advantages to design highly effective nanotheranostics, attractive and needed for development of new therapeutic strategies. Yet changing the particle's very same properties can cause unexpected nano-bio interactions and result in undesired adverse effects. Thus, every new functionalization of a nanoformulation brings additional concerns about its safety and can slow down its translation into clinical practice. The lack of knowledge on nano-bio interactions inside the human body can compromise the prediction of their efficacy/toxicity balance. Understanding whether nanomedicine itself can induce side effects along with the mechanisms of these effects is crucial for the development of safe-in-use theranostic systems. The following part of this chapter aims to describe the major areas where it is highly important to characterize the behavior of nanoformulation in a living organism.

Nanomedicines and Their Physicochemical Properties

Reduction of the particle size to the nanoscale causes an extreme increase of surface area to volume ratio, which results in an increase of potential number of the reactive groups on the NP's surface. Therefore, nano-sized particles have significantly higher biological activity as compared to micro-sized bulk material. The size of the nanoparticles (NPs) cause their intense interaction with biological tissues, increase uptake, and create an opportunity to cross biological barriers.

The current view is that the adverse effects of NPs depend on their physicochemical properties such as size, shape, charge, surface chemistry and site of the particle's administration, since they are considered to define protein and cellular NPs interactions (Nel et al., 2009; Treuel et al., 2013).

In many cases, development nanomedicines for the certain applications requires the data on relation of NP's properties and their adverse effects. For instance, there is a size cut-off for the particles recommended for the intravenous administration – particle's size should not exceed the diameter of fine capillaries (9 μm) to avoid their blockage, which could result in fat embolism and death (Mehnert & Mader, 2001). Of note, this restriction becomes folds higher (a submicron range) for the nanoparticles with limited deformability or particles tending to aggregate, such as lipid-based nanoformulations (Elgart et al., 2012). In the study by Zhao and coauthors, a smaller size range of the nanoparticles was a key factor of their safety(Zhao et al., 2011). Attachment of nanoparticles to the surface of the red blood cells was described as a tool to extend circulation time and to release therapeutic payload (Hall et al., 2007). However, later it was demonstrated that among several surface types and sizes of porous silicon nanoparticles, only small (100-200 μm) nanoparticles of MCM-41-type can adsorb to the red blood cell surface without affecting their membrane morphology. Other nanoparticles, attached to the red blood cells, were size-dependently decreasing membrane deformability of the cells, which is critical for effective blood flow (Zhao et al., 2011).

Nanoformulations and Cell Barriers

Smaller size of nanoparticles (less than 100 μm) makes them similar to physiological molecules and therefore they may utilize the same mechanisms to cross the internal barriers, i.e. blood-brain barrier protecting the brain, the blood-testis barrier protecting the male reproductive system, and placenta protecting the developing embryo (Pietroiusti et al., 2013). Although this is a basis to design nanoparticles for the diagnosis and treatment of diseases in these highly protected organs, at the same time there is a growing concern about unintended access of small nanoparticles to these organs.

There are several main mechanisms for crossing of internal barriers: passive and active transport and endocytosis. Besides being highly protective systems, internal barriers must provide transport of nutrients to the brain, to the fetus and to the testes. Nutrients can cross the internal barriers mainly by two mechanisms – passive diffusion (simple or facilitated) and active diffusion. In simple passive diffusion, crossing occurs by a concentration gradient without energy expenditure. Facilitated passive diffusion involves influx transporters, which allows faster passage of solutes than in a simple passive diffusion. Yet, the other conditions, besides concentration gradient, such as size, hydrophobicity, polarity and protein binding, are necessary for this way of transportation. Active diffusion of solutes occur with the help of influx transporters; however, this way of transportation involves energy expenditure. Endocytosis, one more way through which nanoparticles can cross the internal barriers, is a process of uptake of large polar molecule, which cannot go through the hydrophobic cell membrane.

The direct effects of nanoparticles, crossing the internal barriers, on cells and tissues, involve oxidative stress or DNA damage (Moller et al., 2010). However, Patrick Case and colleagues demonstrated that nanoparticles can induce these effects indirectly: in an *in vitro* model of a multilayer cell barrier they showed that cobalt chromium nanoparticles can cause DNA damage to cells on the other side of the barrier even without passing through this barrier (Bhabra et al., 2009). Other results, coming from this research group revealed that this indirect damage depends on the barrier thickness. Contrary to the logical expectations, signals from the nanoparticles which were damaging DNA, could not be transmitted through monolayer barriers, but were able to go across bilayer and multilayer (Sood et al., 2011). These results were similar irrespective of the cell type near the barrier: for connective tissue cells (fibroblasts), embryonic stem cells, the cells forming the barrier (BeWo cells) or corneal epithelial cells. In all these examples, nanoparticles were able to induce DNA damage when epithelial barrier consisted of more than one cell layer (Huppertz, 2011).

It is known from literature that signaling from nanoparticles through the epithelial barrier to the underlying cells involves – intercellular tube-like communication (gap junctions, mainly formed by protein connexin-43) for transferring small molecules from one cell to another and generation of mitochondrial reactive oxygen species and ATP (Bhabra et al., 2009). Furthermore, the authors observed the release of inflammatory cytokines, belonging to so-called family of senescence-associated secretory phenotype (SASPs). Normally, these molecules are secreted in response to oxidative stress in age-related pathologies and may help tissue reparation or disrupt the normal tissue structure and promote tumor formation, depending on tissue state (Campisi et al., 2011). However, there is no explanation that why the single epithelial layer provides better protection for the cells than a multilayered barrier.

Of note, a route of exposure - i.e. the point of entry of the nanoparticles into the organism (pulmonary, gastro-intestinal, intravenous, intraperitoneal, dermal) plays a critical role in the ability of nanoparticles to cross biological barriers. There is a good example of this statement provided in two subsequent studies on gold nanoparticles. First, it was demonstrated that intravenously administered smaller gold NPs can cross blood-brain barrier 10 times more effectively than bigger NPs (18nm) (Hirn et al., 2011). Later, the authors administered the same NPs gastro-intestinally under the same experimental conditions. In this case the blood concentration of 1.4 nm gold NPs was almost 4 times higher than that of 18 nm of gold NPs. Taking into account the data obtained in the previous intravenous experiment, the authors expected an almost 40 times higher access of 1.4 nm gold NPs through the blood-brain barrier as compared to 18nm gold NPs (Schleh et al., 2012). However, the results were opposite to expectation: 18nm NPs demonstrated 4 times higher access rate into the brain than 1.4 NPs. This is an evidence that initial residence of NPs in gastrointestinal environment before they get to the circulation, can have a significant effect on the translocation rate through the blood-brain barrier.

Thus, one cannot extrapolate the results from one type of studies with a certain administration route to another administration route, i.e. intravenous studies cannot represent the lung or gastrointestinal exposure, even after thorough prediction of the NP dose present in the circulation. Obviously, the physicochemical changes that take place during the residence of NPs in the lungs or gastrointestinal tract can dramatically influence their ability to cross the internal barriers.

Protein Corona

Currently, the so-called "protein corona" –the complex of biomolecules adsorbed on the surface of NPs in physiological conditions– is recognized to be the key factor which affects the transport of nanoparticles in the body and defines their biological fate (Foroozandeh & Aziz, 2015; Treuel et al., 2015). Upon contact with the NPs, the cell perceives protein corona but not the bare NPs surface (Figure 5A). Therefore, understanding of the protein corona formation is important for investigation of physiological as well as toxic responses to NPs.

Due to their large surface-to-volume ratio, NPs have an active surface chemistry compared to bulk materials. Therefore, when NPs are exposed to biological environment, they seek to reduce their high surface energy by adsorbing biomolecules, such as peptides, proteins and glycolipids. This nano-bio interface covers the surface of the nanoparticle and forms its "identity", which defines the interactions of NPs in the biological system and dictates cellular uptake, kinetics, signaling accumulation, transport and toxicity (Foroozandeh & Aziz, 2015).

First, the "soft shell", i.e. loosely bound proteins with short lifetime, forms around NPs. Over time, the composition of "soft" corona evolves to "hard" corona with less dynamic exchange (Foroozandeh & Aziz, 2015; Treuel et al., 2015). Time-dependent composition of a protein layer were described by Vroman in 1962 (Vroman, 1962) and its unexpected complexity were recently confirmed by work of Tenzer and co-workers (Tenzer et al., 2013). Up to 166 plasma proteins were determined within the corona on surface of NPs after half a minute and the number of individual proteins increased to almost 300 in subsequent time-points (up to 480 minutes), depending on the NP type.

Effects of Protein Corona on NP's Fate

Molecular properties of the protein corona are influential factors for the future fate of the NPs in the body (Figure 5A). Firstly, corona formation strongly affects colloidal stability. In physiological conditions, many NPs lose their stability and tend to form agglomerates within seconds (Cho, et al., 2011; Kendall et al., 2015). The stability of native NPs outside biological system can be entirely different from that of NPs under physiological conditions. In fact, some proteins from thousands of individual proteins in the

Figure 5. Protein corona around the nanoformulation. A. Formation of protein corona affects the properties of "bare" nanoparticle and thus can change its biological fate. B. Factors, which govern formation of the "personalized" protein corona.

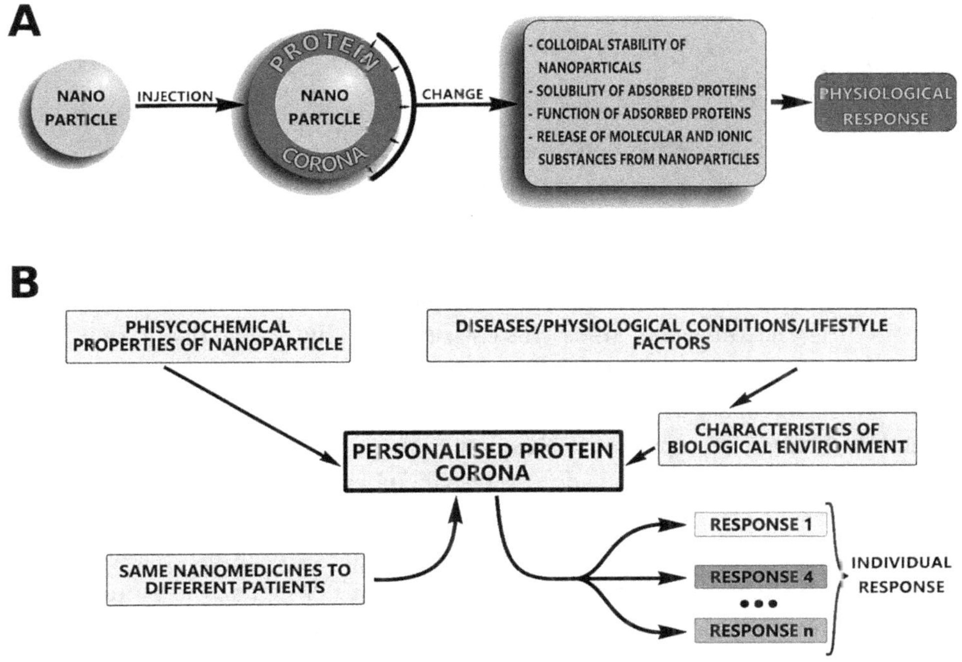

corona exert a stabilizing influence, while other have destabilizing properties. Therefore, it becomes a problem in evaluation of the actual NPs size and dose applied (in both *in vitro* and *in vivo* studies).

Second, structural changes of the proteins adsorbed on the NPs surface may occur and result in altered protein conformations and function. An immune response can be induced in response to this protein denaturation on the NPs surface (Brandes et al, 2006), and define NP's kinetics.

Third possible result of the protein adsorption on NPs surface can be a drastic change in protein's solubility. Since most of the serum proteins are combining optimal function with good solubility, the structural changes, taking place upon their adsorption on the NPs surface can alter their solubility (Treuel et al., 2015).

The change of the surface energy as well as restructuring of NP's surface may cause dissolution of NPs with the release of molecular or ionic substances that can cause their own side effects (Diedrich et al., 2012; Misra et al., 2012).

Thus, protein corona alters the size, surface chemistry, and surface charge of the NPs and thereby affects its cellular uptake and bio-distribution – biological endpoints, where they could not reach without protein cover (Monopoli et al., 2012).

The most common physiological roles, which the complexes of adsorbed proteins play, are lipid and ion transport, complement activation, pathogen recognition and blood coagulation (Foroozandeh & Aziz, 2015).

EFFECT OF NPS PROPERTIES ON COMPOSITION OF PROTEIN CORONA

Both, physicochemical characteristics of the NPs themselves and the characteristics of the biological milieu, where they disperse, affect their unique composition of protein corona for each NP type.

Nanoparticle Size

It was shown that the NP's size alone could be a critical determinant of human blood plasma corona (Tenzer et al., 2011). Many, among the corona proteins, (for example, immunoglobulin G or actin) show no dependence on the NP's size. However, 37% of all identified corona proteins have significantly different binding behavior towards the NPs of the different sizes. Some proteins have higher affinity for larger NPs, while others show higher affinity to smaller NPs. In their work, Tenzer and coauthors showed that as small as 10 nm difference in size of silica NPs can dramatically change the protein corona composition around NPs that are otherwise identical (Tenzer et al., 2011).

Shape of the NPs is another characteristic, which determines the manner of protein adsorption onto NP's surface and the biological responses to NPs. For example, cluster in and apolipoprotein D are only bound to spherical TiO_2 NPs, but not to nanorods or nanotubes (Deng et al., 2009).

Composition and surface properties of NPs strongly determine the proteins that bind to the NPs and the level of the conformational changes of adsorbed proteins. For example, hydrophobic NPs induce more conformational changes than hydrophilic NPs (Buijs et al., 1999) and therefore are likely to induce immune response (Brandes et al., 2006). Surface coating has been demonstrated to influence cytotoxic effects of NPs (Harris et al., 2001), but the core NP composition is also a key parameter. For instance, the cytotoxicity of silver NPs was primarily caused by the release of silver ions even though the NPs were coated by the polymers (Kittler, 2010).

In a recent work, Walkey and coauthors used the fingerprint of protein corona to establish a quantitative model to predict cell associations of various gold NPs types (Walkey et al., 2014). This model was 50% more accurate than the model with application of NP's physicochemical parameters, suggesting that protein corona gives more information of NP's biological fate rather than just its initial properties. Structure of the protein corona can be studied in physiological environment (i.e. *in situ*), or after isolation from this environment (i.e. *ex situ*). The analysis of protein corona includes its different parameters such as thickness, protein identity, protein-NP affinity, protein quantity, density and protein conformation (Kittler, 2010). Thus, the biological responses to the NPs are strongly dependent on the type and amount of associated proteins in protein corona.

"Personalized" Protein Corona

New research findings now demonstrate that the content and properties of plasma proteins significantly vary depending on the type of disease, physiological condition or even lifestyle factors. These plasma alterations include changes in protein stability, concentration and folding. These features can affect the affinity of plasma proteins for NP's surface, influence the protein adsorption on the NPs, hence the difference in corona composition and biological effects of NPs in different patients (Figure 5 B).

In a recent study from Mahmoudi and colleagues (Hajipour et al., 2015), identical graphene oxide sheets were incubated in plasma of patients with different types of diseases/physiological conditions (i.e. hypofibrinogenemia, blood cancer, thalassemia major, thalassemia minor, rheumatism, fauvism, hypercholesterolemia, diabetes and pregnancy). It was demonstrated that the differences in the plasma of these patient groups resulted in formation of personalized, disease/condition specific protein coronas on the surface of NPs. Due to the difference in protein composition and content, these protein coronas induced significantly different cellular toxicity, apoptosis/necrosis, ROS production, lipid peroxidation and inflammation response.

Hence, the biological effects of the same nanomedicine are different in patients with various diseases, in different stages of the same disease and patients with different lifestyles (for example, smokers/non-smokers, etc. (Hajipour et al., 2014).

The experimental evidence described above supports the theory that the presence of concomitant diseases should be one of the primary criteria that is critical for the choice of a suitable nanoformulation for a given patient.

In our recent studies on rats (Vlasova et al., 2014), the adverse hypotension and tachycardia were observed after intravenous administration of several NP types. These effects have been transient in healthy animals; however, they appear to become lethal when combined with inherent disorders such as arterial hypertension and underlying cardiovascular disease (Vlasova et al., unpublished observations). Moreover, these adverse cardiovascular effects turned to be fatal also in rats, pretreated with atenolol - commonly used antihypertensive drug. In addition, the adverse effects of nanomedicine can interfere with the effect of co-administered drug. In our recent publication, we provided a case study, where the nanocarrier and the drug, both affect the same cardiovascular parameters after their intravenous administration. While the drug, Ghrelin antagonist (GhA) increases arterial pressure, thermally hydrocarbonized porous silicon nanoparticles (THCPSi) transiently decrease it. However, intravenous administration of GhA-loaded THCPSi nanoparticles resulted in partial abolishment of the drug activity and the arterial pressure was not increased (Vlasova et al., 2014). Thus, even transient adverse effects induced by the nanocarrier itself can obscure the biological activity of a drug, delivered by this nanocarrier. The described observations once again underline the importance of a patient-specific approach: the nanomedicine, prescribed to a given patient should be compatible with his concomitant diseases and current medication (Figure 6).

Altogether, these findings facilitate the understanding of the reasons behind variety of personal therapeutic and toxic responses induced by exactly the same nanomedicines in different patients, referred to in the beginning of this chapter. The challenge and the beauty of the patient specific and safe-in-use nanotherapeuticsis that their design would be a result of thorough consideration of various factors, such as type, severity and period of disease; individual genetic variation and "personalized protein corona".

SOLUTIONS AND RECOMMENDATIONS

Possible Approaches to Risk Assessment of Nanomedicines

Nanotechnology-specific risk assessment strategies are still a subject of discussion and debate in international scientific community. Current methodologies for the risk assessment of nanomaterials are not sufficient and should be enriched and refined. This would help to create a system of valid tests for quantitative risk evaluation of nanoformulation, developed for a certain drug and administration route. Traditionally nanocarriers undergo tests for cytotoxicity and immunogenic properties, while the determination of their effects on tissues and organs that they are passing by along their administration route remains without attention. However, the severity assessment of these effects is utmost important for

Figure 6. Steps of a patient-specific approach with nanotheranostics

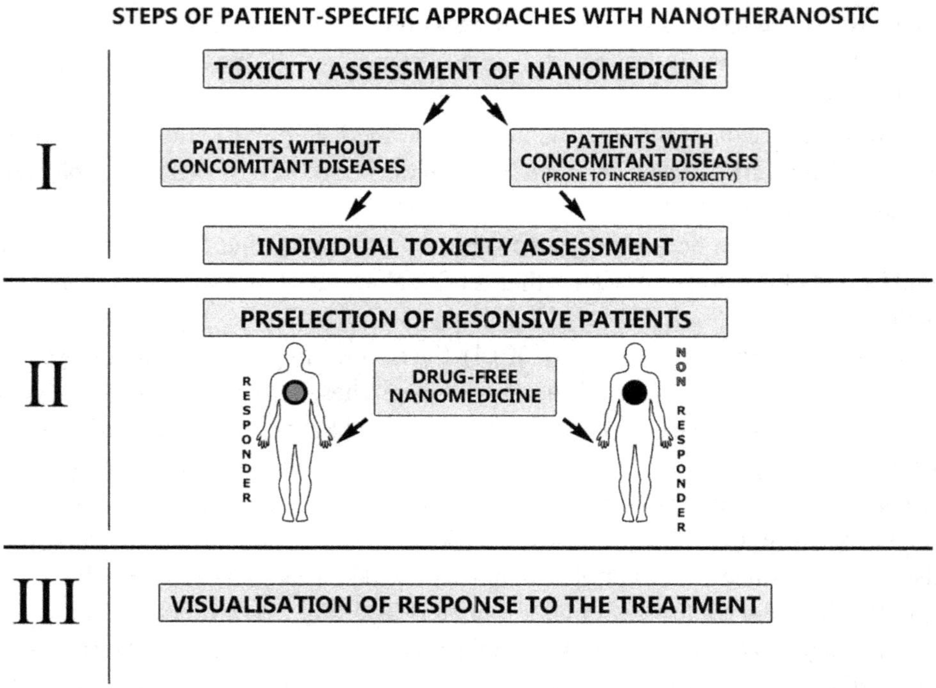

the safe use of nanocarriers. The existing gap in nanotoxicity testing requires a novel approach, which combines the knowledge of several disciplines – physics, chemistry, cell biology and physiology. A novel platform in order to use the full range of methodologies is required. Besides cytotoxicity and immunogenic tests, these methods should include evaluation of NPs effects on physiological systems at cellular, tissue, organ and systemic levels. Combination of both *in vitro* and *in vivo* methods is important to provide objective assessment on biological effects of the NPs. Thus, the scientific community should provide a verified system of rigorous nanotoxicity tests, assessing in detail the NPs safety. These methods should also include the possibility to identify the risk of NPs administration to the groups of patients with comorbidities. Among the patients, prescribed with treatments, involving nanoformulations, there will be a high probability of co-existing widely spread pathologies such as diabetes, cardiovascular disorders and metabolic syndrome. Therefore, it is important to evaluate the risk of NP use in adequate experimental animal models mimicking these disorders. This knowledge, generated by detailed testing of NPs toxicity is ultimately essential in order to select an appropriate nanocarrier for therapy/diagnostics as well as to identify patient groups at risk. Furthermore, this knowledge can be a base for designing of new nanomedicine devices, safe for the certain groups of patients.

Following the idea of personalization, in figure 6, we show an example of consecutive steps for choosing a suitable nanotheranostic for the cancer treatment of a given patient. The first step represents the assessment of individual toxicity to given nanoformulation, based on health status of the patient.

The next step towards patient-specific treatment is to preselect the patients responsive to this therapeutic intervention. In order to explore the level of target site accumulation, at first clinician can apply a drug-free nanocarrier. Patients with low target site accumulation or those who accumulate the nanocarrier in healthy tissues, i.e. “likely non-responders”, are allocated to another therapy, while patients with high to moderate levels of target site accumulation, i.e. “likely responders”, can be treated with drug-loaded nanocarrier. Importantly, the second personalization step of pre-selected patients is based on follow-up monitoring aiming to visualize how well they respond to the treatment (Lammers et al., 2012).

However, this approach has to take into account the fact that pharmacokinetics of drug-free and drug-loaded nanocarrier may be significantly different (Figure 7). Moreover, upon the repeated administration, pharmacokinetics of the nanocarrier after the first injection may differ from the one after subsequent injections (Figure 8).

Firstly, the pharmacokinetics, the biodistribution and the target site accumulation of drug-free and drug-loaded nanocarrier can significantly vary. Here we provide an example, where the conjugation of the nanoparticle with the drug cause this difference. Incorporation of doxorubicin and gemcitabine to iodine-131-labeled HPMA copolymers change the physicochemical properties of the formulation so that its circulation time becomes shorter as compared to drug-free copolymers, while the level of accumulation in kidneys significantly increases (Lammers et al., 2009). Another example illustrates the possible difference in mode and kinetics of clearance between drug-free and drug-loaded nanocarriers. In this case, it is important to consider the functionality of reticuloendothelial system. The majority of drug-free radiolabeled liposomes or polymers most likely end up in macrophages. In case of nanofor-

Figure 7. Schematic example of pharmacokinetic differences between drug-free and drug-loaded nanomedicine

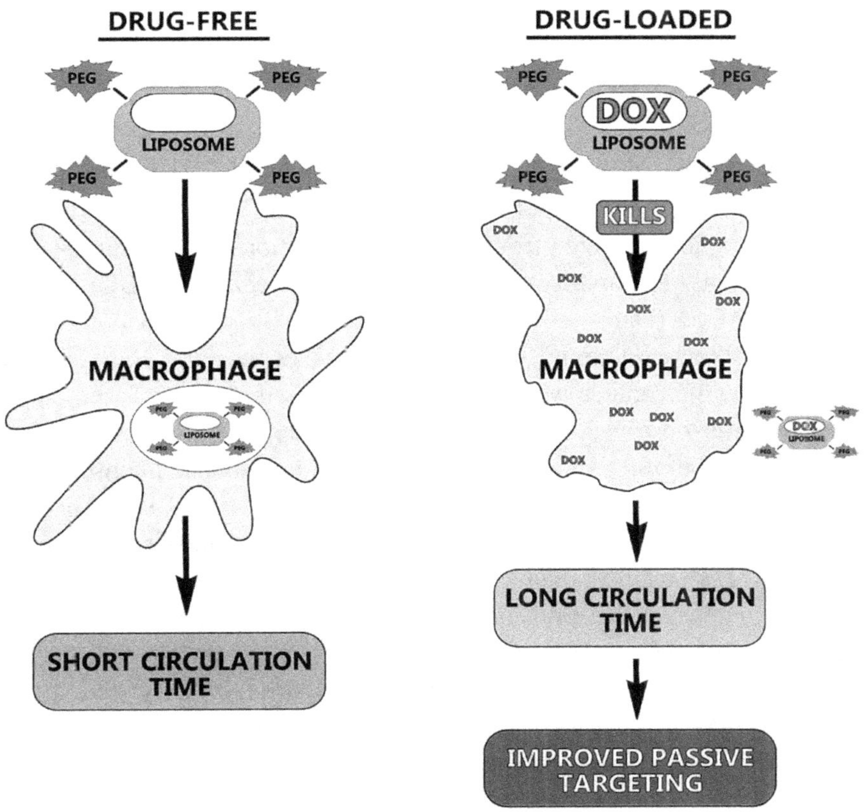

Figure 8. Schematic example of pharmacokinetic differences between single and repeated administration of nanomedicine

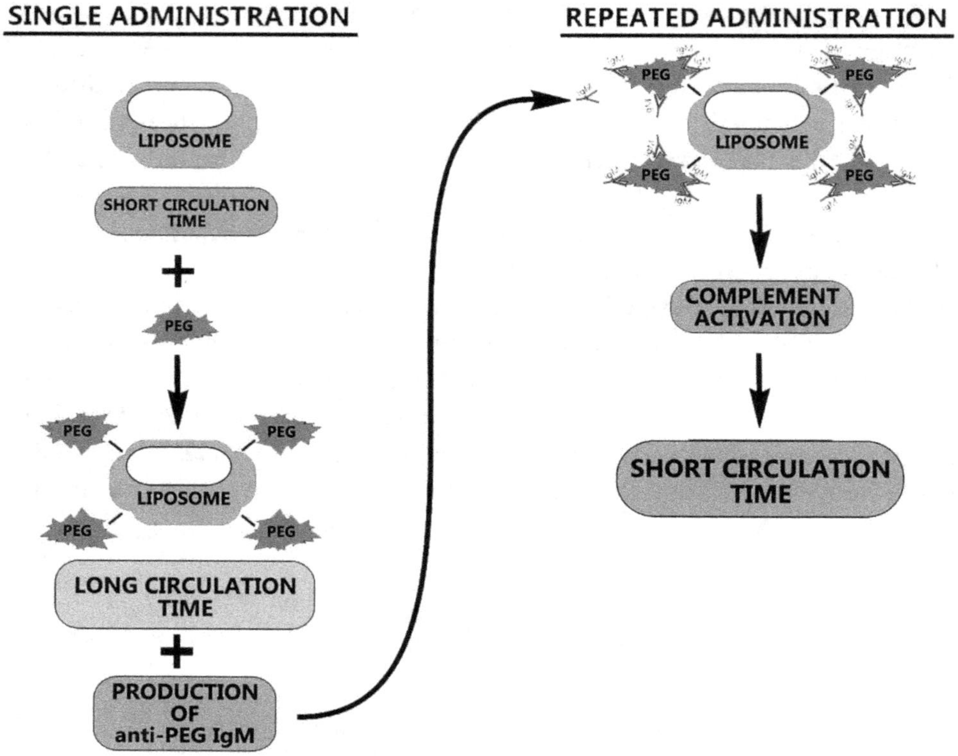

mulation containing chemotherapeutic drug, a large portion of circulating as well as tumor-associated macrophages are killed by this drug, which, in turn, has a major effect on pharmacokinetics, organ distribution and target site accumulation of the drug. It has been shown that radiolabeled PEGylated liposomes are relatively rapidly excreted from systemic circulation even upon repeated administration by the mechanism commonly referred to as accelerated blood clearance (ABC) phenomenon and primarily accumulate in the liver (Dams et al., 2000). However, ABC phenomenon has been absent after administration of doxorubicin-containing PEGylated liposomes, because some part of macrophages, which played a role in rapid clearance were killed by doxorubicin and no decrease in circulation time for the nanoformulation was observed. Thus, attenuation of macrophage-dependent clearance by a chemotherapeutic drug can be helpful for the increase of circulation time and consequently assist passive targeting of the nanomedicine (Figure 7).

Second, the pharmacokinetics of drug-free nanomedicine can significantly change because of its repeated administration. For instance, the increased circulation time achieved by the PEGylation of liposomes was lost due to repeated injections of PEGylated liposomes because the half-life of the second dose, given in a period from 5 days to 4 weeks after the first injection, dramatically decreased (Laverman et al., 2001). Later on Ishida and Kiwada showed that the first dose of PEGylated liposomes induce the production of anti-PEG IgM, which then selectively binds to the surface of subsequently administered PEGylated liposomes, resulting in significant complement activation (Ishida & Kiwada, 2008) (Figure 8).

Therefore, before the above-mentioned pre-selection of "responsive" to nanotherapeutics patients, it is important to obtain really relevant results using both drug-free and drug-loaded nanoformulations with an imaging agent, as well as to have data on nanomedicine behavior upon the repeated administration.

FUTURE RESEARCH DIRECTIONS

The initial point for the risk assessment of the nanomaterial is its physicochemical characterization, which is necessary to understand the relationship between the properties and potential adverse effects. Of note, there is a combination of physical and chemical characteristics, which clearly and uniquely defines each nanomaterial. Currently scientific community aims to unify and harmonize the methodologies used for characterization of the nanoparticles, what is necessary for the possibility to compare different studies. It would be of great importance to obtain new sets of data, which take into account both, physicochemical characteristics of nanomedicine and individual composition of protein corona. The development of new tools to analyze this data and predict nanocarrier's behavior in human body are expected. Furthermore, there is a need for a verified and unified system of tests to assess the risk of different nanomaterial's classes.

CONCLUSION

Development of nanomedicine, especially nanotheranostics, is a promising move towards personalization in clinical practice. However, the knowledge gap regarding adverse effects of nanomedicines on various organs and tissues slows down their application in clinics. New insights on interaction of nanomedicines with human body via "personalized" protein corona would help to create a database for prediction of nanomedicine's adverse effects. As the field of nanomedicine moves from academic findings towards industrial products, new testing systems to assure nanomaterials safety is necessary to make every effort to foresee and alleviate their adverse effects in patients.

REFERENCES

Bhabra, G., Sood, A., Fisher, B., Cartwright, L., Saunders, M., Evans, W. H., & Case, C. P. et al. (2009). Nanoparticles can cause DNA damage across a cellular barrier. *Nature Nanotechnology*, *4*(12), 876–883. doi:10.1038/nnano.2009.313 PMID:19893513

Brandes, N., Welzel, P. B., Werner, C., & Kroh, L. W. (2006). Adsorption-induced conformational changes of proteins onto ceramic particles: Differential scanning calorimetry and FTIR analysis. *Journal of Colloid and Interface Science*, *299*(1), 56–69. doi:10.1016/j.jcis.2006.01.065 PMID:16500671

Buijs, J., Costa Vera, C., Ayala, E., Steensma, E., Hakansson, P., & Oscarsson, S. (1999). Conformational stability of adsorbed insulin studied with mass spectrometry and hydrogen exchange. *Analytical Chemistry*, *71*(15), 3219–3225. doi:10.1021/ac9809433 PMID:10450163

Campisi, J., Andersen, J. K., Kapahi, P., & Melov, S. (2011). Cellular senescence: A link between cancer and age-related degenerative disease? *Seminars in Cancer Biology*, *21*(6), 354–359. PMID:21925603

Carmona-Ribeiro, A. M., & de Melo Carrasco, L. D. (2014). Novel formulations for antimicrobial peptides. *International Journal of Molecular Sciences*, *15*(10), 18040–18083. doi:10.3390/ijms151018040 PMID:25302615

Cho, E. C., Zhang, Q., & Xia, Y. (2011). The effect of sedimentation and diffusion on cellular uptake of gold nanoparticles. *Nature Nanotechnology*, *6*(6), 385–391. doi:10.1038/nnano.2011.58 PMID:21516092

Dams, E. T., Laverman, P., Oyen, W. J., Storm, G., Scherphof, G. L., van Der Meer, J. W., & Boerman, O. C. et al. (2000). Accelerated blood clearance and altered biodistribution of repeated injections of sterically stabilized liposomes. *The Journal of Pharmacology and Experimental Therapeutics*, *292*(3), 1071–1079. PMID:10688625

Deng, Z. J., Mortimer, G., Schiller, T., Musumeci, A., Martin, D., & Minchin, R. F. (2009). Differential plasma protein binding to metal oxide nanoparticles. *Nanotechnology*, *20*(45), 455101. doi:10.1088/0957-4484/20/45/455101 PMID:19822937

Diedrich, T., Dybowska, A., Schott, J., Valsami-Jones, E., & Oelkers, E. H. (2012). The dissolution rates of SiO2 nanoparticles as a function of particle size. *Environmental Science & Technology*, *46*(9), 4909–4915. doi:10.1021/es2045053 PMID:22482930

do Carmo, F. A., Sathler, P. C., Zancan, P., Rodrigues, C. R., Castro, H. C., de Sousa, V. P., & Cabral, L. M. et al. (2014). Therapeutic nanosystems for oral administration of insulin. *Current Pharmaceutical Biotechnology*, *15*(7), 620–628. doi:10.2174/1389201015666140915150826 PMID:25219867

Elgart, A., Cherniakov, I., Aldouby, Y., Domb, A. J., & Hoffman, A. (2012). Lipospheres and pro-nano lipospheres for delivery of poorly water soluble compounds. *Chemistry and Physics of Lipids*, *165*(4), 438–453. doi:10.1016/j.chemphyslip.2012.01.007 PMID:22342324

Foroozandeh, P., & Aziz, A. A. (2015). Merging worlds of nanomaterials and biological environment: Factors governing protein corona formation on nanoparticles and its biological consequences. *Nanoscale Research Letters*, *10*(1), 221. doi:10.1186/s11671-015-0922-3 PMID:25995715

Hajipour, M. J., Laurent, S., Aghaie, A., Rezaee, F., & Mahmoudi, M. (2014). Personalized protein coronas: A "key" factor at the nanobiointerface. *Biomaterials Science*, *2*(9), 1210–1221. doi:10.1039/C4BM00131A

Hajipour, M. J., Raheb, J., Akhavan, O., Arjmand, S., Mashinchian, O., Rahman, M., & Mahmoudi, M. et al. (2015). Personalized disease-specific protein corona influences the therapeutic impact of graphene oxide. *Nanoscale*, *7*(19), 8978–8994. doi:10.1039/C5NR00520E PMID:25920546

Hall, S. S., Mitragotri, S., & Daugherty, P. S. (2007). Identification of peptide ligands facilitating nanoparticle attachment to erythrocytes. *Biotechnology Progress*, *23*(3), 749–754. doi:10.1021/bp0603331 PMID:17469847

Harris, J. M., Martin, N. E., & Modi, M. (2001). Pegylation: A novel process for modifying pharmacokinetics. *Clinical Pharmacokinetics*, *40*(7), 539–551. doi:10.2165/00003088-200140070-00005 PMID:11510630

Hippocrates. (1931). *Nature of man* (vol. 4). Cambridge, MA: Harward University Press.

Hirn, S., Semmler-Behnke, M., Schleh, C., Wenk, A., Lipka, J., Schaffler, M., & Kreyling, W. G. et al. (2011). Particle size-dependent and surface charge-dependent biodistribution of gold nanoparticles after intravenous administration. *European Journal of Pharmaceutics and Biopharmaceutics*, *77*(3), 407–416. doi:10.1016/j.ejpb.2010.12.029 PMID:21195759

Huppertz, B. (2011). Nanoparticles: Barrier thickness matters. *Nature Nanotechnology*, *6*(12), 758–759. doi:10.1038/nnano.2011.206 PMID:22056727

Ishida, T., & Kiwada, H. (2008). Accelerated blood clearance (ABC) phenomenon upon repeated injection of PEGylated liposomes. *International Journal of Pharmaceutics*, *354*(1-2), 56–62. doi:10.1016/j.ijpharm.2007.11.005 PMID:18083313

Jain, R. K., & Stylianopoulos, T. (n.d.). Delivering nanomedicine to solid tumors. *Nature Reviews Clinical Oncology, 7*(11), 653-664.

Kendall, M., Hodges, N. J., Whitwell, H., Tyrrell, J., & Cangul, H. (2015). Nanoparticle growth and surface chemistry changes in cell-conditioned culture medium. *Philosophical Transactions of the Royal Society B: Biological Sciences, 370*(1661), 20140100.

Kim, T. H., Lee, S., & Chen, X. (2013). Nanotheranostics for personalized medicine. *Expert Review of Molecular Diagnostics*, *13*(3), 257–269. doi:10.1586/erm.13.15 PMID:23570404

Kittler, S. G. C., Diendorf, J., Köller, M., & Epple, M. (2010). Toxicity of Silver Nanoparticles Increases during Storage Because of Slow Dissolution under Release of Silver Ions. *Chemistry of Materials*, *22*(16), 4548–4554. doi:10.1021/cm100023p

Lammers, T., Rizzo, L. Y., Storm, G., & Kiessling, F. (2012). Personalized nanomedicine. *Clinical Cancer Research*, *18*(18), 4889–4894. doi:10.1158/1078-0432.CCR-12-1414 PMID:22829203

Lammers, T., Subr, V., Ulbrich, K., Peschke, P., Huber, P. E., Hennink, W. E., & Storm, G. (2009). Simultaneous delivery of doxorubicin and gemcitabine to tumors in vivo using prototypic polymeric drug carriers. *Biomaterials*, *30*(20), 3466–3475. doi:10.1016/j.biomaterials.2009.02.040 PMID:19304320

Laverman, P., Boerman, O. C., Oyen, W. J. G., Corstens, F. H. M., & Storm, G. (2001). In vivo applications of PEG liposomes: Unexpected observations. *Critical Reviews in Therapeutic Drug Carrier Systems*, *18*(6), 551–566. doi:10.1615/CritRevTherDrugCarrierSyst.v18.i6.40 PMID:11789675

Liotta, L., & Petricoin, E. (2000). Molecular profiling of human cancer. *Nature Reviews. Genetics*, *1*(1), 48–56. doi:10.1038/35049567 PMID:11262874

Ma, Q., & Lu, A. Y. (2011). Pharmacogenetics, pharmacogenomics, and individualized medicine. *Pharmacological Reviews*, *63*(2), 437–459. doi:10.1124/pr.110.003533 PMID:21436344

Mehnert, W., & Mäder, K. (2001). Solid lipid nanoparticles: Production, characterization and applications. *Advanced Drug Delivery Reviews*, *47*(2-3), 165–196. doi:10.1016/S0169-409X(01)00105-3 PMID:11311991

Misra, S. K., Dybowska, A., Berhanu, D., Luoma, S. N., & Valsami-Jones, E. (2012). The complexity of nanoparticle dissolution and its importance in nanotoxicological studies. *The Science of the Total Environment*, *438*, 225–232. doi:10.1016/j.scitotenv.2012.08.066 PMID:23000548

Moller, P., Jacobsen, N. R., Folkmann, J. K., Danielsen, P. H., Mikkelsen, L., Hemmingsen, J. G., & Loft, S. et al. (2010). Role of oxidative damage in toxicity of particulates. *Free Radical Research*, *44*(1), 1–46. doi:10.3109/10715760903300691 PMID:19886744

Monopoli, M. P., Aberg, C., Salvati, A., & Dawson, K. A. (2012). Biomolecular coronas provide the biological identity of nanosized materials. *Nature Nanotechnology*, *7*(12), 779–786. doi:10.1038/nnano.2012.207 PMID:23212421

Nel, A. E., Madler, L., Velegol, D., Xia, T., Hoek, E. M., Somasundaran, P., & Thompson, M. (2009). Understanding biophysicochemical interactions at the nano-bio interface. *Nature Materials*, *8*(7), 543–557. doi:10.1038/nmat2442 PMID:19525947

Pietroiusti, A., Campagnolo, L., & Fadeel, B. (2013). Interactions of engineered nanoparticles with organs protected by internal biological barriers. *Small*, *9*(9-10), 1557–1572. doi:10.1002/smll.201201463 PMID:23097249

Sadee, W., & Dai, Z. (2005). Pharmacogenetics/genomics and personalized medicine. *Human Molecular Genetics, 14*(2), R207-214.

Schleh, C., Semmler-Behnke, M., Lipka, J., Wenk, A., Hirn, S., Schaffler, M., & Kreyling, W. G. et al. (2012). Size and surface charge of gold nanoparticles determine absorption across intestinal barriers and accumulation in secondary target organs after oral administration. *Nanotoxicology*, *6*(1), 36–46. doi:10.3109/17435390.2011.552811 PMID:21309618

Sood, A., Salih, S., Roh, D., Lacharme-Lora, L., Parry, M., Hardiman, B., & Keehan, R. C. P. (2011). Signalling of DNA damage and cytokines across cell barriers exposed to nanoparticles depends on barrier thickness. *Nature Nanotechnology*, *6*(12), 824–833. PMID:22056725

Tenzer, S., Docter, D., Kuharev, J., Musyanovych, A., Fetz, V., Hecht, R., & Stauber, R. H. et al. (2013). Rapid formation of plasma protein corona critically affects nanoparticle pathophysiology. *Nature Nanotechnology*, *8*(10), 772–781. doi:10.1038/nnano.2013.181 PMID:24056901

Tenzer, S., Docter, D., Rosfa, S., Wlodarski, A., Kuharev, J., Rekik, A., & Stauber, R. H. et al. (2011). Nanoparticle size is a critical physicochemical determinant of the human blood plasma corona: A comprehensive quantitative proteomic analysis. *ACS Nano*, *5*(9), 7155–7167. doi:10.1021/nn201950e PMID:21866933

Treuel, L., Docter, D., Maskos, M., & Stauber, R. H. (2015). Protein corona - from molecular adsorption to physiological complexity. *Beilstein Journal of Nanotechnology*, *6*, 857–873. doi:10.3762/bjnano.6.88 PMID:25977856

Treuel, L., Jiang, X., & Nienhaus, G. U. (2013). New views on cellular uptake and trafficking of manufactured nanoparticles. *Journal of the Royal Society, Interface*, *10*(82), 20120939. doi:10.1098/rsif.2012.0939 PMID:23427093

Vlasova, M. A., Rytkonen, J., Riikonen, J., Tarasova, O. S., Monkare, J., Kovalainen, M., & Jarvinen, K. et al. (2014). Nanocarriers and the delivered drug: Effect interference due to intravenous administration. *European Journal of Pharmaceutical Sciences*, *63*, 96–102. doi:10.1016/j.ejps.2014.06.011 PMID:24964293

Vlasova, M. A., Tarasova, O. S., Riikonen, J., Raula, J., Lobach, A. S., Borzykh, A. A., & Järvinen, K. et al. (2014). Injected nanoparticles: The combination of experimental systems to assess cardiovascular adverse effects. *European Journal of Pharmaceutics and Biopharmaceutics*, *87*(1), 64–72. doi:10.1016/j.ejpb.2014.02.001 PMID:24530427

Vroman, L. (1962). Effect of absorbed proteins on the wettability of hydrophilic and hydrophobic solids. *Nature*, *196*(4853), 476–477. doi:10.1038/196476a0 PMID:13998030

Walkey, C. D., Olsen, J. B., Song, F., Liu, R., Guo, H., Olsen, D. W., & Chan, W. C. et al. (2014). Protein corona fingerprinting predicts the cellular interaction of gold and silver nanoparticles. *ACS Nano*, *8*(3), 2439–2455. doi:10.1021/nn406018q PMID:24517450

Yang, K., Hu, L., Ma, X., Ye, S., Cheng, L., Shi, X., & Liu, Z. et al. (2012). Multimodal imaging guided photothermal therapy using functionalized graphene nanosheets anchored with magnetic nanoparticles. *Advanced Materials*, *24*(14), 1868–1872. doi:10.1002/adma.201104964 PMID:22378564

Zhang, F., Huang, X., Zhu, L., Guo, N., Niu, G., Swierczewska, M., & Chen, X. et al. (2012). Noninvasive monitoring of orthotopic glioblastoma therapy response using RGD-conjugated iron oxide nanoparticles. *Biomaterials*, *33*(21), 5414–5422. doi:10.1016/j.biomaterials.2012.04.032 PMID:22560667

Zhao, Y., Sun, X., Zhang, G., Trewyn, B. G., Slowing, I. I., & Lin, V. S. (2011). Interaction of mesoporous silica nanoparticles with human red blood cell membranes: Size and surface effects. *ACS Nano*, *5*(2), 1366–1375. doi:10.1021/nn103077k PMID:21294526

KEY TERMS AND DEFINITIONS

Adverse Effects: either harmful or unintended effects of therapeutic agents.

Nanoparticles: particulate drug delivery and/or diagnostic systems of nano-size.

Nanotheranostics: nanoparticulate systems, which combine at least several functions – diagnostic and therapeutic.

Personalized Therapy: medical approach, when the therapy is prescribed according to the detailed health status, physiological condition and genetic data of a patient.

Pharmacokinetics: the fate of pharmaceutical agent from the moment of its administration up to the point at which it is completely eliminated from the body, including its distribution, interactions within a living organism and routes/mechanisms of excretion.

Protein Corona: proteins, peptides and other biomolecules adsorbing to nanoparticles, when they get into biological milieu (intersticial fluid, blood plasma, etc.).

Therapeutic Window: the range of doses, where drug's therapeutic effect is already present and toxic effects are not apparent.

Section 2
Pharmacogenetics

Chapter 2
Drug Delivery Strategies for Tolerogenic Therapy for Autoimmune Diseases in an Antigen-Specific Manner

Kevin J. Peine
The University of North Carolina at Chapel Hill, USA

Eric M. Bachelder
The University of North Carolina at Chapel Hill, USA

Naihan Chen
The University of North Carolina at Chapel Hill, USA

Kristy M. Ainslie
The University of North Carolina at Chapel Hill, USA

ABSTRACT

Autoimmune diseases are the result of an improper immune response towards a self-antigen. Predominantly, autoimmune diseases have been treated using therapies that suppress systemic immune responses, which can result in significant side-effects like increased risk of infection and cancer. Alternatively, induction of immune tolerance through antigen-specific therapies can inhibit disease-associated responses without systemic suppression. Previously, immune tolerance has been accomplished by soluble antigen delivery through oral, nasal or sublingual routes. However, these therapies have shown minimal success in clinical settings. In an attempt to increase the efficacy of these therapies, recent work has utilized microparticulate delivery vehicles for the induction of immune tolerance. Microparticles are capable of increasing the solubility and circulation of cargo. In addition, their ability to passively target macrophages and dendritic cells increases their capacity for modulating the immune response. Recent work has shown microparticles fabricated with disease-associated antigens have limited disease progression and severity in animal models of Multiple Sclerosis, Type 1 Diabetes and Rheumatoid Arthritis. Inhibition of disease progression has corresponded with an antigen-specific decrease in inflammatory responses. The emerging field of inducing tolerance through microparticle-based therapies can limit therapeutic side-effects and increase patient quality of life by providing for long-term suppression of autoimmune disorders without compromising systemic immune function.

DOI: 10.4018/978-1-5225-0754-3.ch002

INTRODUCTION

Autoimmune Diseases

According to the National Institutes of Health (NIH), approximately 23.5 million Americans are living with at least one autoimmune disease. These diseases, which can occur in almost any tissue, are the result of an improper immune response towards self-antigens. In some cases, such as systemic lupus erythematosus (SLE), the immune response mounts a response that targets multiple healthy tissues, while others like Multiple Sclerosis (MS), Type-1 Diabetes (T1D) or Rheumatoid Arthritis (RA) are more organ or site specific. Current therapeutic strategies for autoimmune diseases provide amelioration of symptoms, most commonly through systemic immune suppression, but fail to treat the underlying causes of disease. Although autoimmune diseases manifest themselves very differently, a number of current therapeutics have similar strategies for immune suppression, including inhibition of T cells, B cells, and pro-inflammatory cytokines. This chapter will discuss a number of therapeutic approaches for common autoimmune diseases, as well as the emerging field of nano/microparticulate therapeutics for the treatment of autoimmune diseases.

Multiple Sclerosis

MS is a chronic demyelinating disease of the central nervous system (CNS) and affects nearly 2.5 million people worldwide, at a yearly cost burden of up to $54,000 per patient (Adelman, Rane, & Villa, 2013). T cells targeting auto-antigens in the CNS is believed to be the initial step that drives pathogenesis of MS (Friese, Schattling, & Fugger, 2014). Although the exact mechanism is not clearly known yet, the focal areas of demyelination in the white matter (plaques) are seen as the first site of attack. Immune cells (such as T cells and macrophages) invade across the blood–brain barrier, which further promotes inflammatory responses in the brain parenchyma, leading to demyelination and axonal degeneration (Smith & McDonald, 1999). Current therapies for MS have been successful at decreasing disease symptoms through a wide variety of immunomodulatory, antibody, or small molecule therapies. Interferon beta (IFN-β) (Avonex, Betaseron, Extavia, or Rebif) and glatiramer acetate (GA) (Copaxone) are frontline immunomodulatory therapies for the treatment of MS. IFN-β is a protein that was the first therapy to be accepted for use against MS. This injectable has shown to be effective at decreasing relapse rates, as well as slowing progressive forms of MS. Despite the wide usage of IFN-β, its specific mechanism is yet to be fully understood, though it has been associated with the inhibition of leukocyte migration, decreased inflammatory cytokines, and inhibition of T cell survival and expansion (Dhib-Jalbut & Marks, 2010). It is likely that a combination of these immunomodulatory properties is what makes IFN-β effective for some MS patients. However, a clinical study on IFN-β showed a large number of patients stopped low-dose therapy due to poor efficacy, while the most common causes of stopping high-dose therapy were adverse events, like flu-like symptoms (Ruggieri et al., 2003). Due to these drawbacks, alternative therapies are necessary for a large number of patients. GA is seen as a viable alternative to IFN-β (Vallittu et al., 2005). GA is a daily sub-cutaneous injectable that is a random sequence of four synthetic polypeptides resembling myelin protein. It is thought to be effective against MS by dampening pro-inflammatory responses in the brain, outcompeting endogenous myelin for antigen presentation by antigen presenting cells (APCs), and suppressing responses towards other myelin-associated antigens (Ziemssen & Schrempf, 2007). Though the exact mechanism has yet to be elucidated, GA has been a successful therapy for MS. Over a 5 year study, GA lowered disease progression and disability scores in approximately 70% of patients (Johnson et al., 2000). GA displays a relatively tolerable safety profile, although side-effects including chest tightness and injection site reactions are experienced by ~30% of patients, resulting in them discontinuing GA therapy (Johnson et al., 2000; Vallittu et al., 2005). Although immunomodulatory therapies for MS have shown some clinical success, IFN-β fails to provide long-term protection (Shirani et al., 2012) and a number of patients fail both IFN-β and GA therapy (Vallittu et al., 2005), necessitating the usage of other therapies. Besides IFN-β, IL-10 also plays an important role in the disease progression of MS. Both IFN-β and IL-10 are regulated by NFATc1 (nuclear factor of activated T-cells). It was observed that mice bearing NFATc1$^{-/-}$ B cells showed milder symptoms of EAE (experimental autoimmune encephalomyelitis, a mouse model for human multiple sclerosis) (Bhattacharyya et al., 2011). However, non-specific immune suppression may elicit unwanted side effects, and more research needs to be down using more clinically relevant models.

Both antibody and small molecule therapies have been used in patients that fail frontline immunomodulatory therapeutic regimens. Current antibody and small molecule therapies can inhibit MS symptoms by blocking some of the key immunological processes that lead to disease development. In healthy individuals, the blood brain barrier blocks the migration of inflammatory immune cells into the CNS (Larochelle, Alvarez, & Prat, 2011). However, individuals with MS have a breakdown in this process, allowing leukocyte infiltration, which can induce or exacerbate an inflammatory environment within the CNS. Furthermore, infiltrating lymphocytes proliferating in response to disease-associated antigens further enhance inflammatory responses. Natalizumab (Tysabri), an intravenous monoclonal antibody therapy, is successful in decreasing MS symptoms by blockade of this leukocyte infiltration process. This is accomplished through binding of α4-integrin protein on leukocytes; inhibiting binding of α4-integrin to the endothelial protein, vascular cell adhesion molecule (VCAM)-1. The binding of α4-integrin and VCAM-1 is a necessary step for extravasation of leukocytes into inflamed tissues (D.T. Selewski, 2010), thus blockade decreases the number of extravasating inflammatory cells into the CNS. While this is advantageous for MS therapy, a decrease in leukocyte activity can lead to adverse events. Although Natalizumab was FDA-approved in 2004, it was withdrawn for a 2 year period because of an association to Progressive Multifocal Leukoencephalopathy (PML), a disease with mortality rates reaching 50%. PML is a disease occurring in patients with latent John Cunningham (JC) viral infections. In these patients, Natalizumab may contribute to enhanced viral replication by decreasing infiltration of T cells into the infected areas (Perkins et al., 2012). Furthermore, systemic immune suppression can affect the clearance of other pathogens or limit the ability to destroy cancerous cells. Although Natalizumab is effective against MS, its need for intravenous administration and potential adverse events indicate it should be used only after more desirable therapies have failed.

Orally delivered small molecules like Fingolimod (GILENYA), Teriflunomide (Aubagio), and Dimethyl Fumarate (Tecfidera) are more desirable, partially because of their less invasive delivery routes. Fingolimod is a novel orally delivered small molecule that mimics sphingosine 1-phosphate. It is capable of binding to and down regulating sphingosine 1-phospate receptor1 (Chun & Hartung, 2010). The binding of this lymphocyte receptor to its ligand is a necessary step in the lymphoid egress pathway (Garris et al., 2013), thus its down regulation inhibits lymphocyte activity by inhibiting their ability to exit peripheral lymph nodes (Chun & Hartung, 2010). In addition to blocking lymphocytes from entering the CNS, limiting their proliferation has also shown to lessen MS symptoms. Teriflunomide, an orally delivered small molecule, significantly decreases T and B cell proliferation through inhibition of dihydro-orotate dehydrogenase, and subsequent inhibition of pyrimidine synthesis (Bar-Or, Pachner,

Menguy-Vacheron, Kaplan, & Wiendl, 2014). Inhibition of dihydro-orotate dehydrogenase halts cell cycle progression in G_1 phase (Ruckemann et al., 1998). Although effective at decreasing relapse rates in patients, early clinical data associates Fingolimod (Cohen & Chun, 2011) and Teriflunomide (J. Oh & O'Connor, 2014) with liver damage and an increased risk of infections. This increased risk of infection is likely due to the systemic immune suppression seen with broad-spectrum inhibition of T and B cell function. Both Fingolimod and Teriflunomide received FDA-approval within the previous 5 years, however, a more recently approved orally delivered small molecule is available. Dimethyl Fumarate (Tecfidera) was approved for use by the FDA in 2013. Little is known about the mechanism of action, but animal models have associated it with decreased T cell infiltration and an increase in anti-inflammatory cytokines (Linker & Gold, 2013). Recently, it has been suggested that Dimethyl Fumarate may function through inhibition of NF-κB leading to decreases in cytokines, as well as an inhibition of dendritic cell (DC) maturation (H. Peng et al., 2012). Although a clinical study showed Dimethyl Fumarate outperforms Teriflunomide and has similar efficacy to Fingolimod (Hutchinson et al., 2014), further research should be done on its long-term safety and efficacy profile (English & Aloi, 2015). Immunomodulatory, antibody, and small molecule therapies have all shown clinical success against MS. However, much of this success has occurred at the expense of systemic immune suppression. By limiting T and B cell function, as well as inhibiting inflammatory cytokines, therapies have left patients at risk of infections, cancers, and a number of other side-effects. Emerging therapies should be developed with the goal of decreasing disease-associated immune responses, while keeping the remainder of the immune system functioning. However, this problem is not unique to individuals with MS. Patients receiving treatment for RA and SLE face the same problems from therapy-associated immune suppression.

Rheumatoid Arthritis

RA is a chronic, inflammatory disease resulting in severely debilitating damage to synovial spaces. It is a common autoimmune disorder that affects approximately 1% of the worldwide population (Gibofsky, 2012). The disease initiates by infiltration of fibroblasts and inflammatory cells into the synovial or joint spaces in the hands and feet. This results in an over expression of IL-1 and tumor necrosis factor alpha (TNF-α) (Cunnane, Hummel, Muller-Ladner, Gay, & Gay, 1998). Destructive enzymes, such as serine proteases, matrix metalloproteinases, and the cathepsins, which leads to cartilage and bone destruction. It has been estimated that the economic impact in the United States from RA patients reaches $128 Billion annually (Centers for Disease & Prevention, 2007). The goal of traditional RA therapy is to limit the progression of inflammation and subsequent joint damage, while decreasing joint pain. The most commonly used front-line therapies for RA are oral non-steroidal anti-inflammatory drugs (NSAIDs) (e.g., aspirin, celecoxib, ibuprofen, naproxen). NSAIDs are diverse molecules with classifications based on their chemical structures. These classifications include carboxylic acids (e.g., aspirin, ibuprofen, naproxen), enolic acids, non-acids, and cyclooxygenase (COX)-2 selective inhibitors (e.g., celecoxib) (Crofford, 2013). NSAIDs decrease inflammation through targeting the enzyme COX-2, which subsequently blocks the production of prostaglandins; compounds that are critical for pathogenic inflammatory responses in RA (Ricciotti & FitzGerald, 2011). Although NSAIDs are relatively inexpensive, easy to access, and are tolerated well for short-term use, they fail to halt overall disease progression (Quan, Thiele, Tian, & Wang, 2008). In addition, side-effects for chronic NSAID use include renal, hepatic and cardiovascular problems (Crofford, 2013). An alternative frontline therapy for RA is steroids like corticosteroids (e.g., prednisone, methylprednisolone). These small molecules can be administered orally or as an injectable.

These molecules have shown to slow the progression of RA primarily by binding corticosteroid receptors, activating an intracellular signaling response that results in decreased transcription of genes involved in inflammatory cytokine production (e.g., IL-1, IL-2, TNF-α) and T cell proliferation. Like NSAIDs, steroidal therapies fail to stop long-term disease progression and their sustained dosing can result in side-effects like osteoporosis or gastrointestinal problems (Buchman, 2001). However, short-term usage of NSAIDs and steroidal therapies display excellent efficacy and safety profiles. Due to this, it has been suggested these therapies be used until a more advanced therapeutic is prescribed and becomes effective (Quan et al., 2008).

One of the more advanced classes of therapies is the disease modifying anti-rheumatic drugs (DMARDs). Although DMARDs have been shown to significantly decrease the progression of RA, they can take months to begin to be effective. For these periods, NSAIDs and steroids can provide a stop-gap therapy until efficacy occurs. While a number of DMARDs exist, the fastest acting is methotrexate (MTX) (Trexall), which is an orally delivered or injectable small molecule. MTX provides direct anti-inflammatory effects as well as decreasing inflammatory cytokines in a number of ways (Cutolo, Sulli, Pizzorni, Seriolo, & Straub, 2001). Like Teriflunomide therapy for MS, MTX is capable of decreasing pyrimidine production causing decreased proliferation of T cells. The inhibition of DNA synthesis by MTX has also been associated with an increase in purine metabolism, which subsequently results in increased levels of adenosine secretion from cells, which can limit inflammatory cytokine production (Cutolo et al., 2001). While MTX is effective in controlling RA and has been for decades, it is associated with serious adverse events, and clinical trials have reported patients on MTX are twice as likely to discontinue treatment versus controls (Lopez-Olivo et al., 2014). For these patients, other orally delivered small molecule DMARDs can be used. Leflunomide (Arava) and Sulfasalazine (Azulfidine) have long been used as therapies for RA. Interestingly, the active metabolite of Leflunomide is Teriflunomide, so inhibition of RA symptoms is through decreased T cell proliferation due to inhibition of dihydro-orotate dehydrogenase, and subsequent inhibition of pyrimidine synthesis (Fox et al., 1999). Sulfasalazine also suppresses symptoms in part by decreases in inflammatory cell proliferation. It is a prodrug that, when cleaved by gut bacteria, becomes the functional 5-aminosalicylic acid. This small molecule is capable of decreasing RA symptoms through interaction with a class of nuclear receptors that decrease proliferation, increase apoptosis (Desreumaux & Ghosh, 2006), and contributes to a decrease in inflammatory species (Couto et al., 2010). Decreasing inflammatory responses is an important part of protecting from joint destruction in RA. While these previous DMARDs primarily mediate pro-inflammatory cell inhibition, a newer option, Xeljanz, targets the Janus Kinase (JAK) signaling pathway, thus inhibiting cell signaling that can result in inflammatory cytokine production. While these therapies have worked for a number of patients with RA, a meta-analysis of studies evaluating the effects of DMARDs on RA patients shows a number of individuals withdraw therapy due to high toxicity or low efficacy (Maetzel et al., 2000). Biologics provide an alternative therapeutic option for patients who fail with DMARDs.

Recently, biologics are emerging as a highly researched class of compounds for the treatment of RA. Although biologics are not a new concept, in the past few years a large number of them have gained FDA-approval. The most common biologics for RA treatment are antibody therapies. More specifically, antibodies targeting tumor necrosis factor alpha (TNF-α) (Cimzia, Exemptia, Humira, Remicade, or Simponi) have become exceedingly popular. Of these therapies, all but Remicade are deliverable by sub-cutaneous injection (Remicade by intravenous infusion). TNF-α is a desirable target because it plays a significant role in the pathogenesis of RA, contributing to increased recruitment and proliferation of inflammatory immune cells, as well as regulating pro-inflammatory cytokines and growth factors at sites of inflammation and damage (Feldmann & Maini, 2001). Although a blockade of TNF-α has shown to effectively reduce RA symptoms and progression, TNF-α plays key role in regulating the immune response, therefore its systemic non-specific suppression is capable of causing a number of side-effects. A meta-analysis of TNF-α inhibitors indicates an increased risk of malignancies after use (Bongartz et al., 2006). In fact, the FDA has instituted black box warnings for lymphoma and increased risks of infections while taking TNF blockers. Antibodies blocking TNF-α are not the only ones effective toward treating RA. IL-6 is a potent mediator of joint destruction (Md Yusof & Emery, 2013) and has been inhibited clinically by a monoclonal antibody that blocks IL-6 from binding to the IL-6 receptor (Actemra). Additionally, Rituxin is an intravenously delivered antibody against CD20, which mediates the depletion of B cells. In RA, autoantibodies are present in approximately 60% of patients (Bax, Huizinga, & Toes, 2014) so destruction of B cell populations likely eliminates a major contributor of pathogenesis. Although a large portion of biological therapies are antibody-based, protein-based therapies have been clinically effective for RA.

One major protein-based therapeutic technology is Fc-fusion proteins. These are protein or peptide sequences fused to the Fc region of an immunoglobulin (Czajkowsky, Hu, Shao, & Pleass, 2012). Orencia is a fusion protein that functions to inhibit the progression of RA by halting T cell activation. It is formulated by fusing the Fc region of an antibody with cytotoxic T-lymphocyte associated protein 4 (CTLA4). This formulation can outcompete for binding of CD80/86 on APCs. Patients on Orencia see a normalization of inflammatory mediators, including TNF-α, out to a year from treatment (Herrero-Beaumont, Martinez Calatrava, & Castaneda, 2012). Interestingly, the first anti-TNF agent for RA was the fusion-protein therapy Enbral. Human FC regions are fused to dimeric regions of the TNF-α receptor and administered subcutaneously. Enbral is capable of binding and neutralizing circulating TNF-α through the use of the TNF-α receptor proteins on the FC region (Haraoui & Bykerk, 2007). In addition to fusion-proteins, a protein biologic is available to block an important cytokine in RA pathogenesis. Increased levels of IL-1β in patients is correlated to joint symptoms from RA pathogenesis (Kay & Calabrese, 2004). Kineret is a recombinant version of the IL-1 receptor antagonist and functions by competing with IL-1 for receptor binding. By outcompeting for this binding site, Kineret is able to decrease the pathogenesis caused by IL-1 and its downstream interactions. Although inhibition of cytokines, T cell, and B cell responses has successfully suppressed RA pathogenesis in a number of clinical settings, these therapies can result in severe side-effects. Increased risk of serious infections, as well as an increase in malignancies has been seen, likely due to the wide-suppression of immune functions. Both MS and RA are autoimmune diseases that affect specific tissues however, the wide suppression caused by therapies are evident in the fact that much of this technology can apply to a disease that affects multiple tissues.

Systemic Lupus Erythematosus

Unlike MS and RA, SLE is an autoimmune disease which mounts an immune response to a number of bodily tissues. SLE can damage an individual's brain, skin, kidneys, or joints. Although SLE can affect most tissues and organs, its mechanism of pathogenesis predominantly involves pro-inflammatory cytokines, T cells, and B cells (Mohan & Putterman, 2015). Although the exact mechanism of SLE remains elusive, the disease pathogenesis is believed to involve complicated interactions among various genetic and environmental factors such as sex, ethnicity, and hormone profiles. Defective immune regulations that lead to the loss of immune tolerance toward self-antigens contributes significantly to the development of SLE (Mok & Lau, 2003). Many of the previously described therapies have shown clinical efficacy in

SLE patients. Like therapeutic options for RA; NSAIDs, steroidal therapies, and disease-modifying drugs are established options for limiting the severity of SLE symptoms. Prednisone and methylprednisolone are two of the most common frontline therapies for SLE patients. However, efficacy is tied to high-dose therapy and recently long-term reliance on corticosteroids by SLE patients has been associated with an increased risk of organ failure (Zonana-Nacach, Barr, Magder, & Petri, 2000). The possibility of organ failure, coupled with increased risks from immunosuppression as well as decreased bone density from these therapies, have resulted in a push for dose-sparing therapeutic regimens to be developed.

One method for limiting the amount of corticosteroids administered to SLE patients is through co-therapy with another compound. Due to the ability of MTX to inhibit T cell proliferation and inflammatory cytokines, its co-delivery with steroidal therapies has been explored. However, conflicting results have been established including one study showing no overall reduction in steroid use was achieved (Kipen, Littlejohn, & Morand, 1997), while another indicates MTX co-therapy is able to reduce the number of patients on high dose steroids (Carneiro & Sato, 1999). Aside from co-therapy, the use of an alternative therapy is desirable. Due to its success as an oral small molecule DMARD for RA, Leflunomide has recently been studied as an alternative to steroid-based therapies for SLE. Leflunomide has shown to inhibit disease progression and been effective as a monotherapy, however, its association with its immunological, hepatic, and respiratory side-effects indicate further long-term studies should be performed (Wu, Xu, Huang, & Wu, 2013). Though MTX and Leflunomide are emerging alternatives to corticosteroids for the treatment of SLE, other therapies have long been used to suppress disease progression.

A small molecule that has been used for severe SLE cases is Cyclophosphamide (Cytoxan). Cyclophosphamide is an alkylating agent that causes depletion of immunological cells through inhibition of proliferation, and has been shown to be highly effective at inhibiting organ failure in patients with severe SLE (Petri, 2004). However, cyclophosphamide has severe side-effects that limit its use, including up to 50% of women on cyclophosphamide suffering from ovarian failure (Amissah-Arthur & Gordon, 2010). Predominantly, SLE patients are women so side-effects disproportionally impacting women are problematic. Other small molecule options are available for those patients with less sever SLE. Although its efficacy in severe SLE is minimal (Abu-Shakra & Shoenfeld, 2001), Azathioprine (Imuran, Azasan) is effective at slowing the progression of patients with mild SLE. Azathioprine is a small molecule that becomes incorporated into replicating DNA and blocks purine synthesis, which is likely how it inhibits broad T cell proliferation (Maltzman & Koretzky, 2003). Recently, for patients with mild to severe SLE who have failed steroidal, Cyclophosphamide, or Azathioprine treatments, Mycophenolate (CellCept) has been explored. Mycophenolate inhibits T and B cell proliferation, primarily through preferential depletion of guanosine nucleotides in T and B cells, leading to decreases in proliferation (Allison, 2005). Clinical data shows Mycophenolate is a viable small molecule alternative for patients who have failed previous therapies for SLE (Karim et al., 2002). However, patients in childbearing years should be cautious as it has been associated with increased pregnancy complications including miscarriage (Pisoni & D'Cruz, 2008). Therapies for SLE have varying efficacies, which may depend on toxicity of therapy, organs afflicted, and severity of disease. Many therapies for SLE decrease disease severity through systemic immune suppression, which in-turn can result in a number of side-effects like cancers and infections. In fact, a number of therapies with efficacy in SLE have been used for other autoimmune diseases. The ability for these treatment regimens to suppress broad immune responses is only highlighted by their efficacy across multiple tissues. Emerging therapies should be developed that inhibit tissue or disease-specific autoimmune responses while maintaining an adequate immune response towards other antigens.

Type 1 Diabetes

One autoimmune disease with a unique, although not immunomodulatory, disease-specific therapeutic regimen is T1D. T1D is a T cell mediated autoimmune disease resulting in the destruction of insulin producing pancreatic β-cells (Burn, 2010). Destruction of these insulin producing cells inhibits proper glucose storage and leads to fatal symptoms if left untreated. According to the National Institutes of Health, approximately 80 people are diagnosed in the United States daily, and the disease is reported to account for $14.9 billion in annual healthcare costs (Dall et al., 2009). The first line therapy for T1D is the administration of exogenous insulin to substitute lack of pancreatic production. Insulin administration in T1D patients is accomplished with a daily series of injections or through continuous low dose administration with a pump. Recent studies have suggested patients may respond better using an insulin pump than with sub-cutaneous injections (Atkinson, Eisenbarth, & Michels, 2014). Although insulin therapy has been critical in treatment of patients, multiple daily injections are less than ideal for patients. Unlike the other autoimmune diseases mentioned above, immunomodulatory therapies are for T1D are not clinically used. Recently, clinical studies evaluating monoclonal antibodies targeting CD3 on T cells showed initial efficacy, but ultimately failed clinical endpoints (Atkinson et al., 2014). Additionally, a CTLA-4 (Abatacept) fusion protein showed short-term efficacy in patients, though its long-term efficacy was sub-optimal (Orban et al., 2011). It is apparent that new therapies for T1D, and all other autoimmune diseases, should be developed. These therapies should not only decrease symptoms and protect from long-term disease progression, but also alter the course of disease without severe side-effects from systemic immunosuppression.

Immune Tolerance

Although many of these therapies have increased patient quality of life, and limited autoimmune severity, systemic immune suppression is a significant side-effect. Inhibition of T cell, B cell, and cytokine function can increase the risks of severe infection, certain cancers, and other adverse events. Inhibiting these auto-reactive responses in a disease specific manner may provide a way to inhibit disease-associated responses while maintaining otherwise effective immune function. Eliminating auto-reactive immune responses would more closely resemble the protective effects of a healthy immune system. Healthy individuals are able to avoid autoimmunity in part through immune tolerance; a failure to mount an inflammatory response towards antigens. This tolerance is accomplished in part by processes known as central and peripheral tolerance. Central tolerance selects against auto-reactive T cells in the thymus, and B cells in the bone marrow (Hogquist, Baldwin, & Jameson, 2005), while peripheral tolerance describes the induction of immune tolerance in areas outside the thymus or bone marrow. During central and peripheral tolerance, T cells with reactivity towards self-antigens can be deleted, made anergic, or differentiated into alternative lineages like regulatory T cells (Pacholczyk & Kern, 2008), which actively inhibit effector cell reactivity towards self-antigens. Much of these tolerance mechanisms are mediated through APCs, like DCs. Predominantly, these cellular fates are decided through signaling from DCs that have been tolerized towards self-antigens. Tolerized DCs present self-antigen to T cells, but fail to deliver co-stimulatory signals required for activation and expansion (Xing & Hogquist, 2012). Without co-stimulatory signals, T cells become unreactive towards presented self-antigen. This mechanism naturally protects against responses towards apoptotic debris from healthy tissues (Hawiger et al., 2001), as well food antigens and commensal bacteria (Faria & Weiner, 2005). Much of the peripheral tolerance induction that prevents inflammatory responses towards these antigens occurs at mucosal surfaces. By introducing self-antigens to mucosal surfaces, it may be possible to direct a tolerogenic immune response, which can alter disease-associated immune responses while leaving the remainder of the immune system functional.

Previously, antigen-specific tolerance has been accomplished through the ex-vivo manipulation of cells, as well as by introduction of antigens to mucosal surfaces. The induction of antigen-specific immune tolerance at mucosal sites has occurred through oral (Faria & Weiner, 2005) (Alpan, Bachelder, Isil, Arnheiter, & Matzinger, 2004), nasal (Maassen et al., 2003), and sublingual (Fleischer et al., 2013) delivery routes. In addition to delivering antigens to mucosal sites, ex vivo manipulation of immune cells is possible. Manipulated cells are expanded ex vivo and administration of cells has shown great promise inhibiting autoimmune responses. Ex vivo tolerogenic immune cells have been developed through a number of protocols. T cells receiving tolerogenic cytokine combinations, like Transforming Growth Factor beta (TGF-β) and IL-2, have shown to inhibit graft versus host disease and lupus animal models (Zheng et al., 2004). Tolerogenic T cells can also be created in vitro by blockade of co-stimulatory signals from co-cultured DCs (Taylor, Friedman, Korngold, Noelle, & Blazar, 2002). Although expansion of T cells is promising, alteration of APCs allows administration of a cell subset that can convert a large number of cells in vivo. Prior work has shown educated DCs can in-turn, educate multiple naïve T cell populations (Alpan et al., 2004). Additionally, Yamano et al. showed administration of bone marrow DCs expanded ex vivo with Flt3 ligand were capable of trafficking to the thymus and inducing central tolerance through clonal deletion (Yamano et al., 2011). These cells also functioned in peripheral tolerance by inducing anergy in auto-reactive populations (Yamano et al., 2011). Additional methods use peripheral tolerance mechanisms as well; specifically tolerance towards apoptotic cell debris. Taking advantage of high rates of erythrocyte apoptosis, Kontos et al. formulated antigen constructs that bind erythrocytes in vivo after intravenous administration (Kontos, Kourtis, Dane, & Hubbell, 2013). As the erythrocytes become apoptotic, they present bound auto-antigens to induce tolerance. This theory has also been tested using cells altered ex vivo. Parenteral delivery of ethylcarbodiimide (ECDI) treated splenocytes (Wang et al., 2014) or leukocytes (McCarthy, Bryant, Galvin, Miller, & Luo, 2015) coupled with autoantigens has induced immune tolerance through apoptotic clearance mechanisms. While these studies have all shown tolerance in animal models, and a recent Phase I clinical trial indicated antigen-coupled peripheral blood mononuclear cells were well tolerated (Lutterotti et al., 2013), however, the majority of antigen-specific therapy for autoimmune disease has yet to become clinically useable.

The lack of effectiveness of inducible mucosal tolerance may be occurring for a number of reasons. One possibility for this is that more than one antigen is involved in clinical autoimmunity, so identifying and selecting correct antigens may be a crucial step for tolerance induction (Krause, Blank, & Shoenfeld, 2000). Antigen dosing quantities also play a critical role in immune regulation. Prior evidence suggests that low levels of antigen provide protection through direct regulation, while high doses result in clonal anergy and deletion (Weiner, 2000). This is especially interesting in the gut mucosal environment where a large portion of antigens may be degraded or denatured prior to interaction with APCs (Weiner, 2000). When choosing an antigen, it is important to determine differences between proteins and peptides. Protein administration may mimic disease-state antigens more accurately, but peptide administration is less prone to antibody neutralization or degradation (Peakman & Dayan, 2001). In addition, these differences may impact dose scheduling which has been shown to play a significant role in tolerance induction (Saklayen, Pesce, Pollak, & Michael, 1984). Alternatively, ex vivo expansion of tolerogenic cells eliminates the potential problems with in vivo antigen delivery; however, expansion of these cells can be difficult and generally comes with considerable costs. It is necessary to find new methods for the delivery of tolerogenic therapies that can reduce cost, protect therapeutics from degradation, target immunological cells, and efficiently induce tolerogenic profiles.

BACKGROUND OF DRUG DELIVERY VEHICLES

Drug delivery using nano/microparticulate carriers could provide a solution to a number of problems with tolerance-inducing therapies. Nanoparticles are those particles under 100 nm in size, while those over 100 nm are characterized as microparticles. Particulate vehicles can increase systemic circulation times of molecules and have been shown to increase pharmacokinetics of compounds, especially within plasma (Moghimi, Hunter, & Andresen, 2012). This is important for the delivery of more hydrophobic therapeutics, which require frequent low-dose administration for effective plasma levels (Savjani, Gajjar, & Savjani, 2012). Furthermore, encapsulation of peptides and proteins can also provide protection against systemic clearance mechanisms (e.g., enzymatic degradation, acidic degradation, opsonization). This can mitigate the issues seen with protein denaturation at mucosal sites which would decrease the activity of immunotolerance. Increased circulation and enhanced protection for the encapsulated cargo can decrease the amount of drug/protein required for therapeutic levels to be met. By decreasing the dosing requirements, it is possible to limit toxicity and cost of potential therapeutic regimens. Particle-based delivery of therapies can decrease clearance of cargo and dosing requirements while increasing the chance tolerogenic compounds are delivered within an appropriate therapeutic window.

Another advantage in using particulate vehicles to modulate the immune response is their ability to passively target, and be readily taken up by APCs. Nanoparticles have been shown to interact with APCs by independently trafficking to draining lymph nodes, while microparticles were shown to be phagocytized at local sites of delivery (Manolova et al., 2008). Prior work using polymeric microparticles suggests that 2-3 μm particles are an optimal size for being phagocytized by macrophages (Champion, Walker, & Mitragotri, 2008), whereas 0.5-2 μm particles were more often associated with DCs (Manolova et al., 2008). Although, nanoparticles can be associated with APC uptake, they have also been shown to be taken up through endocytosis by alternative cell types, such as epithelial cells (N. Oh & Park, 2014). Liposomes have also shown uptake by macrophages in a size-dependent fashion. Sub-micron sized liposomes showed increased macrophage uptake with increased size, although this effect was diminished with liposomes greater than 1 μm in size (Chono, Tanino, Seki, & Morimoto, 2007). Although size plays a role in the passive targeting and subsequent uptake of particles by APCs, it is not the only factor that may impact particulate fate in vivo.

Previous studies have suggested particles formulated from more hydrophobic materials have a preferential uptake compared to those formulated with hydrophilic materials (Chen, Langer, & Edwards, 1997; Tabata & Ikada, 1988). Furthermore, particulate shape and orientation relative to the macrophage may also determine if vehicles are phagocytized by macrophages (Champion & Mitragotri, 2006). Uptake by APCs at local sites, and in the lymph nodes, provides a mechanism for efficient delivery of tolerogenic compounds to the sites and cells necessary for tolerance induction. While particulate-based carriers provide a number of advantages for tolerance delivery, there are many types and formulation methods which should be explored.

Particulate drug delivery vehicles have been formulated using a number of materials including polymers, lipids, and inorganics. Inorganic particulate vehicles, like those formulated from iron oxide or gold, have long been studied for drug delivery. Iron oxide nanoparticles can be formulated through multiple methods that enable low-cost production of large quantities and have uniform morphology (Gupta & Gupta, 2005). Iron oxide nanoparticles have been extensively studied and the technology has current approved clinical uses for imaging (Feridex, Feraheme). Similarly, gold nanoparticles (Figure 1) have been used for in vivo imaging, as well as the diagnosis and treatment of disease (Dreaden, Austin, Mackey, & El-Sayed, 2012). Treatment of disease has been accomplished through chemically binding therapeutics to nanoparticle surfaces. Therapies and imaging using gold nanoparticles to treat head/neck cancer (AuroLase, Aurimmune) and solid tumors (Auritol) are currently in clinical trials (Dobrovolskaia & McNeil, 2007). Although much research has been done on these technologies, iron oxide and gold nanoparticles are not biodegradable and can remain in tissues. Due to this, polymeric particles for drug delivery are a very popular alternative.

Polymeric particles (Figure 1) have long been used for drug delivery purposes. Some of the most common particle formulation methods are oil-in-water (O/W) or water-in-oil-in-water (W/O/W) emulsification by processes such as homogenization, probe sonication, nanoprecipitation, solvent displacement (Anton, Benoit, & Saulnier, 2008), or electrohydrodynamic spraying (Duong et al., 2013). These

Figure 1. Examples of gold nanoparticle, polymeric microparticle, or a liposome for delivery of tolerogenic cargo. The right panel shows a gold nanoparticle cartoon depicting the cargo on the surface only with a transmission electron micrograph (TEM) of a gold nanoparticle used for tolerance by Yeste et al. (Yeste, Nadeau, Burns, Weiner, & Quintana, 2012). This TEM is re-printed with permissions from PNAS. The center panel depicts potential cargo locations using polymeric delivery vehicles with a scanning electron micrograph of microparticles formulated by homogenization. The right panel shows a liposome where cargo is incorporated into the core. This is accompanied by a TEM of liposomal delivery vehicles.

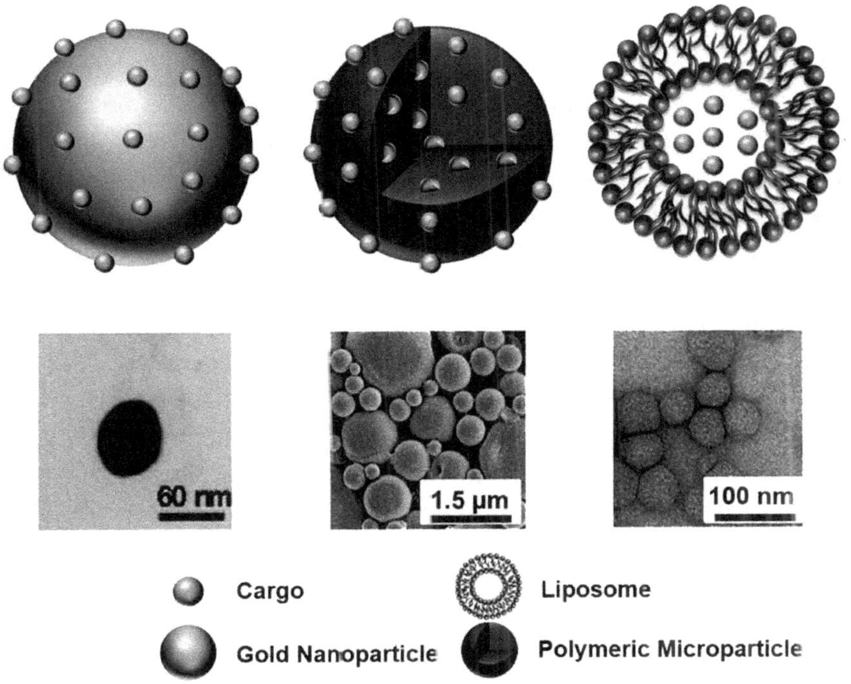

techniques provide a way to encapsulate both hydrophobic and hydrophilic cargo. Much of this work has been performed using polyesters, such as poly(lactic-*co*-glycolic acid) (PLGA), poly-L-lactic acid (PLA) and polycaprolactone (PCL). Polyesters are advantageous because they have FDA-approval for many uses (e.g. sutures and drug delivery), are biodegradable (degradation is on the order of months to years (Labet & Thielemans, 2009; Lu et al., 2000)), and have low toxicity. However, using high concentrations of polyesters, coupled with sustained degradation, can cause accumulation of byproducts. These byproducts are capable of lowering local pH (Lu et al., 2000), which could cause tissue damage or detrimentally alter acid-sensitive cargo (e.g. proteins). In addition to polyesters, polyanhydrides (e.g. sebacic acid, p-(carboxyphenoxy)propane, or p-(carboxyphenoxy)hexane) degrade, are biodegradable, and have been used clinically (e.g., Gliadel). However, polyanhydrides are hydrolytically unstable (Vilar, Tulla-Puche, & Albericio, 2012) and are non-degradable at low pH. Due to the low pH of intracellular phagolysosomes of APCs, Keselowsky et al. have suggested pH-sensitive polymers could provide a number of benefits for delivery of autoimmune therapies (Keselowsky, Xia, & Clare-Salzler, 2011). Unlike polyesters and polyanhydrides, a novel polymer capable of degrading at acidic pH conditions and not producing acidic byproducts is acetalated dextran (Ac-DEX). Ac-DEX is formed by replacing the hydroxyl groups on dextran, a polysaccharide of glucose, with acetal groups (Bachelder et al., 2008). Ac-DEX has a favorable tunable degradation profile and is biocompatible. Other polymer-based therapeutics have been FDA-approved for the treatment of MS (glatiramer acetate; Copaxone) and RA (certolizumab pegol; CIMZIA). Although these therapies are not nano/microparticles, they highlight the increasing interest and potential of polymers for the treatment of autoimmune diseases.

Liposomes (Figure 1), which are composed of a phospholipid bilayer, are another particulate vehicle used for drug delivery. Primarily, manufacturing is done through batch processes using lipid-film hydration, solvent vaporization, or ethanol injection. Like polymeric particles, liposomes have the ability to encapsulate both hydrophobic and hydrophilic cargo. Hydrophobic compounds placed in the lipid phase, or hydrophilic compounds placed within the aqueous buffer, are readily encapsulated within the vesicles. Liposomes are biodegradable and have tolerable degradation products however, a number of issues do exist. Batch processes can increase costs and yield variable particle heterogeneity. To alleviate this, many methods utilize extrusion through membranes to make more homogenous populations (Laouini, Charcosset, Fessi, Holdich, & Vladisavljevic, 2013). Due to drug leaking and particle aggregation, liposomes can also have poor shelf lives (Nounou, El-Khordagui, & Khalafallah, 2005). Despite these drawbacks, a number of liposomal formulations encapsulating therapeutics for cancer (Doxil, Myocet), infectious diseases (AmBisome), and other formulations containing inactivated hepatitis A virus (Epaxal) and inactivated influenza hemaglutinine (Inflexal V) are being used in clinics (Chang & Yeh, 2012). The approval of these formulations highlights the long-term success and potential of this delivery method.

Particulate formulation using inorganic, polymer, or lipid constituents provides a novel method for delivery of tolerizing therapies. These technologies provide protection for sensitive proteins and peptides, as well as increase the circulation time for cargo. In addition, particulate vehicles passively target DCs, which provides a unique mechanism for directing tolerogenic processes. Due to the many advantages seen with nano/microparticulate vehicles, researchers have begun to explore particulate delivery vehicles for the treatment of autoimmune disorders.

NANO/MICROPARTICLES FOR THE TREATMENT OF AUTOIMMUNITY

Current Research in the Field

The most widely used model to study nano/microparticle therapy for autoimmunity is experimental autoimmune encephalomyelitis (EAE). This is an animal model of MS, and can be induced through a number of mechanisms. EAE severity can be measured through assignment of a clinical score, where 0 is a healthy animal and 5 is suffering from full paralysis. Two commonly used methods of induction are immunization against Myelin Basic Protein (MBP) or Myelin Oligodendrocyte Glycoprotein (MOG). MBP is the second most prevalent protein within the CNS and is responsible for efficient signaling along axons (Boggs, 2006), while MOG is less abundant, but is thought to play a significant role in the immune response towards myelin (Reindl, Di Pauli, Rostasy, & Berger, 2013). Immunization of C57Bl/6 mice with either MBP or MOG creates a well characterized form of EAE that has chronic progressive pathogenesis (Miller & Karpus, 2007). The immune response seen in these animals is overwhelmingly antigen specific, therefore making it an excellent model to study antigen specific tolerance. Induction of EAE in Swiss Jim Lambert (SJL) mice, most commonly through immunization with Proteolipid Protein (PLP), results in a relapsing and remitting form of EAE (rr-EAE). PLP is the majority constituent of myelin and the pathogenesis of EAE in SJL mice immunized with PLP is T cell mediated and can influence auto-reactive responses towards multiple antigens (Miller & Karpus, 2007). The SJL rr-EAE model is more closely related to clinical MS manifestations. These mouse models provide well established antigen-specific disease models for which to examine tolerance inductions through the use of particulate carriers.

As a particulate carrier to treat an EAE model, Yeste et al. first used gold nanoparticles to co-deliver MOG with 2-(1'H-indole-3'-carbonyl)-thiazole-4-carboxylic acid methyl ester (ITE), a small mucosal ligand shown to induce anti-inflammatory cytokines and expand FOXp3+ T cells (Figure 1) (Yeste et al., 2012). Gold nanoparticles (60nm) functionalized with surface bound ITE and MOG (MOG/ITE/NPs) were stabilized by a single layer of thiol-polyethylene glycol (thiol-PEG). Initial in vitro studies of MOG/ITE/NPs showed they significantly reduced inflammatory cytokine production and increased FOXp3+ expression in MOG-specific T cells. When MOG/ITE/NPs were administered intra-peritoneally, at the time of disease immunization, they significantly inhibited disease onset. The mechanism, determined by in vitro studies, was supported by the disease model. Mice treated with MOG/ITE/NPs showed decreased levels of IFN-γ and IL-17, as well as increased FOXp3+ T cells. The role of CD4+ FoxP3+ Tregs was confirmed when mice were protected from EAE after receiving T cells isolated from MOG/ITE/NPs treated mice. Furthermore, these nanoparticles lowered the clinical score in SJL mice when administered after symptom onset. The gold nanoparticles used by Yeste et al. provide for a potential antigen-specific therapy that can decrease established symptoms and slow the progression of MS.

Previous work has examined tolerance induction through intravenous delivery of ECDI treated splenocytes (Wang et al., 2014) and leukocytes (McCarthy et al., 2015) coupled with autoantigens. One major drawback to this method of therapy is the difficult and often expensive process of ex vivo modification of cells. Expanding on this clinically relevant research, Getts et al. investigated the ability of antigen-decorated polystyrene beads (PSB) to mimic the effects of ex vivo antigen conjugated cells (Getts et al., 2012). Here, 500 nm PSBs were carboxylated and coupled with $PLP_{139\text{-}151}$ (PLP/PSBs). When administered intravenously, PLP/PSBs protected SJL mice from EAE onset. Mice treated with

PLP/PSBs showed a broad inactivation of myelin-specific CD4+ T cells, as well as decreased leukocyte infiltration into the CNS. Coinciding with Yeste et al., cells treated with PLP/PSBs showed decreased proliferation and production of inflammatory cytokines (IFN-γ and IL-17). However, treatment coupled with CD25-antibody treatment only partially blocked induction of tolerance, suggesting $FOXp3^+$ cells may only play a limited role in this system. Other possible T cell mediate roles are the induction of T cell anergy or T cell deletion. Interestingly, disease inhibition and tolerance induction seemed to be mediated through the splenic marginal zone macrophage receptor with collagenous structure (MARCO). PLP/PSBs co-localized with this subset of macrophages, which are partially responsible for tolerance towards apoptotic proteins (McGaha, Chen, Ravishankar, van Rooijen, & Karlsson, 2011). This result indicates that nano/microparticle delivery has the potential to take the place of expensive and complicated ex vivo therapies.

Although effective, using MOG/ITE/NPs and PLP/PSBs to treat EAE should be improved upon. Both gold nanoparticles and PSBs are biocompatible however; they are not biodegradable and could pose long-term toxicity issues. With this in mind, Hunter et al. used antigen-conjugated PLGA microparticles for both prophylactic and therapeutic treatment of rr-EAE (Hunter et al., 2014). Microparticles were 500 nm in size and coupled with PLP (PLGA-PLP/MPs) at higher efficiencies than commercially available PSBs. When PLGA-PLP/MPs were administered intravenously, they were capable of delaying disease onset and ameliorating symptoms of established EAE. Moreover, PLGA-PLP/MPs treated naïve SJL mice showed enhanced protection after adoptive transfer of auto-reactive T cells and particulate treated mice showed limited demyelination and reduced inflammatory immune cell infiltration into the CNS. Like the previous two studies, protection was at least partially mediated through a decrease in IFN-γ and IL-17. Studies looking at antigen-decorated microparticles administered intravenously show promising results. One drawback to this work is intravenous administration is less desirable compared with subcutaneous delivery, as subcutaneous can be patient administered and intravenous usually requires a medical professional. Unlike Yeste et al., the work done by Getts et al. and Hunter et al. did not use a small molecule known to inhibit APC signaling. Further work looking at subcutaneous delivery methods, and formulations using immunomodulatory drugs would provide more insight into the feasibility of this technology.

This was accomplished in part by Maldonado et al. who formulated PLGA nanoparticles encapsulating rapamycin, a small molecule known to inhibit co-stimulatory signals, and PLP (Rapa/PLP/NPs) (Maldonado et al., 2015). Although the effective delivery route seems to be intravenously for these vehicles, treatment with Rapa/PLP/MPs were able to prophylactically limit clinical scores in rr-EAE mice and intravenous administration ameliorated clinical scores and decreased relapse rates in a therapeutic fashion. Cappellano et al. also formulated 200 nm PLGA microparticles encapsulating MOG and the anti-inflammatory cytokine IL-10 (IL-10/MOG/MPs) (Cappellano et al., 2014). Subcutaneous administered significantly inhibited EAE development in a prophylactic fashion while concomitantly decreasing histopathological lesions in the spinal cord. Like the previous work, these mice showed lower levels of pro-inflammatory cytokines which corresponded with protection from EAE. As was previously discussed, high concentrations of polyesters, coupled with long degradation rates can cause accumulation of acidic byproducts (Lu et al., 2000). Sensitive cargo can be adversely impacted by this environment, and long degradation rates could lead to less optimal delivery of encapsulates (Broaders, Cohen, Beaudette, Bachelder, & Frechet, 2009). Evidence of this may be seen in Bryant et al. who previously showed that donor apoptotic splenocytes could induce long-term donor-specific tolerance to islet allografts, but donor antigen-coupled PLGA microparticles (PLGA-dAg) were sub-optimal compared with splenocytes (Bryant et al., 2014). It is important to explore alternative delivery formulations that could alleviate these issues.

One polymer that could enhance the field of tolerance therapies is Ac-DEX. Ac-DEX is a novel biocompatible and biodegradable polymer with pH neutral byproducts. This polymer is also highly tunable, providing enhanced controlled release of therapeutics. Peine et al. used Ac-DEX to encapsulated MOG and dexamethasone (DXM), another small molecule known to inhibit co-stimulatory signals (Peine et al., 2014). These microparticles (DXM/MOG/MPs) not only contained a tolerogenic compound with an antigen, but were also subcutaneously administered, 3 days after symptom onset, and significantly decreased the clinical score in the chronic progressive C57Bl/6 model. Here, EAE is induced through immunization with Complete Fruend's Adjuvant and MOG peptide, resulting in a mouse model characterized by a high degree of inflammation and high clinical scores. These mice went from an average clinical score of 3.4 to a clinical score of 1.6 after 3 injections. Interestingly, DXM/MOG/MPs significantly decreased clinical scores compared with microparticles encapsulating MOG only, suggesting the role of an immunomodulator is important. Antigen recall assays showed significantly lower levels of IL-17 and GM-CSF in mice treated with DXM/MOG/MPs. Although cytokine data corresponded with other EAE studies, there was no indication that FOXp3$^+$ T cells had an impact on treatment of mice with EAE.

Although most of the current work using particulate vehicles has been performed on EAE models, other autoimmune models provide useful systems to explore the use of nano/microparticles. In RA, T cells and autoantibodies within the synovial space have been implicated in pathogenesis. A number of animal models exist to study RA, including the collagen-induced arthritis (CIA) model, which is induced by immunization towards collagen in a similar fashion as EAE. This model mimics clinical disease through breaking tolerance to endogenous collagen, as well as the development of autoantibodies (Asquith, Miller, McInnes, & Liew, 2009). Although this model is considered the gold-standard for modeling RA, immunization with methylated bovine serum albumin (mBSA) followed by an intra-articular mBSA challenge is also widely used. This model is useful because it allows for extensive studies of T cell mediated responses in the synovial fluid. Capini et al. studied induction of immune tolerance using liposomal vehicles for therapy on the mBSA mouse model (Capini et al., 2009). Here, liposomes encapsulating mBSA and a lipophilic NF-κB inhibitor (curcumin, quercetin, or Bay11-7082) were tested against mice challenged with mBSA-induced inflammatory arthritis. The egg phosphatidylcholine liposomes (400 nm) were prepared by lipid film hydration and delivered by subcutaneous injection. This therapy ameliorated symptoms and lowered disease scores, likely due to the induction of antigen-specific regulatory CD4+ T cells. Liposomes encapsulating antigen and curcumin lowered antigen-specific T cell proliferation, reduced levels of IL-2, TNF, and IFN-γ, and increased secretion of IL-10 in the draining lymph nodes. There was an expanded population of antigen-specific FoxP3+ CD4+ regulatory T cells in the draining lymph nodes in response to the treatment. Therefore, Capini suggested that liposomes, loaded with an antigen and a NF-κB inhibitor, could induce antigen-specific tolerance by inducing development and expansion of FoxP3+ CD4+ Tregs, as well as inhibiting inflammatory cytokines. Particulate platforms have been effective here, and for EAE however, work is also being done to evaluate this technology for rarer diseases.

Another serious but rare, autoimmune disorder is Acquired Hemophilia A (AHA). Here, antibodies are formed against coagulation factor VIII (factor 8). Factor 8 is a necessary protein involved in clotting of blood. In patients with no history of blood disorders, auto-antibodies can form towards factor 8. In addition, hemophiliacs receiving replacement protein therapy may develop inhibitory antibodies towards their therapy (Zhang, Skupsky, & Scott, 2009). Maldonado et al. demonstrated the efficacy PLGA nanoparticles as a delivery platform to treat AHA (Maldonado et al., 2015). Here, inhibition of autoantibodies was accomplished through co-therapy with factor 8 and factor 8/rapamycin loaded PLGA nanoparticles. The AHA model is advantageous because the disease-specific antigen is more clearly defined. This work, and the work previously discussed using EAE and RA models, provides a number of methods to achieve antigen-specific disease suppression. Limiting disease severity in these models provides a framework for new technologies to treat autoimmune diseases. Although these animal models are well established and useful, they are inducible models and may not fully represent the complexity of spontaneous disease onset.

The Non-Obese Diabetic (NOD) model, which provides for reliable spontaneous disease onset mediated mostly by T cell infiltration, is the most common model used to research T1D. T1D is a T cell mediated autoimmune disease destroying insulin producing pancreatic β-cells. Along with the NOD model, T1D is studied using viral-mediated, adoptive transfer, and transgenic models (Van Belle, Taylor, & von Herrath, 2009). NOD models are commonly used because of the spontaneous onset of disease, and the high number of antigens involved in pathogenesis. Importantly, this can mimic clinical T1D and require correct antigen choice for therapies. These antigens include common diabetic-associated proteins like insulin or glutamic decarboxylase (GAD), as well as auto-reactive CD8+ T cells recognizing mimetopes relevant to human disease (Khadra, Tsai, Santamaria, & Edelstein-Keshet, 2010). Among these mimetopes is NRP-V7, which Tsai et al. coupled with MHC (NRP-V7-K^d) and coated on ~100 nm superparamagnetic iron oxide nanoparticles (NRP/NPs) (Tsai et al., 2010). NRP/NPs administered intravenously slowed NOD progression and restored normoglycemia. Recently, NOD-scid mice (lacking T and B cells) have been shown to be able to be populated with human haematolymphoid transplant. This transplant allows the study of human immune responses in an animal model. Tsai et al. utilized humanized NOD mice, treating them with the relevant antigen-coated iron oxide nanoparticles ($hIGRP_{265\text{-}273}$ and insulin $B_{10\text{-}18}$ peptide). These nanoparticles were effective at restoring normoglycemia and increasing the number of regulatory CD8+ T cells. These cells displayed a memory-like phenotype. Tsai et al. also saw fewer numbers of CD11c+ dendritic cells, suggesting the particulate treatment could have altered APC populations. The work by Tsai et al. not only alters the immune profile and disease progression in a spontaneous model of autoimmunity, it also shows a particulate platform is capable of altering the immune response in humanized mice. Utilization of these mice provides enhanced evidence that these therapeutic platforms may be translated into clinically useable therapies.

The use of nano/microparticulate therapy for autoimmune disorders is a new and emerging field. To date, researchers have successfully utilized particulate technologies to alter immune responses in an antigen-specific manner. Alteration of these responses has led to protection against disease in animal models of MS, RA, AHA and T1D. The previously discussed work suggests protective effects by many formulations and delivery routes, across multiple disease models (Table 1). Much of the evidence points to protection stemming from a combination of decreased inflammatory cytokines and expansion of regulatory and tolerized cell populations. Though, there is some disparity between mechanisms in this work. Although the preliminary work looks promising, more work needs be done to progress the field into clinical relevance.

Table 1. Details of publications using particulate carriers for immune tolerance therapies for the treatment of autoimmune diseases.

Particulate Formulation	Approximate Size (nm)	Antigen	Tolerogenic Compound	Disease	Reference
Gold Conjugated	60	Myelin Oligodendrocyte Glycoprotein	ITE Sequence	Multiple Sclerosis	Yeste A. et al., 2012
Polystyrene Beads	500	Proteolipid Protein or Myelin Oligodendrocyte Glycoprotein	n/a	Multiple Sclerosis	Getts DR. et al., 2012
PLG Conjugated	400-500	Proteolipid Protein	n/a	Multiple Sclerosis	Hunter Z. et al., 2014
PLGA Bulk Encapsulated	500	Proteolipid Protein	Rapamycin	Multiple Sclerosis	Maldonado RA. et al., 2014
Ac-DEX Bulk Encapsulated	200	Myelin Oligodendrocyte Glycoprotein	Dexamethasone	Multiple Sclerosis	Peine KJ. et al., 2014
PLGA Bulk Encapsulated	200	Myelin Oligodendrocyte Glycoprotein	rIL-10	Multiple Sclerosis	Cappellano G. et al., 2014
PLGA Bulk Encapsulated	500	Factor VIII	Rapamycin	Acquired Hemophilia A	Maldonado RA. et al., 2014
Iron Oxide Absorbed	100	NRP-V7, hIGRP, or Insulin B10 Peptide	n/a	Type 1 Diabetes	Tsai S. et al., 2010
Liposome	400	Methylated Bovine Serum Albumin	Curcumin, Quercetin, or Bay 11-7082	Antigen-Induced Arthritis	Capini C. et al., 2009
PLG Conjugated	450	Donor Antigen	Rapamycin	Transplant	Bryant J. et al., 2014

FUTURE CHALLENGES AND RECOMMENDATIONS

The autoimmune disorders discussed above are the most prevalent, but the NIH estimates over 80 diseases are caused by the immune system responding to self-antigens. Inflammatory reactions towards healthy tissues can have devastating effects on patients and their quality of life. Current therapies aim to alleviate symptoms of autoimmunity through systemic immune suppression, but this can result in a number of adverse events for patients. Therapeutics for disease-specific suppression is one method that could limit the prevalence of these adverse events. Much work has been done to introduce tolerance therapy into the clinics, however many of these technologies have failed. While delivery of these therapies in particulate vehicles solves many problems seen with tolerance induction, a number of issues should still be addressed.

Incorrect identification of primary disease causing antigens may account for a number of failures seen clinically with tolerance therapies (Krause et al., 2000). While particulate vehicles can increase solubility and deliverability of cargo, they will only function if the correct antigens are selected. Delivering MOG, MBP, or PLP has become a mainstay for research into antigen-specific tolerance for MS. On the other hand, alternative peptides have shown to ameliorate symptoms in animal models induced with multiple myelin antigens (Nicholson, Murtaza, Hafler, Sette, & Kuchroo, 1997). Suppression of an antigen-specific response by an alternative antigen is likely caused through bystander effect, where the anti-inflammatory effect of some cells will alter the phenotype of neighboring cells. Further work should be done to identify key peptides for therapies that have cross-reactivity over multiple antigens. Additionally, autoimmune disorders like MS are localized in specific tissue subsets, while diseases like SLE can have systemic reactivity. Auto-reactivity in SLE has been associated with antigens from self-DNA and nucleosomes, as well as possible foreign pathogen implications. It is vital that research is done to identify crucial antigens for all autoimmune diseases. Enhancing the understanding of antigens involved with autoimmune diseases will lead to the development of better antigen-specific therapies.

While identifying antigens to deliver is important, so too is determining ideal particulate vehicles. While gold and iron oxide nanoparticles showed efficacy in treating autoimmune models, their lack of biodegradability could cause long-term toxicity. Similarly, vehicles with biodegradable properties may degrade at inopportune times, missing optimal delivery windows for cargo. Further work should be done to identify which particulate vehicle has the potential to give tunable release of cargo, while maintaining a reasonable safety profile. Furthermore, previous work using particulate carriers for the treatment of autoimmunity has been performed with protein adsorbed or conjugated to the particle surface, as well as bulk encapsulated within the particle. More research should be done to determine whether or not surface presentation of proteins can alter therapeutic efficacy. Adsorbing proteins to the surface of particles, as well as the interaction of proteins with biological environments, can lead to denaturation while bulk encapsulation provides protection from this (Di Marco et al., 2010). Identifying how denaturation of proteins affects tolerance will provide necessary knowledge to determine which formulation may work. In fact, Peng et al. have suggested that oral tolerance may be abrogated after heat (H. J. Peng, Chang, Tsai, et al., 1998) or chemical (H. J. Peng, Chang, Lin, Han, & Chang, 1998) denaturation. Alternatively, surface bound proteins can increase circulation times and decrease aggregation of particulate carriers within the blood stream. Therefore, surface-bound proteins could benefit intravenous particle delivery (Di Marco et al., 2010). With changes to particulate carriers altering therapeutic efficacy, it is necessary to also examine the effect of particle size and route of delivery on the protective ability of particles.

The prior work on tolerance induction using particulate carriers has been performed using a variety of particle sizes and delivery routes. Yeste et al. accomplished tolerance induction in EAE through injection of antigen-decorated 60 nm nanoparticles injected intraperitoneally, while Getts et al. accomplished this using 500 nm antigen-decorated polymer microparticles intravenously. A great deal of previous work indicates that size and delivery method of particulate vehicles has a significant effect on tissue distribution and clearance rates (Longmire, Choyke, & Kobayashi, 2008). When determining delivery methods, it is also important to take patient quality of life under consideration. Therapies developed with clinical restraints in mind will allow for expeditious translation to marketable therapeutics. While oral delivery is the ideal delivery method, subcutaneous administration is preferable over intravenous delivery. In addition to clinical preferences in delivery methods, the timing of delivery should also be taken under consideration.

Although models like EAE have been vital for drug discovery, administration of these emerging therapeutics should be done with clinically relevant time points in mind. Vesterinen et al. have provided a meta-analysis of EAE papers and shown as low as 30% of studies treat after disease induction, and as little as 5% of studies administer therapeutics after two weeks post-induction (Vesterinen et al., 2010). Diagnosis of MS prior to symptom onset is not yet possible. Therefore, experiments looking into particulate therapies should be performed after onset of EAE. Additionally, much of the current work examines the protective effect of induced FOXp3+ T cells after particulate administration, however much of this work has examined expansions of these cells after prophylactic administration. Inflammation and immune signaling are altered during disease states, so mechanisms of therapeutic protection should be performed in models already afflicted with symptoms. To date, researchers have not provided adequate mechanisms of protection, so it is imperative that further research is done to elucidate a mechanism of protection seen with particulate-based tolerance therapies.

CONCLUSION

Autoimmune disorders are the result of a breakdown in immune tolerance towards self-tissues. Therapies suppressing the immune system have been clinically effective, but the development of therapeutics specifically targeting disease-causing cells provides a more ideal method of treatment. Recent work has utilized organic, inorganic, or lipid-based particles to deliver therapeutics allowing immune suppression in an antigen specific response. This research has shown promising results in well characterized animal models. While this work has shown promise, it is still and emerging field and requires further research. Future work optimizing particle formulation, delivery routes, and elucidating mechanisms will provide much needed data to move forward into clinical settings. A number of particulate-based therapeutics have been FDA-approved for use in recent years and with the proper research and investment, particulate-based therapeutics will soon emerge as a powerful tool to combat autoimmune diseases.

REFERENCES

Abu-Shakra, M., & Shoenfeld, Y. (2001). Azathioprine therapy for patients with systemic lupus erythematosus. *Lupus*, *10*(3), 152–153. doi:10.1191/096120301676669495 PMID:11315344

Adelman, G., Rane, S. G., & Villa, K. F. (2013). The cost burden of multiple sclerosis in the United States: A systematic review of the literature. *Journal of Medical Economics*, *16*(5), 639–647. doi:10.3111/13696998.2013.778268 PMID:23425293

Allison, A. C. (2005). Mechanisms of action of mycophenolate mofetil. *Lupus*, *14*(Suppl 1), s2–s8. doi:10.1177/096120330501400102 PMID:15803924

Alpan, O., Bachelder, E., Isil, E., Arnheiter, H., & Matzinger, P. (2004). 'Educated' dendritic cells act as messengers from memory to naive T helper cells. *Nature Immunology*, *5*(6), 615–622. doi:10.1038/ni1077 PMID:15156140

Amissah-Arthur, M. B., & Gordon, C. (2010). Contemporary treatment of systemic lupus erythematosus: An update for clinicians. *Ther Adv Chronic Dis*, *1*(4), 163–175. doi:10.1177/2040622310380100 PMID:23251736

Anton, N., Benoit, J. P., & Saulnier, P. (2008). Design and production of nanoparticles formulated from nano-emulsion templates-a review. *Journal of Controlled Release*, *128*(3), 185–199. doi:10.1016/j.jconrel.2008.02.007 PMID:18374443

Asquith, D. L., Miller, A. M., McInnes, I. B., & Liew, F. Y. (2009). Animal models of rheumatoid arthritis. *European Journal of Immunology*, *39*(8), 2040–2044. doi:10.1002/eji.200939578 PMID:19672892

Atkinson, M. A., Eisenbarth, G. S., & Michels, A. W. (2014). Type 1 diabetes. *Lancet*, *383*(9911), 69–82. doi:10.1016/S0140-6736(13)60591-7 PMID:23890997

Bachelder, E. M., Beaudette, T. T., Broaders, K. E., Paramonov, S. E., Dashe, J., & Frechet, J. M. (2008). Acid-degradable polyurethane particles for protein-based vaccines: Biological evaluation and in vitro analysis of particle degradation products. *Molecular Pharmaceutics*, *5*(5), 876–884. doi:10.1021/mp800068x PMID:18710254

Bar-Or, A., Pachner, A., Menguy-Vacheron, F., Kaplan, J., & Wiendl, H. (2014). Teriflunomide and its mechanism of action in multiple sclerosis. *Drugs*, *74*(6), 659–674. doi:10.1007/s40265-014-0212-x PMID:24740824

Bax, M., Huizinga, T. W., & Toes, R. E. (2014). The pathogenic potential of autoreactive antibodies in rheumatoid arthritis. *Seminars in Immunopathology*, *36*(3), 313–325. doi:10.1007/s00281-014-0429-5 PMID:24763532

Bhattacharyya, S., Deb, J., Patra, A. K., Thuy Pham, D. A., Chen, W., Vaeth, M., & Serfling, E. et al. (2011). NFATc1 affects mouse splenic B cell function by controlling the calcineurin--NFAT signaling network. *The Journal of Experimental Medicine*, *208*(4), 823–839. doi:10.1084/jem.20100945 PMID:21464221

Boggs, J. M. (2006). Myelin basic protein: A multifunctional protein. *Cellular and Molecular Life Sciences*, *63*(17), 1945–1961. doi:10.1007/s00018-006-6094-7 PMID:16794783

Bongartz, T., Sutton, A. J., Sweeting, M. J., Buchan, I., Matteson, E. L., & Montori, V. (2006). Anti-TNF antibody therapy in rheumatoid arthritis and the risk of serious infections and malignancies: Systematic review and meta-analysis of rare harmful effects in randomized controlled trials. *Journal of the American Medical Association*, *295*(19), 2275–2285. doi:10.1001/jama.295.19.2275 PMID:16705109

Broaders, K. E., Cohen, J. A., Beaudette, T. T., Bachelder, E. M., & Frechet, J. M. (2009). Acetalated dextran is a chemically and biologically tunable material for particulate immunotherapy. *Proceedings of the National Academy of Sciences of the United States of America*, *106*(14), 5497–5502. doi:10.1073/pnas.0901592106 PMID:19321415

Bryant, J., Hlavaty, K. A., Zhang, X., Yap, W. T., Zhang, L., Shea, L. D., & Luo, X. (2014). Nanoparticle delivery of donor antigens for transplant tolerance in allogeneic islet transplantation. *Biomaterials*, *35*(31), 8887–8894. doi:10.1016/j.biomaterials.2014.06.044 PMID:25066477

Buchman, A. L. (2001). Side effects of corticosteroid therapy. *Journal of Clinical Gastroenterology*, *33*(4), 289–294. doi:10.1097/00004836-200110000-00006 PMID:11588541

Burn, P. (2010). Type 1 diabetes. *Nature Reviews. Drug Discovery*, *9*(3), 187–188. doi:10.1038/nrd3097 PMID:20190784

Capini, C., Jaturanpinyo, M., Chang, H. I., Mutalik, S., McNally, A., Street, S., & Thomas, R. et al. (2009). Antigen-specific suppression of inflammatory arthritis using liposomes. *Journal of Immunology (Baltimore, MD.: 1950)*, *182*(6), 3556–3565. doi:10.4049/jimmunol.0802972 PMID:19265134

Cappellano, G., Woldetsadik, A. D., Orilieri, E., Shivakumar, Y., Rizzi, M., Carniato, F., & Dianzani, U. et al. (2014). Subcutaneous inverse vaccination with PLGA particles loaded with a MOG peptide and IL-10 decreases the severity of experimental autoimmune encephalomyelitis. *Vaccine*, *32*(43), 5681–5689. doi:10.1016/j.vaccine.2014.08.016 PMID:25149432

Carneiro, J. R., & Sato, E. I. (1999). Double blind, randomized, placebo controlled clinical trial of methotrexate in systemic lupus erythematosus. *The Journal of Rheumatology*, *26*(6), 1275–1279. PMID:10381042

Centers for Disease Control & Prevention. (2007). National and state medical expenditures and lost earnings attributable to arthritis and other rheumatic conditions--United States, 2003. *MMWR. Morbidity and Mortality Weekly Report*, *56*(1), 4–7. PMID:17218935

Champion, J. A., & Mitragotri, S. (2006). Role of target geometry in phagocytosis. *Proceedings of the National Academy of Sciences of the United States of America*, *103*(13), 4930–4934. doi:10.1073/pnas.0600997103 PMID:16549762

Champion, J. A., Walker, A., & Mitragotri, S. (2008). Role of particle size in phagocytosis of polymeric microspheres. *Pharmaceutical Research*, *25*(8), 1815–1821. doi:10.1007/s11095-008-9562-y PMID:18373181

Chang, H. I., & Yeh, M. K. (2012). Clinical development of liposome-based drugs: Formulation, characterization, and therapeutic efficacy. *International Journal of Nanomedicine*, *7*, 49–60. doi:10.2147/IJN.S26766 PMID:22275822

Chen, H., Langer, R., & Edwards, D. A. (1997). A Film Tension Theory of Phagocytosis. *Journal of Colloid and Interface Science*, *190*(1), 118–133. doi:10.1006/jcis.1997.4865 PMID:9241149

Chono, S., Tanino, T., Seki, T., & Morimoto, K. (2007). Uptake characteristics of liposomes by rat alveolar macrophages: Influence of particle size and surface mannose modification. *The Journal of Pharmacy and Pharmacology*, *59*(1), 75–80. doi:10.1211/jpp.59.1.0010 PMID:17227623

Chun, J., & Hartung, H. P. (2010). Mechanism of action of oral fingolimod (FTY720) in multiple sclerosis. *Clinical Neuropharmacology*, *33*(2), 91–101. doi:10.1097/WNF.0b013e3181cbf825 PMID:20061941

Cohen, J. A., & Chun, J. (2011). Mechanisms of fingolimod's efficacy and adverse effects in multiple sclerosis. *Annals of Neurology*, *69*(5), 759–777. doi:10.1002/ana.22426 PMID:21520239

Couto, D., Ribeiro, D., Freitas, M., Gomes, A., Lima, J. L., & Fernandes, E. (2010). Scavenging of reactive oxygen and nitrogen species by the prodrug sulfasalazine and its metabolites 5-aminosalicylic acid and sulfapyridine. *Redox Report*, *15*(6), 259–267. doi:10.1179/135100010X12826446921707 PMID:21208525

Crofford, L. J. (2013). Use of NSAIDs in treating patients with arthritis. *Arthritis Research & Therapy*, *15*(Suppl 3), S2. doi:10.1186/ar4174 PMID:24267197

Cunnane, G., Hummel, K. M., Muller-Ladner, U., Gay, R. E., & Gay, S. (1998). Mechanism of joint destruction in rheumatoid arthritis. *Archivum Immunologiae et Therapiae Experimentalis*, *46*(1), 1–7. PMID:9510939

Cutolo, M., Sulli, A., Pizzorni, C., Seriolo, B., & Straub, R. H. (2001). Anti-inflammatory mechanisms of methotrexate in rheumatoid arthritis. *Annals of the Rheumatic Diseases*, *60*(8), 729–735. doi:10.1136/ard.60.8.729 PMID:11454634

Czajkowsky, D. M., Hu, J., Shao, Z., & Pleass, R. J. (2012). Fc-fusion proteins: New developments and future perspectives. *EMBO Molecular Medicine*, *4*(10), 1015–1028. doi:10.1002/emmm.201201379 PMID:22837174

Dall, T. M., Mann, S. E., Zhang, Y., Quick, W. W., Seifert, R. F., Martin, J., & Zhang, S. et al. (2009). Distinguishing the economic costs associated with type 1 and type 2 diabetes. *Population Health Management*, *12*(2), 103–110. doi:10.1089/pop.2009.12203 PMID:19361253

Desreumaux, P., & Ghosh, S. (2006). Review article: Mode of action and delivery of 5-aminosalicylic acid - new evidence. *Alimentary Pharmacology & Therapeutics*, *24*(Suppl 1), 2–9. doi:10.1111/j.1365-2036.2006.03069.x PMID:16939423

Dhib-Jalbut, S., & Marks, S. (2010). Interferon-beta mechanisms of action in multiple sclerosis. *Neurology*, *74*(Suppl 1), S17–S24. doi:10.1212/WNL.0b013e3181c97d99 PMID:20038758

Di Marco, M., Shamsuddin, S., Razak, K. A., Aziz, A. A., Devaux, C., Borghi, E., & Sadun, C. et al. (2010). Overview of the main methods used to combine proteins with nanosystems: Absorption, bioconjugation, and encapsulation. *International Journal of Nanomedicine*, *5*, 37–49. PMID:20161986

Dobrovolskaia, M. A., & McNeil, S. E. (2007). Immunological properties of engineered nanomaterials. *Nature Nanotechnology*, *2*(8), 469–478. doi:10.1038/nnano.2007.223 PMID:18654343

Dreaden, E. C., Austin, L. A., Mackey, M. A., & El-Sayed, M. A. (2012). Size matters: Gold nanoparticles in targeted cancer drug delivery. *Ther Deliv*, *3*(4), 457–478. doi:10.4155/tde.12.21 PMID:22834077

Duong, A. D., Sharma, S., Peine, K. J., Gupta, G., Satoskar, A. R., Bachelder, E. M., & Ainslie, K. M. et al. (2013). Electrospray encapsulation of toll-like receptor agonist resiquimod in polymer microparticles for the treatment of visceral leishmaniasis. *Molecular Pharmaceutics*, *10*(3), 1045–1055. doi:10.1021/mp3005098 PMID:23320733

English, C., & Aloi, J. J. (2015). New FDA-Approved Disease-Modifying Therapies for Multiple Sclerosis. *Clinical Therapeutics*, *37*(4), 691–715. doi:10.1016/j.clinthera.2015.03.001 PMID:25846320

Faria, A. M., & Weiner, H. L. (2005). Oral tolerance. *Immunological Reviews*, *206*(1), 232–259. doi:10.1111/j.0105-2896.2005.00280.x PMID:16048553

Feldmann, M., & Maini, R. N. (2001). Anti-TNF alpha therapy of rheumatoid arthritis: What have we learned? *Annual Review of Immunology*, *19*(1), 163–196. doi:10.1146/annurev.immunol.19.1.163 PMID:11244034

Fleischer, D. M., Burks, A. W., Vickery, B. P., Scurlock, A. M., Wood, R. A., Jones, S. M., . . . Consortium of Food Allergy. (2013). Sublingual immunotherapy for peanut allergy: a randomized, double-blind, placebo-controlled multicenter trial. *J Allergy Clin Immunol, 131*(1), 119-127. doi: 10.1016/j.jaci.2012.11.011

Fox, R. I., Herrmann, M. L., Frangou, C. G., Wahl, G. M., Morris, R. E., Strand, V., & Kirschbaum, B. J. (1999). Mechanism of action for leflunomide in rheumatoid arthritis. *Clinical Immunology (Orlando, Fla.)*, *93*(3), 198–208. doi:10.1006/clim.1999.4777 PMID:10600330

Friese, M. A., Schattling, B., & Fugger, L. (2014). Mechanisms of neurodegeneration and axonal dysfunction in multiple sclerosis. *Nat Rev Neurol*, *10*(4), 225–238. doi:10.1038/nrneurol.2014.37 PMID:24638138

Garris, C. S., Wu, L., Acharya, S., Arac, A., Blaho, V. A., Huang, Y., & Han, M. H. et al. (2013). Defective sphingosine 1-phosphate receptor 1 (S1P1) phosphorylation exacerbates TH17-mediated autoimmune neuroinflammation. *Nature Immunology*, *14*(11), 1166–1172. doi:10.1038/ni.2730 PMID:24076635

Getts, D. R., Martin, A. J., McCarthy, D. P., Terry, R. L., Hunter, Z. N., Yap, W. T., & Miller, S. D. et al. (2012). Microparticles bearing encephalitogenic peptides induce T-cell tolerance and ameliorate experimental autoimmune encephalomyelitis. *Nature Biotechnology*, *30*(12), 1217–1224. doi:10.1038/nbt.2434 PMID:23159881

Gibofsky, A. (2012). Overview of epidemiology, pathophysiology, and diagnosis of rheumatoid arthritis. *The American Journal of Managed Care*, *18*(13Suppl), S295–S302. PMID:23327517

Gupta, A. K., & Gupta, M. (2005). Synthesis and surface engineering of iron oxide nanoparticles for biomedical applications. *Biomaterials*, *26*(18), 3995–4021. doi:10.1016/j.biomaterials.2004.10.012 PMID:15626447

Haraoui, B., & Bykerk, V. (2007). Etanercept in the treatment of rheumatoid arthritis. *Ther Clin Risk Manag*, *3*(1), 99–105. doi:10.2147/tcrm.2007.3.1.99 PMID:18360618

Hawiger, D., Inaba, K., Dorsett, Y., Guo, M., Mahnke, K., Rivera, M., & Nussenzweig, M. C. et al. (2001). Dendritic cells induce peripheral T cell unresponsiveness under steady state conditions in vivo. *The Journal of Experimental Medicine*, *194*(6), 769–779. doi:10.1084/jem.194.6.769 PMID:11560993

Herrero-Beaumont, G., Martinez Calatrava, M. J., & Castaneda, S. (2012). Abatacept mechanism of action: Concordance with its clinical profile. *Reumatol Clin*, *8*(2), 78–83. doi:10.1016/j.reuma.2011.08.002 PMID:22104048

Hogquist, K. A., Baldwin, T. A., & Jameson, S. C. (2005). Central tolerance: Learning self-control in the thymus. *Nature Reviews. Immunology*, *5*(10), 772–782. doi:10.1038/nri1707 PMID:16200080

Hunter, Z., McCarthy, D. P., Yap, W. T., Harp, C. T., Getts, D. R., Shea, L. D., & Miller, S. D. (2014). A biodegradable nanoparticle platform for the induction of antigen-specific immune tolerance for treatment of autoimmune disease. *ACS Nano*, *8*(3), 2148–2160. doi:10.1021/nn405033r PMID:24559284

Hutchinson, M., Fox, R. J., Havrdova, E., Kurukulasuriya, N. C., Sarda, S. P., Agarwal, S., & Deniz, B. et al. (2014). Efficacy and safety of BG-12 (dimethyl fumarate) and other disease-modifying therapies for the treatment of relapsing-remitting multiple sclerosis: A systematic review and mixed treatment comparison. *Current Medical Research and Opinion*, *30*(4), 613–627. doi:10.1185/03007995.2013.863755 PMID:24195574

Johnson, K. P., Brooks, B. R., Ford, C. C., Goodman, A., Guarnaccia, J., Lisak, R. P., & Wolinsky, J. S. et al. (2000). Sustained clinical benefits of glatiramer acetate in relapsing multiple sclerosis patients observed for 6 years. Copolymer 1 Multiple Sclerosis Study Group. *Multiple Sclerosis*, *6*(4), 255–266. doi:10.1177/135245850000600407 PMID:10962546

Karim, M. Y., Alba, P., Cuadrado, M. J., Abbs, I. C., D'Cruz, D. P., Khamashta, M. A., & Hughes, G. R. (2002). Mycophenolate mofetil for systemic lupus erythematosus refractory to other immunosuppressive agents. *Rheumatology (Oxford, England)*, *41*(8), 876–882. doi:10.1093/rheumatology/41.8.876 PMID:12154204

Kay, J., & Calabrese, L. (2004). The role of interleukin-1 in the pathogenesis of rheumatoid arthritis. *Rheumatology (Oxford, England)*, *43*(Suppl 3), iii2–iii9. doi:10.1093/rheumatology/keh201 PMID:15150426

Keselowsky, B. G., Xia, C. Q., & Clare-Salzler, M. (2011). Multifunctional dendritic cell-targeting polymeric microparticles: Engineering new vaccines for type 1 diabetes. *Human Vaccines*, *7*(1), 37–44. doi:10.4161/hv.7.1.12916 PMID:21157186

Khadra, A., Tsai, S., Santamaria, P., & Edelstein-Keshet, L. (2010). On how monospecific memory-like autoregulatory CD8+ T cells can blunt diabetogenic autoimmunity: A computational approach. *Journal of Immunology (Baltimore, MD.: 1950)*, *185*(10), 5962–5972. doi:10.4049/jimmunol.1001306 PMID:20962260

Kipen, Y., Littlejohn, G. O., & Morand, E. F. (1997). Methotrexate use in systemic lupus erythematosus. *Lupus*, *6*(4), 385–389. doi:10.1177/096120339700600407 PMID:9175024

Kontos, S., Kourtis, I. C., Dane, K. Y., & Hubbell, J. A. (2013). Engineering antigens for in situ erythrocyte binding induces T-cell deletion. *Proceedings of the National Academy of Sciences of the United States of America*, *110*(1), E60–E68. doi:10.1073/pnas.1216353110 PMID:23248266

Krause, I., Blank, M., & Shoenfeld, Y. (2000). Immunomodulation of experimental autoimmune diseases via oral tolerance. *Critical Reviews in Immunology*, *20*(1), 1–16. PMID:10770268

Labet, M., & Thielemans, W. (2009). Synthesis of polycaprolactone: A review. *Chemical Society Reviews*, *38*(12), 3484–3504. doi:10.1039/b820162p PMID:20449064

Laouini, A., Charcosset, C., Fessi, H., Holdich, R. G., & Vladisavljevic, G. T. (2013). Preparation of liposomes: A novel application of microengineered membranes--from laboratory scale to large scale. *Colloids and Surfaces. B, Biointerfaces*, *112*, 272–278. doi:10.1016/j.colsurfb.2013.07.066 PMID:23999143

Larochelle, C., Alvarez, J. I., & Prat, A. (2011). How do immune cells overcome the blood-brain barrier in multiple sclerosis? *FEBS Letters*, *585*(23), 3770–3780. doi:10.1016/j.febslet.2011.04.066 PMID:21550344

Linker, R. A., & Gold, R. (2013). Dimethyl fumarate for treatment of multiple sclerosis: Mechanism of action, effectiveness, and side effects. *Current Neurology and Neuroscience Reports*, *13*(11), 394. doi:10.1007/s11910-013-0394-8 PMID:24061646

Longmire, M., Choyke, P. L., & Kobayashi, H. (2008). Clearance properties of nano-sized particles and molecules as imaging agents: Considerations and caveats. *Nanomedicine (London)*, *3*(5), 703–717. doi:10.2217/17435889.3.5.703 PMID:18817471

Lopez-Olivo, M. A., Siddhanamatha, H. R., Shea, B., Tugwell, P., Wells, G. A., & Suarez-Almazor, M. E. (2014). Methotrexate for treating rheumatoid arthritis. *Cochrane Database of Systematic Reviews, 6*, CD000957. doi:10.1002/14651858.CD000957.pub2 PMID:24916606

Lu, L., Peter, S. J., Lyman, M. D., Lai, H. L., Leite, S. M., Tamada, J. A., & Mikos, A. G. et al. (2000). In vitro and in vivo degradation of porous poly(DL-lactic-co-glycolic acid) foams. *Biomaterials, 21*(18), 1837–1845. doi:10.1016/S0142-9612(00)00047-8 PMID:10919687

Lutterotti, A., Yousef, S., Sputtek, A., Sturner, K. H., Stellmann, J. P., Breiden, P., & Martin, R. et al. (2013). Antigen-specific tolerance by autologous myelin peptide-coupled cells: A phase 1 trial in multiple sclerosis. *Science Translational Medicine, 5*(188), 188ra175. doi:10.1126/scitranslmed.3006168 PMID:23740901

Maassen, C. B., Laman, J. D., van Holten-Neelen, C., Hoogteijling, L., Groenewegen, L., Visser, L., & Claassen, E. et al. (2003). Reduced experimental autoimmune encephalomyelitis after intranasal and oral administration of recombinant lactobacilli expressing myelin antigens. *Vaccine, 21*(32), 4685–4693. doi:10.1016/S0264-410X(03)00522-X PMID:14585676

Maetzel, A., Wong, A., Strand, V., Tugwell, P., Wells, G., & Bombardier, C. (2000). Meta-analysis of treatment termination rates among rheumatoid arthritis patients receiving disease-modifying anti-rheumatic drugs. *Rheumatology (Oxford, England), 39*(9), 975–981. doi:10.1093/rheumatology/39.9.975 PMID:10986302

Maldonado, R. A., LaMothe, R. A., Ferrari, J. D., Zhang, A. H., Rossi, R. J., Kolte, P. N., & Kishimoto, T. K. et al. (2015). Polymeric synthetic nanoparticles for the induction of antigen-specific immunological tolerance. *Proceedings of the National Academy of Sciences of the United States of America, 112*(2), E156–E165. doi:10.1073/pnas.1408686111 PMID:25548186

Maltzman, J. S., & Koretzky, G. A. (2003). Azathioprine: Old drug, new actions. *The Journal of Clinical Investigation, 111*(8), 1122–1124. doi:10.1172/JCI200318384 PMID:12697731

Manolova, V., Flace, A., Bauer, M., Schwarz, K., Saudan, P., & Bachmann, M. F. (2008). Nanoparticles target distinct dendritic cell populations according to their size. *European Journal of Immunology, 38*(5), 1404–1413. doi:10.1002/eji.200737984 PMID:18389478

McCarthy, D. P., Bryant, J., Galvin, J. P., Miller, S. D., & Luo, X. (2015). Tempering allorecognition to induce transplant tolerance with chemically modified apoptotic donor cells. *American Journal of Transplantation, 15*(6), 1475–1483. doi:10.1111/ajt.13237 PMID:25807873

McGaha, T. L., Chen, Y., Ravishankar, B., van Rooijen, N., & Karlsson, M. C. (2011). Marginal zone macrophages suppress innate and adaptive immunity to apoptotic cells in the spleen. *Blood, 117*(20), 5403–5412. doi:10.1182/blood-2010-11-320028 PMID:21444914

Md Yusof, M. Y., & Emery, P. (2013). Targeting interleukin-6 in rheumatoid arthritis. *Drugs, 73*(4), 341–356. doi:10.1007/s40265-013-0018-2 PMID:23456676

Miller, S. D., & Karpus, W. J. (2007). Experimental autoimmune encephalomyelitis in the mouse. Curr Protoc Immunol. doi:10.1002/0471142735.im1501s77

Moghimi, S. M., Hunter, A. C., & Andresen, T. L. (2012). Factors controlling nanoparticle pharmacokinetics: An integrated analysis and perspective. *Annual Review of Pharmacology and Toxicology*, *52*(1), 481–503. doi:10.1146/annurev-pharmtox-010611-134623 PMID:22035254

Mohan, C., & Putterman, C. (2015). Genetics and pathogenesis of systemic lupus erythematosus and lupus nephritis. *Nature Reviews. Nephrology*, *11*(6), 329–341. doi:10.1038/nrneph.2015.33 PMID:25825084

Mok, C. C., & Lau, C. S. (2003). Pathogenesis of systemic lupus erythematosus. *Journal of Clinical Pathology*, *56*(7), 481–490. doi:10.1136/jcp.56.7.481 PMID:12835292

Nicholson, L. B., Murtaza, A., Hafler, B. P., Sette, A., & Kuchroo, V. K. (1997). A T cell receptor antagonist peptide induces T cells that mediate bystander suppression and prevent autoimmune encephalomyelitis induced with multiple myelin antigens. *Proceedings of the National Academy of Sciences of the United States of America*, *94*(17), 9279–9284. doi:10.1073/pnas.94.17.9279 PMID:9256473

Nounou, M. M., El-Khordagui, L. K., & Khalafallah, N. (2005). Release stability of 5-fluorouracil liposomal concentrates, gels and lyophilized powder. *Acta Poloniae Pharmaceutica*, *62*(5), 381–391. PMID:16459487

Oh, J., & O'Connor, P. W. (2014). Teriflunomide in the treatment of multiple sclerosis: Current evidence and future prospects. *Ther Adv Neurol Disord*, *7*(5), 239–252. doi:10.1177/1756285614546855 PMID:25342978

Oh, N., & Park, J. H. (2014). Endocytosis and exocytosis of nanoparticles in mammalian cells. *International Journal of Nanomedicine*, *9*(Suppl 1), 51–63. doi:10.2147/IJN.S26592 PMID:24872703

Orban, T., Bundy, B., Becker, D. J., DiMeglio, L. A., Gitelman, S. E., Goland, R., & Skyler, J. S. et al. (2011). Co-stimulation modulation with abatacept in patients with recent-onset type 1 diabetes: A randomised, double-blind, placebo-controlled trial. *Lancet*, *378*(9789), 412–419. doi:10.1016/S0140-6736(11)60886-6 PMID:21719096

Pacholczyk, R., & Kern, J. (2008). The T-cell receptor repertoire of regulatory T cells. *Immunology*, *125*(4), 450–458. doi:10.1111/j.1365-2567.2008.02992.x PMID:19128356

Peakman, M., & Dayan, C. M. (2001). Antigen-specific immunotherapy for autoimmune disease: Fighting fire with fire? *Immunology*, *104*(4), 361–366. doi:10.1046/j.1365-2567.2001.01335.x PMID:11899420

Peine, K. J., Guerau-de-Arellano, M., Lee, P., Kanthamneni, N., Severin, M., Probst, G. D., & Ainslie, K. M. et al. (2014). Treatment of experimental autoimmune encephalomyelitis by codelivery of disease associated Peptide and dexamethasone in acetalated dextran microparticles. *Molecular Pharmaceutics*, *11*(3), 828–835. doi:10.1021/mp4005172 PMID:24433027

Peng, H., Guerau-de-Arellano, M., Mehta, V. B., Yang, Y., Huss, D. J., Papenfuss, T. L., & Racke, M. K. et al. (2012). Dimethyl fumarate inhibits dendritic cell maturation via nuclear factor kappaB (NF-kappaB) and extracellular signal-regulated kinase 1 and 2 (ERK1/2) and mitogen stress-activated kinase 1 (MSK1) signaling. *The Journal of Biological Chemistry*, *287*(33), 28017–28026. doi:10.1074/jbc.M112.383380 PMID:22733812

Peng, H. J., Chang, Z. N., Lin, S. Y., Han, S. H., & Chang, C. H. (1998). Chemical denaturation of ovalbumin abrogates the induction of oral tolerance of mouse reaginic antibody responses. *Scandinavian Journal of Immunology*, *47*(5), 475–480. doi:10.1046/j.1365-3083.1998.00333.x PMID:9627132

Peng, H. J., Chang, Z. N., Tsai, L. C., Su, S. N., Shen, H. D., & Chang, C. H. (1998). Heat denaturation of egg-white proteins abrogates the induction of oral tolerance of specific Th2 immune responses in mice. *Scandinavian Journal of Immunology*, *48*(5), 491–496. doi:10.1046/j.1365-3083.1998.00432.x PMID:9822257

Perkins, M. R., Ryschkewitsch, C., Liebner, J. C., Monaco, M. C., Himelfarb, D., Ireland, S., & Douek, D. C. et al. (2012). Changes in JC virus-specific T cell responses during natalizumab treatment and in natalizumab-associated progressive multifocal leukoencephalopathy. *PLoS Pathogens*, *8*(11), e1003014. doi:10.1371/journal.ppat.1003014 PMID:23144619

Petri, M. (2004). Cyclophosphamide: New approaches for systemic lupus erythematosus. *Lupus*, *13*(5), 366–371. doi:10.1191/0961203303lu1028oa PMID:15230294

Pisoni, C. N., & D'Cruz, D. P. (2008). The safety of mycophenolate mofetil in pregnancy. *Expert Opinion on Drug Safety*, *7*(3), 219–222. doi:10.1517/14740338.7.3.219 PMID:18462179

Quan, L. D., Thiele, G. M., Tian, J., & Wang, D. (2008). The Development of Novel Therapies for Rheumatoid Arthritis. *Expert Opin Ther Pat*, *18*(7), 723–738. doi:10.1517/13543776.18.7.723 PMID:19578469

Reindl, M., Di Pauli, F., Rostasy, K., & Berger, T. (2013). The spectrum of MOG autoantibody-associated demyelinating diseases. *Nat Rev Neurol*, *9*(8), 455–461. doi:10.1038/nrneurol.2013.118 PMID:23797245

Ricciotti, E., & FitzGerald, G. A. (2011). Prostaglandins and inflammation. *Arteriosclerosis, Thrombosis, and Vascular Biology*, *31*(5), 986–1000. doi:10.1161/ATVBAHA.110.207449 PMID:21508345

Ruckemann, K., Fairbanks, L. D., Carrey, E. A., Hawrylowicz, C. M., Richards, D. F., Kirschbaum, B., & Simmonds, H. A. (1998). Leflunomide inhibits pyrimidine de novo synthesis in mitogen-stimulated T-lymphocytes from healthy humans. *The Journal of Biological Chemistry*, *273*(34), 21682–21691. doi:10.1074/jbc.273.34.21682 PMID:9705303

Ruggieri, R. M., Settipani, N., Viviano, L., Attanasio, M., Giglia, L., Almasio, P., & Piccoli, F. et al. (2003). Long-term interferon-beta treatment for multiple sclerosis. *Neurological Sciences*, *24*(5), 361–364. doi:10.1007/s10072-003-0190-3 PMID:14716534

Saklayen, M. G., Pesce, A. J., Pollak, V. E., & Michael, J. G. (1984). Kinetics of oral tolerance: Study of variables affecting tolerance induced by oral administration of antigen. *International Archives of Allergy and Applied Immunology*, *73*(1), 5–9. doi:10.1159/000233428 PMID:6693181

Savjani, K. T., Gajjar, A. K., & Savjani, J. K. (2012). Drug solubility: Importance and enhancement techniques. *ISRN Pharm*, *195727*. doi:10.5402/2012/195727 PMID:22830056

Selewski, Segal, Rajdev, & Mukherji. (2010). Natalizumab (Tysabri). *American Journal of Neuroradiology*.

Shirani, A., Zhao, Y., Karim, M. E., Evans, C., Kingwell, E., van der Kop, M. L., & Tremlett, H. et al. (2012). Association between use of interferon beta and progression of disability in patients with relapsing-remitting multiple sclerosis. *Journal of the American Medical Association*, *308*(3), 247–256. doi:10.1001/jama.2012.7625 PMID:22797642

Smith, K. J., & McDonald, W. I. (1999). The pathophysiology of multiple sclerosis: The mechanisms underlying the production of symptoms and the natural history of the disease. *Philosophical Transactions of the Royal Society of London. Series B, Biological Sciences*, *354*(1390), 1649–1673. doi:10.1098/rstb.1999.0510 PMID:10603618

Tabata, Y., & Ikada, Y. (1988). Effect of the size and surface charge of polymer microspheres on their phagocytosis by macrophage. *Biomaterials*, *9*(4), 356–362. doi:10.1016/0142-9612(88)90033-6 PMID:3214660

Taylor, P. A., Friedman, T. M., Korngold, R., Noelle, R. J., & Blazar, B. R. (2002). Tolerance induction of alloreactive T cells via ex vivo blockade of the CD40:CD40L costimulatory pathway results in the generation of a potent immune regulatory cell. *Blood*, *99*(12), 4601–4609. doi:10.1182/blood.V99.12.4601 PMID:12036894

Tsai, S., Shameli, A., Yamanouchi, J., Clemente-Casares, X., Wang, J., Serra, P., & Santamaria, P. et al. (2010). Reversal of autoimmunity by boosting memory-like autoregulatory T cells. *Immunity*, *32*(4), 568–580. doi:10.1016/j.immuni.2010.03.015 PMID:20381385

Vallittu, A. M., Peltoniemi, J., Elovaara, I., Kuusisto, H., Farkkila, M., Multanen, J., & Eralinna, J. P. (2005). The efficacy of glatiramer acetate in beta-interferon-intolerant MS patients. *Acta Neurologica Scandinavica*, *112*(4), 234–237. doi:10.1111/j.1600-0404.2005.00464.x PMID:16146492

Van Belle, T. L., Taylor, P., & von Herrath, M. G. (2009). Mouse Models for Type 1 Diabetes. *Drug Discovery Today. Disease Models*, *6*(2), 41–45. doi:10.1016/j.ddmod.2009.03.008 PMID:20407588

Vesterinen, H. M., Sena, E. S., ffrench-Constant, C., Williams, A., Chandran, S., & Macleod, M. R. (2010). Improving the translational hit of experimental treatments in multiple sclerosis. *Multiple Sclerosis*, *16*(9), 1044–1055. doi:10.1177/1352458510379612 PMID:20685763

Vilar, G., Tulla-Puche, J., & Albericio, F. (2012). Polymers and drug delivery systems. *Current Drug Delivery*, *9*(4), 367–394. doi:10.2174/156720112801323053 PMID:22640038

Wang, S., Zhang, X., Zhang, L., Bryant, J., Kheradmand, T., Hering, B. J., & Luo, X. et al. (2014). Preemptive Tolerogenic Delivery of Donor Antigens for Permanent Allogeneic Islet Graft Protection. *Cell Transplantation*. doi:10.3727/096368914X681027 PMID:24759564

Weiner, H. L. (2000). Oral tolerance, an active immunologic process mediated by multiple mechanisms. *The Journal of Clinical Investigation*, *106*(8), 935–937. doi:10.1172/JCI11348 PMID:11032852

Wu, G. C., Xu, X. D., Huang, Q., & Wu, H. (2013). Leflunomide: Friend or foe for systemic lupus erythematosus? *Rheumatology International*, *33*(2), 273–276. doi:10.1007/s00296-012-2508-z PMID:22961090

Xing, Y., & Hogquist, K. A. (2012). T-cell tolerance: Central and peripheral. *Cold Spring Harbor Perspectives in Biology*, *4*(6), a006957. doi:10.1101/cshperspect.a006957 PMID:22661634

Yamano, T., Watanabe, S., Hasegawa, H., Suzuki, T., Abe, R., Tahara, H., & Kishimoto, H. et al. (2011). Ex vivo-expanded DCs induce donor-specific central and peripheral tolerance and prolong the acceptance of donor skin grafts. *Blood*, *117*(9), 2640–2648. doi:10.1182/blood-2010-07-293860 PMID:21220748

Yeste, A., Nadeau, M., Burns, E. J., Weiner, H. L., & Quintana, F. J. (2012). Nanoparticle-mediated codelivery of myelin antigen and a tolerogenic small molecule suppresses experimental autoimmune encephalomyelitis. *Proceedings of the National Academy of Sciences of the United States of America*, *109*(28), 11270–11275. doi:10.1073/pnas.1120611109 PMID:22745170

Zhang, A. H., Skupsky, J., & Scott, D. W. (2009). Factor VIII inhibitors: Risk factors and methods for prevention and immune modulation. *Clinical Reviews in Allergy & Immunology*, *37*(2), 114–124. doi:10.1007/s12016-009-8122-5 PMID:19199081

Zheng, S. G., Wang, J. H., Koss, M. N., Quismorio, F. Jr, Gray, J. D., & Horwitz, D. A. (2004). CD4+ and CD8+ regulatory T cells generated ex vivo with IL-2 and TGF-beta suppress a stimulatory graft-versus-host disease with a lupus-like syndrome. *Journal of Immunology (Baltimore, MD.: 1950)*, *172*(3), 1531–1539. doi:10.4049/jimmunol.172.3.1531 PMID:14734731

Ziemssen, T., & Schrempf, W. (2007). Glatiramer acetate: Mechanisms of action in multiple sclerosis. *International Review of Neurobiology*, *79*, 537–570. doi:10.1016/S0074-7742(07)79024-4 PMID:17531858

Zonana-Nacach, A., Barr, S. G., Magder, L. S., & Petri, M. (2000). Damage in systemic lupus erythematosus and its association with corticosteroids. *Arthritis and Rheumatism*, *43*(8), 1801–1808. doi:10.1002/1529-0131(200008)43:8<1801::AID-ANR16>3.0.CO;2-O PMID:10943870

Chapter 3
Cancer Drug Delivery:
Pharmacogenetics, Biomarkers, and Targeted Therapies

Jai N. Patel
Levine Cancer Institute, USA

Jeryl Villadolid
Levine Cancer Institute, USA

ABSTRACT

Advancements in cancer drug delivery have led to the development of personalized oncology care through molecularly-driven targeted therapies. Understanding molecular and cellular mechanisms which drive tumor progression and resistance is critical in managing new treatment strategies which have shifted from empiric to biomarker-directed therapy selection. Biomarker-directed therapies have improved clinical outcomes in multiple malignancies as monotherapy and in combination with other treatment modalities, however the changing scope of treatment options presents new opportunities and challenges for research. Furthermore, pharmacogenetics may provide a rationale method of personalizing anticancer drug dosing and supportive care management for oncology patients. This chapter reviews biomarker classifications and pharmacogenetics in anticancer therapy and supportive care. Examples of biomarker-directed therapies and clinical assays, in addition to future directions of molecular profiling in oncology therapy management are discussed.

INTRODUCTION

Novel methods of individualizing cancer drug delivery and selection are critical to improve patient outcomes given the large heterogeneity in drug response that exists across the cancer patient population. Until recently, the majority of genomic cancer research has been in discovery and validation; however, as our knowledge of tumor molecular profiling improves, the implementation of genomic cancer medicine in the clinic becomes increasingly tangible, paralleled with the development of dozens of targeted cancer therapies (Tran et al., 2012). Our current understanding of cancer at the molecular level has resulted in a shift from characterizing tumors solely based on their anatomical location and histology to consideration

DOI: 10.4018/978-1-5225-0754-3.ch003

of their molecular profile, opening an array of possibilities for a targeted approach to cancer therapy (Macconaill, Van Hummelen, Meyerson, & Hahn, 2011).

Pharmacogenetic biomarkers found within the tumor and the host offer valuable information for personalizing anticancer drug delivery. As the number of clinical assays available to test for pharmacogenetic biomarkers increases, it is imperative for clinicians to understand the therapeutic implications of mutations occurring within these molecular pathways to aid in drug selection and delivery. This chapter aims to summarize clinically relevant pharmacogenetic biomarkers, which may be used to personalize cancer therapy selection and dosing, in addition to a review of pharmacogenetics in supportive care management related to the treatment of cancer-related symptoms. Tables 1 and 2 summarize clinically relevant somatic and germ-line pharmacogenetic biomarkers and drug targets, and their respective clinical assays available in practice.

BACKGROUND: BIOMARKERS OVERVIEW

DNA analysis for pharmacogenetic purposes can be performed with either somatic or germ-line DNA. The major difference between somatic and germ-line DNA is the origin of the mutated cell (Patel, Mandock, & McLeod, 2014). While germ-line DNA is found in germ cells (sperm or egg) and therefore inherited and transmitted to the offspring, somatic DNA is found within the tumor after conception and subsequently not passed on to offspring, i.e. acquired after birth. Germ-line DNA is readily obtained by blood samples, and variations, if present, will occur homogenously throughout any randomly drawn blood sample within the same individual. Somatic DNA must be obtained by tumor biopsy and is therefore subject to sample selection. Common practice is to obtain one biopsy from the primary tumor for molecular analysis, as it was assumed that tumors were homogenous and the section sampled accurately represented the complete tumor composition. However, there is evidence to suggest that intra-tumor heterogeneity exists within cancer, where molecular analysis of one biopsy site may differ from another biopsy site (Gerlinger et al., 2012). Additionally, somatic mutations may change or evolve during cancer progression, resulting in a significant challenge in applying routine cancer pharmacogenetics to the clinic. While germ-line DNA is particularly useful for determining the pharmacokinetic behavior of a drug by understanding variations in drug metabolizing enzymes and/or transporters, somatic DNA is particularly useful in determining the pharmacodynamic effect of a drug and ultimately tumor response (Deenen, Cats, Beijnen, & Schellens, 2011).

Cancer biomarkers can be broadly categorized into two classifications: prognostic and predictive. A prognostic biomarker is mainly associated with disease outcome in the absence of treatment (i.e. Oncotype Dx, Mammaprint), while a predictive biomarker is valuable in assessing drug response (i.e. *ALK* [anaplastic lymphoma kinase], *BCR-ABL, EGFR* [epidermal growth factor receptor] (Mandrekar & Sargent, 2009; Patel, 2014).

Alternatively, some biomarkers may be classified as both prognostic and predictive (i.e. human epidermal growth factor receptor-2 [*HER2*], KRAS [Kirsten rat sarcoma viral oncogene homolog], and *BRAF* [v-RAF murine sarcoma viral oncogene homolog B]). Figure 1 highlights several strategic growth pathways, which cancer cells can activate through somatic mutations, and their respective targeted therapies. Pharmacodynamic biomarkers, a subset of predictive biomarkers, are useful in measuring the treatment effects of a drug on the tumor or on the host and can be used to guide dose selection; examples include dihydropyrimidine dehydrogenase (*DPYD*), thiopurine-S-methyltransferase (*TPMT*) and uridine diphosphate glucuronosyl transferase 1A1 (*UGT1A1*) amongst others (Patel, 2014; Sawyers, 2008).

Figure 1. Summary of somatic biomarkers and targeted therapies

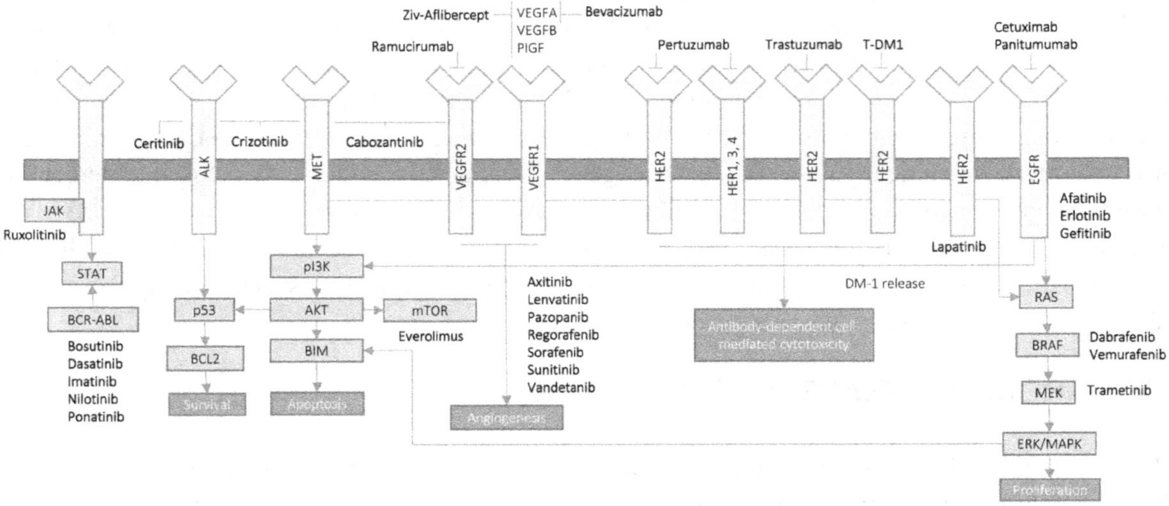

ALK: anaplastic lymphoma kinase; BCL2: B-cell lymphoma 2; BCR-ABL: breakpoint cluster region – Abelson tyrosine kinase; BRAF: v-RAF murine sarcoma viral oncogene homolog B; EGFR: epidermal growth factor receptor; HER2: human epidermal growth factor receptor-2; JAK: Janus kinase; KRAS: Kirsten rat sarcoma viral oncogene homolog; mTOR: mammalian target of rapamycin; PIGF: phosphatidylinositol-glycan biosynthesis class F (placental growth factor); pI3K: phosphoinositide 3-kinase; TDM-1: ado-trastuzumab emtansine; VEGFA: vascular endothelial growth factor ligand A; VEGFB: vascular endothelial growth factor ligand B; VEGFR: vascular endothelial growth factor receptor

[This figure depicts examples of key signaling pathways and downstream effects of somatic biomarker molecular targets. One example pathway is the inhibition of vascular endothelial growth factor (VEGF) which can disrupt tumor angiogenesis through multiple mechanisms. Bevacizumab inhibits VEGF ligand A, ziv-aflibercept acts as a decoy receptor for VEGF ligands A and B and placental growth factor (PIGF), and ramucirumab inhibits the interaction between VEGF receptor 2 and its ligands. Although small molecule tyrosine kinase inhibitors such as axitinib, lenvatinib, pazopanib, regorafenib, sorafenib, sunitinib, and vandetanib all target VEGF, these agents also have additional targets that differentiate indications and potential adverse effects. Other signaling pathways include inhibition of anaplastic lymphoma kinase (ALK), HER2, and EGFR which can lead to changes in tumor survival, apoptosis, antibody-dependent cell-mediated cytotoxicity, and proliferation.]

SOMATIC PHARMACOGENETIC BIOMARKERS

ALK

Anaplastic lymphoma kinase (ALK) is a member of the insulin receptor tyrosine kinase family (RTK), first found to be associated with the (2;5)(p23;q35) chromosome translocation in Ki-1 lymphoma or anaplastic large cell lymphoma. The fusion of the echinoderm microtubule-associated protein like-4 (*EML4*) gene with the *ALK* gene was identified in 2007 from an inversion in chromosome 2 that juxtaposes the 5' end of the *EML4* gene with the 3' end of the *ALK* gene. This protein allows activations of the RAS-MEK-ERK, Janus kinase 3 (JAK3)-STAT3, and PI3K-AKT pathways (Iragavarapu et al., 2015).

The *ALK* translocation is detected using fluorescence in situ hybridization (FISH) as the gold standard assay in the United States. Other assays include, immunohistochemistry (IHC) and reverse transcription polymerase reaction of cDNA (RT-PCR). The overall incidence of *ALK* translocations reported in the NSCLC population ranges from 2 to 7% and occurs independently of *EGFR* or *KRAS* mutations. Similar to *EGFR* mutations, *ALK* rearrangements in NSCLC are associated with clinical and histopathologic features. Patients with *ALK* gene rearrangements are relatively younger, male, and never or light smokers (<10 pack years) (Iragavarapu et al., 2015).

Crizotinib is a small molecular tyrosine kinase inhibitor (TKI) that competitively binds to and inhibits *ALK* and is approved by the Food and Drug Administration (FDA) for the treatment of locally advanced or metastatic *ALK*–positive NSCLC. In a phase III trial with treatment-naïve patients, crizotinib showed a statistically significant improvement in progression-free survival (PFS) (10.9 vs. 7 months), response rate (74 vs. 45%), and quality of life compared to standard chemotherapy with pemetrexed plus either cisplatin or carboplatin (Solomon et al., 2014). In a phase III trial with patients previously treated with one prior platinum-based chemotherapy regimen, crizotinib improved PFS (7.7 vs. 3 months, $p<0.05$) and objective response rate (ORR) (65% vs. 20%; $p <0.05$) compared to single-agent pemetrexed or docetaxel (Shaw et al., 2013). Crizotinib is generally continued until there is evidence of disease progression or unacceptable toxicity. The most common toxicities include visual disturbances, nausea, diarrhea, edema, and fatigue.

Although the majority of patients with *ALK*-positive NSCLC derive substantial benefit from crizotinib, the majority of patients will develop resistance to crizotinib during the first year. Mechanisms of resistance to crizotinib may be due to the development of new, secondary *ALK* mutations, amplification of the *ALK* fusion gene, or activation of alternating pathways that bypass the *ALK* pathway. Secondary *ALK* mutations include *L1196M*, which results from the substitution of leucine by methionine at position 1196 of the *ALK* kinase domain and alters the ATP-binding site of *ALK*, and *C1156Y*, which results in the substitution of a cysteine by tyrosine at position 1156. *KIT* gene amplification has been identified as a potential bypass-signaling pathway (Iragavarapu et al., 2015).

More recently, ceritinib, a second generation *ALK*-inhibitor that is approximately 20 times more potent than crizotinib received accelerated FDA approval for the treatment of patients with metastatic *ALK*-positive NSCLC who are resistant or unable to tolerate crizotinib. The efficacy of ceritinib was established in a multicenter, single-arm, open-label clinical trial where patients with metastatic *ALK*-positive NSCLC who progressed while receiving or were intolerant to crizotinib had an improvement in ORR of 58% and 56% in crizotinib naïve and resistant cases, respectively (Shaw et al., 2014). Both agents have similar adverse effects and are metabolized by the cytochrome P450 enzyme system.

As evident by crizotinib and ceritinib, the drug development paradigm for highly targeted therapies is changing, allowing earlier, accelerated approval of exceedingly effective therapies, years before phase III randomized studies are completed. Alectinib is a second generation *ALK* inhibitor that was approved in Japan for the treatment of patients with recurrent or relapsed *ALK*-positive NSCLC, and is now FDA approved following Breakthrough Therapy Designation by the United States for patients who progressed on crizotinib. Clinical trials of new *ALK* inhibitors that can potentially overcome resistance mechanisms in addition to combination targeted therapy with EGFR, TRK, FAK, and ROS1 are ongoing (Iragavarapu et al., 2015; Seto et al., 2013).

BCR-ABL

The *BCR-ABL* chromosomal abnormality is formed by a translocation between chromosomes 9 and 22, resulting in a fusion between the breakpoint cluster region (*BCR*) and the *c-ABL* oncogene (the Philadelphia chromosome, t(9;22) (q34.1;q11.21)) (Heisterkamp, Stam, Groffen, de Klein, & Grosveld, 1985). The chimeric *BCR-ABL* tyrosine kinase (TK) is constitutively active, triggering signal transduction pathways associated with cell survival. The translocation occurs in >95% of chronic myeloid leukemia (CML) cases, 25% of adult acute lymphocytic leukemia (ALL) cases, and 3% of pediatric ALL cases (de Klein et al., 1982; Fielding, 2011). The discovery of the TKIs, imatinib, nilotinib, dasatinib and most recently, bosutinib and ponatinib, have resulted in mean cytogenetic response rates > 90% (Jabbour et al., 2011). Although these TKIs have slightly different mechanisms, they primarily exert their activity by binding to the *ABL* domain of the TK and preventing the binding of ATP, thereby preventing phosphorylation and subsequent activation of various downstream substrates. Imatinib, nilotinib, and ponatinib all bind to the inactive conformation of the *ABL* kinase, preventing the conformational switch to the active form. Dasatinib inhibits both the active and inactive conformations and bosutinib inhibits both *SRC* and *ABL*. Nilotinib has a higher affinity for the *ABL* kinase domain than imatinib, resulting in greater potency and selectivity (Bixby & Talpaz, 2009). Both nilotinib and dasatinib are >100-fold more potent than imatinib in vitro.

Roughly 10% of patients will initially present with resistance to TKIs, and close to 20% will develop resistance within five years (Mauro, 2006). Primary resistance is observed when a patient fails to achieve a desired response to treatment (up to 25% of patients in the chronic phase of CML) and secondary resistance occurs when patients with an initial response ultimately relapse (up to 80, 50, and 15% at around two years for patients in blast crisis, accelerated phase or chronic phase of CML, respectively). The principal mechanisms of resistance to TKIs are point mutations in the kinase domain of the *BCR-ABL* protein, resulting in the inability of the TKI to bind to the *BCR-ABL* protein. The T315I mutation of the *ABL* gene represents the highest magnitude of resistance, as current TKIs require threonine at position 315 in order to bind to their targets (Gorre et al., 2001).

A newer compound, ponatinib (a pan-*BCR-ABL* inhibitor), is the only TKI shown to be effective in overcoming resistance mediated by the T315I mutation. Although ponatinib received accelerated approval by the FDA for the treatment of CML in adults with resistance or intolerance to prior tyrosine kinase inhibitor therapy, its indication has been narrowed due to the risk for life-threatening vascular complications, thrombosis, and hepatotoxicity (Bixby & Talpaz, 2009; T. Zhou et al., 2011).

BRAF

BRAF mutations have been identified in a wide range of cancers including 40 to 60% of malignant melanomas, 45% of papillary thyroid cancer, 10% of colorectal cancers, and 3-5% of lung cancers and gynecologic cancers. Mutations result in a substitution of glutamic acid at amino acid 600 (*V600E*) in 80 to 90% of cases or a substitution of lysine for valine (*V600K*) in 10 to 20% of cases, causing downstream signaling through the mitogen-activated protein kinase (MAPK) pathway (Chapman et al., 2011). Inhibition of the MAPK pathway in patients whose tumors contain a *BRAF V600* mutation using either a *BRAF* inhibitor and/or a *MEK* inhibitor is a targeted therapeutic approach to the treatment of advanced melanoma. As such, all patients with advanced melanoma should have their tumors assayed for the presence of a *BRAF* mutation. *BRAF* mutations are more frequent in patients with early age at tumor onset, truncal primary, and lack of chronic skin damage. Patients with a *BRAF V600* mutation and bulky disease, visceral metastases, elevated serum LDH, or a poor performance status are more likely to have rapidly progressive disease and a shorter overall survival (Chapman et al., 2011).

BRAF inhibitors have been shown to have a shorter time to response for the treatment of advanced melanoma compared to immunotherapy such as ipilimumab, however, the duration of response is short and almost all patients eventually have disease progression. There are currently two *BRAF* inhibitors that are FDA approved for the treatment of advanced melanoma, vemurafenib and dabrafenib. In a phase III trial comparing vemurafenib to dacarbazine in previously untreated, *BRAF* V600E mutation-positive patients, vemurafenib improved overall survival (OS) compared to dacarbazine (13.6 vs. 9.7 months, HR 0.70, 95% CI 0.57-0.87) (McArthur et al., 2014). Dabrafenib increased median PFS compared to dacarbazine (median 5.1 vs. 2.7 months, HR 0.33, 95% CI 0.20-0.54, $p<0.0001$) (Hauschild et al., 2012). Similar to vemurafenib, the most frequent grade 2 or greater toxicities were dermatologic. Dabrafenib must be taken on an empty stomach and has active metabolites, less squamous cell carcinoma, rash, photosensitivity, and increased pyrexia, hyperglycemia, and hypophosphatemia compared to vemurafenib (Trinh, Davis, Anderson, & Kim, 2014).

Resistance quickly develops in roughly 20-25% of *BRAF* mutant, metastatic melanoma patients treated with vemurafenib, with a mean time to diagnosis of first lesion at approximately 10 weeks. A number of mechanisms have been elucidated, including the paradoxical activation of the MAPK pathway through *RAS* mutations, elevation of pERK, and additional acquired mutations (*NRASQ61, MEK1*) (Su et al., 2012).

A potent inhibitor of *MEK1* and *MEK2*, trametinib, has been studied as monotherapy and in combination with dabrafenib to overcome resistance due to downstream effects in the MAPK pathway. Blocking a paradoxical activation of the MAPK pathway with *MEK* inhibition may also reduce the incidence of skin toxicity. The combination of dabrafenib and trametinib resulted in prolonged PFS (median 11.0 vs. 8.8 months, HR 0.67, 95% CI 0.53-0.84), higher ORR (69 vs. 53%) and prolonged OS (median 25.1 vs. 18.7 months, HR 0.71, 95% CI 0.55-0.92) compared with dabrafenib alone. The combination is also associated with less toxicity, but increased pyrexia and chills (Flaherty et al., 2012). OS was significantly increased in the combination when compared against vemurafenib in previously untreated patients with *BRAF V600* mutation-positive melanoma (one-year survival rate 72 vs. 65%, HR for death 0.69, 95% CI 0.53-0.89) (Robert, Karaszewska, et al., 2015).

Patients with *BRAF*-mutated colorectal tumors tend to have significantly shorter PFS and OS compared to wild-type patients, and also have the potential to impair the effects of EGFR-inhibitor therapy in *KRAS* wild-type patients (Di Nicolantonio et al., 2008). The benefit observed with vemurafenib in melanoma patients was not evident in colorectal cancer (CRC) patients harboring the *BRAF* mutation, indicating the significant influence of tumor origin and microenvironment on treatment response. Early phase studies suggest EGFR inhibition in addition to vemurafenib may overcome the resistance mechanisms demonstrated in CRC (Prahallad et al., 2012). The data for BRAF inhibition in lung cancer is scarce, although case reports have demonstrated clinical activity with vemurafenib (Peters, Michielin, & Zimmermann, 2013). Interim results of a phase II study of dabrafenib in *BRAF* V600E-positive NSCLC patients who failed at least one line of chemotherapy showed early antitumor activity with an ORR of 54% (Planchard et al., 2013).

C-KIT

The CD117 antigen is almost universally expressed by gastrointestinal tumors (GISTs) and is part of the KIT transmembrane receptor tyrosine kinase (RTK) that is the product of the KIT proto-oncogene, *c-KIT* (Rubin, Fletcher, & Fletcher, 2000). The *c-KIT* proto-oncogene encodes a receptor TK, which binds to stem cell factor ligand, allowing for the development of melanocytes, erythrocytes, germ cells, and mast cells, ultimately resulting in dimerization, autophosporylation, and signal transduction (Yasuda et al., 2007). More than 80% of GISTs express a mutation in the *c-KIT* gene that leads to oncogenic signaling in the cell; 75% of the *c-KIT* mutations affect exon 11, while other mutations affect exon 9, 13, or 17. However, uncontrolled *c-KIT* activation may be present in the absence of *c-KIT* mutations, which occurs in 4 to 5% of cases. *C-KIT*-negative GISTs may be attributed to transcriptional silencing mechanisms or different activating mutations (e.g. platelet-derived growth factor receptor alpha [*PDGFRA*]) (Emile et al., 2004). Adult patients with confirmed GIST that are *c-KIT* or *PDGFRA* mutation-negative usually have tumors localized the stomach, whereas GISTs expressing *c-KIT* mutations are often larger in size and more frequently invade adjacent tissues (Heinrich et al., 2003).

Imatinib inhibits several targets including *BCR-ABL, c-KIT,* EPHA2, PDGFR, and *SRC*. By binding to the ATP-binding pocket required for phosphorylation and activation of *c-KIT* and PDGFR, imatinib has induced dramatic clinical benefit for the treatment of GIST (Balachandran et al., 2011). The partial response rate for GISTs harboring exon 11 *c-KIT* mutations is approximately 80-85% when administering imatinib, whereas patients with tumors containing an exon 9 *c-KIT* mutation, or no detectable mutation, have partial response rates closer to 45-50% (Heinrich et al., 2003). Studies show a rapid response as early as 24 hours after the first dose of imatinib. Long-term follow-up studies show an estimated 10-year survival rate of 22% (Demetri et al., 2014).

Although imatinib is highly effective in GIST, patients may acquire resistance through secondary mutations in *c-KIT* with an average median time to progression of about 2 to 3 years. Use of more potent or multi-targeted inhibitors that target other receptors like PDGFR such as sunitinib can help overcome resistance (Demetri et al., 2006; Reichardt et al., 2012). Regorafenib was most recently approved in 2013 for patients who are no longer responsive to imatinib and sunitinib (Demetri et al., 2013).

EGFR

Epidermal growth factor receptor (EGFR, also called dHER1 or erbB-1) tyrosine kinases are cell surface receptors that dimerize to activate and control intracellular signaling via the PI3K-AKT and RAS-MEK-ERK pathways (Yarden & Shilo, 2007). *EGFR* mutations are present in about 15% of NSCLC adenocarcinoma in the United States and occur more frequently in Asians and non-smoking females (Shepherd et al., 2005; Thatcher et al., 2005). Deletions in exon 19 and a missense mutation at exon 21, resulting in an arginine to leucine substitution (*L858R*), account for 90% of all *EGFR* mutations and are associated with a higher response rate to EGFR TKIs (gefitinib, erlotinib, afatinib) compared to traditional chemotherapy (Lynch et al., 2004).

Currently, screening for *EGFR* mutations is used to select stage IV NSCLC patients who may receive erlotinib in the first-line setting. In 2013, the FDA approved a companion diagnostic test for erlotinib and authorized expanded approval for first-line use in patients with metastatic NSCLC that test positive for the *EGFR* activating mutation. Data from 13 phase III trials comparing EGFR TKIs and platinum-based chemotherapy show prolonged PFS in patients with *EGFR*-positive advanced NSCLC, however, no significant increase in OS was noted (Lee et al., 2013). Erlotinib improved PFS (13.1 vs. 4.6 months, HR 0.16; 95% CI 0.10-0.26) and ORR (83 vs. 36%) compared with standard gemcitabine plus carboplatin in patients receiving initial therapy for advanced NSCLC with *EGFR* mutations (C. Zhou et al., 2011). Compared to platinum-based doublet therapy, erlotinib also increased PFS (median 9.7 vs. 5.2 months, HR 0.37, 95% CI 0.25-0.54) with no significant difference in OS (Rosell et al., 2012).

Afatinib was FDA approved in 2013 for first-line therapy of metastatic NSCLC in *EGFR* mutation-positive patients. It covalently binds to the kinase domains of EGFR (ErbB1), HER2 (ErbB2), and HER4 (ErbB4) and irreversibly inhibits tyrosine kinase autophosphorylation, resulting in downregulation of ErbB signaling. This irreversible binding allows for enhanced activity in resistant tumors that have progressed after initial *EGFR* inhibitor therapy (Miller et al., 2012). Data from two phase III trials did not show a statistically significant increase in OS when comparing afatinib to chemotherapy for NSCLC (median 25.8 vs. 24.5 months, HR 0.91, 95% CI 0.75-1.11). Mutation analysis showed a significant benefit in OS and PFS in patients with exon 19 deletion and a significant benefit in PFS but not OS for patients with *L858R* mutations (Yang et al., 2015).

Patients initially responding to EGFR TKIs can subsequently develop disease progression due to acquired resistance. Two primary mechanisms of resistance to EGFR inhibitors include a secondary point mutation in *EGFR* (*T790M*) that blocks the capacity for erlotinib to inhibit the receptor, and the amplification of *MET*, which activates similar downstream signaling pathways. *MET* amplification is thought to account for resistance in 5 to 20% of patients who progressed after treatment with erlotinib or gefitinib (Bean et al., 2007). Multiple agents have also been developed for patients that have acquired a resistance mutation with *T790M* and have limited benefit from EGFR tyrosine kinase inhibition, including AZD9291 (61% response rate in *T790M* mutation-positive patients) and rociletinib (59% response rate in *T790M* mutation-positive patients) (Sequist et al., 2015; Yang et al., 2015). Combination therapy may be beneficial in patients whose tumors contain an *EGFR* driver mutation (Herbst et al., 2011).

HER2

HER2 is a transmembrane glycoprotein EGFR that belongs to a family of four receptors EGFR/HER1, HER2, HER3, HER4) responsible for cell growth, survival and differentiation through signal transduction activation of the PI3K/Akt and RAS/RAF/MEK/MAPK pathways (Arteaga et al., 2012).

HER2 status represents both a prognostic and predictive biomarker. Amplification of HER2 occurs in about 20% of patients with early stage breast cancer. Prior to the introduction of HER2-directed therapies, HER2 overexpression was associated with high recurrence rates and increased mortality. A high level of HER2 overexpression by either 3+ immunohistochemical staining (IHC) for the HER2 protein or evidence of *HER2* gene amplification by fluorescence in situ hybridization (FISH >2.0), is a strong predictive factor for sensitivity to HER2-targeted agents (Arteaga et al., 2012).

Trastuzumab binds to the extracellular domain of the HER2 receptor and is thought to work by several potential mechanisms including antibody-dependent-cell-mediated cytotoxicity (ADCC), inhibition of cleavage of the extracellular domain of the receptor, inhibition of ligand-dependent dimerization, and inhibition of downstream signaling pathways (Arteaga et al., 2012). Trastuzumab is recommended in the adjuvant setting as monotherapy after completion of chemotherapy, in combination with paclitaxel or docetaxel or given concurrently with carboplatin and docetaxel. A meta-analysis including eight randomized clinical trials showed that the combination of trastuzumab with adjuvant chemotherapy produced a significant benefit in disease-free survival (DFS) (HR 0.60, 95% CI 0.50-0.71), OS (0.66, 95% CI 0.57-0.77), locoregional recurrence (OR = 0.53), and distant recurrence (OR = 0.62), as compared to chemotherapy alone (Moja et al., 2012). Trastuzumab in the neoadjuvant setting also improves pathological complete response rates and event-free survival in patients with locally advanced or early stage breast cancer. In addition, it is approved in metastatic *HER2*-positive disease in combination with paclitaxel, docetaxel or as monotherapy.

Mechanisms of resistance to trastuzumab include loss of or increased HER2 expression, increased ligand (TGF-α) expression, steric hindrance of the antibody interaction, inhibition of binding by extracellular domain fragments cleaved from the HER2 receptor, and alternate signaling pathways. Incomplete HER family blockade could allow another HER receptor to compensate when one receptor is blocked. *PIK3CA* and *PTEN* expression may affect the sensitivity of tumor cells to trastuzumab and lapatinib. Variability of human breast cancer cell lines with regard to growth factor receptors, co-amplification of other genes, and acquired drug resistance phenotypes may be limitations to correlating resistance and HER2 overexpression (Arteaga et al., 2012).

Lapatinib is a small molecule TKI that reversibly inhibits intracellular HER2 and EGFR (HER1) by suppressing tyrosine autophosphorylation and downstream pathways. Studies have demonstrated that lapatinib may have additive or synergistic activity if combined with trastuzumab with better central nervous system penetration. Use of lapatinib has led to significant improvements in time to progression in metastatic HER2 positive breast cancer in combination with capecitabine compared to capecitabine alone (HR=0.49; P<0.001) (Geyer et al., 2006). Resistance to lapatinib may include survival pathways leading to upregulation of transcription factors leading to increased estrogen receptor signaling and an estrogen receptor-independent mechanism of acquired autoresistance (Arteaga et al., 2012).

Pertuzumab is a monoclonal antibody that binds the extracellular dimerization domain of HER2 and prevents it from binding to itself or other members of the EGFR family. It is administered in combination with trastuzumab for more complete HER2 inhibition. The combination of trastuzumab, pertuzumab, and a taxane showed an improvement in median PFS compared with placebo (19 vs. 12 months; HR 0.62, 95% CI 0.51-0.75), improvement in overall response rate (80 vs. 69%), and median OS (56.5 vs. 40.8 months, HR 0.68, 95% CI 0.56-0.84) (Baselga et al., 2012).

Most recently, ado-trastuzumab emtansine (TDM-1), an antibody-drug conjugate composed of trastuzumab, a thioether link, and an extremely potent antimicrotubule agent, DM1, was approved for the treatment of metastatic breast cancer. Compared with trastuzumab plus docetaxel, ado-trastuzumab emtansine showed a longer median PFS (14 vs. 9 months, HR 0.58, 95% CI 0.36-0.97) and higher ORR of 64 vs. 58% (Hurvitz et al., 2013).

KRAS

KRAS belongs to a group of small GTP-binding proteins, known as the RAS superfamily or RAS-like GTPases. More than 150 *RAS*-like genes have been identified in mammalian genomes. Activating mutations in the *KRAS* gene impair the ability of the KRAS protein to switch between active and inactive states, leading to cell transformation and increased resistance to chemotherapy and biological therapies targeting EGFR. *KRAS* gene point mutations have been detected in pancreatic carcinomas (>80%), colon carcinomas (40–50%), and lung carcinomas (30–50%), but are also present in biliary tract malignancies, myeloid leukemias, endometrial, cervical, bladder, liver, and breast cancers. The Qiagen Therascreen *KRAS* RCQ PCR kit is FDA-approved to detect seven different mutations of the *KRAS* gene within exon

2, however testing for all *RAS* mutations may be preferred (Jancik, Drabek, Radzioch, & Hajduch, 2010). The National Comprehensive Cancer Network (NCCN) recommends testing for *KRAS* and *NRAS* exons 2, 3, and 4 in patients being considered for an anti-EGFR agent.

The *KRAS* genes associated with colon cancer appear most often in codons 12 (28%) and 13 (8%) of exon 1 and less frequently in codon 61. Mutations in codon 12 are more frequent in primary metastatic carcinoma, suggesting a more aggressive phenotype. A mutation in codon 13 has been shown to be associated with reduced survival rates. Expression of *KRAS*, mainly on exon 2 (codons 12 and 13) has been associated with upregulated carcinoembryonic antigen (CEA) expression, disturbance of epithelial cell polarization, and increased adhesiveness of colon cancer cells (Jancik, Drabek, Radzioch, & Hajduch, 2010). *KRAS* mutation status is the most important predictor of resistance to EGFR-inhibitors used in colon cancer, cetuximab or panitumumab; both the median PFS of cetuximab-treated patients and OS found to be superior in a *KRAS* wild-type group than in a *KRAS* mutant group (31 vs. 10 weeks, and 16 vs. 7 months, respectively) (Lievre et al., 2008).

Cetuximab is approved for use in combination with FOLFIRI (fluorouracil, leucovorin, irinotecan) for first-line treatment of patients with *KRAS* wild-type CRC. Patients with wild-type *KRAS* treated with cetuximab had a median OS of 23.5 vs. 20 months and PFS of 9.9 vs. 8 months compared to those patients who did not receive cetuximab (Van Cutsem et al., 2009). Cetuximab is also approved for squamous head and neck cancer.

In 2006, a humanized monoclonal anti-EGFR1 IgG2 antibody, panitumumab, was approved for the treatment of patients with metastatic CRC who progressed after chemotherapy. Patients with metastatic CRC who were previously untreated and had *KRAS* mutations had a predicted response to panitumumab when added to FOLFOX (fluorouracil, leucovorin, oxaliplatin) compared to FOLFOX alone. The mutations were associated with inferior PFS and OS (Douillard et al., 2013). In a phase III trial, panitumumab monotherapy was compared to best supportive care and *KRAS* mutations were detected using polymerase chain reaction on DNA from tumor. PFS of patients with wild-type compared to mutant *KRAS* gene tumors was 12 vs. 7 weeks, showing that panitumumab monotherapy efficacy in metastatic CRC is confined to patients with wild-type *KRAS* tumors and *KRAS* status should be considered in patients who may be candidates for therapy. (Amado et al., 2008). Mutations in the *KRAS* gene in codons 12 and 13 were detected in 21% of NSCLC. *RAS* gene (exon 1: codons 12, 13, or 61) with or without increases in *EGFR* copy numbers did not derive benefit from erlotinib in NSCLC and had about a 96% chance of disease progression (Massarelli et al., 2007).

PD-1

Programmed death 1 protein (PD-1) is an immune checkpoint receptor that is expressed by activated T cells and binds to its ligands, PD-L1 and PD-L2, to provide a negative signal for T cell activation and proliferation. Anti-PD-1 monoclonal antibodies such as nivolumab and pembrolizumab disrupt the interaction between PD-1 and its ligands to provide an immune antitumor response. In contrast to CTLA-4-mediated inhibition, which is a central event, PD-1-mediated inhibition can occur peripherally in the tumors, providing a potential mechanism for adaptive immune resistance. Checkpoint inhibitor pathways have a mechanism of action that is not limited to one tumor or tissue type. Tumor expression of PD-L1 in early trials appears to predict a higher response rate, longer PFS and OS compared to tumors that do not express PD-L1; however, sensitivity of assays and appropriate cutoff values for expression are heavily debated (Pardoll, 2012).

Pembrolizumab was studied in patients with advanced melanoma in three dose cohorts and showed an overall ORR of 33%, one-year OS of 66%, and median PFS 4.4 months (Duad, Ribas, Robert, & al., 2015). Pembrolizumab regimens (10 mg/kg every 2 or 3 weeks) also significantly prolonged PFS when compared to ipilimumab (47.3% and 46.6% for pembrolizumab, respectively, and 26.5% for ipilimumab) with an OS HR of 0.63-0.69 at one year (Robert, Schachter, et al., 2015).

Nivolumab received accelerated FDA-approval in December 2014 based on tumor response and durability of response in patients with previously treated metastatic melanoma. In a phase III trial comparing nivolumab to investigators choice chemotherapy (dacarbazine or carboplatin and paclitaxel) in patients with unresectable or metastatic melanoma who progressed on ipilimumab and a *BRAF*-inhibitor (if *BRAF* mutation-positive), nivolumab improved ORR compared with chemotherapy (32% vs. 10%, 95% CI 3.5-23.1) with a longer duration of response (median not reached vs. 3.5 months with chemotherapy) (Weber et al., 2015). In previously untreated patients with wild-type *BRAF* mutations, OS was significantly increased in patients treated with nivolumab compared to dacarbazine (one-year OS rate 73% vs. 42%, HR 0.42, 99.8% CI 0.25-0.73) (Robert, Long, et al., 2015). The combination of nivolumab and ipilimumab in patients with wild-type *BRAF* mutations showed an improved ORR of 61% vs. 11% ($P<0.001$) compared to ipilimumab monotherapy, however a higher rate of grade 3 to 4 drug-related adverse effects occurred with combination therapy (54% vs. 24%) compared to monotherapy (Postow et al., 2015).

Based on current published clinical trials, both pembrolizumab and nivolumab seem to be more effective than ipilimumab in patients regardless of *BRAF* mutation status, with a more tolerable safety profile, and a possible biomarker for response (anti-PD-L1), however additional studies are ongoing to determine their place in therapy.

The FDA indication for nivolumab was expanded to include the treatment of metastatic, squamous NSCLC in March 2015 based on a single-arm trial in patients who progressed after receiving platinum-doublet therapy with an ORR of 14.5% (95% CI 8.7-22.2) (Rizvi et al., 2015). There have also been positive preliminary results in the second-line non-squamous NSCLC setting after failure of platinum-based doublet chemotherapy and TKI with a 27% risk reduction in death with nivolumab compared to docetaxel (Spigel et al., 2015). PD-1 inhibition continues to be a target of interest for new cancer drug development for both hematologic and oncologic tumor types, in addition to identifying novel combinations of chemotherapy and/or targeted therapy with immunotherapy.

VEGF

Vascular endothelial growth factor (VEGF) promotes angiogenesis through endothelial cell proliferation and migration. The biological effects of VEGF are mediated by two receptor tyrosine kinases, VEGFR-1 and VEGFR-2 (Ferrara, Gerber, & LeCouter, 2003). Genetic variability in the promoter regions of VEGF affects the activity and expression of the VEGF protein, which may impact the benefit of targeted VEGF inhibitor therapy (Schneider, Radovich, & Miller, 2009). No biomarkers have been validated to date to identify patients who are more likely to benefit from VEGF inhibitor therapy, however many agents have been recently approved in multiple malignancies (Gerger, LaBonte, & Lenz, 2011).

The VEGF family contains VEGF-A, VEGF-B, VEGF-C, VEGF-D, VEGF-E, and placental growth factor (PLGF). VEGF-A was the first pharmacologically targeted VEGF family member and acts selectively on vascular endothelial cells. VEGF-A expression is regulated by hypoxia, whereby the promotion of new blood vessel formation occurs to respond to reduced tissue oxygenation. The pro-angiogenic role of VEGF is inhibited by anti-VEGF and anti-VEGF-receptor antibodies, soluble VEGF "decoy" receptors, and small molecule TKIs (Ferrara, Gerber, & LeCouter, 2003).

Bevacizumab is a humanized monoclonal antibody directed against VEGF that targets VEGF-A. A pooled analysis of trials comparing chemotherapy with and without bevacizumab in the first-line setting of metastatic CRC showed a 19% reduction in risk of death (HR 0.81, 95% CI 0.70-0.93), however OS improvement was modest (median 19.8 vs. 17.6 months) (Hurwitz et al., 2013). Bevacizumab is FDA approved for the treatment of metastatic CRC, both as first-line in combination with fluorouracil-based chemotherapy and as second-line after progression on a first-line bevacizumab-containing regimen (Bennouna et al., 2013). Bevacizumab is also FDA approved in cervical cancer, glioblastoma, NSCLC, ovarian, and renal cell cancer.

Soluble "decoy" receptors consisting of native VEGFR sequences can bind to VEGF and prevent its interaction with VEGFRs on tumor or endothelial cells. Aflibercept is a recombinant fusion protein that contains the VEGF-binding domains of VEGFR1 and VEGFR2 fused to the Fc domain of human IgG1 and acts as a decoy receptor for VEGF, inactivating receptor binding to VEGF-A and VEGF-B (Holash et al., 2002). Aflibercept has a higher affinity for VEGF-A than bevacizumab and is approved for use in combination with FOLFIRI for the treatment of metastatic CRC that is resistant to or has progressed on an oxaliplatin-containing regimen. Patients who progressed during or within six months of receiving oxaliplatin-containing chemotherapy with or without bevacizumab had longer OS and PFS if treated with FOLFIRI plus aflibercept compared to FOLFIRI plus placebo (13.5 vs. 12.1 months and 6.9 vs. 4.7 months, respectively), regardless of bevacizumab exposure (Van Cutsem et al., 2012).

More recently, an antibody that targets the cell surface receptor for VEGF (VEGFR) has been approved to block VEGF signaling. Ramucirumab is a recombinant IgG1 monoclonal antibody that prevents the interaction of VEGF receptor 2 (VEGFR2) and its ligands. Two trials have shown survival benefit for treatment of second-line advanced or metastastic gastric or gastroesophageal junction adenocarcinoma for ramucirumab as monotherapy or in combination with paclitaxel. In one trial, patients with previously treated advanced or metastatic gastric or gastroesophageal junction adenocarcinoma and treated with either ramucirumab had an improved median PFS (2.1 vs 1.3 months) and OS (5.2 vs. 3.8 months, HR 0.78, 95% CI 0.60-0.998) compared to placebo (Fuchs et al., 2014). In another trial, weekly paclitaxel plus ramucirumab in patients who had disease progression after first-line platinum fluropyrimidine-based combination therapy for metastatic gastric or gastroesophageal junction adenocarcinoma had an OS benefit of 9.6 vs. 7.4 months (HR 0.807, 95% CI 0.768-0.962), PFS (4.4 vs. 2.9 months), and ORR (28 vs. 16%) compared to placebo (Wilke et al., 2014). Based on these results, the FDA approved ramucirumab both as a single agent and in combination with paclitaxel for advanced or metastatic gastric or gastroesophageal junction adenocarcinoma in the second-line setting. This indication was also expanded to include treatment of second-line NSCLC (median OS 10.5 vs. 9.1 months in patients treated with docetaxel plus ramucirumab compared to docetaxel plus placebo after progression on platinum doublet therapy for NSCLC) and second-line treatment of metastatic colorectal cancer (median OS 13.3 vs. 11.7 months and PFS 5.7 vs 4.5 months in patients receiving FOLFIRI plus ramucirumab compared to FOLFIRI plus placebo) (Garon et al., 2014; Tabernero et al., 2015).

Oral, small molecule VEGF inhibitors are available, but may have targets in addition to VEGF. The broader specificity is due to the structural similarity of the catalytic ATP-binding site region. This broad activity may enhance the action of VEGF inhibitors by allowing inhibition of multiple signaling pathways, however there could be additional toxicity based on other targets. These agents typically have shorter half-lives compared to monoclonal antibodies. Some examples of multi-targeted VEGF inhibitors and their targets include: axitinib (VEGFR1-3), lenvatinib (VEGFR, RET, FGFR), pazopanib (VEGFR1-3, PDGFR, FGFR1 and 3, c-KIT), sorafenib (VEGFR2, FLT3, PDGFR, FGFR-1), sunitinib (c-KIT, VEGFR1-3, PDGFR-α, PDGFR-β, FLT3, CSF-1R, RET), regorafenib (VEGFR1-3, RET, c-KIT, PDGFR, FGFR), and vandetanib (VEGFR, RET, EGFR). These agents have approvals for the treatment of multiple malignancies such as renal cell carcinoma and thyroid carcinoma (Zhang, Tan, Ding, Xin, & Jiang, 2012; Zhong & Bowen, 2011).

Although VEGF inhibitors have been shown to prolong survival in multiple malignancies, the benefit often does not last longer than a few months, potentially due to tumor resistance or adaptation. Tumor production of alternative angiogenic factors, such as fibroblast growth factor (FGF) and human growth factor (HGF), may contribute to resistance to VEGF inhibition (Ebos, Lee, & Kerbel, 2009).

GERM-LINE PHARMACOGENETIC BIOMARKERS

CYP2D6 and Tamoxifen

Tamoxifen is a selective estrogen receptor modulator and is widely used to treat hormone receptor positive breast cancer. Tamoxifen is a prodrug that requires bioactivation to the more active metabolite, endoxifen, via the hepatic enzyme cytochrome P450 2D6 (CYP2D6). The gene coding for this enzyme, *CYP2D6*, is highly polymorphic, where the **1* allele is the wild-type allele resulting in normal enzyme activity (i.e. extensive metabolizers [EM]), while **3*, **4*, and **5* result in null enzyme activity (i.e. poor metabolizers [PM]), and the **9*, **10*, and **17* alleles result in reduced enzyme activity (i.e. intermediate metabolizers [IM]). Patients with multiple copies of the functional allele are considered ultrarapid metabolizers (UM). The most common variant allele, **4*, is present in roughly 18% of Caucasians, moderately present in African Americans (7-9%), and rarely present in Asians (<1%) (Jin et al., 2005). The intermediate **10* allele is present in 40% of patients of Japanese origin, while the **17* allele is present in about 25% of patients of African origin (Bradford, 2002; Jin et al., 2005).

A retrospective cohort study of over 1300 patients demonstrated higher recurrence rates for PMs and IMs compared to EMs (29% and 20.9% vs. 14.9%, respectively) (Schroth et al., 2009). Subsequently, a prospective, genotype-guided study demonstrated a significant increase in endoxifen exposure in PMs/IMs as the dose was increased from 20 mg to 40 mg daily. While a significant difference in endoxifen levels was observed between EMs and IMs at the standard dose, this difference was diminished after doubling the dose in IMs, whereas concentrations in PMs were still significantly lower compared to IMs/EMs even at the 40 mg dose (Irvin et al., 2011). The influence of endoxifen exposure on response was not addressed in this study, limiting the clinical translation of these findings on breast cancer recurrence. However, studies have demonstrated that patients with the lowest endoxifen concentrations have the highest risk of relapse, suggesting that a therapeutic threshold may be needed for optimal benefit (Madlensky et al., 2011; Saladores et al., 2014). This data further implies that PMs and IMs may be unable to achieve this therapeutic threshold at standard tamoxifen doses.

Controversy exists on the clinical utility of *CYP2D6* testing as two of the largest studies investigating the *CYP2D6*-tamoxifen relationship and breast cancer recurrence demonstrated no association between genotype and recurrence rates (Rae et al., 2012; Regan et al., 2012); however, flaws in the genomic study design, such as use of tumor DNA as opposed to germ-line DNA, have been noted by pharmacogenetic experts (Nakamura et al., 2012). Subsequently, Rae et al. identified concordance rates >95% between

CYP2D6 genotypes obtained from tumor-derived and germ-line DNA from 122 breast cancer patients (Rae et al., 2013). Alternatively, Goetz et al. genotyped nearly 1200 breast tumor samples and demonstrated loss of heterozygosity (LOH) in over a third of samples, while also documenting that non-malignant tissue did not exhibit LOH (Goetz et al., 2015). Investigators also reported that while there was approximately 20% discordance between tumor and buccal cell genotypes, there was 100% concordance between non-malignant and buccal cell genotypes (Goetz et al., 2015), suggesting that breast tumor tissue should not be used to genotype for *CYP2D6* and may result in false genotypes. Lastly, the development of oral endoxifen may bypass the pharmacogenetic issues presented (Ahmad, Ali, Ahmad, Sheikh, & Ahmad, 2010). Advocates of *CYP2D6* genetic testing indicate that until prospective, adjuvant trial data is available, the current evidence is sufficient to accept the *CYP2D6*-tamoxifen pharmacogenetic relationship in postmenopausal women (Brauch et al., 2013); however, the appropriate dose adjustment and ultimate impact on breast cancer recurrence appear to be unclear.

DPYD and 5-Fluorouracil

Dihydropyrimidine dehydrogenase (DPD), the rate-limiting enzyme involved in the metabolism of 5-fluorouracil (5-FU) to 5,6-dihydrofluorouracil, has been shown to exhibit polymorphic potential (Toffoli & Cecchin, 2007). Given that 80% of 5-FU is metabolized by DPD, a loss of enzyme activity has the potential to extend the half-life of 5-FU by up to 100-fold, enhancing the prolonged cytotoxic effect of the agent, including side effects such as severe neutropenia and diarrhea. However, the frequency of null enzyme activity is very low at <1%, while about 5-7% have intermediate enzyme activity (Saif, Ezzeldin, Vance, Sellers, & Diasio, 2007). More than 30 variants of *DPYD*, the gene coding for DPD, have been identified and result in functional changes in enzyme activity (Van Kuilenburg, Meinsma, Zoetekouw, & Van Gennip, 2002). The polymorphic variant most commonly associated with DPD deficiency is a splice-site mutation, *IV14+1G>A* (also referred to as *DPYD*2A*), located on the exon 14-flanking region and causing skipping of 165 base pairs (Toffoli & Cecchin, 2007).

In a multicenter trial, approximately 700 patients with various cancers and treated with 5-FU were genotyped for *DPYD*. Investigators observed a positive predictive value of 0.46 for overall toxicity in patients carrying the *DPYD*2A* variant; however, of interest was a gene/sex-interaction resulting in an OR for overall toxicity of 41.8 ($P<0.0001$) for male patients but only 1.33 ($P>0.05$) for female patients (Schwab et al., 2008). A smaller study demonstrated that 60% of 60 patients who had experienced severe 5-FU-related toxicity had decreased DPD enzyme activity, independently of genotype (Van Kuilenburg, Meinsma, Zoetekouw, & Van Gennip, 2002). In a prospective genotype-guided clinical trial, investigators administered an initial 5-FU dose reduction of $\geq$ 50% with subsequent dose titration based on clinical tolerance in CRC patients carrying the *DPYD*2A* allele. Safety was compared with 45 historical *DPYD*2A* controls having administered 5-FU at the full dose. Of 1,700 patients screened, only 17 were heterozygous for the variant allele. Results demonstrated that the risk of grade $\geq$ 3 toxicity was reduced from 68% in historical controls to 15% and drug-induced death was reduced from 10 to 0% in patients receiving genotype-guided dosing. Furthermore, 5-FU exposure in *DPYD*2A* carriers at reduced doses was comparable to fully dosed non-carriers, supporting the role of genotype-guided therapy to decrease drug toxicity (M.J. Deenen et al., 2011). Most recently, a systematic review of candidate genes associated with capecitabine (the oral prodrug of 5-FU) toxicity in 927 CRC patients demonstrated that global toxicity was associated with the *DPYD* alleles *2846T>A* and **2A* (combined OR, 5.51; P = 0.0013) (Rosmarin et al., 2014).

Based on the available literature, it is evident that patients with *DPYD* variants (or DPD deficiency) are at an increased risk of 5-FU induced toxicity; however, measuring catalytic DPD activity in peripheral blood mononuclear cells is challenging. Standardized cut-offs for deficient DPD activity are not readily available and different laboratories may use different thresholds for activity (Yen & McLeod, 2007). Furthermore, there are implications on cost and resources as the minor allele frequency is very low resulting in a high number of patients needed to screen to prove a beneficial impact on reducing toxicity. Additionally, experimental protocols for genotyping are often laborious, intensive and limit the number of patients who can be tested (Yen & McLeod, 2007), ultimately limiting the utility of genetic testing in clinical practice. Nonetheless, the Clinical Pharmacogenetics Implementation Consortium (CPIC) guidelines provide recommendations for dosing based on DPD enzyme activity: patients with normal enzyme activity require no dose adjustment; patients with decreased enzyme activity require at least a 50% dose reduction, followed by titration of dose based on toxicity or exposure, and patients with complete enzyme deficiency should receive an alternative drug (Caudle et al., 2013).

TPMT and 6-Mercaptopurine

Thiopurine-S-methyltransferase (TPMT) is a cytosolic enzyme ubiquitously expressed in the human body and catalyzes the S-methylation of thiopurines, including 6-mercaptopurine (6-MP), into inactive compounds. 6-MP is one of the backbone agents used to treat ALL in both children and adults. It inhibits the formation of purine ribonucleotides, ultimately leading to cell death (McLeod, Lin, Scott, Pui, & Evans, 1994). Severe hematological toxicity, including myelosuppression, is the most common adverse effect associated with 6-MP (McLeod, Krynetski, Relling, & Evans, 2000). The *TPMT* locus is subject to genetic polymorphisms with roughly 6-11% of the population being heterozygous and 0.2%-0.6% being homozygous for the variant allele. *TPMT *2* and **3* alleles account for approximately 95% of the defective TPMT activity (Stanulla et al., 2005). The risk of myelosuppression is significantly elevated in patients who harbor *TPMT* genetic variants, given elevated circulating thioguanine nucleotide levels (Stanulla et al., 2005).

A study of 180 children with ALL treated with a 6-MP-based regimen demonstrated that wild-type, heterozygous, and homozygous-deficient patients were able to tolerate the full dose of 6-MP for 84%, 65%, and 7%, of the total weeks of therapy, respectively. Additionally, a statistically significant inverse relationship between thioguanine nucleotide concentrations and *TPMT* was observed, with an average concentration (pmol/8 $\times$ 10^8 erythrocytes) of 417, 963, and 3,565 in *TPMT* homozygous wild type, heterozygous, and homozygous deficient patients, respectively (Relling et al., 1999). In a prospective study, investigators determined that the OR for patients with at least one variant allele and receiving a 30-70% dose reduction based on genotype was 1.30 (equivalent to the risk seen in wild type patients receiving full dose 6-MP), whereas the OR of toxicity for patients with at least one variant allele and receiving standard 6-MP dosages (no dose adjustment for genotype) was 4.0 (Stocco et al., 2009). In a comprehensive phenotype-genotype study of 1214 healthy volunteers, investigators identified a clearly defined trimodal distribution of TPMT activity with 0.6% deficient, 9.9% intermediate and 89.5% normal to high. Four novel variants were identified resulting in 17 individuals with intermediate TPMT activity discordant to genotype. Taking these variants into account, the overall concordance rate between genotype and phenotype was 98.4% (Schaeffeler et al., 2004).

Given the available data, *TPMT* genetic testing is routinely utilized to identify ALL patients with defective enzyme activity (Relling et al., 2011). CPIC guidelines recommend an initial 10-fold dose reduction of 6-MP in patients with two inactive alleles and reduced doses (30-70% of the full dose) in heterozygous patients (Relling et al., 2013).

TYMS and 5-Fluorouracil

Thymidylate synthase (TS), a critical enzyme involved in DNA synthesis, serves as the primary target of 5-FU. *TYMS*, the gene coding for TS, contains 28-base pair tandem repeat units found in the 5' untranslated region (UTR), acting as an enhancer to the *TYMS* promoter (Toffoli & Cecchin, 2007). As 5-FU is involved with the inhibition of TS, low *TYMS* expression induced by *TYMS 2R* (two repeats) or the 6-base pair (bp) deletion in the *TYMS* 3'-UTR would subsequently increase the cytotoxic effects of 5-FU, whereas high expression induced by *TYMS 3R* (three repeats) or 6-bp insertion in the 3'-UTR would decrease the efficacy of 5-FU [73].Approximately 25% of European patients are homozygous for *TYMS 3R/3R*, 20% are homozygous for *2R/2R*, and 55% are heterozygous for *2R/3R*.

In a study of 65 patients with rectal cancer treated with 5-FU-based preoperative chemoradiotherapy, patients harboring the *TYMS 3R/3R* genotype achieved a 22% down-staging rate, whereas *2R/2R* patients achieved a 60% down-staging rate (Villafranca et al., 2001). In a genotype-guided clinical trial of 135 patients with rectal cancer, investigators administered 5-FU chemoradiation plus irinotecan to patients with the *TYMS 3R/3R* or *3R/4R* genotypes, i.e. the poor-risk group (27.4%), and administered standard 5-FU chemoradiation alone to those with *2R/2R, 2R/3R*, and *2R/4R*, i.e. the good-risk group (72.6%). Down-staging and complete tumor response rates were 64.4% and 20% for good risk and 64.5% and 42% for poor-risk patients, respectively, suggesting that the addition of irinotecan may help overcome 5-FU resistance. However, the addition of irinotecan in good risk patients was not addressed (Tan et al., 2011). Lastly, in a large analysis of 927 colorectal cancer patients treated with capecitabine or another 5-FU-based regimen, investigators identified that global toxicity (grades 0/1/2 vs. grades 3/4/5) was associated with the common polymorphisms *TYMS 2R/3R* and *3'UTR 6bp ins-del* (combined OR, 1.31; $P = 9.4 \times 10^{-5}$) (Rosmarin et al., 2014). A large number of studies support the association between *TYMS* and 5-FU response/toxicity (Patel, Fuchs, Owzar, Chen, & McLeod, 2013); however, a paucity of prospective, interventional clinical trials exists, owing to the current lack of clinical utility. Despite availability of clinical assays, large prospective, interventional trials are warranted to confirm *TYMS* as a predictive biomarker for 5-FU therapy.

UGT1A1 and Irinotecan

Uridine diphosphate glucuronosyltransferase 1A1 (UGT1A1) conjugates SN-38, the active component of irinotecan, a topoisomerase I inhibitor, to a glucuronide inactive metabolite, SN-38G. More than 60 polymorphisms in *UGT1A1* have been identified, most of which result in TA (thymine-adenine) repeats in the promoter region of the gene. The wild type allele is referred to as *UGT1A1*1*, while the most common and studied variant, *UGT1A1*28*, results in up to a 70% reduction in enzyme activity (other less frequent variants include **6*, **60*, and **93*). The frequency of the **28* allele is 39% in patients of European, 16% of Asian, and 43% of African origins. Roughly 10–20% of Caucasians and African Americans are homozygous for **28*, while less than 5% of Asians are homozygous for **28* (Perera, Innocenti, & Ratain, 2008). A meta-analysis demonstrated a significant increase in grade 3/4 neutropenia for **28/*28* patients at medium (150-250 mg/m^2) and high doses (>250 mg/m^2) (OR=3.22, P=0.008 and OR=27.8,

P=0.005, respectively) (Hoskins, Goldberg, Qu, Ibrahim, & McLeod, 2007). The current U.S. FDA approved package insert includes the *UGT1A1 *28/*28* genotype as a risk factor for severe neutropenia.

Given the genetic basis for irinotecan intolerance, investigators performed a prospective, genotype-guided phase I study in metastatic colorectal cancer patients receiving FOLFIRI. Patients were stratified by *UGT1A1* genotype and received dose escalations to the maximum tolerated dose (MTD). Results demonstrated that the MTDs of irinotecan were 370 and 310 mg/m^2 in **1/*1* and **1/*28*, respectively, suggesting higher tolerable doses in wild-type and heterozygous patients compared to the standard 180 mg/m^2 dose currently administered to all patients as part of the routine FOLFIRI regimen (Toffoli et al., 2010). A subsequent and similar genotype-guided dose escalation study determined the MTD to be 390, 340, and 150 mg/m^2 in **1/*1*, **1/*28*, and **28/*28*, respectively (Marcuello et al., 2011). Although not powered to detect differences in clinical outcome, the first study identified a significantly higher response rate in patients treated at doses ≥ MTD vs. those treated at doses < MTD (65% vs. 25%; P<0.05) (Toffoli et al., 2010). Similarly, the second study demonstrated significantly higher response rates in patients treated at ≥ 260 mg/m^2 (median dose) compared to those receiving < 260 mg/m^2 (67% vs. 24%; P<0.05), in addition to a significant difference in time to disease progression (16 vs. 7 months, respectively; P<0.05) (Marcuello et al., 2011). A similar trial of patients receiving irinotecan monotherapy demonstrated fixed MTDs of 850 mg, 700 mg, and 400 mg in **1/*1*, **1/*28* and **28/*28* patients. Interestingly, at the MTD for each genotype, dosing by genotype resulted in similar SN-38 areas under the curve (AUCs; r^2 = 0.0003; P=0.97), while the irinotecan AUC was correlated with the actual dose (r^2 = 0.39; P<0.001) (Innocenti et al., 2014).

While it is evident that *UGT1A1 *28/*28* patients are at an increased risk of toxicity and dose reduction to ≤150 mg/m^2 in these patients is appropriate, the optimal irinotecan dose in **1/*1* and **1/*28* patients is unknown and is currently under investigation in a phase II genotype-guided study of irinotecan dosing in metastatic CRC patients receiving FOLFIRI plus bevacizumab (Clinicaltrials.gov: NCT02138617).

SUPPORTIVE CARE PHARMACOGENETIC BIOMARKERS

Antidepressants

Antidepressant drugs are widely prescribed to cancer patients to treat depression and anxiety disorders, however, only one-third of these patients exhibit a beneficial therapeutic response (Rush et al., 2006). Potential reasons for lack of drug response include clinical heterogeneity, diagnostic uncertainty, environmental and social factors, and genetic factors.

The heterogenous response to antidepressant drugs, particularly tricyclic antidepressants (TCAs) and selective serotonin reuptake inhibitors (SSRIs), may be in part due to differences in cytochrome P450 activity, by which the majority of antidepressants are metabolized by. The main enzymes involved in antidepressant drug metabolism are CYP2D6, CYP2C9, CYP2C19, CYP3A4 and CYP1A2, with CYP2D6 involved in the metabolism of approximately half of the commonly prescribed psychotropic drugs (Staddon, Arranz, Mancama, Mata, & Kerwin, 2002). Studies with nortriptyline showed that *CYP2D6* poor metabolizers (PMs) reached therapeutic plasma levels with initial starting doses, whereas escalated doses would result in a higher risk of toxicity. Alternatively, patients with functional (extensive metabolizers [EMs]) or ultra-rapid metabolizer (UM) phenotypes required higher doses to reach therapeutic plasma levels (Bertilsson, Dahl, Dalen, & Al-Shurbaji, 2002). Another study also identified an association between *CYP2D6* genotype and plasma level concentrations of venlafaxine, however, did not find any such association for desvenlafaxine. When subjects received venlafaxine 75 mg, the area under the concentration-time curve (AUC) and maximum concentration (Cmax) of O-desmethylvenlafaxine (the primary active metabolite) were 445% and 434% higher, respectively, in *CYP2D6* EMs compared with PMs ($P \leq 0.001$) (Nichols, Focht, Jiang, Preskorn, & Kane, 2011).

Variations in the *CYP2C19* gene have also been shown to be associated with antidepressant response, including citalopram, imipramine and clomipramine. Additionally, tertiary amines (e.g. amitriptyline) are mainly metabolized by CYP2C19 to desmethyl metabolites (e.g., nortriptyline). Therefore, variations in CYP2C19 metabolism may modulate antidepressant activity and side effects through the pharmacological actions of the tertiary amines. Serotonin reuptake inhibition has been shown to be more pronounced in *CYP2C19* PMs due to the decreased conversion to nortriptyline (Hicks et al., 2013). In addition, *CYP2C19* alleles have been shown to affect escitalopram metabolism (Jin et al., 2010; Noehr-Jensen et al., 2009) including a positive association in the European consortium project Genome-Based Therapeutic Drugs for Depression (GENDEP) (Huezo-Diaz et al., 2012). Investigators identified that those homozygous for the *CYP2C19*17* allele (UM phenotype) had a significantly lower mean escitalopram concentrations (approximately 2-fold, $P = 0.0001$) and a higher mean metabolic ratio ($P = 0.0003$) than EMs, while those homozygous for alleles conferring the PM phenotype had a higher mean escitalopram concentration than EMs (1.55-fold, $P = 0.008$). Furthermore, the side-effect profile of amitriptyline appears to be dependent on a combination of alleles coding for *CYP2D6* and *CYP2C19* (Huezo-Diaz et al., 2012).

A larger analysis combined samples from four studies and found an association between *CYP2D6* alleles and treatment response to venlafaxine (Lobello et al., 2010). Specifically, investigators identified that, compared with PMs, EMs had significantly greater mean changes from baseline on 4 of 5 depression rating scales (all 4 comparisons, $P \leq .020$) and a greater percentage experiencing response or remission ($P \leq .015$) (Lobello et al., 2010). However, other studies have found no such association for either *CYP2D6* or *CYP2C19* alleles (Grasmader et al., 2004; Serretti et al., 2009). Particularly, an analysis in the large STAR*D sample set did not find an association with either *CYP2D6* or *CYP2C19* and response to citalopram (Fava et al., 2003). As a result, the clinical translation and use of these genes in practice has been limited and larger prospective studies are needed to fully elucidate these effects. Nonetheless, CPIC guidelines provide dosing recommendations for amitriptyline, desipramine, doxepin, imipramine, nortriptyline and trimipramine (see https://www.pharmgkb.org/page/cpic). Other genetic determinants of response to antidepressant therapies include variations in p-glycoprotein, monoamine metabolic enzymes, 5-HT genes, dopamine genes, and norepinephrine genes; however, these have not been validated and further research is needed to elucidate the role of these genes in response to therapy (Narasimhan & Lohoff, 2012).

Antiemetics

Chemotherapy-induced nausea and vomiting (CINV) is one of the most debilitating adverse drug effects experienced by patients treated with cytotoxic chemotherapy (Blower, 2002; Rojas & Slusher, 2012). Ineffective CINV control occurs in ≥ 25% of all cancer patients despite antiemetic administration (Feyer & Jordan, 2011). Three classes of medications are considered standard to treat CINV: 5-hydroxytryptamine (5HT; serotonin) type 3 (5HT3) receptor antagonists (5HT3-RAs), neurokinin 1 receptor antagonists, and corticosteroids (Basch et al., 2011; Roila et al., 2010). Variability in emetic control with 5HT3-RAs has resulted in the examination of the genetic variance in 5HT3 receptor subunits, genetic differences in cytochrome P450 metabolism of the various 5HT3-RAs, and polymorphisms associated with drug transporters (Blower, 2002; Fasching et al., 2008; Tremblay et al., 2003; Yaakob, Malone, Exintaris, & Irving, 2011).

The five subunits that make up the 5HT3 receptor pentamer have been identified as 5HT3A, 5HT3B, 5HT3C, 5HT3D, and 5HT3E (Bruss et al., 2000; Krzywkowski, Jensen, Connolly, & Brauner-Osborne, 2007; Yaakob, Malone, Exintaris, & Irving, 2011). The subunits and the genes coding for them have become the target of studies of genetic variation to explain suboptimal control with 5HT3-RAs (de Wit, Aapro, & Blower, 2005; Gandara et al., 1998; Machu, 2011; Ward, Kotasek, & McKinnon, 2008; Yaakob, Malone, Exintaris, & Irving, 2011). A study demonstrated that patients who were homozygous for the polymorphism, -100_-120delAAG promoter region deletion in the start codon of 5HT3B, had a much higher frequency of vomiting than other patients (Tremblay et al., 2003). Multivariate analysis further identified that poor CINV control associated with the deletion was not due to the level of chemotherapeutic emetic risk or co-administered medications (Tremblay et al., 2003). Another study assessed 5HT3C receptor gene polymorphisms and CINV incidence post ondansetron and dexamethasone administration in 110 breast cancer patients treated with anthracyclines. Results identified a SNP in the gene *K163N*, which was associated with increased incidence of poorly controlled CINV in 50% of *CC* homozygous patients (P=0.009) as compared with 22% of *AA* or *AC* patients (Fasching et al., 2008). The clinical implications of the genetic variability within the individual subunits of the 5HT3 receptor remain to be seen. Using genetic variations in 5HT3 receptors to predict efficacy from 5HT3-RAs is limited owing to the need for validation across larger and more diverse populations. The 3C, 3D, and 3E subunits have failed to produce any statistically significant variations that could impact clinical decision making.

CYP2D6 is notable as a major metabolic pathway for several of the 5HT3-RAs. The 5HT3-RAs ondansetron, palonosetron, tropisetron, and dolasetron rely on CYP2D6 metabolism in differing degrees, whereas granisetron does not rely on CYP2D6 metabolism. Therefore, the identification of a patient's *CYP2D6* phenotype may help guide clinician choices in antiemetic therapy. The weakest control of CINV with 5HT3-RAs is seen in the UM population who rapidly metabolize these medications resulting in loss of efficacy (de Wit, Aapro, & Blower, 2005; Ingelman-Sundberg, 2004; Tzvetkov et al., 2012). A study reported that UM patients had a significantly higher mean number of vomiting episodes compared to IMs, PMs, and EMs receiving cyclophosphamide, cisplatin, or carboplatin (2.3 ± 2.5 vs 0.2 ± 1.0 (P<0.001) episodes of vomiting, respectively). In addition, UM patients have experienced severe nausea despite use of ondansetron or tropisetron (Kaiser et al., 2002). Other antiemetic options remain for suspected UM patients with poor CINV control. Granisetron is the only 5HT3-RA that does not involve CYP2D6 in its metabolism; thus, conferring a reasonable option in a suspected UM patient (Bloomer et al., 1994), in addition to other antiemetics such as dexamethasone, lorazepam, prochlorperazine, etc.

Lastly, the ATP-binding cassette subfamily B member 1 (ABCB1) transporter (also known as p-glycoprotein, a multi-drug-resistant protein) functions as an efflux pump for a variety of substances, including ondansetron (Babaoglu et al., 2005; Ishikawa, Hirano, Onishi, Sakurai, & Tarui, 2004). Given that ABCB1 is thought to be an active component of the blood brain barrier, the potential of genetic variations to influence antiemetic activity is of importance. The *ABCB1 3435C>T* variant has been correlated with significantly reduced expression of ABCB1, resulting in increasing concentrations of medications that require ABCB1 for drug efflux (Babaoglu et al., 2005; Ishikawa, Hirano, Onishi, Sakurai, & Tarui, 2004). A study demonstrated that 93%, 48% and 56% of patients who were treated with granisetron and were homozygous for the *TT*, *CT* and *CC* genotypes, for the *3435C>T* variant experienced a significantly higher rate of CINV control (P<0.05), respectively. The presence of the *3435*

C>T variant did not significantly improve CINV control in the ondansetron group, and had no effect in the tropisetron group (Babaoglu et al., 2005). Lastly, a study of 215 children with acute myeloid leukemia (AML) treated with high-dose cytarabine and pre- and post-chemotherapy ondansetron identified a significant association between *ABCB1* polymorphisms and antiemetic efficacy in the acute phase, but not in the delayed phase (He et al., 2014). Specifically, the *CG* haplotype (*C3435T* and *G2677T*) was associated with a higher risk of grade 3/4 nausea and vomiting (P=0.003 and P= 0.026, respectively). After adjustment for patient-specific clinical factors in a multivariate analysis, the *CG* haplotype was identified as a predictive marker of grade 3/4 CINV (P = 0.003 and P = 0.039, respectively). In addition, a significant association between the *3435CC* genotype and grade 3/4 vomiting in AML patients was observed (P = 0.016) (He et al., 2014).

Although polymorphisms exist that may explain variability in 5HT3-RA efficacy, the only current clinically actionable gene may be *CYP2D6*, given the test is readily available in practice and may be used to guide 5HT3-RA regimen choices. Further prospective studies are needed to replicate remaining polymorphisms, such as those in the 5HT3 receptor and drug transporters (i.e. ABCB1).

Opioids

CYP2D6 is the primary metabolic enzyme responsible for the activation of weaker opioids (codeine, tramadol, oxycodone and hydrocodone) into stronger opioids (morphine, o-desmethyltramadol, oxymorphone and hydromorphone, respectively). As mentioned previously, the **3*, **4*, and **5* alleles account for approximately 95% of the poor metabolizer (PM) phenotype, while multiple copies of a functional allele result in the ultra-rapid metabolizer (UM) phenotype (most often occurring with **1* or **2* duplications) (Bernard, Neville, Nguyen, & Flockhart, 2006).

Codeine and tramadol rely almost exclusively on CYP2D6 for activation to their active metabolites, morphine and O-desmethyltramadol, respectively. The clinical analgesic effect of codeine is mainly attributed to its conversion to morphine, which has a 200 times higher affinity and 50 times higher intrinsic activity at the mu-opioid receptor than codeine itself (Mignat, Wille, & Ziegler, 1995). Case reports of codeine fatalities in *CYP2D6* UMs (Ciszkowski, Madadi, Phillips, Lauwers, & Koren, 2009; Gasche et al., 2004; Koren, Cairns, Chitayat, Gaedigk, & Leeder, 2006; Madadi et al., 2011; Madadi et al., 2010; Madadi & Koren, 2008) resulted in a black box warning being issued in 2013, stating that codeine use in certain children with the UM phenotype may result in life-threatening adverse events or death. As a result, several U.S. institutions require preemptive *CYP2D6* genotyping prior to codeine administration. Similarly, a case report of tramadol-induced respiratory depression was reported in a UM patient who also had renal impairment (Stamer, Stuber, Muders, & Musshoff, 2008). Alternatively, it has been demonstrated that the analgesic activity of tramadol in PM patients is significantly reduced (Musshoff, Madea, Stuber, & Stamer, 2006; Stamer et al., 2003; Stamer et al., 2007; Stamer, Stuber, Muders, & Musshoff, 2008). In a prospective study of nearly 300 patients recovering from abdominal surgery, the percentage of non-responders was significantly higher in the PM group (46.7%) compared with the EM group (21.6%; p=0.005) (Stamer et al., 2003).

Oxycodone and hydrocodone are metabolized by CYP2D6 to more potent metabolites, oxymorphone and hydromorphone, respectively, and by CYP3A4 to inactive metabolites, noroxycodone and norhydrocodone (Stauble et al., 2014). In one study, *CYP2D6* PMs required significantly larger cumulative oxycodone doses for equianalgesic effect compared to EMs (25 mg vs. 16 mg; P=0.005) (Stamer et al., 2013). Similarly, a study showed that PMs achieved 8-fold lower hydromorphone concentrations vs.

UMs, which significantly correlated with pain relief (Stauble et al., 2014). Another study demonstrated that *CYP2D6* UMs experienced 40% higher pain tolerance thresholds compared to EMs, while PMs had a 20-30-fold lower pain tolerance compared to EM/IMs (Samer et al., 2010). Furthermore, drug-gene and drug-drug interactions may overlap, resulting in additive effects on drug disposition and ultimately therapeutic response and/or toxicity.

Catechol-O-methyltransferase (COMT) is responsible for the inactivation of catecholamines (dopamine, adrenaline and norepinephrine), which are involved in pain modulation. As a result, genetic variability in *COMT* can contribute to pain sensitivity. It has been shown that a common variant allele (*1947G>A*) (allele frequency 48%) results in a three- to four-fold reduction in COMT enzyme activity (Lotta et al., 1995). A study of 207 Caucasian cancer patients demonstrated that patients with the *GG* genotype required significantly more morphine (155 mg/24 hours) compared to *AG* (117 mg/24 hours) and *AA* genotypes (95 mg/ 24 hours) ($P<0.05$) (Rakvag et al., 2005).

Lastly, the mu-opioid receptor, the primary site of action of opioids, is encoded by the gene opioid receptor-like 1 (*OPRM1*). The *OPRM1 118A>G* polymorphism (allele frequency 8-17%) results in less effective opioid analgesia. One study demonstrated that cancer patients with the *GG* genotype required higher morphine doses for pain relief compared to *AA* patients (Klepstad et al., 2004). Another study showed that patients undergoing total knee arthroplasty with the *GG* genotype consumed approximately 60% more morphine than patients who were heterozygous or homozygous wild-type (Chou et al., 2006).

CPIC guidelines (Crews et al., 2014) provide pharmacogenetic-based dosing recommendations for codeine, while the Dutch Pharmacogenetics Working Group (DPWG) (Samer, Lorenzini, Rollason, Daali, & Desmeules, 2013) provides guidelines for codeine, oxycodone and tramadol (amongst other classes of drugs metabolized by CYP2D6, such as antidepressants). Understanding genetic variations in *CYP2D6*, *COMT* and *OPRM1* may allow for better analgesia selection and dosing.

Voriconazole

Voriconazole is a triazole antifungal agent commonly used to treat and prevent invasive fungal infections (IFIs) in patients undergoing allogeneic hematopoietic stem cell transplant (HSCT) and other hematological conditions. The half-life of voriconazole is estimated to be approximately 6 to 9 hours; however, this may be highly variable due to the drug's non-linear saturable pharmacokinetics, which results in high inter-patient variability in exposure. Voriconazole steady state concentrations are estimated to reach at 5-7 days, with an optimal therapeutic concentration of 1.0-5.5 mg/L. Overall, only 50% of patients achieve the pre-defined therapeutic range by 5-7 days (Hicheri, Cook, & Cordonnier, 2012; Troke, Hockey, & Hope, 2011), while as many as 50% of patients treated with prophylactic doses of 200 mg twice daily have sub-therapeutic levels (<1.0 mg/L) (Trifilio et al., 2007).

Therapeutic drug monitoring (TDM) of voriconazole is useful due to unpredictable pharmacokinetics, the drug's narrow therapeutic index, and serum concentrations that are associated with both efficacy and toxicity (Troke, Hockey, & Hope, 2011). Furthermore, drug interactions and genetic polymorphisms in *CYP2C19,* the gene coding for the drug metabolizing enzyme of voriconazole which inactivates the parent compound, have an effect on serum concentrations (Mikus, Scholz, & Weiss, 2011). Sub-therapeutic voriconazole trough concentrations (<1.0 mg/L) have been associated with therapeutic failure (Hamada, Seto, Yago, & Kuroyama, 2012). In a prospective treatment trial, patients randomized to receive TDM-guided dosing had a significantly greater percentage of complete or partial response compared to the non-TDM group (81% vs. 57%, respectively; $P=0.04$) (Park et al., 2012). However, another study demonstrated a significant association between IFI-related mortality and initial trough concentrations ≤0.35 mg/L at day 5 (OR 11.0; P=0.004), even when TDM was subsequently utilized to target a therapeutic concentration, suggesting TDM alone may have limitations such as low initial trough concentrations and better methods of preemptive dose individualization are warranted (Miyakis, van Hal, Ray, & Marriott, 2010).

The greatest risk of voriconazole failure due to inadequate drug concentrations is in *CYP2C19 *1/*17* and **17/*17* UMs who rapidly inactivate voriconazole (Hamada, Seto, Yago, & Kuroyama, 2012; Hassan et al., 2011; Hicks et al., 2014; Owusu Obeng, Egelund, Alsultan, Peloquin, & Johnson, 2014; Pieper et al., 2012; Wang et al., 2014). *CYP2C19 *1/*1* (extensive metabolizer; EM) patients are expected to metabolize voriconazole normally, whereas patients homozygous for **2* and/or **3* are considered PMs and may achieve higher voriconazole concentrations (although the correlation between high concentrations and toxicity is inconsistent, and toxicity is often reversible). The frequency of UMs, EMs, IMs and PMs in the European population is approximately 31%, 42%, 19% and 3%, respectively (Owusu Obeng, Egelund, Alsultan, Peloquin, & Johnson, 2014). A study demonstrated that nearly 20% of 747 routine TDM samples had voriconazole concentrations ≤0.2 mg/L, and 80% of subjects with these sub-therapeutic concentrations harbored at least one *CYP2C19*17* allele (Hassan et al., 2011). Therefore, the greatest concern for voriconazole is sub-therapeutic concentrations in UM patients. A population pharmacokinetic model was used to simulate various dosage regimens in order to optimize therapeutic dosing according to *CYP2C19* status and found that voriconazole dosed 200 mg by mouth twice daily in PM patients was comparable to 300 mg by mouth twice daily in non-PM patients (Wang et al., 2014). Although there is a paucity of data on the direct influence of *CYP2C19* genotype-guided voriconazole dosing on clinical outcomes, substantial evidence exists to support the relationship between both genotype-exposure and exposure-response (Owusu Obeng, Egelund, Alsultan, Peloquin, & Johnson, 2014). Studies examining the clinical utility of prospective, *CYP2C19*-guided voriconazole dosing are currently underway.

Figure 2. Example of personalized cancer medicine: translating pharmacogenomic results into actionable prescribing decisions

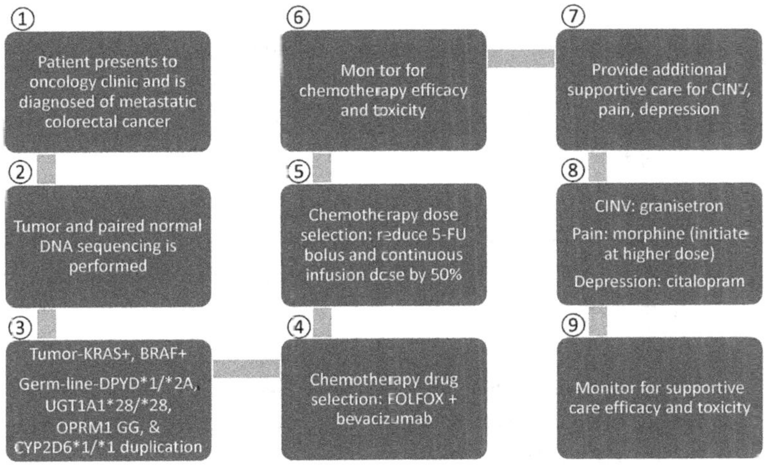

DPYD-dihydropyrimidine dehydrogenase; UGT1A1-uridinediphosphate glucuronosyl transferase 1A1; OPRM1-mu-opioid receptor gene; CYP2D6-cytochrome P450 2D6; 5-FU-5-fluorouracil; FOLFOX- 5-FU, oxaliplatin, leucovorin; CINV-chemotherapy-induced nausea and vomiting;

FUTURE RESEARCH DIRECTIONS

More than 100 drugs approved by the U.S. FDA include pharmacogenetic biomarkers in the drug label, the majority of which are related to cancer therapies. With declining costs and faster turnaround times for next generation sequencing, enormous amounts of molecular data will be generated for each patient. The results from thousands of patients being profiled from around the world will provide critical information on drug-gene associations and clinical outcomes. Future research on clinical implementation of these molecular results will be pivotal in translating molecular profiling from bench to bedside. However, for pharmacogenetic tests to be adopted in clinical practice, it must provide reliable, actionable and predictive information that the clinician would not have otherwise known. Figure 2 summarizes an example of personalized cancer medicine and how a clinician can translate pharmacogenetic test results into actionable prescribing decisions.

[This diagram summarizes how pharmacogenomic information, including both somatic and germ-line, can be used to personalize anticancer and supportive care pharmacotherapy.

1. The patient presents to clinic, a biopsy is obtained, and the pathologist reviews the results with the multidisciplinary team.
2. The patient has confirmed metastatic CRC and both tumor and paired normal DNA are sent for DNA sequencing.
3. Next generation sequencing identifies a KRAS and BRAF mutation in the tumor, in addition to a DPYD, UGT1A1, OPRM1 and CYP2D6 mutation in the germ-line DNA.
4. Because the patients' tumor has a KRAS mutation, EGFR inhibitor therapy is ruled out, and because the patient has a UGT1A1 mutation, they would be at an increased risk for irinotecan-induced toxicity, therefore, FOLFIRI is ruled out. The recommendation is to initiate first-line therapy with FOLFOX plus bevacizumab.
5. Because the patient has a DPYD mutation, the 5-FU bolus and continuous infusion dose are reduced by 50% to avoid excessive toxicity.
6. The patient is closely monitored for drug efficacy and toxicity.]
7. The patient experiences CINV, pain and depression, therefore, supportive care is needed.
8. Given the CYP2D6 duplication, the optimal choice of a serotonin receptor antagonist would be granisetron for CINV, morphine (or another opioid not metabolized by CYP2D6) for pain (consider higher dose due to OPRM1 GG genotype, which confers increased pain sensitivity), and citalopram (or another antidepressant not metabolized by CYP2D6).
9. Finally, monitor closely for supportive care efficacy and toxicity.

Reliance on prospective, randomized controlled clinical trials (RCTs) as the sole method of justifying implementation may not be realistic. While RCTs are generally considered the gold standard, the delay in conducting and interpreting results may potentially deprive patients of life-saving or extending therapies. Initiatives such as the American Society of Oncology's (ASCO) CancerLinq (http://cancerlinq.org/), NCI Match (http://www.cancer.gov/about-cancer/treatment/clinical-trials/nci-supported/nci-match), ASCO's TAPUR study (http://www.asco.org/practice-research/targeted-agent-and-profiling-utilization-registry-study) and other biomarker-driven basket trials will provide critical information to better assign targeted therapies to molecular aberrations and ultimately allow evaluation of clinical outcomes for eventual translation into clinical practice. Furthermore, germ-line DNA from patients enrolled into cancer clinical trials and the drug development process should be exploited to retrospectively discover and validate germ-line pharmacogenetic associations, with subsequent pilot studies to investigate the clinical implementation of promising variants.

CONCLUSION

A concerted effort should be made by researchers and clinicians to implement pharmacogenetic and biomarker-driven therapies in clinical practice. The examples outlined in this chapter provide evidence for the use of both somatic and germ-line DNA to personalize anticancer therapy and supportive care management. As more driver mutations are being discovered and the pharmaceutical industry continues to develop more and more targeted therapies, clinicians must be aware of the molecular mechanisms which perpetuate tumor growth, and an understanding of how molecularly targeted therapies can be effective in slowing or stopping cancer progression. National and institutional treatment pathways should make a focused effort to incorporate molecular profiling and biomarker driven therapies where appropriate, which will allow for the promise of personalized drug delivery in the oncology patient population.

REFERENCES

Ahmad, A., Ali, S. M., Ahmad, M. U., Sheikh, S., & Ahmad, I. (2010). Orally administered endoxifen is a new therapeutic agent for breast cancer. *Breast Cancer Research and Treatment*, *122*(2), 579–584. doi:10.1007/s10549-009-0704-7 PMID:20052538

Amado, R. G., Wolf, M., Peeters, M., Van Cutsem, E., Siena, S., Freeman, D. J., & Chang, D. D. et al. (2008). Wild-type KRAS is required for panitumumab efficacy in patients with metastatic colorectal cancer. *Journal of Clinical Oncology*, *26*(10), 1626–1634. doi:10.1200/JCO.2007.14.7116 PMID:18316791

Arteaga, C. L., Sliwkowski, M. X., Osborne, C. K., Perez, E. A., Puglisi, F., & Gianni, L. (2012). Treatment of HER2-positive breast cancer: Current status and future perspectives.[Review]. *Nature Reviews Clinical Oncology*, *9*(1), 16–32. doi:10.1038/nrclinonc.2011.177 PMID:22124364

Babaoglu, M. O., Bayar, B., Aynacioglu, A. S., Kerb, R., Abali, H., Celik, I., & Bozkurt, A. (2005). Association of the ABCB1 3435C>T polymorphism with antiemetic efficacy of 5-hydroxytryptamine type 3 antagonists. *Clinical Pharmacology and Therapeutics*, *78*(6), 619–626. doi:10.1016/j.clpt.2005.08.015 PMID:16338277

Balachandran, V. P., Cavnar, M. J., Zeng, S., Bamboat, Z. M., Ocuin, L. M., Obaid, H., & DeMatteo, R. P. et al. (2011). Imatinib potentiates antitumor T cell responses in gastrointestinal stromal tumor through the inhibition of Ido. *Nature Medicine*, *17*(9), 1094–1100. doi:10.1038/nm.2438 PMID:21873989

Basch, E., Prestrud, A. A., Hesketh, P. J., Kris, M. G., Feyer, P. C., & Somerfield, M. R. et al. American Society of Clinical, O. (2011). Antiemetics: American Society of Clinical Oncology clinical practice guideline update. *Journal of Clinical Oncology*, *29*(31), 4189–4198. PMID:21947834

Baselga, J., Cortes, J., Kim, S. B., Im, S. A., Hegg, R., Im, Y. H., & Group, C. S. et al. (2012). Pertuzumab plus trastuzumab plus docetaxel for metastatic breast cancer. *The New England Journal of Medicine*, *366*(2), 109–119. doi:10.1056/NEJMoa1113216 PMID:22149875

Bean, J., Brennan, C., Shih, J. Y., Riely, G., Viale, A., Wang, L., & Pao, W. et al. (2007). MET amplification occurs with or without T790M mutations in EGFR mutant lung tumors with acquired resistance to gefitinib or erlotinib. *Proceedings of the National Academy of Sciences of the United States of America*, *104*(52), 20932–20937. doi:10.1073/pnas.0710370104 PMID:18093943

Bennouna, J., Sastre, J., Arnold, D., Osterlund, P., Greil, R., Van Cutsem, E., & Investigators, M. L. S. et al. (2013). Continuation of bevacizumab after first progression in metastatic colorectal cancer (ML18147): A randomised phase 3 trial. *The Lancet Oncology*, *14*(1), 29–37. doi:10.1016/S1470-2045(12)70477-1 PMID:23168366

Bernard, S., Neville, K. A., Nguyen, A. T., & Flockhart, D. A. (2006). Interethnic differences in genetic polymorphisms of CYP2D6 in the U.S. population: Clinical implications. *The Oncologist*, *11*(2), 126–135. doi:10.1634/theoncologist.11-2-126 PMID:16476833

Bertilsson, L., Dahl, M. L., Dalen, P., & Al-Shurbaji, A. (2002). Molecular genetics of CYP2D6: Clinical relevance with focus on psychotropic drugs. *British Journal of Clinical Pharmacology*, *53*(2), 111–122. doi:10.1046/j.0306-5251.2001.01548.x PMID:11851634

Bixby, D., & Talpaz, M. (2009). *Mechanisms of resistance to tyrosine kinase inhibitors in chronic myeloid leukemia and recent therapeutic strategies to overcome resistance*. Hematology American Society of Hematology Education Program.

Bloomer, J. C., Baldwin, S. J., Smith, G. J., Ayrton, A. D., Clarke, S. E., & Chenery, R. J. (1994). Characterisation of the cytochrome P450 enzymes involved in the in vitro metabolism of granisetron. *British Journal of Clinical Pharmacology*, *38*(6), 557–566. doi:10.1111/j.1365-2125.1994.tb04397.x PMID:7888294

Blower, P. R. (2002). 5-HT3-receptor antagonists and the cytochrome P450 system: Clinical implications. *Cancer Journal (Sudbury, Mass.)*, *8*(5), 405–414. doi:10.1097/00130404-200209000-00012 PMID:12416899

Bradford, L. D. (2002). CYP2D6 allele frequency in European Caucasians, Asians, Africans and their descendants. *Pharmacogenomics*, *3*(2), 229–243. doi:10.1517/14622416.3.2.229 PMID:11972444

Brauch, H., Schroth, W., Goetz, M. P., Murdter, T. E., Winter, S., Ingle, J. N., & Eichelbaum, M. et al. (2013). Tamoxifen use in postmenopausal breast cancer: CYP2D6 matters. *Journal of Clinical Oncology*, *31*(2), 176–180. doi:10.1200/JCO.2012.44.6625 PMID:23091108

Bruss, M., Barann, M., Hayer-Zillgen, M., Eucker, T., Gothert, M., & Bonisch, H. (2000). Modified 5-HT3A receptor function by co-expression of alternatively spliced human 5-HT3A receptor isoforms. *Naunyn-Schmiedeberg's Archives of Pharmacology*, *362*(4-5), 392–401. doi:10.1007/s002100000342 PMID:11111833

Caudle, K. E., Thorn, C. F., Klein, T. E., Swen, J. J., McLeod, H. L., Diasio, R. B., & Schwab, M. (2013). Clinical Pharmacogenetics Implementation Consortium guidelines for dihydropyrimidine dehydrogenase genotype and fluoropyrimidine dosing. *Clinical Pharmacology and Therapeutics*, *94*(6), 640–645. doi:10.1038/clpt.2013.172 PMID:23988873

Chapman, P. B., Hauschild, A., Robert, C., Haanen, J. B., Ascierto, P., Larkin, J., & McArthur, G. A. et al. (2011). Improved survival with vemurafenib in melanoma with BRAF V600E mutation. *The New England Journal of Medicine*, *364*(26), 2507–2516. doi:10.1056/NEJMoa1103782 PMID:21639808

Chou, W. Y., Yang, L. C., Lu, H. F., Ko, J. Y., Wang, C. H., Lin, S. H., & Hsu, C. J. et al. (2006). Association of mu-opioid receptor gene polymorphism (A118G) with variations in morphine consumption for analgesia after total knee arthroplasty. *Acta Anaesthesiologica Scandinavica*, *50*(7), 787–792. doi:10.1111/j.1399-6576.2006.01058.x PMID:16879459

Ciszkowski, C., Madadi, P., Phillips, M. S., Lauwers, A. E., & Koren, G. (2009). Codeine, ultrarapid-metabolism genotype, and postoperative death. *The New England Journal of Medicine*, *361*(8), 827–828. doi:10.1056/NEJMc0904266 PMID:19692698

Crews, K. R., Gaedigk, A., Dunnenberger, H. M., Leeder, J. S., Klein, T. E., Caudle, K. E., . . . Skaar, T. C. (2014). Clinical Pharmacogenetics Implementation Consortium Guidelines for Cytochrome P450 2D6 Genotype and Codeine Therapy: 2014 Update. *Clinical Pharmacology and Therapeutics*.

de Klein, A., van Kessel, A. G., Grosveld, G., Bartram, C. R., Hagemeijer, A., Bootsma, D., & Stephenson, J. R. et al. (1982). A cellular oncogene is translocated to the Philadelphia chromosome in chronic myelocytic leukaemia. *Nature*, *300*(5894), 765–767. doi:10.1038/300765a0 PMID:6960256

de Wit, R., Aapro, M., & Blower, P. R. (2005). Is there a pharmacological basis for differences in 5-HT3-receptor antagonist efficacy in refractory patients?. *Cancer Chemotherapy and Pharmacology*, *56*(3), 231–238. doi:10.1007/s00280-005-1033-0 PMID:15838653

Deenen, M. J., Cats, A., Beijnen, J. H., & Schellens, J. H. (2011). Part 1: Background, methodology, and clinical adoption of pharmacogenetics. *The Oncologist*, *16*(6), 811–819. doi:10.1634/theoncologist.2010-0258 PMID:21632456

Deenen, M. J., Cats, A., Sechterberger, M. K., Severens, J. L., Smits, P. H. M., Bakker, R., . . . Schellens, J. H. M. (2011). Safety, pharmacokinetics (PK), and cost effectiveness of upfront genotyping of DPYD in fluoropyrimidine therapy. *Journal of Clinical Oncology, 29*.

Demetri, G. D., Rankin, C.J., Benjamin, R. S., Boreden, E.C., Ryan, C.W., Priebat, D.A., . . . Blanke, C.D. (2014). Long-term disease control of advanced gastrointestinal stromal tumors (GIST) with imatinib (IM): 10-year outcomes from SWOG phase III intergroup trial S0033. *Journal of Clinical Oncology, 32*(5).

Demetri, G. D., Reichardt, P., Kang, Y. K., Blay, J. Y., Rutkowski, P., Gelderblom, H., & Casali, P. G et al.. (2013). Efficacy and safety of regorafenib for advanced gastrointestinal stromal tumours after failure of imatinib and sunitinib (GRID): An international, multicentre, randomised, placebo-controlled, phase 3 trial. *Lancet*, *381*(9863), 295–302. doi:10.1016/S0140-6736(12)61857-1 PMID:23177515

Demetri, G. D., van Oosterom, A. T., Garrett, C. R., Blackstein, M. E., Shah, M. H., Verweij, J., & Casali, P. G. et al. (2006). Efficacy and safety of sunitinib in patients with advanced gastrointestinal stromal tumour after failure of imatinib: A randomised controlled trial. *Lancet, 368*(9544), 1329–1338. doi:10.1016/S0140-6736(06)69446-4 PMID:17046465

Di Nicolantonio, F., Martini, M., Molinari, F., Sartore-Bianchi, A., Arena, S., Saletti, P., & Bardelli, A. et al. (2008). Wild-type BRAF is required for response to panitumumab or cetuximab in metastatic colorectal cancer. *Journal of Clinical Oncology, 26*(35), 5705–5712. doi:10.1200/JCO.2008.18.0786 PMID:19001320

Douillard, J. Y., Oliner, K. S., Siena, S., Tabernero, J., Burkes, R., Barugel, M., & Patterson, S. D. et al. (2013). Panitumumab-FOLFOX4 treatment and RAS mutations in colorectal cancer. *The New England Journal of Medicine, 369*(11), 1023–1034. doi:10.1056/NEJMoa1305275 PMID:24024839

Duad, A., Ribas, A., & Robert, C. (2015). Long-term efficacy of pembrolizumab (pembro; MK-3475) in a pooled analysis of 655 patients (pts) with advanced melanoma (MEL) enrolled in KEYNOTE-001. *Journal of Clinical Oncology.*

Ebos, J. M., Lee, C. R., & Kerbel, R. S. (2009). Tumor and host-mediated pathways of resistance and disease progression in response to antiangiogenic therapy. *Clinical Cancer Research, 15*(16), 5020–5025. doi:10.1158/1078-0432.CCR-09-0095 PMID:19671869

Emile, J. F., Theou, N., Tabone, S., Cortez, A., Terrier, P., Chaumette, M. T., & Lemoine, A. et al. (2004). Clinicopathologic, phenotypic, and genotypic characteristics of gastrointestinal mesenchymal tumors. *Clinical Gastroenterology and Hepatology, 2*(7), 597–605. doi:10.1016/S1542-3565(04)00243-5 PMID:15224284

Fasching, P. A., Kollmannsberger, B., Strissel, P. L., Niesler, B., Engel, J., Kreis, H., & Strick, R. et al. (2008). Polymorphisms in the novel serotonin receptor subunit gene HTR3C show different risks for acute chemotherapy-induced vomiting after anthracycline chemotherapy. *Journal of Cancer Research and Clinical Oncology, 134*(10), 1079–1086. doi:10.1007/s00432-008-0387-1 PMID:18389280

Fava, M., Rush, A. J., Trivedi, M. H., Nierenberg, A. A., Thase, M. E., Sackheim, H. A., & Kupfer, D. J. et al. (2003). Background and rationale for the sequenced treatment alternatives to relieve depression (STAR*D) study. *The Psychiatric Clinics of North America, 26*(2), 457–494. doi:10.1016/S0193-953X(02)00107-7 PMID:12778843

Ferrara, N., Gerber, H. P., & LeCouter, J. (2003). The biology of VEGF and its receptors. *Nature Medicine, 9*(6), 669–676. doi:10.1038/nm0603-669 PMID:12778165

Feyer, P., & Jordan, K. (2011). Update and new trends in antiemetic therapy: The continuing need for novel therapies. *Annals of Oncology, 22*(1), 30–38. doi:10.1093/annonc/mdq600 PMID:20947707

Fielding, A. K. (2011). Current treatment of Philadelphia chromosome-positive acute lymphoblastic leukemia. *Hematology, 2011*(1), 231–237. doi:10.1182/asheducation-2011.1.231 PMID:22160039

Flaherty, K. T., Infante, J. R., Daud, A., Gonzalez, R., Kefford, R. F., Sosman, J., & Weber, J. et al. (2012). Combined BRAF and MEK inhibition in melanoma with BRAF V600 mutations. *The New England Journal of Medicine, 367*(18), 1694–1703. doi:10.1056/NEJMoa1210093 PMID:23020132

Fuchs, C. S., Tomasek, J., Yong, C. J., Dumitru, F., Passalacqua, R., Goswami, C., & Investigators, R. T. et al. (2014). Ramucirumab monotherapy for previously treated advanced gastric or gastro-oesophageal junction adenocarcinoma (REGARD): An international, randomised, multicentre, placebo-controlled, phase 3 trial. *Lancet*, *383*(9911), 31–39. doi:10.1016/S0140-6736(13)61719-5 PMID:24094768

Gandara, D. R., Roila, F., Warr, D., Edelman, M. J., Perez, E. A., & Gralla, R. J. (1998). Consensus proposal for 5HT3 antagonists in the prevention of acute emesis related to highly emetogenic chemotherapy. Dose, schedule, and route of administration. *Supportive Care in Cancer*, *6*(3), 237–243. doi:10.1007/s005200050160 PMID:9629876

Garon, E. B., Ciuleanu, T. E., Arrieta, O., Prabhash, K., Syrigos, K. N., Goksel, T., & Perol, M. et al. (2014). Ramucirumab plus docetaxel versus placebo plus docetaxel for second-line treatment of stage IV non-small-cell lung cancer after disease progression on platinum-based therapy (REVEL): A multicentre, double-blind, randomised phase 3 trial. *Lancet*, *384*(9944), 665–673. doi:10.1016/S0140-6736(14)60845-X PMID:24933332

Gasche, Y., Daali, Y., Fathi, M., Chiappe, A., Cottini, S., Dayer, P., & Desmeules, J. (2004). Codeine intoxication associated with ultrarapid CYP2D6 metabolism. *The New England Journal of Medicine*, *351*(27), 2827–2831. doi:10.1056/NEJMca041888 PMID:15625333

Gerger, A., LaBonte, M., & Lenz, H. J. (2011). Molecular predictors of response to antiangiogenesis therapies. *Cancer Journal (Sudbury, Mass.)*, *17*(2), 134–141. doi:10.1097/PPO.0b013e318212db3c PMID:21427557

Gerlinger, M., Rowan, A. J., Horswell, S., Larkin, J., Endesfelder, D., Gronroos, E., & Swanton, C. et al. (2012). Intratumor heterogeneity and branched evolution revealed by multiregion sequencing. *The New England Journal of Medicine*, *366*(10), 883–892. doi:10.1056/NEJMoa1113205 PMID:22397650

Geyer, C. E., Forster, J., Lindquist, D., Chan, S., Romieu, C. G., Pienkowski, T., & Cameron, D. et al. (2006). Lapatinib plus capecitabine for HER2-positive advanced breast cancer. *The New England Journal of Medicine*, *355*(26), 2733–2743. PMID:17192538

Goetz, M. P., Sun, J. X., Suman, V. J., Silva, G. O., Perou, C. M., Nakamura, Y., & Yelensky, R. et al. (2015). Loss of heterozygosity at the CYP2D6 locus in breast cancer: Implications for germline pharmacogenetic studies. *Journal of the National Cancer Institute*, *107*(2). PMID:25490892

Gorre, M. E., Mohammed, M., Ellwood, K., Hsu, N., Paquette, R., Rao, P. N., & Sawyers, C. L. (2001). Clinical resistance to STI-571 cancer therapy caused by BCR-ABL gene mutation or amplification. *Science*, *293*(5531), 876–880. doi:10.1126/science.1062538 PMID:11423618

Grasmader, K., Verwohlt, P. L., Rietschel, M., Dragicevic, A., Muller, M., Hiemke, C., & Rao, M. L. et al. (2004). Impact of polymorphisms of cytochrome-P450 isoenzymes 2C9, 2C19 and 2D6 on plasma concentrations and clinical effects of antidepressants in a naturalistic clinical setting. *European Journal of Clinical Pharmacology*, *60*(5), 329–336. doi:10.1007/s00228-004-0766-8 PMID:15168101

Hamada, Y., Seto, Y., Yago, K., & Kuroyama, M. (2012). Investigation and threshold of optimum blood concentration of voriconazole: A descriptive statistical meta-analysis. *Journal of Infection and Chemotherapy*, *18*(4), 501–507. doi:10.1007/s10156-011-0363-6 PMID:22231601

Hassan, A., Burhenne, J., Riedel, K. D., Weiss, J., Mikus, G., Haefeli, W. E., & Czock, D. (2011). Modulators of very low voriconazole concentrations in routine therapeutic drug monitoring. *Therapeutic Drug Monitoring, 33*(1), 86–93. doi:10.1097/FTD.0b013e31820530cd PMID:21192313

Hauschild, A., Grob, J. J., Demidov, L. V., Jouary, T., Gutzmer, R., Millward, M., & Chapman, P. B. et al. (2012). Dabrafenib in BRAF-mutated metastatic melanoma: A multicentre, open-label, phase 3 randomised controlled trial. *Lancet, 380*(9839), 358–365. doi:10.1016/S0140-6736(12)60868-X PMID:22735384

He, H., Yin, J. Y., Xu, Y. J., Li, X., Zhang, Y., Liu, Z. G., . . . Liu, Z. Q. (2014). Association of ABCB1 polymorphisms with the efficacy of ondansetron in chemotherapy-induced nausea and vomiting. *Clinical Therapeutics, 36*(8), 1242-1252.

Heinrich, M. C., Corless, C. L., Demetri, G. D., Blanke, C. D., von Mehren, M., Joensuu, H., & Fletcher, J. A. et al. (2003). Kinase mutations and imatinib response in patients with metastatic gastrointestinal stromal tumor. *Journal of Clinical Oncology, 21*(23), 4342–4349. doi:10.1200/JCO.2003.04.190 PMID:14645423

Heisterkamp, N., Stam, K., Groffen, J., de Klein, A., & Grosveld, G. (1985). Structural organization of the bcr gene and its role in the Ph' translocation. *Nature, 315*(6022), 758–761. doi:10.1038/315758a0 PMID:2989703

Herbst, R. S., Ansari, R., Bustin, F., Flynn, P., Hart, L., Otterson, G. A., & Hainsworth, J. et al. (2011). Efficacy of bevacizumab plus erlotinib versus erlotinib alone in advanced non-small-cell lung cancer after failure of standard first-line chemotherapy (BeTa): A double-blind, placebo-controlled, phase 3 trial. *Lancet, 377*(9780), 1846–1854. doi:10.1016/S0140-6736(11)60545-X PMID:21621716

Hicheri, Y., Cook, G., & Cordonnier, C. (2012). Antifungal prophylaxis in haematology patients: The role of voriconazole. *Clinical Microbiology and Infection, 18*(Suppl 2), 1–15. doi:10.1111/j.1469-0691.2012.03772.x PMID:22409648

Hicks, J. K., Crews, K. R., Flynn, P., Haidar, C. E., Daniels, C. C., Yang, W., & Relling, M. V. et al. (2014). Voriconazole plasma concentrations in immunocompromised pediatric patients vary by CYP2C19 diplotypes. *Pharmacogenomics, 15*(8), 1065–1078. doi:10.2217/pgs.14.53 PMID:25084200

Hicks, J. K., Swen, J. J., Thorn, C. F., Sangkuhl, K., Kharasch, E. D., Ellingrod, V. L., & Stingl, J. C. et al. (2013). Clinical Pharmacogenetics Implementation Consortium guideline for CYP2D6 and CYP2C19 genotypes and dosing of tricyclic antidepressants. *Clinical Pharmacology and Therapeutics, 93*(5), 402–408. doi:10.1038/clpt.2013.2 PMID:23486447

Holash, J., Davis, S., Papadopoulos, N., Croll, S. D., Ho, L., Russell, M., & Rudge, J. S. et al. (2002). VEGF-Trap: A VEGF blocker with potent antitumor effects. *Proceedings of the National Academy of Sciences of the United States of America, 99*(17), 11393–11398. doi:10.1073/pnas.172398299 PMID:12177445

Hoskins, J. M., Goldberg, R. M., Qu, P., Ibrahim, J. G., & McLeod, H. L. (2007). UGT1A1*28 genotype and irinotecan-induced neutropenia: Dose matters. *Journal of the National Cancer Institute, 99*(17), 1290–1295. doi:10.1093/jnci/djm115 PMID:17728214

Huezo-Diaz, P., Perroud, N., Spencer, E. P., Smith, R., Sim, S., Virding, S., & Aitchison, K. J. et al. (2012). CYP2C19 genotype predicts steady state escitalopram concentration in GENDEP. *Journal of Psychopharmacology (Oxford, England)*, *26*(3), 398–407. doi:10.1177/0269881111414451 PMID:21926427

Hurvitz, S. A., Dirix, L., Kocsis, J., Bianchi, G. V., Lu, J., Vinholes, J., & Perez, E. A. et al. (2013). Phase II randomized study of trastuzumab emtansine versus trastuzumab plus docetaxel in patients with human epidermal growth factor receptor 2-positive metastatic breast cancer. *Journal of Clinical Oncology*, *31*(9), 1157–1163. doi:10.1200/JCO.2012.44.9694 PMID:23382472

Hurwitz, H. I., Tebbutt, N. C., Kabbinavar, F., Giantonio, B. J., Guan, Z. Z., Mitchell, L., & Tabernero, J. et al. (2013). Efficacy and safety of bevacizumab in metastatic colorectal cancer: Pooled analysis from seven randomized controlled trials. *The Oncologist*, *18*(9), 1004–1012. doi:10.1634/theoncologist.2013-0107 PMID:23881988

Ingelman-Sundberg, M. (2004). Pharmacogenetics of cytochrome P450 and its applications in drug therapy: The past, present and future. *Trends in Pharmacological Sciences*, *25*(4), 193–200. doi:10.1016/j.tips.2004.02.007 PMID:15063083

Innocenti, F., Schilsky, R. L., Ramirez, J., Janisch, L., Undevia, S., House, L. K., & Ratain, M. J. et al. (2014). Dose-finding and pharmacokinetic study to optimize the dosing of irinotecan according to the UGT1A1 genotype of patients with cancer. *Journal of Clinical Oncology*, *32*(22), 2328–2334. doi:10.1200/JCO.2014.55.2307 PMID:24958824

Iragavarapu, C., Mustafa, M., Akinleye, A., Furqan, M., Mittal, V., Cang, S., & Liu, D. (2015). Novel ALK inhibitors in clinical use and development. *Journal of Hematology and Oncology*, *8*(1), 17. PMID:25888090

Irvin, W. J. Jr, Walko, C. M., Weck, K. E., Ibrahim, J. G., Chiu, W. K., Dees, E. C., & Carey, L. A. et al. (2011). Genotype-guided tamoxifen dosing increases active metabolite exposure in women with reduced CYP2D6 metabolism: A multicenter study. *Journal of Clinical Oncology*, *29*(24), 3232–3239. doi:10.1200/JCO.2010.31.4427 PMID:21768473

Ishikawa, T., Hirano, H., Onishi, Y., Sakurai, A., & Tarui, S. (2004). Functional evaluation of ABCB1 (P-glycoprotein) polymorphisms: High-speed screening and structure-activity relationship analyses. *Drug Metabolism and Pharmacokinetics*, *19*(1), 1–14. doi:10.2133/dmpk.19.1 PMID:15499164

Jabbour, E., Kantarjian, H., O'Brien, S., Shan, J., Quintas-Cardama, A., Faderl, S., & Cortes, J. et al. (2011). The achievement of an early complete cytogenetic response is a major determinant for outcome in patients with early chronic phase chronic myeloid leukemia treated with tyrosine kinase inhibitors. *Blood*, *118*(17), 4541–4546, quiz 4759. doi:10.1182/blood-2011-04-348110 PMID:21803854

Jancik, S., Drabek, J., Radzioch, D., & Hajdúch, M. (2010). Clinical relevance of KRAS in human cancers. *Journal of Biomedicine & Biotechnology*, *2010*, 150960. doi:10.1155/2010/150960 PMID:20617134

Jin, Y., Desta, Z., Stearns, V., Ward, B., Ho, H., Lee, K. H., & Flockhart, D. A. et al. (2005). CYP2D6 genotype, antidepressant use, and tamoxifen metabolism during adjuvant breast cancer treatment. *Journal of the National Cancer Institute*, *97*(1), 30–39. doi:10.1093/jnci/dji005 PMID:15632378

Jin, Y., Pollock, B. G., Frank, E., Cassano, G. B., Rucci, P., Muller, D. J., & Bies, R. R. et al. (2010). Effect of age, weight, and CYP2C19 genotype on escitalopram exposure. *Journal of Clinical Pharmacology*, *50*(1), 62–72. doi:10.1177/0091270009337946 PMID:19841156

Kaiser, R., Sezer, O., Papies, A., Bauer, S., Schelenz, C., Tremblay, P. B., & Brockmoller, J. et al. (2002). Patient-tailored antiemetic treatment with 5-hydroxytryptamine type 3 receptor antagonists according to cytochrome P-450 2D6 genotypes. *Journal of Clinical Oncology*, *20*(12), 2805–2811. doi:10.1200/JCO.2002.09.064 PMID:12065557

Klepstad, P., Rakvag, T. T., Kaasa, S., Holthe, M., Dale, O., Borchgrevink, P. C., & Skorpen, F. et al. (2004). The 118 A > G polymorphism in the human mu-opioid receptor gene may increase morphine requirements in patients with pain caused by malignant disease. *Acta Anaesthesiologica Scandinavica*, *48*(10), 1232–1239. doi:10.1111/j.1399-6576.2004.00517.x PMID:15504181

Koren, G., Cairns, J., Chitayat, D., Gaedigk, A., & Leeder, S. J. (2006). Pharmacogenetics of morphine poisoning in a breastfed neonate of a codeine-prescribed mother. *Lancet*, *368*(9536), 704. doi:10.1016/S0140-6736(06)69255-6 PMID:16920476

Krzywkowski, K., Jensen, A. A., Connolly, C. N., & Brauner-Osborne, H. (2007). Naturally occurring variations in the human 5-HT3A gene profoundly impact 5-HT3 receptor function and expression. *Pharmacogenetics and Genomics*, *17*(4), 255–266. doi:10.1097/FPC.0b013e3280117269 PMID:17496724

Lee, C. K., Brown, C., Gralla, R. J., Hirsh, V., Thongprasert, S., Tsai, C. M., & Yang, J. C. et al. (2013). Impact of EGFR inhibitor in non-small cell lung cancer on progression-free and overall survival: A meta-analysis. *Journal of the National Cancer Institute*, *105*(9), 595–605. doi:10.1093/jnci/djt072 PMID:23594426

Lievre, A., Bachet, J. B., Boige, V., Cayre, A., Le Corre, D., Buc, E., & Laurent-Puig, P. et al. (2008). KRAS mutations as an independent prognostic factor in patients with advanced colorectal cancer treated with cetuximab. *Journal of Clinical Oncology*, *26*(3), 374–379. doi:10.1200/JCO.2007.12.5906 PMID:18202412

Lobello, K. W., Preskorn, S. H., Guico-Pabia, C. J., Jiang, Q., Paul, J., Nichols, A. I., & Ninan, P. T. et al. (2010). Cytochrome P450 2D6 phenotype predicts antidepressant efficacy of venlafaxine: A secondary analysis of 4 studies in major depressive disorder. *The Journal of Clinical Psychiatry*, *71*(11), 1482–1487. doi:10.4088/JCP.08m04773blu PMID:20441720

Lotta, T., Vidgren, J., Tilgmann, C., Ulmanen, I., Melen, K., Julkunen, I., & Taskinen, J. (1995). Kinetics of human soluble and membrane-bound catechol O-methyltransferase: A revised mechanism and description of the thermolabile variant of the enzyme. *Biochemistry*, *34*(13), 4202–4210. doi:10.1021/bi00013a008 PMID:7703232

Lynch, T. J., Bell, D. W., Sordella, R., Gurubhagavatula, S., Okimoto, R. A., Brannigan, B. W., & Haber, D. A. et al. (2004). Activating mutations in the epidermal growth factor receptor underlying responsiveness of non-small-cell lung cancer to gefitinib. *The New England Journal of Medicine*, *350*(21), 2129–2139. doi:10.1056/NEJMoa040938 PMID:15118073

Macconaill, L. E., Van Hummelen, P., Meyerson, M., & Hahn, W. C. (2011). Clinical implementation of comprehensive strategies to characterize cancer genomes: Opportunities and challenges. *Cancer Discovery*, *1*(4), 297–311. doi:10.1158/2159-8290.CD-11-0110 PMID:21935500

Machu, T. K. (2011). Therapeutics of 5-HT3 receptor antagonists: Current uses and future directions. *Pharmacology & Therapeutics*, *130*(3), 338–347. doi:10.1016/j.pharmthera.2011.02.003 PMID:21356241

Madadi, P., Ciszkowski, C., Gaedigk, A., Leeder, J. S., Teitelbaum, R., Chitayat, D., & Koren, G. (2011). Genetic transmission of cytochrome P450 2D6 (CYP2D6) ultrarapid metabolism: Implications for breast-feeding women taking codeine. *Current Drug Safety*, *6*(1), 36–39. doi:10.2174/157488611794479991 PMID:21241245

Madadi, P., Joly, Y., Avard, D., Chitayat, D. C., Smith, M. A., Ross, C. J., & Koren, G. et al. (2010). Communicating pharmacogenetic research results to breastfeeding mothers taking codeine: A pilot study of perceptions and benefits. *Clinical Pharmacology and Therapeutics*, *88*(6), 792–795. doi:10.1038/clpt.2010.125 PMID:20739920

Madadi, P., & Koren, G. (2008). Pharmacogenetic insights into codeine analgesia: Implications to pediatric codeine use. *Pharmacogenomics*, *9*(9), 1267–1284. doi:10.2217/14622416.9.9.1267 PMID:18781855

Madlensky, L., Natarajan, L., Tchu, S., Pu, M., Mortimer, J., Flatt, S. W., & Pierce, J. P. et al. (2011). Tamoxifen metabolite concentrations, CYP2D6 genotype, and breast cancer outcomes. *Clinical Pharmacology and Therapeutics*, *89*(5), 718–725. doi:10.1038/clpt.2011.32 PMID:21430657

Mandrekar, S. J., & Sargent, D. J. (2009). Clinical trial designs for predictive biomarker validation: Theoretical considerations and practical challenges. *Journal of Clinical Oncology*, *27*(24), 4027–4034. doi:10.1200/JCO.2009.22.3701 PMID:19597023

Marcuello, E., Paez, D., Pare, L., Salazar, J., Sebio, A., del Rio, E., & Baiget, M. (2011). A genotype-directed phase I-IV dose-finding study of irinotecan in combination with fluorouracil/leucovorin as first-line treatment in advanced colorectal cancer. *British Journal of Cancer*, *105*(1), 53–57. doi:10.1038/bjc.2011.206 PMID:21654688

Massarelli, E., Varella-Garcia, M., Tang, X., Xavier, A. C., Ozburn, N. C., Liu, D. D., & Wistuba, I. I. et al. (2007). KRAS mutation is an important predictor of resistance to therapy with epidermal growth factor receptor tyrosine kinase inhibitors in non-small-cell lung cancer. *Clinical Cancer Research*, *13*(10), 2890–2896. doi:10.1158/1078-0432.CCR-06-3043 PMID:17504988

Mauro, M. J. (2006). Defining and managing imatinib resistance. Hematology American Society of Hematology Education Program.

McArthur, G. A., Chapman, P. B., Robert, C., Larkin, J., Haanen, J. B., Dummer, R., & Hauschild, A. et al. (2014). Safety and efficacy of vemurafenib in BRAF(V600E) and BRAF(V600K) mutation-positive melanoma (BRIM-3): Extended follow-up of a phase 3, randomised, open-label study. *The Lancet Oncology*, *15*(3), 323–332. doi:10.1016/S1470-2045(14)70012-9 PMID:24508103

McLeod, H. L., Krynetski, E. Y., Relling, M. V., & Evans, W. E. (2000). Genetic polymorphism of thiopurine methyltransferase and its clinical relevance for childhood acute lymphoblastic leukemia. *Leukemia*, *14*(4), 567–572. doi:10.1038/sj.leu.2401723 PMID:10764140

McLeod, H. L., Lin, J. S., Scott, E. P., Pui, C. H., & Evans, W. E. (1994). Thiopurine methyltransferase activity in American white subjects and black subjects. *Clinical Pharmacology and Therapeutics*, *55*(1), 15–20. doi:10.1038/clpt.1994.4 PMID:8299312

Mignat, C., Wille, U., & Ziegler, A. (1995). Affinity profiles of morphine, codeine, dihydrocodeine and their glucuronides at opioid receptor subtypes. *Life Sciences*, *56*(10), 793–799. doi:10.1016/0024-3205(95)00010-4 PMID:7885194

Mikus, G., Scholz, I. M., & Weiss, J. (2011). Pharmacogenomics of the triazole antifungal agent voriconazole. *Pharmacogenomics*, *12*(6), 861–872. doi:10.2217/pgs.11.18 PMID:21692616

Miller, V. A., Hirsh, V., Cadranel, J., Chen, Y. M., Park, K., Kim, S. W., & Yang, J. C. et al. (2012). Afatinib versus placebo for patients with advanced, metastatic non-small-cell lung cancer after failure of erlotinib, gefitinib, or both, and one or two lines of chemotherapy (LUX-Lung 1): A phase 2b/3 randomised trial. *The Lancet Oncology*, *13*(5), 528–538. doi:10.1016/S1470-2045(12)70087-6 PMID:22452896

Miyakis, S., van Hal, S. J., Ray, J., & Marriott, D. (2010). Voriconazole concentrations and outcome of invasive fungal infections. *Clinical Microbiology and Infection*, *16*(7), 927–933. doi:10.1111/j.1469-0691.2009.02990.x PMID:19845698

Moja, L., Tagliabue, L., Balduzzi, S., Parmelli, E., Pistotti, V., Guarneri, V., & D'Amico, R. (2012). Trastuzumab containing regimens for early breast cancer. *Cochrane Database of Systematic Reviews*, *4*, CD006243. PMID:22513938

Musshoff, F., Madea, B., Stuber, F., & Stamer, U. M. (2006). Enantiomeric determination of tramadol and O-desmethyltramadol by liquid chromatography- mass spectrometry and application to postoperative patients receiving tramadol. *Journal of Analytical Toxicology*, *30*(7), 463–467. doi:10.1093/jat/30.7.463 PMID:16959140

Nakamura, Y., Ratain, M. J., Cox, N. J., McLeod, H. L., Kroetz, D. L., & Flockhart, D. A. (2012). Re: CYP2D6 genotype and tamoxifen response in postmenopausal women with endocrine-responsive breast cancer: the Breast International Group 1-98 trial. *Journal of the National Cancer Institute*, *104*(16), 1264, author reply 1266–1268. doi:10.1093/jnci/djs304 PMID:22851270

Narasimhan, S., & Lohoff, F. W. (2012). Pharmacogenetics of antidepressant drugs: Current clinical practice and future directions. *Pharmacogenomics*, *13*(4), 441–464. doi:10.2217/pgs.12.1 PMID:22380000

Nichols, A. I., Focht, K., Jiang, Q., Preskorn, S. H., & Kane, C. P. (2011). Pharmacokinetics of venlafaxine extended release 75 mg and desvenlafaxine 50 mg in healthy CYP2D6 extensive and poor metabolizers: A randomized, open-label, two-period, parallel-group, crossover study. *Clinical Drug Investigation*, *31*(3), 155–167. doi:10.2165/11586630-000000000-00000 PMID:21288052

Noehr-Jensen, L., Zwisler, S. T., Larsen, F., Sindrup, S. H., Damkier, P., Nielsen, F., & Brosen, K. (2009). Impact of CYP2C19 phenotypes on escitalopram metabolism and an evaluation of pupillometry as a serotonergic biomarker. *European Journal of Clinical Pharmacology*, *65*(9), 887–894. doi:10.1007/s00228-009-0657-0 PMID:19404631

Owusu Obeng, A., Egelund, E. F., Alsultan, A., Peloquin, C. A., & Johnson, J. A. (2014). CYP2C19 polymorphisms and therapeutic drug monitoring of voriconazole: Are we ready for clinical implementation of pharmacogenomics? *Pharmacotherapy*, *34*(7), 703–718. doi:10.1002/phar.1400 PMID:24510446

Pardoll, D. M. (2012). The blockade of immune checkpoints in cancer immunotherapy. *Nature Reviews. Cancer*, *12*(4), 252–264. doi:10.1038/nrc3239 PMID:22437870

Park, W. B., Kim, N. H., Kim, K. H., Lee, S. H., Nam, W. S., Yoon, S. H., & Yu, K. S. et al. (2012). The effect of therapeutic drug monitoring on safety and efficacy of voriconazole in invasive fungal infections: A randomized controlled trial. *Clinical Infectious Diseases*, *55*(8), 1080–1087. doi:10.1093/cid/cis599 PMID:22761409

Patel, J. N. (2014). Application of genotype-guided cancer therapy in solid tumors. *Pharmacogenomics*, *15*(1), 79–93. doi:10.2217/pgs.13.227 PMID:24329193

Patel, J. N., Fuchs, C. S., Owzar, K., Chen, Z., & McLeod, H. L. (2013). Gastric cancer pharmacogenetics: Progress or old tripe? *Pharmacogenomics*, *14*(9), 1053–1064. doi:10.2217/pgs.13.88 PMID:23837480

Patel, J. N., Mandock, K., & McLeod, H. L. (2014). Clinically relevant cancer biomarkers and pharmacogenetic assays. *Journal of Oncology Pharmacy Practice*, *20*(1), 65–72. doi:10.1177/1078155212473862 PMID:23353710

Perera, M. A., Innocenti, F., & Ratain, M. J. (2008). Pharmacogenetic testing for uridine diphosphate glucuronosyltransferase 1A1 polymorphisms: Are we there yet? *Pharmacotherapy*, *28*(6), 755–768. doi:10.1592/phco.28.6.755 PMID:18503403

Peters, S., Michielin, O., & Zimmermann, S. (2013). Dramatic response induced by vemurafenib in a BRAF V600E-mutated lung adenocarcinoma. *Journal of Clinical Oncology*, *31*(20), e341–e344. doi:10.1200/JCO.2012.47.6143 PMID:23733758

Pieper, S., Kolve, H., Gumbinger, H. G., Goletz, G., Wurthwein, G., & Groll, A. H. (2012). Monitoring of voriconazole plasma concentrations in immunocompromised paediatric patients. *The Journal of Antimicrobial Chemotherapy*, *67*(11), 2717–2724. doi:10.1093/jac/dks258 PMID:22796890

Planchard, D., Mazieres, J., Riely, G. J., Rudin, C. M., Barlesi, F., Quoix, E. A., & Souquet, M. A. (2013). Interim results of phase II study BRF113928 of dabrafenib in BRAF V600E mutation–positive non-small cell lung cancer (NSCLC) patients. *Journal of Clinical Oncology*.

Postow, M. A., Chesney, J., Pavlick, A. C., Robert, C., Grossmann, K., McDermott, D., & Hodi, F. S. et al. (2015). Nivolumab and ipilimumab versus ipilimumab in untreated melanoma. *The New England Journal of Medicine*, *372*(21), 2006–2017. doi:10.1056/NEJMoa1414428 PMID:25891304

Prahallad, A., Sun, C., Huang, S., Di Nicolantonio, F., Salazar, R., Zecchin, D., & Bernards, R. et al. (2012). Unresponsiveness of colon cancer to BRAF(V600E) inhibition through feedback activation of EGFR. *Nature*, *483*(7387), 100–103. doi:10.1038/nature10868 PMID:22281684

Rae, J. M., Drury, S., Hayes, D. F., Stearns, V., Thibert, J. N., Haynes, B. P., & Dowsett, M. et al. (2012). CYP2D6 and UGT2B7 genotype and risk of recurrence in tamoxifen-treated breast cancer patients. *Journal of the National Cancer Institute*, *104*(6), 452–460. doi:10.1093/jnci/djs126 PMID:22395643

Rae, J. M., Regan, M. M., Thibert, J. N., Gersch, C., Thomas, D., Leyland-Jones, B., & Van Poznak, C. et al. (2013). Concordance between CYP2D6 genotypes obtained from tumor-derived and germline DNA. *Journal of the National Cancer Institute*, *105*(17), 1332–1334. doi:10.1093/jnci/djt204 PMID:23958736

Rakvag, T. T., Klepstad, P., Baar, C., Kvam, T. M., Dale, O., Kaasa, S., & Skorpen, F. et al. (2005). The Val158Met polymorphism of the human catechol-O-methyltransferase (COMT) gene may influence morphine requirements in cancer pain patients. *Pain*, *116*(1-2), 73–78. doi:10.1016/j.pain.2005.03.032 PMID:15927391

Regan, M. M., Leyland-Jones, B., Bouzyk, M., Pagani, O., Tang, W., Kammler, R., & Viale, G. et al. (2012). CYP2D6 genotype and tamoxifen response in postmenopausal women with endocrine-responsive breast cancer: The breast international group 1-98 trial. *Journal of the National Cancer Institute*, *104*(6), 441–451. doi:10.1093/jnci/djs125 PMID:22395644

Reichardt, P., Blay, J. Y., Gelderblom, H., Schlemmer, M., Demetri, G. D., Bui-Nguyen, B., & Rutkowski, P. et al. (2012). Phase III study of nilotinib versus best supportive care with or without a TKI in patients with gastrointestinal stromal tumors resistant to or intolerant of imatinib and sunitinib. *Annals of Oncology*, *23*(7), 1680–1687. doi:10.1093/annonc/mdr598 PMID:22357255

Relling, M. V., Gardner, E. E., Sandborn, W. J., Schmiegelow, K., Pui, C. H., Yee, S. W., & Klein, T. E. et al. (2011). Clinical Pharmacogenetics Implementation Consortium guidelines for thiopurine methyltransferase genotype and thiopurine dosing. *Clinical Pharmacology and Therapeutics*, *89*(3), 387–391. doi:10.1038/clpt.2010.320 PMID:21270794

Relling, M. V., Gardner, E. E., Sandborn, W. J., Schmiegelow, K., Pui, C. H., Yee, S. W., & Klein, T. E. et al. (2013). Clinical pharmacogenetics implementation consortium guidelines for thiopurine methyltransferase genotype and thiopurine dosing: 2013 update. *Clinical Pharmacology and Therapeutics*, *93*(4), 324–325. doi:10.1038/clpt.2013.4 PMID:23422873

Relling, M. V., Hancock, M. L., Rivera, G. K., Sandlund, J. T., Ribeiro, R. C., Krynetski, E. Y., & Evans, W. E. et al. (1999). Mercaptopurine therapy intolerance and heterozygosity at the thiopurine S-methyltransferase gene locus. *Journal of the National Cancer Institute*, *91*(23), 2001–2008. doi:10.1093/jnci/91.23.2001 PMID:10580024

Rizvi, N. A., Mazieres, J., Planchard, D., Stinchcombe, T. E., Dy, G. K., Antonia, S. J., & Ramalingam, S. S. et al. (2015). Activity and safety of nivolumab, an anti-PD-1 immune checkpoint inhibitor, for patients with advanced, refractory squamous non-small-cell lung cancer (CheckMate 063): A phase 2, single-arm trial. *The Lancet Oncology*, *16*(3), 257–265. doi:10.1016/S1470-2045(15)70054-9 PMID:25704439

Robert, C., Karaszewska, B., Schachter, J., Rutkowski, P., Mackiewicz, A., Stroiakovski, D., & Schadendorf, D. et al. (2015). Improved overall survival in melanoma with combined dabrafenib and trametinib. *The New England Journal of Medicine*, *372*(1), 30–39. doi:10.1056/NEJMoa1412690 PMID:25399551

Robert, C., Long, G. V., Brady, B., Dutriaux, C., Maio, M., Mortier, L., & Ascierto, P. A. et al. (2015). Nivolumab in previously untreated melanoma without BRAF mutation. *The New England Journal of Medicine*, *372*(4), 320–330. doi:10.1056/NEJMoa1412082 PMID:25399552

Robert, C., Schachter, J., Long, G. V., Arance, A., Grob, J. J., Mortier, L., & Ribas, A. et al. (2015). Pembrolizumab versus Ipilimumab in Advanced Melanoma. *The New England Journal of Medicine*, *372*(26), 2521–2532. doi:10.1056/NEJMoa1503093 PMID:25891173

Roila, F., Herrstedt, J., Aapro, M., Gralla, R. J., Einhorn, L. H., Ballatori, E., & Group, E. M. G. W. et al. (2010). Guideline update for MASCC and ESMO in the prevention of chemotherapy- and radiotherapy-induced nausea and vomiting: Results of the Perugia consensus conference. *Annals of Oncology*, *21*(Suppl 5), v232–v243. doi:10.1093/annonc/mdq194 PMID:20555089

Rojas, C., & Slusher, B. S. (2012). Pharmacological mechanisms of 5-HT(3) and tachykinin NK(1) receptor antagonism to prevent chemotherapy-induced nausea and vomiting. *European Journal of Pharmacology*, *684*(1-3), 1–7. doi:10.1016/j.ejphar.2012.01.046 PMID:22425650

Rosell, R., Carcereny, E., Gervais, R., Vergnenegre, A., Massuti, B., Felip, E., & Associazione Italiana Oncologia, T. et al. (2012). Erlotinib versus standard chemotherapy as first-line treatment for European patients with advanced EGFR mutation-positive non-small-cell lung cancer (EURTAC): A multicentre, open-label, randomised phase 3 trial. *The Lancet Oncology*, *13*(3), 239–246. doi:10.1016/S1470-2045(11)70393-X PMID:22285168

Rosmarin, D., Palles, C., Church, D., Domingo, E., Jones, A., Johnstone, E., & Tomlinson, I. et al. (2014). Genetic markers of toxicity from capecitabine and other fluorouracil-based regimens: Investigation in the QUASAR2 study, systematic review, and meta-analysis. *Journal of Clinical Oncology*, *32*(10), 1031–1039. doi:10.1200/JCO.2013.51.1857 PMID:24590654

Rubin, B. P., Fletcher, J. A., & Fletcher, C. D. (2000). Molecular Insights into the Histogenesis and Pathogenesis of Gastrointestinal Stromal Tumors. *International Journal of Surgical Pathology*, *8*(1), 5–10. doi:10.1177/106689690000800105 PMID:11493959

Rush, A. J., Trivedi, M. H., Wisniewski, S. R., Nierenberg, A. A., Stewart, J. W., Warden, D., & Fava, M. et al. (2006). Acute and longer-term outcomes in depressed outpatients requiring one or several treatment steps: A STAR*D report. *The American Journal of Psychiatry*, *163*(11), 1905–1917. PMID:17074942

Saif, M. W., Ezzeldin, H., Vance, K., Sellers, S., & Diasio, R. B. (2007). DPYD*2A mutation: The most common mutation associated with DPD deficiency. *Cancer Chemotherapy and Pharmacology*, *60*(4), 503–507. doi:10.1007/s00280-006-0392-5 PMID:17165084

Saladores, P., Murdter, T., Eccles, D., Chowbay, B., Zgheib, N. K., Winter, S., & Brauch, H. et al. (2014). Tamoxifen metabolism predicts drug concentrations and outcome in premenopausal patients with early breast cancer. *The Pharmacogenomics Journal*. PMID:25091503

Samer, C. F., Daali, Y., Wagner, M., Hopfgartner, G., Eap, C. B., Rebsamen, M. C., & Desmeules, J. A. et al. (2010). Genetic polymorphisms and drug interactions modulating CYP2D6 and CYP3A activities have a major effect on oxycodone analgesic efficacy and safety. *British Journal of Pharmacology*, *160*(4), 919–930. doi:10.1111/j.1476-5381.2010.00709.x PMID:20590588

Samer, C. F., Lorenzini, K. I., Rollason, V., Daali, Y., & Desmeules, J. A. (2013). Applications of CYP450 testing in the clinical setting. *Molecular Diagnosis & Therapy*, *17*(3), 165–184. doi:10.1007/s40291-013-0028-5 PMID:23588782

Sawyers, C. L. (2008). The cancer biomarker problem. *Nature*, *452*(7187), 548–552. doi:10.1038/nature06913 PMID:18385728

Schaeffeler, E., Fischer, C., Brockmeier, D., Wernet, D., Moerike, K., Eichelbaum, M., & Schwab, M. et al. (2004). Comprehensive analysis of thiopurine S-methyltransferase phenotype-genotype correlation in a large population of German-Caucasians and identification of novel TPMT variants. *Pharmacogenetics*, *14*(7), 407–417. doi:10.1097/01.fpc.0000114745.08559.db PMID:15226673

Schneider, B. P., Radovich, M., & Miller, K. D. (2009). The role of vascular endothelial growth factor genetic variability in cancer. *Clinical Cancer Research*, *15*(17), 5297–5302. doi:10.1158/1078-0432.CCR-08-2576 PMID:19706811

Schroth, W., Goetz, M. P., Hamann, U., Fasching, P. A., Schmidt, M., Winter, S., & Brauch, H. et al. (2009). Association between CYP2D6 polymorphisms and outcomes among women with early stage breast cancer treated with tamoxifen. *Journal of the American Medical Association*, *302*(13), 1429–1436. doi:10.1001/jama.2009.1420 PMID:19809024

Schwab, M., Zanger, U. M., Marx, C., Schaeffeler, E., Klein, K., Dippon, J., & German, F. U. T. S. G. et al. (2008). Role of genetic and nongenetic factors for fluorouracil treatment-related severe toxicity: A prospective clinical trial by the German 5-FU Toxicity Study Group. *Journal of Clinical Oncology*, *26*(13), 2131–2138. doi:10.1200/JCO.2006.10.4182 PMID:18299612

Sequist, L. V., Soria, J. C., Goldman, J. W., Wakelee, H. A., Gadgeel, S. M., Varga, A., & Camidge, D. R. et al. (2015). Rociletinib in EGFR-mutated non-small-cell lung cancer. *The New England Journal of Medicine*, *372*(18), 1700–1709. doi:10.1056/NEJMoa1413654 PMID:25923550

Serretti, A., Calati, R., Massat, I., Linotte, S., Kasper, S., Lecrubier, Y., & Souery, D. et al. (2009). Cytochrome P450 CYP1A2, CYP2C9, CYP2C19 and CYP2D6 genes are not associated with response and remission in a sample of depressive patients. *International Clinical Psychopharmacology*, *24*(5), 250–256. doi:10.1097/YIC.0b013e32832e5b0d PMID:19593158

Seto, T., Kiura, K., Nishio, M., Nakagawa, K., Maemondo, M., Inoue, A., & Tamura, T. et al. (2013). CH5424802 (RO5424802) for patients with ALK-rearranged advanced non-small-cell lung cancer (AF-001JP study): A single-arm, open-label, phase 1-2 study. *The Lancet Oncology*, *14*(7), 590–598. doi:10.1016/S1470-2045(13)70142-6 PMID:23639470

Shaw, A. T., Kim, D. W., Mehra, R., Tan, D. S., Felip, E., Chow, L. Q., & Engelman, J. A. et al. (2014). Ceritinib in ALK-rearranged non-small-cell lung cancer. *The New England Journal of Medicine*, *370*(13), 1189–1197. doi:10.1056/NEJMoa1311107 PMID:24670165

Shaw, A. T., Kim, D. W., Nakagawa, K., Seto, T., Crino, L., Ahn, M. J., & Janne, P. A. et al. (2013). Crizotinib versus chemotherapy in advanced ALK-positive lung cancer. *The New England Journal of Medicine*, *368*(25), 2385–2394. doi:10.1056/NEJMoa1214886 PMID:23724913

Shepherd, F. A., Rodrigues Pereira, J., Ciuleanu, T., Tan, E. H., Hirsh, V., Thongprasert, S., & Seymour, L. et al. (2005). Erlotinib in previously treated non-small-cell lung cancer. *The New England Journal of Medicine*, *353*(2), 123–132. doi:10.1056/NEJMoa050753 PMID:16014882

Solomon, B. J., Mok, T., Kim, D. W., Wu, Y. L., Nakagawa, K., Mekhail, T., & Investigators, P. et al. (2014). First-line crizotinib versus chemotherapy in ALK-positive lung cancer. *The New England Journal of Medicine*, *371*(23), 2167–2177. doi:10.1056/NEJMoa1408440 PMID:25470694

Spigel, D.R., Reckamp, K.L., Rizvi, N.A., Poddubskaya, E., West, H.J, Eberhardt, W.E.E, . . . Brahmer, J.R. (2015). A phase III study (CheckMate 017) of nivolumab (NIVO; anti-programmed death-1 [PD-1]) versus docetaxel (DOC) in previously treated advanced or metastatic squamous cell non-small cell lung cancer. *Journal of Clinical Oncology*.

Staddon, S., Arranz, M. J., Mancama, D., Mata, I., & Kerwin, R. W. (2002). Clinical applications of pharmacogenetics in psychiatry. *Psychopharmacology*, *162*(1), 18–23. doi:10.1007/s00213-002-1084-4 PMID:12107612

Stamer, U. M., Lehnen, K., Hothker, F., Bayerer, B., Wolf, S., Hoeft, A., & Stuber, F. (2003). Impact of CYP2D6 genotype on postoperative tramadol analgesia. *Pain*, *105*(1-2), 231–238. doi:10.1016/S0304-3959(03)00212-4 PMID:14499440

Stamer, U. M., Musshoff, F., Kobilay, M., Madea, B., Hoeft, A., & Stuber, F. (2007). Concentrations of tramadol and O-desmethyltramadol enantiomers in different CYP2D6 genotypes. *Clinical Pharmacology and Therapeutics*, *82*(1), 41–47. doi:10.1038/sj.clpt.6100152 PMID:17361124

Stamer, U. M., Stuber, F., Muders, T., & Musshoff, F. (2008). Respiratory depression with tramadol in a patient with renal impairment and CYP2D6 gene duplication. *Anesthesia and Analgesia*, *107*(3), 926–929. doi:10.1213/ane.0b013e31817b796e PMID:18713907

Stamer, U. M., Zhang, L., Book, M., Lehmann, L. E., Stuber, F., & Musshoff, F. (2013). CYP2D6 genotype dependent oxycodone metabolism in postoperative patients. *PLoS ONE*, *8*(3), e60239. doi:10.1371/journal.pone.0060239 PMID:23555934

Stanulla, M., Schaeffeler, E., Flohr, T., Cario, G., Schrauder, A., Zimmermann, M., & Schwab, M. et al. (2005). Thiopurine methyltransferase (TPMT) genotype and early treatment response to mercaptopurine in childhood acute lymphoblastic leukemia. *Journal of the American Medical Association*, *293*(12), 1485–1489. doi:10.1001/jama.293.12.1485 PMID:15784872

Stauble, M. E., Moore, A. W., Langman, L. J., Boswell, M. V., Baumgartner, R., McGee, S., & Jortani, S. A. et al. (2014). Hydrocodone in postoperative personalized pain management: Pro-drug or drug? *Clinica Chimica Acta*, *429*, 26–29. doi:10.1016/j.cca.2013.11.015 PMID:24269714

Stocco, G., Cheok, M. H., Crews, K. R., Dervieux, T., French, D., Pei, D., & Evans, W. E. et al. (2009). Genetic polymorphism of inosine triphosphate pyrophosphatase is a determinant of mercaptopurine metabolism and toxicity during treatment for acute lymphoblastic leukemia. *Clinical Pharmacology and Therapeutics*, *85*(2), 164–172. doi:10.1038/clpt.2008.154 PMID:18685564

Su, F., Viros, A., Milagre, C., Trunzer, K., Bollag, G., Spleiss, O., & Marais, R. et al. (2012). RAS mutations in cutaneous squamous-cell carcinomas in patients treated with BRAF inhibitors. *The New England Journal of Medicine*, *366*(3), 207–215. doi:10.1056/NEJMoa1105358 PMID:22256804

Tabernero, J., Yoshino, T., Cohn, A. L., Obermannova, R., Bodoky, G., Garcia-Carbonero, R., & Investigators, R. S. et al. (2015). Ramucirumab versus placebo in combination with second-line FOLFIRI in patients with metastatic colorectal carcinoma that progressed during or after first-line therapy with bevacizumab, oxaliplatin, and a fluoropyrimidine (RAISE): A randomised, double-blind, multicentre, phase 3 study. *The Lancet Oncology*, *16*(5), 499–508. doi:10.1016/S1470-2045(15)70127-0 PMID:25877855

Tan, B. R., Thomas, F., Myerson, R. J., Zehnbauer, B., Trinkaus, K., Malyapa, R. S., & McLeod, H. L. et al. (2011). Thymidylate synthase genotype-directed neoadjuvant chemoradiation for patients with rectal adenocarcinoma. *Journal of Clinical Oncology*, *29*(7), 875–883. doi:10.1200/JCO.2010.32.3212 PMID:21205745

Thatcher, N., Chang, A., Parikh, P., Rodrigues Pereira, J., Ciuleanu, T., von Pawel, J., & Carroll, K. et al. (2005). Gefitinib plus best supportive care in previously treated patients with refractory advanced non-small-cell lung cancer: Results from a randomised, placebo-controlled, multicentre study (Iressa Survival Evaluation in Lung Cancer). *Lancet*, *366*(9496), 1527–1537. doi:10.1016/S0140-6736(05)67625-8 PMID:16257339

Toffoli, G., & Cecchin, E. (2007). Pharmacogenetics and stomach cancer: An update. *Pharmacogenomics*, *8*(5), 497–505. doi:10.2217/14622416.8.5.497 PMID:17465714

Toffoli, G., Cecchin, E., Gasparini, G., D'Andrea, M., Azzarello, G., Basso, U., & Innocenti, F. et al. (2010). Genotype-driven phase I study of irinotecan administered in combination with fluorouracil/leucovorin in patients with metastatic colorectal cancer. *Journal of Clinical Oncology*, *28*(5), 866–871. doi:10.1200/JCO.2009.23.6125 PMID:20038727

Tran, B., Dancey, J. E., Kamel-Reid, S., McPherson, J. D., Bedard, P. L., Brown, A. M., & Siu, L. L. et al. (2012). Cancer genomics: Technology, discovery, and translation. *Journal of Clinical Oncology*, *30*(6), 647–660. doi:10.1200/JCO.2011.39.2316 PMID:22271477

Tremblay, P. B., Kaiser, R., Sezer, O., Rosler, N., Schelenz, C., Possinger, K., & Brockmoller, J. et al. (2003). Variations in the 5-hydroxytryptamine type 3B receptor gene as predictors of the efficacy of antiemetic treatment in cancer patients. *Journal of Clinical Oncology*, *21*(11), 2147–2155. doi:10.1200/JCO.2003.05.164 PMID:12775740

Trifilio, S., Pennick, G., Pi, J., Zook, J., Golf, M., Kaniecki, K., & Mehta, J. et al. (2007). Monitoring plasma voriconazole levels may be necessary to avoid subtherapeutic levels in hematopoietic stem cell transplant recipients. *Cancer*, *109*(8), 1532–1535. doi:10.1002/cncr.22568 PMID:17351937

Trinh, V. A., Davis, J. E., Anderson, J. E., & Kim, K. B. (2014). Dabrafenib therapy for advanced melanoma. *The Annals of Pharmacotherapy*, *48*(4), 519–529. doi:10.1177/1060028013513009 PMID:24259661

Troke, P. F., Hockey, H. P., & Hope, W. W. (2011). Observational study of the clinical efficacy of voriconazole and its relationship to plasma concentrations in patients. *Antimicrobial Agents and Chemotherapy*, *55*(10), 4782–4788. doi:10.1128/AAC.01083-10 PMID:21768513

Tzvetkov, M. V., Saadatmand, A. R., Bckelmann, K., Meineke, I., Kaiser, R., & Brockmoller, J. (2012). Effects of OCT1 polymorphisms on the cellular uptake, plasma concentrations and efficacy of the 5-HT(3) antagonists tropisetron and ondansetron. *The Pharmacogenomics Journal, 12*(1), 22–29. doi:10.1038/tpj.2010.75 PMID:20921968

Van Cutsem, E., Kohne, C. H., Hitre, E., Zaluski, J., Chang Chien, C. R., Makhson, A., & Rougier, P. et al. (2009). Cetuximab and chemotherapy as initial treatment for metastatic colorectal cancer. *The New England Journal of Medicine, 360*(14), 1408–1417. doi:10.1056/NEJMoa0805019 PMID:19339720

Van Cutsem, E., Tabernero, J., Lakomy, R., Prenen, H., Prausova, J., Macarulla, T., & Allegra, C. et al. (2012). Addition of aflibercept to fluorouracil, leucovorin, and irinotecan improves survival in a phase III randomized trial in patients with metastatic colorectal cancer previously treated with an oxaliplatin-based regimen. *Journal of Clinical Oncology, 30*(28), 3499–3506. doi:10.1200/JCO.2012.42.8201 PMID:22949147

Van Kuilenburg, A. B., Meinsma, R., Zoetekouw, L., & Van Gennip, A. H. (2002). High prevalence of the IVS14 + 1G>A mutation in the dihydropyrimidine dehydrogenase gene of patients with severe 5-fluorouracil-associated toxicity. *Pharmacogenetics, 12*(7), 555–558. doi:10.1097/00008571-200210000-00007 PMID:12360106

Villafranca, E., Okruzhnov, Y., Dominguez, M. A., Garcia-Foncillas, J., Azinovic, I., Martinez, E., & Brugarolas, A. et al. (2001). Polymorphisms of the repeated sequences in the enhancer region of the thymidylate synthase gene promoter may predict downstaging after preoperative chemoradiation in rectal cancer. *Journal of Clinical Oncology, 19*(6), 1779–1786. PMID:11251009

Wang, T., Zhu, H., Sun, J., Cheng, X., Xie, J., Dong, H., & Dong, Y. et al. (2014). Efficacy and safety of voriconazole and CYP2C19 polymorphism for optimised dosage regimens in patients with invasive fungal infections. *International Journal of Antimicrobial Agents, 44*(5), 436–442. doi:10.1016/j.ijantimicag.2014.07.013 PMID:25239277

Ward, M. B., Kotasek, D., & McKinnon, R. A. (2008). Investigation of HTR3C mutations for association with 5HT(3) receptor antagonist anti-emetic efficacy. *Pharmacogenomics, 9*(8), 1027–1033. doi:10.2217/14622416.9.8.1027 PMID:18681779

Weber, J. S., D'Angelo, S. P., Minor, D., Hodi, F. S., Gutzmer, R., Neyns, B., & Larkin, J. et al. (2015). Nivolumab versus chemotherapy in patients with advanced melanoma who progressed after anti-CTLA-4 treatment (CheckMate 037): A randomised, controlled, open-label, phase 3 trial. *The Lancet Oncology, 16*(4), 375–384. doi:10.1016/S1470-2045(15)70076-8 PMID:25795410

Wilke, H., Muro, K., Van Cutsem, E., Oh, S. C., Bodoky, G., Shimada, Y., & Group, R. S. et al. (2014). Ramucirumab plus paclitaxel versus placebo plus paclitaxel in patients with previously treated advanced gastric or gastro-oesophageal junction adenocarcinoma (RAINBOW): A double-blind, randomised phase 3 trial. *The Lancet Oncology, 15*(11), 1224–1235. doi:10.1016/S1470-2045(14)70420-6 PMID:25240821

Yaakob, N., Malone, D. T., Exintaris, B., & Irving, H. R. (2011). Heterogeneity amongst 5-HT(3) receptor subunits: Is this significant? *Current Molecular Medicine, 11*(1), 57–68. doi:10.2174/156652411794474392 PMID:21189117

Yang, J. C., Wu, Y. L., Schuler, M., Sebastian, M., Popat, S., Yamamoto, N., & Sequist, L. V. et al. (2015). Afatinib versus cisplatin-based chemotherapy for EGFR mutation-positive lung adenocarcinoma (LUX-Lung 3 and LUX-Lung 6): Analysis of overall survival data from two randomised, phase 3 trials. *The Lancet Oncology*, *16*(2), 141–151. doi:10.1016/S1470-2045(14)71173-8 PMID:25589191

Yarden, Y., & Shilo, B. Z. (2007). SnapShot: EGFR signaling pathway. *Cell*, *131*(5), 1018. doi:10.1016/j.cell.2007.11.013 PMID:18045542

Yasuda, A., Sawai, H., Takahashi, H., Ochi, N., Matsuo, Y., Funahashi, H., & Manabe, T. et al. (2007). Stem cell factor/c-kit receptor signaling enhances the proliferation and invasion of colorectal cancer cells through the PI3K/Akt pathway. *Digestive Diseases and Sciences*, *52*(9), 2292–2300. doi:10.1007/s10620-007-9759-7 PMID:17410437

Yen, J. L., & McLeod, H. L. (2007). Should DPD analysis be required prior to prescribing fluoropyrimidines? *European Journal of Cancer*, *43*(6), 1011–1016. doi:10.1016/j.ejca.2007.01.030 PMID:17350823

Zhang, C., Tan, C., Ding, H., Xin, T., & Jiang, Y. (2012). Selective VEGFR inhibitors for anticancer therapeutics in clinical use and clinical trials. *Current Pharmaceutical Design*, *18*(20), 2921–2935. doi:10.2174/138161212800672732 PMID:22571661

Zhong, H., & Bowen, J. P. (2011). Recent advances in small molecule inhibitors of VEGFR and EGFR signaling pathways. *Current Topics in Medicinal Chemistry*, *11*(12), 1571–1590. doi:10.2174/156802611795860924 PMID:21510831

Zhou, C., Wu, Y. L., Chen, G., Feng, J., Liu, X. Q., Wang, C., & You, C. et al. (2011). Erlotinib versus chemotherapy as first-line treatment for patients with advanced EGFR mutation-positive non-small-cell lung cancer (OPTIMAL, CTONG-0802): A multicentre, open-label, randomised, phase 3 study. *The Lancet Oncology*, *12*(8), 735–742. doi:10.1016/S1470-2045(11)70184-X PMID:21783417

Zhou, T., Commodore, L., Huang, W. S., Wang, Y., Thomas, M., Keats, J., & Zhu, X. et al. (2011). Structural mechanism of the Pan-BCR-ABL inhibitor ponatinib (AP24534): Lessons for overcoming kinase inhibitor resistance. *Chemical Biology & Drug Design*, *77*(1), 1–11. doi:10.1111/j.1747-0285.2010.01054.x PMID:21118377

ENDNOTE

[1] Estimated frequency in the European/Caucasian population for most frequently reported variants

APPENDIX

Table 1. Summary of FDA-approved targeted therapies, biomarkers and clinical assay availability.

Biomarker	Therapy	FDA-Approved Indication(s)	Clinical Assay(s) Available
ALK	ceritinib	NSCLC	Vysis ALK Break Apart FISH probe kit
	crizotinib	NSCLC	
BCR-ABL	bosutinib	CML	BCR-ABL Mutation Analysis test
	dasatinib	ALL, CML	
	imatinib	ALL, CML, GIST	
	nilotinib	CML	
	ponatinib	ALL, CML	
BRAF	dabrafenib	Melanoma	Cobas 4800 V600E THxID BRAF test
	vemurafenib	Melanoma	
BTK	ibrutinib	MCL, CLL, WM	No Clinical Assay Available
CDK 4/6	palbociclib	Breast	No Clinical Assay Available
c-KIT	imatinib	ALL, CML, GIST	c-KIT pharmDX
	regorafenib	CRC, GIST	
	sunitinib	RCC, GIST, pNET	
CTLA-4	ipilimumab	Melanoma	No Clinical Assay Available
EGFR	afatinib	NSCLC	EGFR pharmDx Cobas EGFR Mutation Assay
	erlotinib	NSCLC	
ER/PR	anastrazole	Breast	ER/PR pharmDx TargetPrint
	exemestane	Breast	
	letrozole	Breast	
	tamoxifen	Breast	
HER2	ado-trastuzumab emtansine	Breast	HercepTest[1], Pathway Insite PathVysion SPOT-Light HER2 CISH
	lapatinib	Breast	
	pertuzumab	Breast	
	trastuzumab	Breast, Gastric	
JAK	ruxolitinib	Myelofibrosis, PCV	JAK2 V617F Mutation Detection Assay HTScan JAK2 Kinase Assay Kit
KRAS	cetuximab	CRC, NSCLC, HNC	Cobas KRAS Mutation Test Therascreen KRAS RGQ PCR Kit DxS KRAS Mutation Test Kit, Genzyme's KRAS Mutation Analysis
	panitumumab	CRC	
MEK	trametinib	Melanoma	No Clinical Assay Available
mTOR	everolimus	Breast, pNET, RCC	No Clinical Assay Available
	temsirolimus	RCC	
PARP	olaparib	BRCA-mutated ovarian	No Clinical Assay Available
PD-1	pembrolizumab	Melanoma	No Clinical Assay Available
	nivolumab	Melanoma, NSCLC	

continued on following page

Table 1. Continued

Biomarker	Therapy	FDA-Approved Indication(s)	Clinical Assay(s) Available
SMO	vismodegib	BCC	No Clinical Assay Available
VEGF	aflibercept	CRC	No Clinical Assay Available
	axitinib	RCC	
	bevacizumab	Cervical, CRC, GBM, NSCLC, Ovarian, RCC	
	cabozantinib	MTC	
	lenvatinib	Thyroid	
	pazopanib	RCC, STS	
	ramucirumab	Gastric	
	regorafenib	CRC, GIST	
	sorafenib	RCC, HCC, DTC	
	sunitinib	RCC, GIST, pNET	
	vandetanib	MTC	

BBT: basal cell carcinoma; CLL: chronic lymphocytic leukemia; CML: chronic myeloid leukemia; CRC: colorectal; DTC: differentiated thyroid cancer; GBM: glioblastoma; GIST: gastrointestinal stromal tumor; HCC: hepatocellular carcinoma; HNC: head and neck cancer; MCL: mantle cell lymphoma; MTC: medullary thyroid carcinoma; NSCLC: non-small cell lung cancer; PCV: polycythemia vera; pNET: pancreatic neuroendocrine tumor; RCC: renal cell carcinoma; STS: soft-tissue sarcoma; WM: Waldenstrom's macroglubulinemia

Table 2. Overview of select germ-line biomarkers used for personalized cancer medicine

Biomarker	Therapy	Tumor	Clinical Assay(s) Available	Frequency of Variant/ Biomarker[1]
CYP450 2D6	tamoxifen amitriptyline nortriptyline clomipramine desipramine fluoxetine paroxetine venlafaxine imipramine codeine oxycodone hydrocodone tramadol ondansetron	Breast (tamoxifen) Any (for antidepressants and opioids)	AmpliChip Cytochrome P450 Genotyping test, xTAG CYP2D6, P450-Glo	*4 allele – 18% *10 allele – 6% Gene duplication (ultrarapid metabolizer) – 5%
DPYD	5-fluorouracil capecitabine	CRC, gastric, breast	Theraguide 5-FU DPD Enzyme Assay	*2A variant – 2%
TPMT	6-mercaptopurine	ALL	TPMT Enzyme diagnostic test, Prometheus TPMT genetic test	*2 allele – 0.4% *3A allele – 5% *3C allele – 0.5%
TYMS	5-fluorouracil	CRC	Theraguide 5-FU	2R – 46% 3R – 54%
UGT1A1	irinotecan nilotinib	Leukemia, CRC	Invader UGT1A1 Molecular Assay, INFINITI UGT1A1 Assay	*28 – 38%
CYP2C19	amitriptyline citalopram clomipramine imipramine voriconazole	Any	CYP2C19 Testing Spartan Rx Verigene CYP2C19 Test INFINITI CYP2C19 Assay xTAG CYP2C19	*2 allele – 15% *3 allele – <1% *17 allele – 25%

Section 3
Proteomics and Genomics

Chapter 4
Genomics and Proteomic Approach in the Treatment of Various Human Diseases:
Applications of Genomics and Proteomics

Urmila Jarouliya
Jiwaji University, India

Raj K. Keservani
Rajiv Gandhi Proudyogiki Vishwavidyalaya, India

ABSTRACT

World wise genomic analysis is beginning to move from the laboratories of basic investigators to large-scale clinical trials. The potential of this technology is to improve diagnosis and tailored treatment of various human diseases. In addition, new data from the emerging proteomics platforms add another layer of molecular information to the study of human disease, as scientists attempt to catalogue a complete list of the proteins encoded by the genome and to establish a 'bio-signature' profile of human health and disease. In the medical sciences identification of human genome sequence is a significant milestone for all the genes and their regulatory regions which provides the required framework for the genetic blueprint of humankind and that will make possible to recognize the molecular premise of disease. It is accepted that, together, these technologies genomic and proteomic will make easier to study all aspects of genes, gene products and signaling pathways so that the objective of personalised molecular medicine can be achieved.

INTRODUCTION

Genomics is an area within genetics that concerns the sequencing and analysis of an organism's genome. Our genomes hold the information and instructions that define how our bodies function. But sometimes there are mistakes, mutations, or variations in our genome that predisposes us to or cause disease. Clini-

DOI: 10.4018/978-1-5225-0754-3.ch004

cal genomics is the practice of using DNA sequencing to find these variations to help diagnose disease and find the best treatment or to identify patients at risk for disease to help with prevention.

Gene therapy may provide some clues in the efficient delivery of biologics. For this reason, several studies have focussed to design the vectors, promoter or target gene and testing them in animal models of arthritis, cancer and hepatitis C, and the obtained results concludes that gene therapy can be a convenience procedure in the treatment of provocative and ruinous rheumatoid arthritis as well as in cancer and hepatitis C. Gene therapy is defined as an introduction of nucleic acids into a host cell for therapeutic purposes; one option may be the over expression of a therapeutic gene, another option consist in the repression of a target gene highly expressed in disease {small interfering RNA (siRNA)}. Another approach in gene expression is that it profiles the entire analysis of thousands of gene and its isolation to generate a global picture of biological functions in a specific cell or tissue or even organ. Gene expression profiling has recently been at the forefront of advance in personalized medicine, especially in the field of cancer for the prediction of tumour behaviour in several types of cancer, in arthritis and for hepatitis (Walsh et al., 2004; Tak & Bresnihan, 2000; Bessis et al., 1998; Kim et al., 2002).

The term proteome was introduced in the 1990s, referring to an entire complement of proteins produced. Several metabolic diseases and genetic abnormalities are known to impair the cellular transcription and translation status and thereby creating a variation in proteome (Di Girolamo et al. 2012). These alterations in proteome are an opportunity for development of diagnosis of molecular signatures for several diseases and lead to the development of a new segment of research called 'clinical proteomics'. Proteomics is a study of the structures and functions of the proteins and refers to a large-scale experimental analysis of proteins available in low abundance (Ceciliani et al., 2014). While clinical proteomics is defined as clinical and analytical validation and implementation of novel therapy or diagnosis related markers that originate from preclinical studies designed to identify leads in analogy to drug screening studies (Apweiler et al., 2009).

Early detection, control and prevention of various diseases are difficult (Wulfkuhle et al., 2003). Proteomics provide powerful approach to identify and analyse the normal and transformed cell function from complex mixture (Roy & Shukla, 2008). It is very strong tool for both biomarker discovery and for the observation of biochemical processes involved in diseases. Simply can be said that proteomics includes the inclusive regulation of protein expression levels and consequently allows the regulated pathway for cellular processes. Now a day's three types of proteomics approach have been recognized, (a) Structural proteomics: it analyze the protein structure in large scale, it compares protein structure and help to identify the function of newly discovered gene. (b) Expression proteomics: analysis of protein structure at large scale, it helps identify proteins in normal and diseased condition sample such as healthy vs. diseased tissue. (c) Interaction proteomics: analysis of protein interactions at larger scale, it includes protein-protein analysis or protein-DNA/RNA interactions (Andy et al., 2003). Proteomics and their applications were shown in Figure 1.

The study of human gene and protein helps to identify the new drug for the treatment of diseases. Computer software uses a target for new drugs proteins which are associated with a disease, identified by proteome information. If some of the protein mixed with then its three dimensional (3D) structures provides information to design the drugs to interfere with the action of protein (Vaidyanathan, 2012). Specific proteins as biomarkers were used to diagnose the diseases. Various techniques employed to test for protein produce during a disease and help to diagnose the disease instantly. The proteomics techniques includes secretomics, western blot, ELISA (enzyme linked immuno-sorbent assay) or mass spectrometry, immunohistochemical staining (Klopfleisch et al., 2010; Klopfleisch et al., 2009). Proteomics studied

Figure 1. Types of Proteomics and their applications

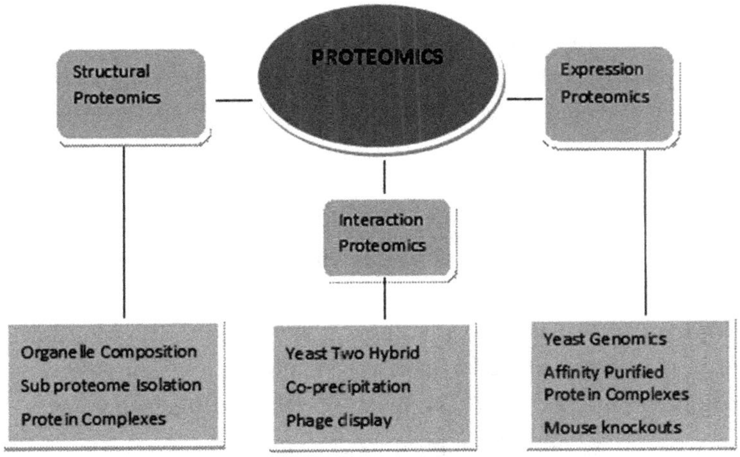

secretion pathway and secreted proteins via its approach and recently it emerged as a biomarker tool for the discovery of various human associated diseases (Hathout, 2007). In this chapter we discuss the currently used gene therapy approaches and gene expression profiling and the proteomic approach that are applied for the treatment of rheumatoid arthritis (RA), Cancer and Hepatitis C trials.

Rheumatoid Arthritis

Rheumatoid arthritis (RA) approximately affects up to 1% of the general adult population worldwide. It affects mostly women in between forty and sixty years old. The causes of rheumatoid arthritis are still unknown and no cure has been discovered to treat the disease. However, genetic methods and approaches can be used to identify the genes that are responsible for the disease and to cure the disease. This disease is an autoimmune disorder and systemic means it affects the entire body rather than a single organ or body part but mainly it affects the joints, designated by long term inflammation that is chronic with an increase in cell numbers leading to the destruction of cartilage and bone, inspite of joints the hematologic, respiratory, and cardiovascular system commonly are also affected. This disease is related with a reduction in life probability and standard. The initiator of the disease is still unknown, but after the long period of research over the last two decades has make it clear that the immunological reactions such as inflammation of the synovial membrane due to the combination of genetic and environmental factors may be the cause of this disease (Walsh et al., 2004; Tak & Bresnihan, 2000). In a study by Glant et al. (2014) they concluded that a large number of studies show that apart from the inherited genetic structure (that is, genomic DNA), various environmental factors notably leads to the physiology of rheumatoid arthritis. Epigenetic factors (those interact with genetic material like DNA, but do not change their sequence. Instead, they act as chemical tags for the gene regulation) react to external stimuli and form bridges between the environment and the genetic information-harboring DNA. Epigenetic mechanisms are involved in the concluding explanation of the encoded genetic information by regulating gene expression and alterations in their profile effects the activity of the immune system. Overall, further epigenetic process increase the complications of rheumatoid arthritis by providing additional ultra fine contributions to its protection, it is becoming obvious that the two systems (genetic and epigenetic) interact with each other and are ultimately responsible for rheumatoid arthritis development.

Large number of peoples with RA produces a group of auto-antibodies (an antibody produced by an organism in response to a constituent of its own tissues), called rheumatoid factors (RF), that are reactive with determinants in the Fc region of IgG. RF is an IgM antibody and such auto-antibodies bind to normal circulating IgG, forming IgG-IgM complexes that are deposited in the joints. These complexes can activate the complement cascade, resulting in a type III (immune complex mediated) hypersensitive reaction, which leads to chronic inflammation of the joints. The primary symptoms indicate joints swelling, tenderness and stiffness that results in weakened movement. In RA, with time multiple joints are affected like joints of hand, shoulder, knee, and feet and sometimes cervical spine are also features usually not found in other forms of arthritis (Muller-Ladner et al., 2005; Majithia & Geraci 2007). Vitamin D deficiency is more common characteristic in RA subjects. Although a variety of cells play a role in RA disease development but specifically significance cell are macrophages.

Macrophages are rich sources and major producers of pro-inflammatory cytokines including TNF-α (tumor necrosis factor alpha), IL-1 (interleukin-1), IL-6 (interleukin-6), IL-8 (interleukin-8), and GMCSF (Granulocyte macrophage colony stimulating factor). These cytokines further stimulate the macrophage, as well as other cells in the micro-environment, including fibroblasts and osteoclasts, and finally at distant sites in the body through cell surface. Macrophages are also producers of prostaglandins and leukotrienes, nitric oxide, and other pro-inflammatory mediators with local and systemic effects (Kang et al., 2010).

Macrophages, the main functional cell of the synovial in synovial tissue are efficient of antigen presentation and T-cell activation. They remain inactive in the healthy joint and become activated in the swollen (inflamed) joints, regulates the secretion of pro-inflammatory cytokines (IL-1, IL-6, IL-8 and TNF-α). These cytokines are produced in excess in joints of patients with RA and triggers elevation in synoviocyte expansion and a flow of secondary mediators involved in the neophytement of inflammatory cells and in the process of joint destruction (Camussi & Lupia, 1998). Synovial macrophages are present within the sub-lining and lining layer at the cartilage–pannus junction and arbitrate articular smashing. These sub-lining macrophages are now also regarded as the most authentic biomarker for disease extremity and response to treatment in rheumatoid arthritis (RA).

Therapy for RA

However, in the past decade treatment pattern have been dramatically changed by the introduction of biologic therapies which specifically target molecules involved in disease pathogenesis. Biologic therapies for RA have mutinized clinical outcomes where disease remission has become a realistic goal for individuals with an average to severe RA. Disease modifying anti-rheumatic drugs (DMARDs) has been used for decades to manage rheumatic Diseases such as Methotrexate (MTX), it is an anti-metabolite and a folate analog designed to compete for folate receptors, which affects the de novo synthesis of purine and pyrimidine precursors of DNA and RNA. MTX also has anti-inflammatory effects at low doses. MTX inhibits T-cell activation and proliferation, down-regulates the expression of some activation and adhesion molecules, decreases immunoglobulin production, inhibits cyclooxygenases (COX) and lipo-oxygenases, and modulates the secretion of various cytokines by monocytes and macrophages. MTX, administrated alone or in combination with either synthetic or biologic DMARDs remains the first drug of choice for patients with RA (Katchamart et al., 2009). Current biologics available or/in development for RA has mechanisms of action which interfere with pivotal chemical mediators or cell types which are involved in the RA inflammatory response. These include those directed against cytokine actions such as anti-TNF, anti-IL-1 and anti-IL-6 and also those directed against cell surface receptors involved in T and B cell activation, such as anti-CD28 and anti CD-20 respectively. An early outcome prognosis of remarkable DMARD therapies offers an option for independently modified medications and may therefore prevent serious side effects of current RA and reduce costs for treatment strategies.

To describe the related biomarkers for MTX monotherapy, specific response marker genes such as CD11c for anti-TNF monotherapy leads to a valuable interest (Stuhlmüller et al., 2010). Moreover, the association of those markers is a way to calculate the outcome of the standard fusion therapy with both drugs. In addition, supplemental correlation analyses of the presented gene expression profiles with the expression of specific micro-RNAs could ameliorate the predictive power of the selected markers and might also provide a more facts to understand the pathological process of RA.

Gene Therapy

Another way for systemic protein delivery is gene therapy. Two strategies may be proposed for therapeutic gene transfer into rheumatic joints: either in vitro transduction of synovial cells before injection (ex vivo cell-mediated approach) or local injection of the therapeutic vector (in vivo approach)

Ex Vivo Gene Transfer

In ex-vivo gene transfer method the cells are inserted in culture coursed by the injection of these modified cells into the target tissue. The cells used for ex vivo gene therapy should be easy to obtainable and without changing their observable characteristics are capable to live for longer periods. This can be achieved by using genetically modified fibroblasts cells such as- synoviocytes, myoblasts, mesenchymal stromal cells, as well as immune cells like- T cells, B cells and dendritic cells (Morita et al., 2001; Annenkov & Chernajovsky, 2000). The cells which are genetically redesigned secrete the required protein at the site of injection. The benefit of this method is (a) it controls the standard of injected material, particularly when using a vector, (b) resolving the problem of transduced cells so they should not be inserted reverse and (c) attaining accurate amount of expressed transgene, and genetically modified cells that are injected clinically for the desired transgene.

In Vivo Gene Transfer

Another method for gene transfer is in vivo, in which gene is directly delivered to target tissues by using commonly recombinant viral (AAV, HSV, retrovirus, lentivirus, adenovirus) and non-viral (plasmid) vectors. From the resident or parenchymal cells therapeutically important agents can be achieved directly in a single injection, with minimum risk of modification of the targeted cells and expanding of the vector. This method does not require complicated medical procedures like surgery or anaesthesia and it enabled the treatment of as many joints as requisite. Before using for human surgery the vector and transgene used for the gene delivery in RA treatment has been successfully proofed by many groups, for RA trials in various animal models.

These methods also used nucleic acid associated with chemical (liposome and polymers) or mechanical (gene gun). Although, preclinical observation of the vector proliferation and the immune-response initiation against the vector following intra-articular administration showed that the technique is free from any drawback. To keep away from any kind of adverse affect (setback) from this method needs a close follow up for gene therapy approach in the future application. Finally the objective of gene therapy will be the injection of a vector that has a particular aimed cell.

Gene Expression Profiling

Lots of descriptive methods have been employed for the expression of thousands of genes. Some of them are massively parallel signature sequencing (MPSS), serial analysis of gene expression (SAGE) and microarrays (oligonucleotide and cDNA).

- **MPSS (Massively Parallel Signature Sequencing):** In this method direct quantification of definite number of mRNA's are observed in a tissue or cell. By employing this technique cDNA libraries are created from the desired tissue or cells and the obtained cDNAs are expanded by PCR (polymerase chain reaction). This technique is as favourable as SAGE, need not to purify and sequence every clone, also in advance there is no necessitate recognizing the sequences of the transcripts expressed in the tissue or cell. The outcome of the investigation can be directly compared by calculating. So it is said that this technique allows in detail profiling of gene expression, but the draw back with this is that it requires some specific equipments (Brenner et al., 2000).
- **SAGE (Serial Analysis of Gene Expression):** In this method polyadenylated mRNA is separated from biotinylated oligo-dT and precipitated with streptavidin-coupled magnetic beads used in combination with biotin. The mRNA is then reversed transcribed by reverse transcriptase and the double stranded cDNA is created. The created cDNA's are cuts at the restriction sites by Hin1II (Nla III) and gives rise to 15bp fragments or tags. These fragments are ligated by ligase, amplified with PCR and the achieved clones are sequenced. The profit of this method is that the large quantity of transcripts can be quantitated and the restriction is that huge number of purified and sequenced clones is needed. This can be expensive and the rate of production that is throughout is limited (Shah et al., 2002).

The most commonly used technology to profile the expression of thousands of transcripts at a time is microarrays.

- **Microarrays:** A microarray is a set of short Expressed Sequence Tags (ESTs) made from a cDNA library of a set of known (or partially known) gene loci. The ESTs are spotted onto a cover-slip-sized glass plate; microarrays of many thousand ESTs are possible. The main advantages of microarray technology are high throughput, parallelism, miniaturization, speed and automation. The most often used microarrays are cDNA and oligonucleotide arrays. cDNA microarray is the strongest tool for studying gene expression in many various organisms and has been successfully employed to the operation of many thousands of genes expression and to large-scale gene discovery, as well as polymorphism screening and mapping of genomic DNA clones. It also allows the quantitative analysis of RNAs transcribed from both known and unknown genes. This technique provides diagnostic fingerprints by comparing gene expression patterns in normal and pathological cells, and because it can simultaneously track expression levels of many genes, it provides a source of operational context for inference and predication about complex cell control systems.

The second type of microarray uses oligonucleotides. In oligonucleotide microarrays, short DNA oligonucleotides are spotted onto the array. The main feature of oligonucleotide microarray is that each gene is normally represented by more than one probe.

In a study by Sugino et al (2010) they described that for the past many years, through genome-wide association studies (GWAS) six high-risk rheumatoid arthritis (RA) susceptibility genes – namely, CD244, PADI4, SLC22A2, PTPN22, CTLA4, and STAT4 was recognized and in their research they finalized that the association of microarray analysis and GWAS would be a more successful step for gene identification than the analysis of individual datasets and both methods would allow for more precise recognition of RA genes in humans.

In 2003, van der Pouw Kraan et al. studied gene expression in RA synovium and found proof for adaptive immune responses in some patients with RA, and fibroblast abnormalities in others. Gene expression profiling is also beginning to show potential clinical utility for RA in the area of predicting responses to therapy, specifically to tumor necrosis factor alpha (TNF-α) blockers. In a study by Meugmer et al. (2011), they had identified gene expression in RA patient's peripheral blood mononuclear cells (PBMCs), and observed that genes identified in these cells having varying gene expression pattern. The evolvement of inhibitors of tumor necrosis factor (TNF-α) has led to major approaches in the management of RA. The potential of this therapy highlights the key role of TNF-α in the pathological process of RA. TNF-α have its effects on immune system, inflammation, or apoptosis, and controls the expression of gene networks through the activation of intracellular signalling pathways and specific transcription factors (Hehlgans & Pfeffer, 2005). The identification of these transcriptional events using microarrays and large-scale gene expression analysis can therefore help to better understand the mechanisms of action of therapeutic agents, as successfully performed in various chronic inflammatory diseases (Laukens et al., 2006; Ospelt & Gay, 2007).

Anti-TNF-α Therapy

The genetic approach for the treatment of RA includes gene studies and genome wide association studies (GWAS). Genes study in RA explains that which gene has been related to RA (such as disease risk/susceptibility genes) or pathways involved in the RA process or pathogenesis. Scientific research investigated that gene function and signaling pathways of cytokines (mainly TNF-α) involved in RA pathogenesis (McGeough & Bjourson, 2012). TNF-α is a cytokine that plays an important role in joint inflammation. TNF-α inhibitors (namely etanercept, infliximab, and adalimumab) have been used successfully to treat RA patients. Anti-TNF-α therapy leads to significant useful development in the large number of RA patients and down-regulates inflammatory cytokines stimulated by TNF-α. The effects of a TNF-α blockade are moderately based on synovial TNF-α expression and infiltration by TNF-α-producing inflammatory cells. TNF- α inhibitors (Infliximab, etanercept and adalimumab) have been knows available commercially more than fifteen years. They bind and block TNF-α by different mechanisms, and etanercept additionally binds to lymphotoxin. Inspite of their quite short lived days, many studies have been reported treating these agents. The mechanisms of action, efficacy and safety of these compounds have been demonstrated in clinical trials, which allow physicians to use them more efficiently (Jin et al., 2010). Signalling pathways such as Toll- like receptor (TLR), NF kappa B (NFκB) and P38 mitogen activated protein kinase (MAPK) are involved in the propagation of chronic inflammatory processes and are also potential sources of biomarkers for response to anti-inflammatory therapies that include mechanisms driving and regulating the immune cell responses.

Proteomics as Biomarker in RA

Proteomics were also used in study of rheumatoid arthritis and osteoarthritis. We mainly discuss here only the rheumatoid arthritis. For the diagnosis of RA proteomic technology is used as a biomarker (Gobezie et al., 2006; Ruiz-Romero CBlanco FJ, 2013). Several proteomic approaches have been applied to the investigation of autoimmune disorders including (i) autoantigen and biomarker discovery by 2-dimensional gel electrophoresis (2-DE) based separation of proteins and subsequent protein identification by mass spectrometry (MS); (ii) protein microarrays for the characterisation of antibody responses; (iii) reverse phase protein arrays to analyze protein phosphorylation (iv) antibody array technologies to profile cytokines and other biomolecules; and (v) flow cytometric analysis of phosphoproteins (Dasilva et al., 2012; Hueber & Robinson, 2006). As earlier discussed the tumor necrosis factor-α (TNF-α) and interleukin-1 (IL-1) is the main cytokine related to the pathogenesis of RA. 2-DE (2-dimensional gel electrophoresis) separates complex protein mixtures based on their isoelectric points (pI) and molecular weights and various combinations of liquid chromatography. Mass spectroscopy of individual proteins has enabled us to develop the ability to identify almost any protein, analyze the protein for the presence of post-translational modifications (PTM's), characterize its protein-protein interactions and provide structural information about the specific protein. The various methods of ionization in MS are electrospray ionisation (ESI), matrix-assisted laser desorption/ionisation (MALDI) or the surface- enhanced laser desorption ionisation (SELDI) (Ying-Chou Chen et al., 2008). Peptide multiple reactions monitoring (MRM) assays have emerged as an alternative to affinity-based measurement of proteins and allow reproducible protein quantification (Hüttenhain et al., 2012). Richard et al. (2009) reported that the use of proteomics in the field of arthritis gave more important information's. Calgranulin-A is a unique biomarker which differentiate the rheumatoid arthritis, its protein is better known by its gene identification S100A8 or MRP8 in the field of rheumatology. The expression of this protein is specific for cells like monocytes, granulocytes and macrophages and released during the interaction of monocytes with the inflammatory activated endothelium. This marker has been identified in several proteome analyses (Page et al., 2007). Mateos et al. (2012) studied and identify some proteins, which are more abundant in the synovial fluid (SF) of patients suffering from rheumatoid arthritis (RA) and osteoarthritis (OA) by using high performance liquid chromatography coupled to mass spectrometry (Tilleman et al., 2005).

Cancer

Theodor Boveri initially proposed in 1902 that a single cell with scrambled chromosomes and hence uncontrolled cell division was the origin of a cancerous tumor. Currently, treatments for basic, translational, and clinical cancer research are essentially designed based on the organ of the body in which the cancer is originally observed (Javier Cortes et al., 2014). However, gene expression and genomic analyses using high-throughput technologies have helped to elucidate the molecular characteristics of cancer, providing a new angle to oncology.

The primary treatment for early stages of cancer was surgery (De Vita et al., 2012). Later in 1943, nitrogen mustard and in 1948 folic acid antagonists was used in the management of patients with lymphoma (Goodman et al., 1984) and for the childhood leukaemia. After that, there has been a sudden evolution in chemotherapy exploration for cancer. Further viruses have been studied more intensely in humans, with the successive discovery of gene therapy. Later on in 1987, immunotherapy was initiated in the control of cancer patients (Kelly et al., 2007). In the United States the first FDA (Food and Drug Administration) approved gene therapy was appeared in 1990 for a patient with severe combined immunodeficiency (SCID) syndrome (Sheridan et al., 2011). After that, lots of experimental work has been done for cancer patients, using various methods in gene therapy, with fruitful outcomes mentioned in victims with chronic lymphocytic leukaemia, acute lymphocytic leukaemia, brain tumors, and some others (Chiocca et al., 2004).

Genomics and proteomics are becoming increasingly important therapeutic pillars in cancer research. The last few decades have seen increasingly deeper knowledge of the pathogenesis of cancer and specific aberrations in the genome and proteome of cancer cells. For example, an aberrant gene often translates into an abnormal protein, capable of driving malignant behaviour of the cells. Profiling abnormal genes may help us better classify cancers and select the optimal treatment, and profiling abnormal proteins holds even greater potential. Although cancer genomics can help and predict what may happen in cancer cells while cancer proteomics can determine what actually happens because it focuses on final gene function. The approach of scientific methodologies such as SNP (Single-nucleotide polymorphism) analysis, DNA microarray, and tissue microarray investigation will indubitably make some changes radically or fundamentally for cancer treatment. Very soon it will be able to achieve and recognize the patients who response or unsuccessful to response to cancer therapy early in the clinical drug making procedure. Facts provided from these technologies would give a remarkable step in separating cancer therapy for various types of cancer and expanding the advantage of treatment by adapting these therapies. The use of polymorphic markers, particularly single nucleotide polymorphisms (SNPs), promises to make available a complete tool for examining the human genome and identifying those genes and genomic regions presenting to the cancer phenotype. Gene expression studies in human cancer can identify genetic markers of malignant transformation. DNA microarray-based gene expression pro-filing depends on nucleic acid hybridization and the use of nucleic acid polymers, immobilized on a solid surface, as probes for complementary gene sequences. This Expression profiling techniques have been used to simultaneously monitor the expression of thousands of genes from both tumour and normal tissues. They are relatively easy to use and can be applied to large numbers of samples in parallel. These are some important technologies that provide the basic understanding of the genetic complexities involved in cancer and have important clinical suggestions for exhibiting the pathways and novel targets associated with the uncontrolled growth process of tumor cells. Single-nucleotide polymorphism analysis, combined with cDNA microarrays and tissue microarrays, should help to disclose the peculiar genetic profiles and novel molecular targets that have significant effect on drug effectiveness and virulence. By combining all these technologies research can proceed towards in developing widely and fastly therapeutic agents that are specifically targets for particular tumour patient. Proteomic methods, for example, 2-dimensional electrophoresis and mass spectrometry, are now commonly used to evaluate the expression profiles of genes and proteins in cancer cells, their surrounding tissues, and body fluids (kim, 2007).

Gene Therapy

Cancer is a process in which cells grow aberrantly. The growth of cancer cells leads to damage of normal tissues, causing loss of function and often pain. Many types of tumors shed cells that migrate to other distant sites in the body, establish a base there, and grow continuously. These secondary cancer sites, called metastases, cause local destruction, loss of normal tissue function and can acquire an even greater propensity to shed. Multiple cumulative genetic and/or epigenetic changes are needed to cause cancer. Those genes on which the maintenance of the cancer process depends are called "driver genes" which, unlike passenger genes, are key targets although non-driver genes can also contribute to cancer growth. A number of gene therapy strategies are being evaluated in patients with cancer and these include manipulating cells to gain or lose function. For example, half of all cancers have a mutated p53 protein that interferes with the ability of tumor cells to self-destruct by a process called apoptosis. Furthermore, other tumor suppressor genes are being placed in gene cassettes for expression in tumor cells, which can similarly render them more sensitive to apoptosis, or the process of programmed cell death. Other investigators are utilizing gene therapy approaches to induce expression of immune stimulating proteins called cytokines which in turn may increase the ability of the patient's own immune system to recognize and kill these cancer cells. Another immune modulating alternative entering the clinic is the use of RNA interference (RNAi) silencing of endogenous cancer intracellular immune suppressor proteins, e.g., TGF beta, as a component of immunotherapy. Beside this gene silencing has been designed to inhibit the expression of specific genes which are activated or over expressed in cancer cells and can drive tumor growth (with particular attention to presumptive driver genes), blood vessel formation, seeding of tumor cells to other tissues, and allow for resistance to chemotherapy. Several such genes, termed oncogenes, are often expressed continuously at high concentrations in cancer cells and express proteins that increase cell growth and/or division. Alternatively, tumor growth requires new blood vessel formation to survive, a process known as angiogenesis, which is mediated by an array of interacting proteins. A number of approaches to gene silencing have been or are being explored in the clinic including antisense oligonucleotides (ASO), short interfering RNA (siRNA) and short hairpin RNA (shRNA) that target post-transcription mRNA, and bi-functional shRNA which has both post-transcriptional silencing and translation-inhibitory effects. Gene therapy approaches may be designed to directly kill tumor cells using tumor-killing viruses, or through the introduction of genes termed suicide genes into the tumor cells. Scientists have generated viruses, termed oncolytic viruses, which grow selectively in tumor cells as compared to normal cells. For example, an expanding number of human viruses such as measles virus, vesticular stomatitis virus, reovirus, adenovirus, and herpes simplex virus (HSV) can be genetically modified to grow in tumor cells which in result kills the tumor cell, but very poorly in normal cells thereby establishing a therapeutic advantage. Various commercially accepted drugs for gene therapy were liberated, such as ONYX-15 (Onyx Pharmaceuticals) for refractory head and neck cancer (2005); human papilloma virus vaccine (Gardasil) (Merck Sharp & Dohme) for the preclusion of cervix cancer (2006); and modified dendritic cells, sipuleucel-T (Provenge) (Dendreon Corporation, Seattle, WA), for minimally symptomatic, metastatic prostate cancer (2010). The main aim of cancer gene therapy is to introduce new genetic material into target cells without toxicity to non-target tissues.

Several techniques have been invented to make possible the entry of genetic materials (transgenes) into target cells, using diverse vectors. They are mainly separated into two major categories: viral (Adenoviruses, Herpes simplex virus, Lentiviruses, Reovirus) and non-viral (Electroporation, nanoparticles, hydrodynamics, cationic liposomes, transposon, synthetic viruses) vectors. Viruses generally attach to target cells and insert their genetic materials into the host cell as a part of their replication process. For nonviral vectors different approaches have been utilized, using physical, chemical modes of genetic transfer. Non-viral approaches have the advantage of safety and easy modifiability, but have a lower transfection efficiency compared to viral vectors (Shirley et al., 2013).

Physical Methods of Gene Transfer

The physical methods of gene transfer such as gene gun, jet injection, hydrodynamic injection, sonoporation based on ultrasound, magnetofection based on magnetic field and electroporation or electropermeabilization induces reversible alterations in the plasma membrane to allow the direct passage of the molecules of interest into the target cell followed by the release of DNA into its nucleus, ensuring its integrity against enzymes. These methods are mainly applied for gene delivery in tissue or for gene vaccination (Baranyi et al., 2013). Electroporation is presently being tested in several clinical trials, especially on patients with malignant melanoma, prostate cancer, colorectal cancer and leukemia (Shirley et al., 2013).

Chemical Methods of Gene Transfer

Gene transfer via the non-viral vectors or by chemicals is called chemical transfection. In this method DNA is introduced by calcium phosphate, lipid, or protein complexes. Calcium phosphate, DEAE-dextran, liposomes, and lipoplexes for oral delivery of gene; surfactants and perfluro chemical liquids for aerosol delivery of gene. Lipid vector or liposome is generated by a combination of plasmid DNA and a lipid solution. This fuses with the cell membranes of a variety of cell types, introducing the plasmid DNA into the cytoplasm and nucleus, where it is transiently expressed. Gene transfer efficacy to target cell is comparatively high for liposome than other chemical methods with lack of severe side effects (Tagami et al., 2012). Pegylated liposomes have been shown to localize to solid cancers and may deliver radio sensitizing agents preferentially to tumor tissue, potentially improving the therapeutic ratio of chemotherapy. Some artificial viral vectors have been also chemically synthesized with the properties of liposomes (Wagner et al., 1992). Transposons the 'jumping genes' another gene transfer material that can insert the desire gene in the cell as well as into the nucleus without changing its metabolic and genetic properties.

Bacterial Vectors in Gene Transfer

Bactofection or the method in which bacteria is used as a vector for the delivery of therapeutic genes to target cells because of it's the innate (non-specific) biological property that allows the effective DNA delivery to cells or tissues. Some bacteria (includes *E. coli, S. typhimurium, Bifidobacterium* and *Clostridium*) have the capacity to target particular tumor cells with the obstruction of RNA functions, including cellular metabolism and protein synthesis. Bacterial vectors can carries pro-drug converting enzymes and cytotoxic agents into tumor cells, and can arbitrate the host immune reaction. These bacteria can be engineered to carry magnetic or fluorescent material to increase the advantage in diagnosing and localising the tumors within cell, such as with magnetic resonance imaging (MRI) (Benoit et al., 2009), and also in the making of cancer vaccines (Baban et al., 2010). These vaccines can be administered orally.

Viral Vectors in Gene Transfer

Proper gene expression and the entry of therapeutic genes is the critical problem in gene therapy. Viruses are naturally developed vehicles which can effectively transfer their genetic material into the host cells. Their genetic material is either ribonucleic acid (RNA) or deoxyribonucleic acid (DNA), and can be single-stranded (ss) or double-stranded (ds). The ability of gene transfer in host cell had made them advantageous for engineering virus vector for the delivery of therapeutically important genes. The clinically used viral vectors are based on RNA and DNA viruses with different genomic structures and host limits. Particular viruses have been selected as gene delivery vehicles because of their capacities to carry foreign genes and their ability to efficiently deliver these genes associated with efficient gene expression. Many of these gene transfer vectors are modified viruses that retain the capability of the virus for efficient gene delivery but are safer than the inhabitant virus due to alternations that remove or modify one or more necessary viral functions. Non-infectious viruses can be modified genetically and they also work in the same manner as unmodified viruses, they can carry genetic material for delivery into a host cell's cytoplasm, and later on into the nucleus.

The important viral vectors are obtained from retroviruses; adenovirus, adeno-associated virus, herpes virus and poxvirus, these are involved worldwide in clinical gene therapy trials. Among these vector systems, retrovirus vectors represent the most important gene transfer system, since these vectors have high gene transfer efficiency and mediate high expression of therapeutic genes. The advantage of viral vectors in gene therapy is that they can be simply purified, and genes are expressed for long time with negligible side effects. Retroviruses involving lenti-viruses can incorporate themselves into host cell genome at the nucleus, while adenoviruses and adeno related viruses mainly remain stay as extra-chromosomal episomes (Yuan et al., 2013). Some of the virus vectors are detailed here.

Adenovirus

This virus has an icosahedral protein capsid that encompasses a linear duplex genetic material in the form of double stranded DNA. Adenovirus vectors can be replication-defective; certain essential viral genes are deleted and replaced by a cassette that expresses a foreign therapeutic gene. So the vector can be used for gene transfer in cancer therapy and as vaccines. Adenoviruses are ubiquitous, can infect a wide area of human cells and obtains high levels of gene transfer, less pathogenic to humans, can carry large segments of DNA (up to 7.5 kilobase pairs [kb]), integrity of the inserted foreign genes are usually conserved without any change through consecutive rounds of viral replication. Finally, adenoviral vectors are relatively easy to manipulate using recombinant DNA techniques.

In present some artificially synthesized oncolytic adenoviruses are examined in various patients, mainly in patients with astrocytoma of the brain along with radiation and/or temozolomide chemotherapy. ONYX-015 (Onyx Pharmaceuticals) is an artificially synthesized oncolytic adenovirus that was before accepted by the Chinese Food and Drug Administration (2005) in the management of refractory head and neck cancer along with cisplatinum (Chiocca et al., 2004). This was also examined in managing of other malignant tumors. Other oncolytic adenoviruses include Ad5-D24, recombinant H103, Ad5-CD/TKrep, CG7870, KH901, and OBP-301 (Telomelysin). The recently discovered adenoviral vectors are the gutless adenovirus; it is protective and genes are expressed comfortably for long-term (Yuan et al., 2013). So the genetically modified viruses have reduce antivirus immunity, reduced possibility for genomic toxicity because of insertional mutagenesis, and have the ability to carry genes inside the nucleus (Bryson et al., 2013).

Retrovirus

Retroviruses have a positive-strand non-segmented RNA as genetic material that undergoes reverse transcription (carried out by enzyme reverse transcriptase) to a double-stranded DNA. Further integrates its genome with host genome by enzyme integrase. Retroviral vectors have been the most preferred gene transfer systems in clinical gene therapy. Stable incorporation of retroviral viral DNA into the host genome is in itself advantageous, as long-term expression of the transgene is possible for achieving therapeutic efficacy. In recent year's gamma-retroviruses is the second most used gene transfer system. As long as they are actively dividing, these vectors are able to transduce most cell types. Although, most of these retroviral vectors lacking replication, thus results in vivo in defective transduction effect. Because of this factor there is lack of therapeutic success perceived in clinical trials for cancer. Thus, nowadays, replication-deficient retroviral vectors are mainly used in ex vivo gene transfer for the treatment of cancer, rather than in vivo tumor therapy.

Herpes Virus

Herpes simplex virus type 1 (HSV-1) is currently the most extensively engineered virus for gene transfer, consists of large linear double stranded DNA genome of 150kb in length. Oncolytic herpes simplex virus type 1 (HSV-1) vectors are emerging as an effective and powerful therapeutic approach for cancer. Phase I clinical traits of three vectors, G207, 1716, and NV1020, are either ongoing or completed, with no adverse events attributed to the virus. These and other HSV-1 vectors are effective against a myriad of solid tumors in mice, including glioma, melanoma, breast, prostate, colon, ovarian, and pancreatic cancer. Enhancement of activity was observed when HSV-1 vectors were used in combination with traditional therapies such as radiotherapy and chemotherapy, providing an attractive strategy to pursue in the clinic.

Adeno-Associated Virus

Among the currently developed virus vectors, the adeno-associated virus (AAV) vector is reviewed as one of the complete vector for cancer gene therapy. It is better than other gene vectors because it is with reduced host immune response, less toxic, and expresses the gene for long time. To impede the tumour growth and metastasis AAV vector have been used to carry and transport a variety of therapeutic genes (suicide genes, anti-angiogenic genes and immune-related genes) to cancer cells. In a study by Lu et al, they observed that a single intravenous dose of AAV/VEGF (Vascular endothelial growth factor)-Trap not only suppresses the primary growth tissue but also prevented the pulmonary metastasis along with long-term efficiency (Lu et al., 2012). In excess expression of the particular antagonist of hepatocyte growth factor (HGF) NK4, can antagonize the HGF/c-Met system completely by inhibiting c-Met signaling and tumor metastasis, which is also an AAV mediated anti-angiogenic gene therapy. Another therapy is AAV-mediated immune gene therapy it activates the host immune when therapeutic genes such as cytokines, immunogenic cell surface molecules, and tumor antigens are transferred to targets cells. Lv et al. (2011) had investigated and showed that an in vitro and in vivo tumour growth was inhibited by AAV-based anti-DR5 mouse-human chimeric antibody. Xiaojiang et al. (2010) observed that AAV-mediated NT4-Antshepherdin prevents the growth of the lung cancer cell line A549 by inducing apoptosis. So far, exact delivery of AAV mediated therapeutic genes can be improved by adding tumor-specific promoters to AAV vectors, such as extracellular domain of tumor necrosis factor-related apoptosis-inducing ligand (sTRAIL), human telomerase reverse transcriptase (hTERT), tumor-targeting motif, including RGD, and tenascin C (TnC) (Zhang et al., 2008; Wang et al., 2008; He et al., 2009; Ma et al., 2005; Lee et al., 2011). To enhance the antitumor activity, AAV in association with other therapies such as chemotherapy, radiation therapy and ultrasound therapy can significantly elevate the cytotoxicity to tumor cells.

Since it is safe to use, the virus is being used in several clinical trials, as oncolytic reovirus monotherapy, administered intratumoral, intravenously, or intraperitoneally; or as polytherapy, in combination with radiation therapy or chemotherapy (Comins et al., 2013).

RNA interference (RNAi) is a therapeutic biological tool in different cancers. Several types of non-encoding RNAs (siRNAs, shRNAs, and artificial microRNAs) have been used in preclinical studies. The proper design of siRNA, is hypothetically viable for contributing a greater therapeutic prospective in cancer therapy, as well as in the management of other medical disorders such as the hepatitis B virus, human papilloma virus, hypercholesterolemia and liver cirrhosis (Gujrati and Lu, 2013; Sato et al., 2008). Mostly siRNAs are particular for target genes, having less toxicity, and does not generate multidrug resistance. They also not converse with chromosomal DNA, and having a very minimum risk of target cell gene modifications and mutagenesis. Further, these genes can cause strong gene silencing of a large number of cancer related genes, which regrets the tumour but do not destroys the abnormal genes. siRNA therapy can be delivered directly into tumors; to secure them from enzymatic mortification several delivery systems for siRNA have been developed that make possible their effect in silencing specific genes.

Once the genetic materials are moved into the host cell through any of the above mention methods, it incorporates with genetic DNA in nucleus and induces metabolic signaling cascade like gene silencing, gene alteration, down regulation or repair mechanism. Rely on the potency of the gene expression, it can lead to cell death and tumour necrosis (as with the suicide gene), or impaired cell growth with tumor regression (as with the silencing gene). Modified gene can better respond to upcoming cancer therapies such as chemotherapy, immunotherapy and radiation therapy. Further cancer related problems such as thrombosis and the malignancy of the tissues can be prevented by target gene repair mechanism. In future repair mechanism can also be helpful in preventing hereditary cancer syndromes.

Gene Profiling

Gene-expression profiling has been used to develop genomic tests that may provide better predictions of clinical outcome than the traditional clinical and pathological standards. Earlier discussed there are many methods for gene profiling, but the most commonly used is microarray. Microarrays are a well-established technique for genomic research and have proven an important tool for delving into the complex genetic basis of cancer. In the study by Aarøe et al. (2009) for early detection of breast cancer by using microarray they concluded that the gene signature identified in their study in whole blood is being further refined to improve the diagnostic accuracy.

The development of gene expression pattern of patients with known clinical outcomes is compared to identify genes that are associated with prognosis without any prior biologic assumption. Later gene-expression patterns that are associated with a specific biologic phenotype or a deregulated molecular pathway are first identified and then subsequently correlated with the clinical outcome. Quantitative reverse-transcriptase–polymerase chain-reaction (RT-PCR) display the expressed RNA, or subtractive hybridization, which involves the enrichment of genes preferentially expressed in one tissue compared with a second were observed.

Proteomics as Biomarker in Cancer Disease

A proteomics approach is being used for the early detection of a variety of cancers, as well as non-neoplastic diseases such as infectious diseases, autoimmune diseases, vascular diseases, prenatal diagnosis and transplantation rejection. Proteomics is served as biomarkers for detection and monitoring the various cancers via checking the physiological status of cells in normally and diseased conditions (Srinivas et al., 2001). Cancers like lung, breast, prostate, liver and bladder cab be identified and detected by using various techniques such as two-dimensional electrophoresis, Laser capture micro dissection (LCM), surface enhanced laser desorption ionization time-of-flight mass spectrometry (SELDI-TOF MS), MALDI, Protein microarray and tissue array (Vaidyanathan et al., 2012; Klopfleisch et al., 2010).

Lung cancer has long been a significant worldwide public health issue. Lung cancer is the common cause of cancer which leads to death in men and women. Lung cancer is of two types (a) Non small cell lung cancer, represents 85% of cases (b) small cell lung cancer, which represents 15% of the cases. Cigarette smoking is the main cause of lung cancer. More than 800 lung adeno-carcinoma have been found by NCI's-LCMC (National cancer institute's lung cancer mutation consortium) due to the mutations in lung cancer driven genes such as (*egfr, braf, kras, akt1, her2, pik3ca, mek1, eml4-alk, met* amplification) (Kris et al., 2011). Xiao H. and his colleagues studied lung cancer by proteomics approach like (2-DGE) 2-dimensional difference gel electrophoresis and mass spectrometry (Xiao et al., 2012). Petricoin et al. (2002) by using mass spectroscopy coupled with an artificial intelligence computer algorithm developed a system of low molecular weight serum protein profiling and identified a specific protein signature that was associated with ovarian cancer from asymptomatic women with a high risk of developing the disease.

In United States the second most death dealing cancer in men is prostate cancer (Jemal et al., 2010). Micro RNAs is involved in progression and metastasis of human prostate cancer (Shi et al., 2008). Peng and his co-worker reported that expressions of five microRNAs (miRs-508-5p, -145, -143, -33a and -100) was significantly reduced in bone metastasis than that of primary prostate tumor (Peng et al., 2011).

Worldwide the third most usually occurring cancer is colorectal cancer and it is also the major cause of death. During diagnosis it was observed that about 25% patient's organs are affected by cancer, and about 40-50% evolves secondary metastasis. In a study by Yang et al. (2009), they reported about 100 miRNAs that are associated with colorectal cancer, such as miR-21, miR 17-92 cluster, miR-135a/b, miR-471 and miR-675 are the most regulated, while, reduced expression of miR-143, miR-14, let-7 and miR-101 was shown in colorectal cancer. These miRNAs mostly target the transcription factor such as STAT, c-MYC, SOX, OCT4, E2F1, ZEB1, ZEB2, NFIB and some kinases, like ERK and YES1, and proteins involved in matrix metallo-proteinases regulation that works as metastasis suppressors like RECK and TIMP3 (Schetter et al., 2011).

Ma and colleagues from Robert Weinberg's group evidenced that up-regulation of miR-10b suppressed homeobox D10 (HOXD10) expression, allowing the activation of the prometastatic gene RHOC and initiation of breast cancer invasion and metastasis (Ma et al., 2007). The miR-10b was highly expressed in metastatis of MDA-MB-231 cell line than the tumerogenic nonmetastatic MCF7 cells. MiR-10b suppressed the breast cancer in tumor bearing mice and increased the level of its target HOXD10 reported by researchers (Ma et al., 2010).

Many studies have been performed showing that 2DGE can detect differences between normal and cancer cell proteomes, although the extent of these changes appears quite variable. For instance, in breast cancer only few differences were observed in some studies (Hondermarck, 2003). The membrane protein compartment is of high interest, especially in cancer research, where many alterations affect cell-surface proteins and receptors. Improvements in 2DGE of membrane proteins have been made (Molloy, 2000), and alternative methods have been developed. It is a promising approach is MudPIT (multidimensional protein identification technology) (Wu & Yates, 2003). The application of this technology to compare micro dissected hepatocellular carcinoma with normal hepatocytes demonstrated its feasibility for the analysis of clinical samples. Another area of intense research is the development of protein arrays that, similar to gene arrays, would allow us to study changes in protein expression or modification on a global scale without much of the specialist and expensive equipment required by MS-based proteomics. Another technique SELDI (surface-enhanced laser desorption– ionization)-TOF (time-of-flight) MS has been applied to analyze cancers of the prostate, ovary, breast, lung, kidney, bladder, pancreas, liver, colon, endometrium, cervix, melanoma and Lymphoma (Walter Kolch et al., 2005). Although proteomics has established itself as a valuable tool for basic cancer research, it is less clear how it can best be implemented in clinical research.

Current methods for protein quantification mostly involve the use of electrospray ionization (ESI), matrix-assisted laser desorption ionization (MALDI), isotope-coded affinity tags (ICAT and iTRAQ), isotope-coded protein labeling (ICPL), tandem mass tags (TMT) and 15N/14N metabolic labeling, and so forth. These methods provide valuable flexibility to study protein changes in complex samples, and can measure the slight changes (<2-fold) between samples (Roe and Griffin, 2006).

The autoantibody signature method, known as Serological proteomic analysis (SERPA), is one of such technologies that combine proteomic strategies pooled in the MAPPing (multiple affinity protein profiling) strategy. The SERPA associates two-dimensional liquid chromatography followed by immune-detection of proteins. This combination can be performed in serum samples and helps to identifying specific auto-antibodies produced in response to tumor antigens.

The use of fine procedures aiming to purify protein complexes before mass-spectrometry analysis has provided impacting findings regarding tumor biology at the level of protein-protein interactions (Jain, 2008). Some oncogenic pathways have been targeted by functional proteomic analysis that is reviewed by Kolch and Pitt (2010). In the review study by Carolina (2014), they reviewed three major cancer pathways – epidermal growth factor receptor (EGFR), breakpoint cluster region (BCR)-ABL1 and ERK pathway under the prism of proteomic-based approaches for cancer treatment.

Hepatitis C

About 170 million people worldwide are currently living with chronic hepatitis C virus (HCV) infection (Getchell, 2013). Statistically, it is the fifth most prevalent cancer in the world with a continuous increase in the total number of its victim's. Many factors can increase the risk of developing hepatocellular carcinoma (HCC); these factors can be categorized into two major groups, namely toxins and viral infections. Both categories can induce liver cirrhosis and dysfunction. Persistent virus infection with HCV often leads to cirrhosis and hepatocellular carcinoma (HCC). Among those with chronic HCV infection, 15–40% will develop cirrhosis and/or hepatocellular carcinoma. Hepatitis C virus (HCV) is a small (~55 to 65 nm), spherical, enveloped, hepatotropic RNA virus that causes acute and chronic hepatitis in humans. Hepatitis C virus (HCV) is a single-stranded RNA virus containing a structured internal ribosomal entry site (IRES) in the 5′-noncoding region of the viral RNA. The virus is transmitted between people primarily by blood and blood products. Current combination therapy with pegylated interferon (peg-IFN-α) and ribavirin has improved the clinical outcome, but less than half of the patients with chronic hepatitis C can be expected to respond to these available agents. These presently available therapies are expensive, prolonged and associated with significant adverse effect. As such, there is a clear need for the development of additional agents that act through alternate mechanisms (Motavaf et al., 2012). RNAi is thought to be a natural defense mechanism that evolved to protect organisms from RNA viruses, such as hepatitis C virus and it is an effective nucleic acid-based gene silencing tool to target highly conserved or functionally important regions within the HCV genome (Pan et al., 2007).

There are some of the HCV vaccines that are used in the treatment. The recombinant proteins vaccine candidates induce an immune response to a limited number of viral epitopes which are cloned in bacteria, yeast or mammalian cells is sufficient to develop protective immunity (Duan et al., 2010). According to the genetic variability of the HCV viral envelope glycoprotein, this protein is the main target for anti-HCV antibodies. Peptide-based vaccines induce HCV-specific T-cell immunity with the presentation of peptide to T-cell receptor by HLA molecules. DNA delivery such as using a gene gun for DNA vaccination, electroporation with electrical impulses which creates pores in living cells and puts DNA through the cell membrane (Desjardins et al., 2009). Another HCV DNA-based vaccine is a T cell vaccine based on HCV non-structural 3/4A which expressed under the control of the Cytomegalovirus immediate early promoter (ChronVac-C has recently been developed by TripepAB Sweden) used electroporation to inject plasmid expressing HCV antigens NS3/4a.

Nowever, days using viral vector for the delivery of HCV RNA is the aim of vaccine choice. Adenoviral vectors have complete viral genes, so it can deliver HCV proteins and induces T-cell responses and reduce HCV viremia during primary infection. A therapeutic vaccine (TG4040) is a recombinant polyantigenic T cell vaccine base on highly attenuated poxvirus strain, Modified vaccinia Ankara (MVA) which expresses NS3/4/5B proteins (Hossein Keyvani, 2012).

Gene Therapy for Hepatitis C

Discoveries achieved through Genome-wide association studies (GWAS) have recently identified that it is very tough to predict host genetic variation, treatment response and spontaneous clearance in patients infected with hepatitis C virus (HCV). HCV virus has seven major viral genotypes with different geographical distributions and susceptibilities to interferon-α treatment. HCV genotype 1 is the most common genotype worldwide and one of the most difficult to treat (Hayes et al., 2012). Single-nucleotide polymorphisms (SNPs) in the region of the IL28B gene on chromosome 19, coding for the interferon (IFN)- λ-3 or IL28B gene, are strongly associated with treatment response to pegylated IFN and ribavirin in patients infected with genotype 1 HCV (Paul et al., 2011). In the study by Ge et al. (2009) observed and identified that rs12979860 (3 kilobases upstream of the IL28B gene encoding the type III interferon IFN-l3) in patients with HCV genotype (GT) 1 infections with the strongest association to therapy response. The meta-analysis study by Jiménez-Sousa et al. (2013) found remarkable consistency among the studies on IL28B SNPs and treatment of chronic HCV infection. Studies on IL28B genotype based therapy shortening are currently ongoing. The predictive value for IL28B polymorphisms was not limited to treatment with Peg-INF (pegylated-Interferon)/RBV (ribavirin), but could be confirmed also in receiving triple therapy with telaprevir.

Direct acting antiviral drugs are currently replacing antiviral therapy for hepatitis C infection but the treatment causes anaemia as side effect. The genome-wide association approach was successfully used in the search for determinants of drug-induced anaemia, which occurs in most treated patients of hepatitis C infection and is essentially ascribed to ribavirin (RBV) associated red blood cell destruction. In the study by Andri & Jacques (2011), they genotyped the inosine triphosphatase (ITPA) genetic variants associated with differences in susceptibility to anaemia were identified in the (ITPA) gene region (Thompson et al., 2010; Fellay et al., 2010). The association signal was entirely explained by two functional polymorphisms that cause ITPA deficiency, a benign enzymopathy that turns out to play a significant protective role in the particular context of HCV treatment. Genotyping of the genetic variants allows the identification of a minority of patients who are highly unlikely to suffer from severe anaemia during peg-IFN/RBV therapy. So IL28 and ITPA are able to predict treatment response and degree of ribavirin related anaemia for hepatitis C virus infection in humans.

Proteomics as Biomarker in Hepatitis C

Liver biopsies of hepatitis C virus (HCV) infected patient's offers the unique opportunity to study the in vivo human liver biology and disease. Functional analysis of proteins suggests that reduction of key mitochondrial processes including fatty acid oxidation and oxidative phosphorylation, and response to oxidative stress and reactive oxygen species occurs during advanced stage of fibrosis. Clinical study proteomics provides oxidative stress and hepatic mitochondrial dysfunction is due to HCV pathogenesis (Diamond et al., 2007). Protein and peptide can either be separated by 2D PAGE (2-dimentional Polyacrylamide gel electrophoresis) or by liquid chromatography (Chang et al., 2009). Examination of the coupling of some of the identified proteins to IRES function or Hepatitis C Virus (HCV) replication, by overexpression or by specific deletion of individual proteins using siRNA, may identify drug targets for hepatitis C (Lu et al., 2004).

Gonçalves et al. (2014) studied comparative salivary proteome of hepatitis B- and C-infected patients and described salivary protein alterations associated with hepatitis B and C. These findings may provide novel insight into salivary protein differences between HBV- and HCV-infected patients and help to identify candidate biomarkers that may lead to more efficient hepatitis diagnosis in an epidemiological setting. Gangadharan and his co-workers identify 20 novel fibrosis biomarker candidates. The proteins identified may help to assess hepatic fibrosis and eliminate the need for invasive liver biopsies (Gangadharan et al., 2014).

In a study by Dillon et al. (2015), they observed the proteins like moesin (MSN), retinol-binding protein (RBP4), and transgelin (TAGL) have been intricated in viral induced HCC. Other identified proteins that functions as cellular migration, invasion and metastasis of HCC includes Filamin A (FLNA), Moesin (MOES), Caldesmon (CALD1) and tropomyosin alpha-4 (TYB4) (Leung et al., 2010; Huang et al., 2011). Other proteins such as Apolipoprotein A1 (APOA1), and Serotransferrin (TF) that are involved in lipid metabolism and molecular transport were identified as Differentially Expressed Proteins (DEP). Both of these proteins have been shown to be associated with HCV-induced HCC (Mancone et al. 2011; Thi et al., 2009; Tseng et al., 2009).

Liver cells are very active and continuously secrete various metabolites within the circulation. Therefore, screening human serum for potential biomarkers is an attractive option for early diagnosis of liver cancer. It should be noted that biomarkers can also be substances secreted by other organs in response to the growth of the tumor. Many publications have evaluated potential serum biomarkers that can be more sensitive than AFP, such as des-Ácarboxyprothrombin (Okuda et al., 2001), which consists of variant forms depending on the severity of liver damage (Uehara et al., 2005). More recently, Golgi Protein-73 (GP73) was shown to be upregulated within diseased livers (Kladney et al., 2002) and was evaluated as a biomarker candidate. It was suggested that GP73 is a better marker than AFP (alpha fetoprotein) within early stage HCC (Marrero et al., 2005).

Mass spectrometry (MS) has been the center piece of proteomic research and has rapidly evolved during the past 20 years with its various applications extending into every discipline within the life and health sciences. The introduction of soft ionization techniques, namely Electrospray Ionization (ESI) and Matrix Assisted Laser Desorption Ionization (MALDI), has enabled researchers to study biological compounds, such as proteins and DNA. A new technology known as SELDI (surface enhanced laser desorption ionization). SELDI is intended to detect proteins in the sample (biomarkers); its combination with ToF will be beneficial. The goal of using SELDI-ToF in cancer-related applications is to detect a specific biomarker associated with cancer for further identification or to generate mass spectrometric fingerprints. Protein microarrays were first described in the late 1990s and since then, this technology has flourished and hundreds of proteins can now be detected simultaneously on the same array. Protein microarrays can be used to study protein-protein/ protein-DNA interactions (functional arrays); the probe for such an array can be either a protein or oligonucleotides.

In a study by Holly et al. (2015) they used affinity purification/mass spectrometry to define the host interactions of all HCV proteins in hepatoma cells. They combined these studies with RNAi knockdown of corresponding genes using a two-step scoring approach to generate a map of 139 high-confidence HCV-host protein-protein interactions and found mitochondrial proteins highly involved in HCV infection and characterized an interaction between the viral core protein and host protein within bgcn homolog (WIBG). Expression of core prevents WIBG from binding its regular interaction partners Y14 and Magoh, two known mediators of the nonsense-mediated mRNA decay pathway. They also find that surveillance pathway is disrupted in HCV-infected cells, causing potentially harmful transcripts to accumulate.

CONCLUSION

Genetically for the treatment of previously discussed diseases like Rheumatoid arthritis, Cancer, and Hepatitis C host factors are hereby essential to implement an individual's treatment. Apart from this the integration between proteomics, genomics, transcriptomics, bioinformatics and biostatistics has allowed for the development of an important instrument for translational aspects of modern molecular medicine.

ACKNOWLEDGMENT

We the authors of this chapter are very thankful to the publisher and editors of this book for giving opportunity and considering our chapter for publication.

REFERENCES

Aarøe, J., Torbjørn, L., & Vanessa, D. (2010). Gene expression profiling of peripheral blood cells for early detection of breast cancer. *Breast Cancer Research*, *12*, R7. PMID:20078854

Ai, J., Huang, H., Lv, X., Tang, Z., Chen, M., Chen, T., & Zhou, Q. et al. (2011). FLNA and PGK1 are two potential markers for progression in hepatocellular carcinoma. *Cellular Physiology and Biochemistry*, *27*, 207–216. PMID:21471709

Andri, R., & Jacques, F. (2011). Personalized hepatitis C therapy: Opportunities and pitfalls. *Expert Review of Molecular Diagnostics*, *11*(2), 127–129. PMID:21405961

Andy, L. T. Y., Quing-Yu, H. E., & Jen, F. U. C. (2003). Proteomic technology and its biomedical application. *Acta Biochimica et Biophysica Sinica*, *35*, 965–975. PMID:14614532

Annenkov, A., & Chernajovsky, Y. (2000). Engineering mouse T lymphocytes specific to type II collagen by transduction with a chimeric receptor consisting of a single chain Fv and TCR zeta. *Gene Therapy*, *7*, 714–722. PMID:10800096

Apweiler, R., Aslanidis, C., Deufel, T., Gerstner, A., Hansen, J., Hochstrasser, D., & Maser, E. et al. (2009). Approaching clinical proteomics: Current state and future fields of application in cellular proteomics. *Cytometry. Part A*, *75*, 816–832. PMID:19739086

Baban, C. K., Cronin, M., O'Hanlon, D., O'Sullivan, G. C., & Tangney, M. (2010). Bacteria as vectors for gene therapy of cancer. *Bioengineered Bugs*, *1*(6), 385–394. PMID:21468205

Baranyi, L., Slepushkin, V., & Dropulic, B. (2013). Ex vivo gene therapy: utilization of genetic vectors for the generation of genetically modified cell products for therapy. In *Gene Therapy of Cancer* (3rd ed.; pp. 3–18). San Diego, CA: Elsevier.

Benoit, M. R., Mayer, D., Barak, Y., Chen, I. Y., Hu, W., Cheng, Z., & Matin, A. et al. (2009). Visualizing implanted tumors in mice with magnetic resonance imaging using magnetotactic bacteria. *Clinical Cancer Research*, *15*(16), 5170–5177. PMID:19671860

Bessis, N., Chiocchia, G., & Kollias, G. (1988). Modulation of pro-inflammatory cytokine production in tumour necrosis factor alpha (TNF-alpha)-transgenic mice by treatment with cells engineered to secrete IL-4, IL-10 or IL-13. *Clinical and Experimental Immunology*, *111*, 391–396. PMID:9486409

Bryson, P., & Wang, P. (2013). Lentivector vaccines. In *Gene Therapy of Cancer* (3rd ed.; pp. 345–361). San Diego, CA: Elsevier.

Camussi, G., & Lupia, E. (1998). The future role of anti-tumor necrosis factor (TNF) products in the treatment of rheumatoid arthritis. *Drugs*, *55*(5), 613–620. PMID:9585859

Carolina, P. (2014). Proteomic Tools for Cancer Research: Updating the Oncoproteomics. *Journal of Proteomics &. Bioinformatics (Oxford, England)*, S3.

Ceciliani, F., Eckersall, D., Burchmore, R., & Lecchi, C. (2014). Proteomics in veterinary medicine: Applications and trends in disease pathogenesis and diagnostics. *Veterinary Pathology*, *51*(2), 351–362. PMID:24045891

Comins, C., Simpson, G., Relph, K., Harrington, K., Melcher, A., & Pandha, H. (2013). Reoviral therapy for cancer: strategies for improving antitumor efficacy using radio- and chemotherapy. In *Gene Therapy of Cancer* (3rd ed.; pp. 185–198). San Diego, CA: Elsevier.

Dasilva, N., Diez, P., Matarraz, S., Gonzalez-Gonzalez, M., Paradinas, S., Orfao, A., & Fuentes, M. (2012). Biomarker Discovery by Novel Sensors Based on Nanoproteomics Approaches. *Sensors (Basel, Switzerland)*, *12*(2), 2284–2308. PMID:22438764

Desjardins, D., Huret, C., & Dalba, C. (2009). Recombinant retrovirus-like particle forming DNA vaccines in prime-boost immunization and their use for hepatitis C virus vaccine development. *The Journal of Gene Medicine*, *11*, 313–325. PMID:19248137

DeVita, V. T. Jr, & Rosenberg, S. A. (2012). Two hundred years of cancer research. *The New England Journal of Medicine*, *366*(23), 2207–2214. PMID:22646510

Di, G. F., Del, C. F., Caenaro, G., Lante, I., & Muraca, M. (2012). Human serum proteome analysis: New source of markers in metabolic disorders. *Biomarkers in Medicine*, *6*, 759–773. PMID:23227840

Diamond, D. L., Jacobs, J. M., Paeper, B., Proll, S. C., Gritsenko, M. A., Carithers, R. L., & Katze, M. G. et al. (2007). Proteomic profiling of human liver biopsies: Hepatitis C virus-induced fibrosis and mitochondrial dysfunction. *Hepatology (Baltimore, Md.)*, *46*(3), 649–657. PMID:17654742

Duan, H., Struble, E., & Zhong, L. (2010). Hepatitis C virus with a naturally occurring single amino-acid substitution in the E2 envelope protein escapes neutralization by naturally-induced and vaccine-induced antibodies. *Vaccine*, *28*, 4138–4144. PMID:20433800

Gangadharan, B., Bapat, M., Rossa, J., & Antrobus, R. (2014). Discovery of novel biomarker candidates for liver fibrosis in hepatitis C patients using proteomics. *Journal of Molecular Biomarkers & Diagnosis*, *5*, 106.

Ge, D., Fellay, J., Thompson, A. J., Simon, J. S., Shianna, K. V., Urban, T. J., & Muir, A. J. et al. (2009). Genetic variation in il28b predicts Hepatitis C treatmentinduced viral clearance. *Nature*, *461*, 399–401. PMID:19684573

Geng, J., Xiao, S., Zhang, S., Liu, C., Li, Y., Ji, J., & Xu, B. et al. (2014). Clinical effectiveness of recombinant adenovirus-p53 combined with radiotherapy in advanced soft tissue sarcoma: A report of 37 cases. *Journal of Clinical Oncology*, 32.

Getchell, J. P. (2013). Testing for HCV infection: An update of guidance for clinicians and laboratorians. *Morbidity and Mortality Weekly Report*, *62*, 362–365. PMID:23657112

Gobezie, R., Millett, P. J., Sarracino, D. S., Evans, C., & Thornhill, T. S. (2006). Proteomics: Applications to the study of rheumatoid arthritis and osteoarthritis. *The Journal of the American Academy of Orthopaedic Surgeons*, *14*(6), 325–332. PMID:16757672

Goncalves, L. D. R., Campanhon, I. B., Domingues, R. R., Leme, A. F. P., & Dasilva, M. R. S. (2014). Comparative salivary proteome of hepatitis B- and C-infected patients. *PLoS ONE*, 1–13.

Goodman, L. S., Wintrobe, M. M., Dameshek, W., Goodman, M. J., Gilman, A., & McLennan, M. T. (1984). Landmark article Sept. 21, 1946: nitrogen mustard therapy: use of methyl-bis(betachloroethyl) amine hydrochloride and tris(beta-chloroethyl)amine hydrochloride for Hodgkin's disease, lymphosarcoma, leukemia and certain allied and miscellaneous disorders by Louis S. Goodman, Maxwell M. Wintrobe, William Dameshek, Morton J. Goodman, Alfred Gilman and Margaret T. McLennan. *Journal of the American Medical Association*, *251*(17), 2255–2261. PMID:6368885

Gujrati, M., & Lu, Z. (2013). Targeted systemic delivery of therapeutic siRNA. In *Gene Therapy of Cancer* (3rd ed.; pp. 47–65). San Diego, CA: Elsevier.

Hathout, Y. (2007). Approaches to the study of the cell secretome. *Expert Review of Proteomics*, *4*(2), 239–248. PMID:17425459

Hayes, C. N., Imamura, M., Aikata, H., & Chayama, K. (2012). Genetics of IL28B and HCV response to infection and treatment. Nature Reviews. *Gastroenterologia y Hepatologia*, *9*, 406–417.

He, L. F., Wang, Y. G., Xiao, T., Zhang, K. J., Li, G. C., & Gu, J. F. (2009). Suppression of cancer growth in mice by adeno-associated virus vector-mediated IFN-beta expression driven by hTERT promoter. *Cancer Letters*, *286*, 196–205. PMID:19564073

Hehlgans, T., & Pfeffer, K. (2005). The intriguing biology of the tumour necrosis factor/tumour necrosis factor receptor superfamily: Players, rules and the games. *Immunology*, *115*, 1–20. PMID:15819693

Hidehiko, S., Hooi-Ming, L., & Norihiro, N. (2010). DNA microarray analysis of rheumatoid arthritis susceptibility genes identified by genome-wide association studies. *Arthritis Research & Therapy*, *12*, 401. PMID:20346099

Holly, R., Ramage, G., Renuka, K., Erik, V., Jeffrey, R. J., John, V. D., & Billy, N. et al. (2015). A Combined Proteomics/Genomics Approach Links Hepatitis C Virus Infection with Nonsense-Mediated mRNA Decay. *Molecular Cell*, *57*(2), 329–340. PMID:25616068

Hondermarck, H. (2003). Breast cancer: When proteomics challenges biological complexity. *Molecular & Cellular Proteomics*, *2*, 281–291. PMID:12775769

Hossein, K., Mehdi, F., Seyed, H. R. M., & Hamid, R. M. (2012). Hepatitis C Virus - Proteins, Diagnosis, Treatment and New Approaches for Vaccine Development. *Asian Pacific Journal of Cancer Prevention*, *13*, 5917–5935. PMID:23464383

Hu, S. X., Kyulo, N. L., Xia, V. W., Hillebrand, D. J., & Hu, K. Q. (2009). Factors associated with hepatic fibrosis in patients with chronic hepatitis C: A retrospective study of a large cohort of US patients. *Journal of Clinical Gastroenterology*, *43*, 758–764. PMID:19238091

Hueber, W., & Robinson, W. (2006). Proteomic biomarkers for autoimmune disease. *Proteomics*, *6*(14), 4100–4105. PMID:16786488

Hüttenhain, R., Soste, M., Selevsek, N., Rãist, H., Sethi, A., Carapito, C., … Moritz, R.L. (2012). Reproducible Quantification of Cancer-Associated Proteins in Body Fluids Using Targeted Proteomics. *Science Translational Medicine, 4*(142).

Jain, K. K. (2008). Innovations, challenges and future prospects of oncoproteomics. *Molecular Oncology*, *2*, 153–160. PMID:19383334

Javier, C., Emiliano, C., Ana, V., Jose, P. G., Juan, A. R., & Joan, S. (2014). New Approach to Cancer Therapy Based on a Molecularly Defined Cancer Classification. *CA: a Cancer Journal for Clinicians*, *64*, 70–74. PMID:24249308

Jemal, A., Siegel, R., Xu, J., & Ward, E. (2010). Cancer statistics 2010. *CA: a Cancer Journal for Clinicians*, *60*, 277–300. PMID:20610543

Jiménez-Sousa, M., Fernández-Rodríguez, A., & Guzmán-Fulgencio, M., García-Álvarez, M., & Resino, S. (2013). Meta-analysis: Implications of interleukin-28B polymorphisms in spontaneous and treatment-related clearance for patients with hepatitis C. *BMC Medicine*, *11*, 6. PMID:23298311

Juan, J., & Yan, C., & Wei, W. (2010). Clinical application and evaluation of anti-TNF-alpha agents for the treatment of rheumatoid arthritis. *Acta Pharmacologica Sinica*, *31*, 1133–1140. PMID:20711219

Kang, S. Y., Kim, M. H., & Lee, W. I. (2010). Measurement of inflammatory cytokines in patients with rheumatoid arthritis. *The Korean Journal of Laboratory Medicine*, *30*, 301–306. PMID:20603592

Katchamart, W., Trudeau, J., Phumethum, V., & Bombardier, C. (2009). Efficacy and toxicity of methotrexate (MTX) monotherapy versus MTX combination therapy with nonbiological disease-modifying antirheumatic drugs in rheumatoid arthritis: A systematic review and meta-analysis. *Annals of the Rheumatic Diseases*, *68*, 1105–1112. PMID:19054823

Kelly, E., & Russell, S. J. (2007). History of oncolytic viruses: Genesis to genetic engineering. *Molecular Therapy*, *15*(4), 651–659. PMID:17299401

Kim, S. H., Kim, S., & Oligino, T. J. (2002). Effective treatment of established mouse collagen-induced arthritis by systemic administration of dendritic cells genetically modified to express FasL. *Molecular Therapy*, *6*, 584–590. PMID:12409256

Kim, S. Y., & Hahn, W. C. (2007). Cancer genomics: Integrating form and function. *Carcinogenesis*, *28*(7), 1387–1392. PMID:17434922

Kladney, R. D., Cui, X., Bulla, G. A., Brunt, E. M., & Fimmel, C. J. (2002). Expression of GP73, a resident Golgi membrane protein, in viral and nonviral liver disease. *Hepatology (Baltimore, Md.)*, *35*, 1431–1440. PMID:12029628

Klopfleisch, R., & Gruber, A. D. (2009). Increased expression of BRCA2 and RAD51 in lymph node metastases of canine mammary adenocarcinomas. *Veterinary Pathology*, *46*(3), 416–422. PMID:19176491

Klopfleisch, R., Klose, P., Weise, C., Bondzio, A., Multhaup, G., Einspanier, R., & Gruber, A. D. (2010). Proteome of metastatic canine mammary carcinomas: Similarities to and differences from human breast cancer. *Journal of Proteome Research*, *9*(12), 6380–6391. PMID:20932060

Kolch, W., & Pitt, A. (2010). Functional proteomics to dissect tyrosine kinase signalling pathways in cancer. *Nature Reviews. Cancer*, *10*, 618–629. PMID:20720570

Kris, M. G., Johnson, B. E., Kwiatkowski, D. J., & Iafrate, A. J. (2011). Identification of driver mutations in tumor specimens from 1000 patients with lung adenocarcinoma: The NCI's lung cancer mutation consortium (LCMC). *Journal of Clinical Oncology*, 29.

Kyungsoo, C., Tianyi, W., & Guangxiang, L. (2009). Proteomics Study of the Hepatitis C Virus Replication Complex. *Methods in Molecular Biology (Clifton, N.J.)*, *510*, 185–193. PMID:19009262

Laukens, D., Peeters, H., Cruyssen, B.V., Boonefaes, T., & Elewaut, D., De, K. F., … Rottiers, P. (2006). Altered gut transcriptome in spondyloarthropathy. *Annals of the Rheumatic Diseases*, *65*, 1293–1300. PMID:16476712

Lee, H. S., Kim, J. Y., Lee, W. I., Kim, S. J., Ko, M. J., & Jeong, S. (2011). Acquisition of selective anti-tumoral effects of recombinant adeno-associated virus by genetically inserting tumor-targeting peptides into capsid proteins. *Oncology Letters*, *2*, 1113–1119. PMID:22848276

Leung, W. K., Ching, A. K., & Wong, N. (2010). Phosphorylation of caldesmon by PFTAIRE1 kinase promotes actin binding and formation of stress fibers. *Molecular and Cellular Biochemistry*, *350*, 201–206. PMID:21184254

Lu, H., Li, W., Noble, W. S., Payan, D., & Anderson, D. C. (2004). Riboproteomics of the Hepatitis C Virus Internal Ribosomal Entry Site. *Journal of Proteome Research*, 1–9. PMID:15473682

Lu, L., Luo, S. T., Shi, S. H., Li, M., Zhang, H. L., & He, S. S. (2012). AAV2-mediated gene transfer of VEGF-Trap with potent suppression of primary breast tumor growth and spontaneous pulmonary metastases by long-term expression. *Oncology Reports*, *28*, 1332–1338. PMID:22824831

Lv, F., Qiu, Y., Zhang, Y., Liu, S., Shi, J., & Liu, Y. (2011). Adeno-associated virus-mediated anti-DR5 chimeric antibody expression suppresses human tumor growth in nude mice. *Cancer Letters*, *302*, 119–127. PMID:21306822

Ma, H., Liu, Y., Liu, S., Xu, R., & Zheng, D. (2005). Oral adeno-associated virus-sTRAIL gene therapy suppresses human hepatocellular carcinoma growth in mice. *Hepatology (Baltimore, Md.)*, *42*, 1355–1363. PMID:16317690

Ma, L., Reinhardt, F., Pan, E., Soutschek, J., Bhat, B., Marcusson, E. G., & Weinberg, R. A. et al. (2010). Therapeutic silencing of miR-10b inhibits metastasis in a mouse mammary tumor model. *Nature Biotechnology*, *28*, 341–347. PMID:20351690

Ma, L., Teruya-Feldstein, J., & Weinberg, R. A. (2007). Tumour invasion and metastasis initiated by microRNA-10b in breast cancer. *Nature*, *449*, 682–688. PMID:17898713

Majithia, V., & Geraci, S. A. (2007). Rheumatoid arthritis: Diagnosis and management. *The American Journal of Medicine*, *120*(11), 936–939. PMID:17976416

Mancone, C., Steindler, C., Santangelo, L., Simonte, G., Vlassi, C., Longo, M. A., & Alonzi, T. et al. (2011). Hepatitis C virus production requires apolipoprotein A-I and affects its association with nascent low-density lipoproteins. *Gut*, *60*, 378–386. PMID:20940285

Marrero, J. A. (2005). GP73, a resident Golgi glycoprotein, is a novel serum marker for hepatocellular carcinoma. *Journal of Hepatology*, *43*, 1007–1012. PMID:16137783

Maruotti, N., Cantatore, F. P., Crivellato, E., Vacca, A., & Ribatti, D. (2007). Macrophages in rheumatoid arthritis. *Journal of Histology &. Histopathology*, *22*(5), 581–586.

Mateos, J., Lourido, L., Patricia, F. P., Valentina, C., Carlos, F. L., Natividad, O., & Blanco, F. J. et al. (2012). Differential protein profiling of synovial fluid from rheumatoid arthritis and osteoarthritis patients using LC–MALDI TOF/TOF. *Journal of Proteomics*, *75*(10), 2869–2878. PMID:22245418

McGeough, C.M., & Bjourson, A.J. (2012). Diagnostic, Prognostic and Theranostic Genetic Biomarkers for Rheumatoid Arthritis. *Journal of* Clinical *& Cellular Immunology, S6*.

Molloy, M. P. (2000). Two-dimensional electrophoresis of membrane proteins using immobilized pH gradients. *Analytical Biochemistry*, *280*, 1–10. PMID:10805514

Morita, Y., Yang, J., & Gupta, R. (2001). Dendritic cells genetically engineered to express IL-4 inhibit murine collagen-induced arthritis. *The Journal of Clinical Investigation*, *107*, 1275–1284. PMID:11375417

Motavaf, M., Safari, S., & Alavian, S. M. (2012). Therapeutic potential of RNA interference: A new molecular approach to antiviral treatment for hepatitis C. *Journal of Viral Hepatitis*, *19*, 757–765. PMID:23043382

Muller-Ladner, U., Pap, T., Gay, R. E., Neidhart, M., & Gay, S. (2005). Mechanisms of disease: The molecular and cellular basis of joint destruction in rheumatoid arthritis. *Nature Clinical Practice. Rheumatology*, *1*(2), 102–110. PMID:16932639

Okuda, H. (2001). Comparison of clinicopathological features of patients with hepatocellular carcinoma seropositive for alphafetoprotein alone and those seropositive for des-gamma-carboxy prothrombin alone. *Journal of Gastroenterology and Hepatology*, *16*, 1290–1296. PMID:11903749

Ospelt, C., & Gay, S. (2007). Antirheumatic drugs and gene signatures. *Current Opinion in Investigational Drugs (London, England)*, *8*, 385–389. PMID:17520867

Page, T. H., Brown, A. C., Timms, E. M., Brennan, F. M., Ray, K. P., & Foxwell, B. M. J. (2007). Treatment with Non-steroidal Anti-inflammatory Drugs Increases TNF Production in Rheumatoid Arthritis. *Cytokine*, *39*(1), 32–32. PMID:17544674

Pan, Q. W., Henry, S. D., Scholte, B. J., Tilanus, H. W., Janssen, H. L., & van der Laan, L. J. (2007). New therapeutic opportunities for hepatitis C based on small RNA. *World Journal of Gastroenterology*, *13*(33), 4431–4436. PMID:17724797

Paul, J. C., Alex, J. T., & John, G. McHutchison. (2011). IL28B Genomic-Based Treatment Paradigms for Patients with Chronic Hepatitis C Infection: The Future of Personalized HCV Therapies. *The American Journal of Gastroenterology*, *106*, 38–45. PMID:20924369

Peng, X., Guo, W., Liu, T., Wang, X., Tu, X., Xiong, D., & Zou, X. et al. (2011). Identification of miRs-143 and -145 that is associated with bone metastasis of prostate cancer and involved in the regulation of EMT. *PLoS ONE*, *6*(5), e20341. PMID:21647377

Petricoin, E. F., Ardekani, A. M., & Hitt, B. A. (2002). 'Use of proteomic patterns in serum to identify ovarian cancer'. *Lancet*, *359*, 572–577. PMID:11867112

Chen, Chen, & Pan. (2008). Proteomics in rheumatoid arthritis. *Formosan Journal of Rheumatology*, *22*, 4–11.

Roe, M. R., & Griffin, T. J. (2006). Gel-freemass spectrometry-based high throughput proteomics: Tools for studying biological response of proteins and proteomes. *Proteomics*, *6*(17), 4678–4687. PMID:16888762

Roy, P., & Shukla, Y. (2008). Applications of proteomic techniques in cancer research. *Cancer Therapy*, *6*, 841–856.

Ruiz-Romero, & Blanco, F.J. (2013). Achievements and challenges of proteomics in the study of rheumatoid arthritis. *Current Topics in Medicinal Chemistry*, *13*(6), 732–742. PMID:23574522

Saha, S., Sparks, A. B., Rago, C., Akmaev, V., Wang, C. J., Vogelstein, B., & Velculescu, V. E. et al. (2002). Using the transcriptome to annotate the genome. *Nature Biotechnology*, *20*, 508–512. PMID:11981567

Sato, Y., Murase, K., Kato, J., Kobune, M., Sato, T., Kawano, Y., & Niitsu, Y. et al. (2008). Resolution of liver cirrhosis using vitamin A-coupled liposomes to deliver siRNA against a collagen-specific chaperone. *Nature Biotechnology*, *26*(4), 431–442. PMID:18376398

Schetter, A. J., & Harris, C. C. (2011). Alterations of microRNAs contribute to colon carcinogenesis. *Seminars in Oncology*, *38*, 734–742. PMID:22082759

Sheridan, C. (2011). Gene therapy finds its niche. *Nature Biotechnology*, *29*(2), 121–128. PMID:21301435

Shi, X. B., Tepper, C. G., White, R. W., Krichevsky, A. M., & Gabriely, G. (2008). MicroRNAs and prostate cancer. *Journal of Cellular and Molecular Medicine*, *5A*, 1456–1465. PMID:18624768

Shirley, S., Heller, R., & Heller, L. (2013). Electroporation gene therapy. In E. C. Lattime & S. L. Gerson (Eds.), *Gene Therapy of Cancer* (3rd ed.; pp. 93–106). San Diego, CA: Elsevier.

Stuhlmüller, B., Häupl, T., Hernandez, M. M., Grützkau, A., Kuban, R. J., Tandon, N., & Burmester, G. R. et al. (2010). CD11c as a transcriptional biomarker to predict response to anti-TNF monotherapy with adalimumab in patients with rheumatoid arthritis. *Clinical Pharmacology and Therapeutics*, *87*, 311–321. PMID:20032971

Tak, P. P., & Bresnihan, B. (2000). The pathogenesis and prevention of joint damage in rheumatoid arthritis: Advances from synovial biopsy and tissue analysis. *Arthritis &. Rheumatology*, *43*, 2619–2633. PMID:11145019

Tibor, T. G., Katalin, M., & Tibor, A. R. (2014). Epigenetics in the pathogenesis of rheumatoid arthritis. *BMC Medicine*, *12*, 35. PMID:24568138

Tilleman, K., Van Beneden, K., Dhondt, A., Hoffman, I., De Keyser, F., Veys, E., & Deforce, D. et al. (2005). Chronically inflamed synovium from spondyloarthropathy and rheumatoid arthritis investigated by protein expression profiling followed by tandem mass spectrometry. *Proteomics. Clinical Applications*, *5*(8), 2247–2257. PMID:15846842

Tseng, H. H., Chang, J. G., Hwang, Y. H., Yeh, K. T., Chen, Y. L., & Yu, H. S. (2009). Expression of hepcidin and other iron-regulatory genes in human hepatocellular carcinoma and its clinical implication. *Journal of Cancer Research and Clinical Oncology*, *135*, 1413–1420. PMID:19387685

Uehara, S., Gotoh, K., Handa, H., Tomita, H., & Senshuu, M. (2005). Distribution of the heterogeneity of des-gamma-carboxyprothrombin in patients with hepatocellular carcinoma. *Journal of Gastroenterology and Hepatology*, *20*, 1545–1552. PMID:16174072

Vaidyanathan, G. (2012). Redefining clinical trials: The age of personalized medicine. *Cell*, *148*(6), 1079–1080. PMID:22424218

Van der Pouw Kraan, T. C. T. M., Van Gaalen, F. A., Huizinga, T. W. J., Pieterman, E., Breedveld, F. C., & Verweij, C. L. (2003). Discovery of distinctive gene expression profiles in rheumatoid synovium using cDNA microarray technology: Evidence for the existence of multiple pathways of tissue destruction and repair. *Genes and Immunity*, *4*, 187–196. PMID:12700593

Wagner, E., Plank, C., Zatloukal, K., Cotton, M., & Birnstiel, M. L. (1992). Influenza virus hemagglutinin HA-2 N-terminal fusogenic peptides augment gene transfer by transferrin-polylysine-DNA complexes: Toward a synthetic virus-like gene-transfer vehicle. *Proceedings of the National Academy of Sciences of the United States of America*, *89*(17), 7934–7938. PMID:1518816

Walsh, N. C., & Gravallese, E. M. (2004). Bone loss in inflammatory arthritis: Mechanisms and treatment strategies. *Current Opinion in Rheumatology*, *16*, 419–427. PMID:15201606

Walter, K., Harald, M., & Andrew, R. P. (2005). The molecular make-up of a tumour: Proteomics in cancer research. *Clinical Science*, *108*, 369–383. PMID:15831087

Wang, Y., Huang, F., Cai, H., Zhong, S., Liu, X., & Tan, W. S. (2008). Potent antitumor effect of TRAIL mediated by a novel adeno-associated viral vector targeting to telomerase activity for human hepatocellular carcinoma. *The Journal of Gene Medicine*, *10*, 518–526. PMID:18338833

Wilson, R., Whitelock, J. M., & Bateman, J. F. (2009). Proteomics makes progress in cartilage and arthritis research. *Matrix Biology*, *28*(3), 121–128. PMID:19379666

Wu, C. C., & Yates, J. R. III. (2003). The application of mass spectrometry to membrane proteomics. *Nature Biotechnology*, *21*, 262–267. PMID:12610573

Wulfkuhle, J. D., Liotta, L. A., & Petricoin, E. F. (2003). proteomic applications for the early detection of cancer. *National Review*, *3*, 267–275. PMID:12671665

Xiao, H., Zhang, L., Zhou, H., Lee, J. M., Garon, E. B., & Wong, D. T. W. (2012). Proteomic analysis of human saliva from lung cancer patients using two-dimensional difference gel electrophoresis and mass spectrometry. *Molecular & Cellular Proteomics*, *11*(2), 1–12. PMID:22096114

Xiaojiang, T., Jinsong, Z., Jiansheng, W., Chengen, P., Guangxiao, Y., & Quanying, W. (2010). Adeno-associated virus harboring fusion gene NT4-ant-shepherdin induce cell death in human lung cancer cells. *Cancer Investigation*, *28*, 465–471. PMID:19968500

Yang, L., Belaguli, N., & Berger, D. H. (2009). MicroRNA and colorectal cancer. *World Journal of Surgery*, *33*, 638–646. PMID:19123024

Yuan, Z., Pastoriza, J., Quinn, T., & Libutti, S. (2013). Targeting tumor vasculature using adenoassociated virus page vector coding tumor necrosis factor-a. In E. C. Lattime & S. L. Gerson (Eds.), *Gene Therapy of Cancer* (3rd ed.; pp. 19–33). San Diego, CA: Elsevier.

Zhang, Y., Ma, H., Zhang, J., Liu, S., Liu, Y., & Zheng, D. (2008). AAV-mediated TRAIL gene expression driven by hTERT promoter suppressed human hepatocellular carcinoma growth in mice. *Life Sciences*, *82*, 1154–1161. PMID:18485417

Section 4
Bioinformatics

Chapter 5
Bioinformatics and Its Therapeutic Applications

Sarvesh Kumar Gupta
IIIT Allahabad, India

Kamal Kumar Chaudhary
IIIT Allahabad, India

Nidhi Mishra
IIIT Allahabad, India

ABSTRACT

Bioinformatics has emerged as a major element in contemporary biomedical and pharmaceutical region. Bioinformatics deals with growth in biological data and has led to development of many databases. Bioinformatics deals with collection of data that is relevant clinically and these days separate term clinical information has come up. Data mimics are another field which is gaining importance. This chapter shall deal with introduction of bioinformatics and its applications in medicine and health care.

INTRODUCTION

Bioinformatics is an applied science including computer science and Biological related research area. There is model change in biological research approach used in computer application (Bayat, 2002) many software tools and computational mathematics model in different field experiment in a high labeled (Cohen, 2004). Bioinformatics introduces the exponential development in life science including chemical and biological data development of primary database and secondary database protein sequencing, nucleic acid sequencing and many structures (Altman, 1998). Some of the known database including Protein database, gene database, zinc database, Swissprot database, CATH database, SCOP database and PIR database etc. These databases are easily available in many private internet Server Company and government domain information. Essential research and protein modeling is completed using these database with helpful for the protein sequencing analysis tool like FASTA, BLAST,CLUSTALW etc. and the protein modeled structure are visualized in using (Russo, 2000) Bioinformatics work as im-

DOI: 10.4018/978-1-5225-0754-3.ch005

Figure 1. Interaction of disciplines that have contributed to the formation of bioinformatics (source- Science, medicine, and the future: Bioinformatics, a new interdisciplinary science, is essential to managing, understanding, and harnessing clinical benefit from new genetic data.)

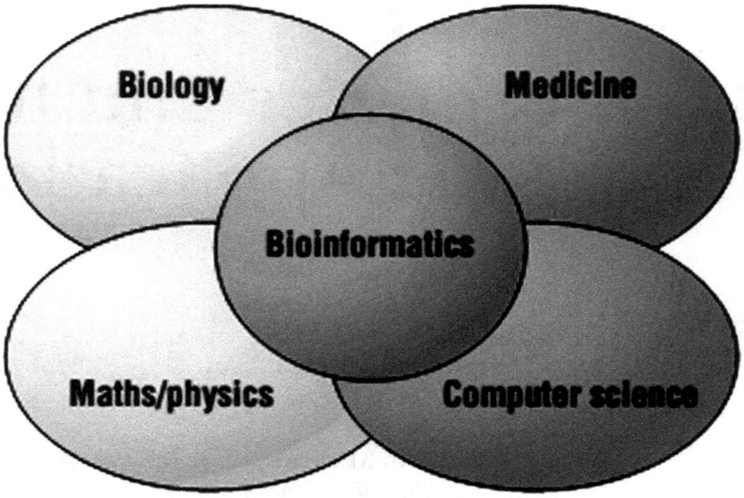

portant role in mixture of broad disciplines of biological organ/tissue to understand the organ complex mechanisms of the body cell. Bioinformatics is also the way in which Pharmaceutical investigation, biomedical investigation and health science use the information technology in their testing proof. The complete process of biological and information data collection to analysis of the proof result such testing may be classified under the specific area named –cheminformatics, Pharma co-informatics and clinical information (Wooley, 1999) (Figure 1).

WHAT IS BIO-INFORMATICS

Bioinformatics research and development studies two important information technology steps in modern biology. The first is the step of proteomic &genomics information from the DNA and RNA of an individual *Homo sapiens* organism up to the characteristics of a population growth of such organisms (Altman, 1998). The second is the steps of practical information from observed biological activity phenomena to models that explain them and then to new experiments in order to test these models. The discipline of bioinformatics has its roots in a number of activities, including the body organization of DNA & RNA sequence and protein three-dimensional structural data collections in the 1960's and 1970's (Langridge, 1974). It has become a booming academic and industrial enterprise with the introduction of biological experiments that rapidly produce massive amounts of data (such as the multiple genome sequencing projects, the large scale analysis of gene expression, and the large scale analysis of protein-protein interactions). Basic biological science has always had an impact on clinical medicine& pharmaceutical (information systems), and is creating a new generation of epidemiologic, diagnostic, prognostic, and treatment modalities. Bioinformatics efforts that appear to be wholly geared towards basic science are likely to become relevant to clinical informatics & pharmaco informatics in the coming decade. For example, DNA sequence information and sequence annotations will appear in the medical chart with increasing frequency. The algorithms developed for research in bioinformatics will soon become part of clinical information and chemo informatics systems.

Bioinformatics is a discipline/sub discipline has been recognized for less than 10 years. The first efforts in bioinformatics can be traced back to the early application of computers to biology in the 1950's and 1960's. The early applications of computers to molecular biology were for graphical rendering of three-dimensional molecular structures and the creation of databases of molecular sequence and three-dimensional structure information. Bioinformatics can generally be defined as the study of how information technologies are used to solve problems in biology. The precise definition of bioinformatics is a matter of some debate. The most narrow usage of the term refers to the creation and management of biological databases in support of genomic sequences. The most broad usage includes essentially all applications of computers and information sciences to problems in biology. Bioinformatics is based on the fundamental example of molecular biology: genomics and proteomics information is stored in sequences of DNA bases. Finally this concept of molecule sequencing including molecule storage and analysis is important and central biological data and does not occur in many other area of information technology.

Bioinformatics and its Scope

Bioinformatics uses modern approaches in the area of life science, computer science and information science including communication technology, computer technology and information technology to problem defined in one or more area in pharmaceutical chemistry, biotechnology and life science. Bioinformatics is data stored in big amount and find out data analysis in data mining have occur main issues for pharma analyst and biological scientists due to fast development in quantitative data in life science such as complete proteomic and genomics of life science species including homo sapiens (human) genome, protein 3-D structure, metabolic pathway and protein sequencing database related information. Advances in bioinformatics particularly the internet source and approach ever increasing information in life science and biotechnology. Functional genomics and proteomics development of new pharmaceutical target and vaccine other pharmacogenomics and biochemical molecule diagnostic kit are many of the field in which bioinformatics has developed in essential part of research and development. The knowledge of multi database, tool to carry out data analysis and design of pharmaceutical molecule and life science system in computer work place as well as in network atmosphere has occur important for any candidate of bioinformatics. Bioinformatics is the multi-disciplinary field and has developed so more than one divides it into Biochemical molecular bioinformatics, sepsis bioinformatics and organelle bioinformatics. Therefore bioinformatics research and development unit are being founded in many pharmaceutical industry, biotechnology laboratory and even in other traditional company introduced in life science (biological). Bioinformatics is thus determined in many numbers of opportunities in this field.

Bioinformatics is introduced with database design, data modeling and data analysis. Data creating is done not only for copy material but also from networking source. Database in life science are mainly multi organized in affiliated database development.

Bioinformatics Tool

The main tools of bioinformatics function are online various related server and computer software like Schrodinger, Auto dock. The fundamental action of molecule sequencing of protein and DNA molecule using different types of software program and biological database easily available on the web server. Bioinformatics is a developed science and every day there is improvement in every branch of life science and computer science, and today bioinformatics expert use in various complex software programs for recovering, molecule prediction, molecule analysis, molecule protein and DNA sequencing data (NCBI, http://www.ncbi.nlm.nih.gov).These are major class of bioinformatics tool they are using data Ming software and genomics & proteomics sequencing database tool, homology and protein functional analysis tool:

- Homology and Similarity Tools
- Protein Function Analysis
- Structure Analysis
- Sequencing Analysis

Some Example of Bioinformatics Tool

- BLAST (Basic Local Alignment Search Tool)
- FASTA
- EMBOSS (European Molecular Biology Open Software Site)
- crustal W
- RasMol
- Prospect
- Pattern Hunter
- COPIA (Consensus Pattern Identification and Analysis)

Application of Programmers in Bioinformatics

- Bio Java
- Bio Perl
- Bio XML
- Bio cobra
- Ensemble
- Bio Perl-db
- Bio Python & Bio Java

CONVERSION OF 2D TO 3D

Chemsketch and CORINA are easy conversion software's and biological data based program system. They create natural data base library in SDF File format convert into 3D for screening which is taken as input. And hydrogen atoms are added (e.g. Ions in salts) and all molecules are neutralized. Structures that couldn't be converted are excluded from the 3D output file but written to a find out error file. The output file is also formatted in MDL SDF File format.

DOCKING TOOL

Schrodinger Software

Schrödinger software arrangement in drug design is software applied for ligand molecule and structure molecule based methods. Schrödinger deliver actual, creditable and high achievement computational dependent technology to solution in life science and other applied science research. Maestro is the unified interface for all Schrödinger software products. Schrodinger software are Supplier L.L.C., US. Following software products of Schrödinger are usually installed.

- Glide
- Desmond
- Q Site
- Maestro
- Site Map

Glide

Glide is all about the ligand and receptor complex docking studies. Glide tool response has good speed and accuracy for virtual screening of compounds. Virtual screening is performed by the help of various phases such as HTVS, SP and XP. Glide tool is most common advanced scoring energy function.

Desmond

Desmond tool performs molecular dynamic simulation for ligand complex molecule of proposed ligand and protein. Molecular simulation dynamics provides natural environment and finds out biological system movement at atmospheric condition. Technical and Pharmaceutical industries take up molecular dynamic simulations from time to time to study computational simulations for knowing stability of bound protein.

Q-Site

Q Site is applied for Quantum mechanism studies, to demonstrate the interaction point of a target, active site and protein molecule interaction function to the comfort of the system. Classical molecular mechanism (MM) process cannot be defined by the electrostatic force change condition of reaction and finding out ligand receptor interaction. Quantum mechanism (QM) is expected to study active chemical molecule affect of transition metal with a protein in atmospheric conditions.

Maestro

Maestro tool is the undivided interaction for all Schrodinger tool and most commonly selected analysis tool. Maestro tool has been developed for chemical molecule simulation and is used in pharmaceutical company and research institute. Maestro tool is computational technology visualization function. Maestro tool is used to find out chemical molecule properties with intramolecular interaction. Maestro tool are used in advanced computational science in drug discovery.

Site Map

Site map is a tool for identification of binding site and characteristic visualization tool. It is easy to use and finds out good ligand binding site corresponding to that area of drug design. Site map is based on proven algorithm for active bind position identification and assessment and can help in research associated to actual point of binding site.

ORGANISM INFORMATION BIOINFORMATICS DATA

The concept of under based many research development procedure in bioinformatics is that big database can be created side by side depending on chemical and biological analogs, for example proteomic and genomic DNA and protein sequence gene (Pedersen, Jensen, Brunak, Staerfeldt, & Ussery, 2000).An essential aspect of management of big amount of database is in developing procedure for doing comparative study between different molecules in biological data and identifying related bimolecular data. We introduced major data base that provide primary source of bioinformatics and introduced in secondary data base in order to colony the data. These are classified correlation between genomic, proteomics and its derivative product (Luscombe, Greenbaum & Gerstein, 2001). There are common term to define the correlation between pair of protein sequence and gene sequence. The two classes can be some time difficult to different especially if the relation between the two proteins is distance (Russell, Saqi, Sayle, Bates & Sternberg, 1997, 1998). Protein that are relation between gene duplication and genome (Fitch, 1970). Normally orthologs contain the same work (Tatusov, Koonin, & Lipman, 1997).The important notation of these area observations is limited for different organism (Gerstein & Hegyi, 1998; Skolnick & Fetrow, 2000) (Table 1).

MOLECULE INFORMATION BIOINFORMATICS DATA

The type of bioinformatics data that are analysed in range of subject and that are consider to relative to that area. We also give near about value introduced in size of biological data base being discussed. Source of information in bio informatics may be defined to raw material in DNA sequencing, genome molecule sequencing, macromolecule protein structure and all other genome bioinformatics data. Basic DNA molecule sequencing is initial stage four base character comparing gene base pair, each generally more than 1000 base pair large. The gene bank stock of nucleic acid sequence latest holds a 9.5 million base pair data base. The protein sequencing strings of 20 amino acids. At time presented 300,000 known protein sequence, with a typical bacteria protein contenting near about 300 amino acids. Macro molecular data represents more information. Latest the big data base for bacteria has made near about 20 times analysis for 6000 gene (Holstege et al., 1998) (Table 2).

ACCOMPLISHMENTS OF BIOINFORMATICS

There are two categories of accomplishments of bioinformatics that can be credited to bioinformatics. The first categories are an empirical principal that have become accepted by this field and generate context

Table 1. List of URLs for the Bioinformatics databases that are cited in the review.

Bioinformatics Data Base	URL
Protein sequence (primary) SWISS-PROT PIR-International	 www.expasy.ch/sprot/sprot-top.html www.mips.biochem.mpg.de/proj/protseqdb
Protein sequence (composite) OWL NRDB	 www.bioinf.man.ac.uk/dbbrowser/OWL www.ncbi.nlm.nih.gov/entrez/query.fcgi?db=Protein
Integrated databases Inter Pro Sequence retrieval system (SRS) Entrez	 www.ebi.ac.uk/interpro www.expasy.ch/srs5 www.ncbi.nlm.nih.gov/Entrez
Genome sequences Entrez genomes Gene Census COGs	 www.ncbi.nlm.nih.gov/entrez/query.fcgi?db=Genome bioinfo.mbb.yale.edu/genome www.ncbi.nlm.nih.gov/COG
Protein sequence (secondary) PROSITE PRINTS Pfam	 www.expasy.ch/prosite www.bioinf.man.ac.uk/dbbrowser/PRINTS/PRINTS.html www.sanger.ac.uk/Pfam/
Macromolecular structures Protein Data Bank (PDB) Nucleic Acids Database (NDB) HIV Protease Database ReLiBase PDB sum CATH SCOP FSSP	 www.rcsb.org/pdb ndbserver.rutgers.edu/ www.ncifcrf.gov/CRYS/HIVdb/NEW_DATABASE www2.ebi.ac.uk:8081/home.html www.biochem.ucl.ac.uk/bsm/pdbsum www.biochem.ucl.ac.uk/bsm/cath scop.mrc-lmb.cam.ac.uk/scop www2.embl-ebi.ac.uk/dali/fssp
Nucleotide sequences Gen Bank EMBL DDBJ	 www.ncbi.nlm.nih.gov/Genbank www.ebi.ac.uk/embl www.ddbj.nig.ac.jp

(source-What is bioinformatics? An introduction and overview" Yearbook of Medical Informatics 2001")

which guides both training and research development. The second categories are particular biological database and algorithm that have been evolved and which are service to Biological science.

1. The molecular structure of protein in evolution contains more changes like mutation, dilation and insertion of building blocks amino acid protein to the sequence. There are many similar chemical and biological structures with many different sequences (Lesk & Chothia, 1980).
2. Chemical and biological sequence can be aligned using algorithm based dynamic program. These mathematically choice alignment are most reliable when the similarity between sequences is high (>30% identical), but become less reliable in the range below 25% (Chung & Subbiah, 1996).
3. Probabilistic model of protein sequencing model known as hidden markov model can sensitively characterize a class of related sequence (Durbin, Eddy, Krogh, & Mitchison, 1998).
4. Different in both host and DNA pathogen genetic information can be used to comprehend which proteins are involved in diseases.

Table 2. Sources of data used in bioinformatics, the quantity of each type of data that is currently

Biological Data Source	Biological Data Size	Bioinformatics Topics
Raw DNA sequence	8.2 million sequences (9.5 billion bases)	Separating coding and non-coding regions Identification of introns and exons Gene product prediction Forensic analysis
Protein sequence	300,000 sequences (~300 amino acids each)	Sequence comparison algorithms Multiple sequence alignments algorithms Identification of conserved sequence motifs
Macromolecular Structure	13,000 structures (~1,000 atomic coordinates each)	Secondary, tertiary structure prediction 3D structural alignment algorithms Protein geometry measurements Surface and volume shape calculations Intermolecular interactions Molecular simulations (force-field calculations, molecular movements, docking predictions)
Genomes	40 complete genomes (1.6 million – 3 billion bases each)	Characterization of repeats Structural assignments to genes Phylogenetic analysis Genomic-scale censuses (characterization of protein content, metabolic pathways) Linkage analysis relating specific genes to diseases
Gene expression	largest: ~20 time point measurements for ~6,000 genes	Correlating expression patterns Mapping expression data to sequence, structural and biochemical data
Other data Literature Metabolic pathways	11 million citations	Digital libraries for automated bibliographical searches Knowledge databases of data from literature Pathway simulations

(2000) available, and bioinformatics subject areas that utilize this data.
(Source-What is bioinformatics? An introduction and overview" Yearbook of Medical Informatics 2001")

The effect of bioinformatics has also been made with the improvement of algorithm and biological database that are generally used some of which were developed by bioinformatics developer/researcher and other important bioinformatics resources and modern bioinformatics tool. The physician is not decided which symptom the patient may have and conformed to go on the web site server to investigate the known genetic syndrome related with disease. Today physician cross web site server to gather biological information in the following manner.

1. The physician first goes to the NCBI (National center for Biotechnology Information) web site server page. Today NCBI maintains a large number of biological database and molecular medicine database.
2. The molecule genetic gen data bank is then approach forms the molecule protein sequence to see the detailed molecular sequence of DNA base that encoded for the gene.

THERAPEUTIC APPLICATION

Bioinformatics has several therapeutic applications. Some of which are discussed below. The application of bioinformatics is in - Preventative medicine, Gene therapy, Antibiotic resistance, Evolutionary studies, Waste cleanup, Biotechnology, Climate change Studies, Alternative energy sources, Crop improvement, Forensic analysis, Bio-weapon creation, Insect resistance, Improve nutritional quality, Development of Drought resistant varieties and Vetinary Science.

BIOINFORMATICS USED IN DATA MINING

In bioinformatics there is huge amount of data to deal, in order to deal with this huge amount of data some techniques are required to sustain this huge amount of data properly. In this sense DATA MINING software provide huge contribution.

Some of the applications are as follow –

1. Finding the gene in large DNA molecule.
2. Domain Finding
3. Protein and gene interaction recognition
4. Motif Detection

For example Microarray technology is used to predict the patient health behavior. On the basis of genotypic behavior of patient, the survival time of the patient and the disease in the patient is recognized i.e. very useful in disease estimation or analyzing. The data mining tool provide machine learning technology for analyzing massive amount of data i.e. peptide identification of mass spectroscopy.

These are main task of data mining:

- **Classification:** provide tools for classification of data based on requirement of experimental purpose i.e. Classes are predefined in it.
- **Estimation:** Given some input data, it helps in estimating the value of some unknown parameter.
- **Prediction:** it is similar to the classification and estimation but the records are classified based on the behavior of future.
- **Association Rules:** this rule helps to determine the dependency between the records so that the similar thing can come up together.
- **Clustering:** is a process of dividing the large population into small-small group containing the similar feature?

Description & visualization the above classified data is now is shown by using the some of visualization technique.

Learning by using these tool fall out under two categories

- Supervised learning
- Unsupervised learning

The classification, estimation, prediction are the example of supervised learning. Supervised means there is guideline to perform the task.

The next three task – association rules, clustering and description & visualization comes under the the categories of unsupervised learning .Unsupervised learning means there is no any definite guideline to perform the task.

BIOINFORMATICS AND DRUG DISCOVERY

Today various type of disease is now known. Today more than 14 to 15 million death every year occur in developing countries as per WHO report. Most death from infectious disease occurs in developing countries like Ebola, malaria, H1N1 etc. (Clark & Pickett, 2000). Such drugs are high in cost and not easily available for developing world. The drug development of low cost and good quality drug for a different type of diseases is one of the most common problems faced by pharmaceutical industry or research institute. The solution to problem drug design is use of bioinformatics. Pharmaceutical company research and development of new drug using bioinformatics tool and various techniques reduces time and cost of pharmacological agent. Computational procedure are used for the forecast of drug similarity which is nothing but the molecules identification of hit molecule that will probably prove to be drug in later stage of drug discovery and development (Shortliffe & Blois, 2000). The pharmaceutical research institute and pharma industry's point of view bioinformatics is a key to drug design. It reduces the number of molecule trial in the screening of drug molecule and identifies potential drug receptor for the specific diseases using computational server workstation and bioinformatics tool. The application of bioinformatics in genomic and proteomic sequence has opened up a new area in pharma co informatics, pharmacogenomics which is the study of molecular genetics basis for the different type of drug design (Figure 2).

Figure 2. Above is a schematic outlining how scientists can use bioinformatics to aid rational drug discovery.
(Source-What is bioinformatics? An introduction and overview "Yearbook of Medical Informatics 2001")

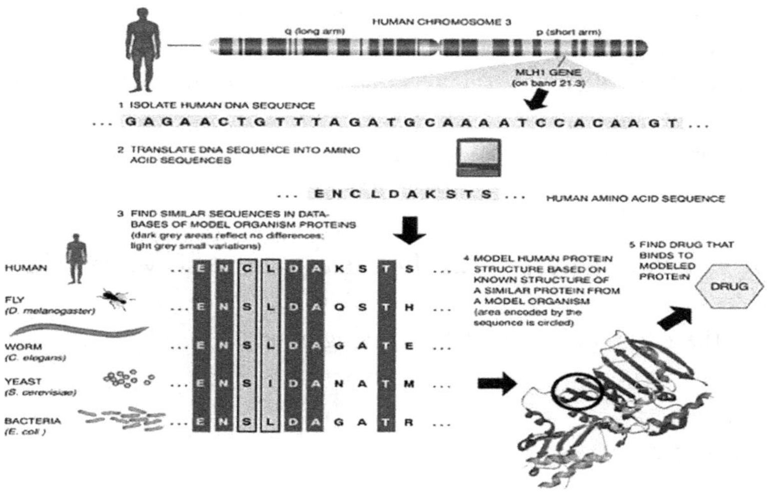

BRIEF HISTORY OF COMPUTER AIDED DRUG DESIGN

2000's: Vast information handling technology (pharmacogenomics)
1990's: First Computer based genomic assembly or Genomics based target selection
1900: Human Genome Project, Bioinformatics, Combinational chemistry and HTVS (High throughput virtual Screening)
1900: Receptor based and locks and key principal [(1909) P. Ehrich and (1894) E. Fisher]
1980: Beginning of Computer aided drug design, Computer graphics, X-ray crystallography, and Multi-dimensional NMR, Molecular Modeling and Molecular computational biology.
1980's: First computer based docking
1980's: Data based combinatorial libraries including information technology
1970: QSAR (Quantitative Structure Activity Relationship) including 2-Dimentional and retrospective analysis.
1960's: Review the target or drug interaction

COMPUTER AIDED DRUG DESIGN

Computer based drug design including Structure or ligand based drug design; rational drug design and intelligent drug design are very typical and longtime processes developed in last 12to15 years (Richards, 1994). Today computer aided drug design (CADD) works on various types of algorithm based software and working technology in a very short time for drug development and gives a hypothetical result. And it has led to development of a branch called Bioinformatics (applied science). (Clark & Pickett, 2000). Today entire scientific community, most pharmaceutical research and development companies including biotechnology research development laboratories and research institute use computational based design software tools. Because of low cost involved by their use in drug development (Zeng, 2000). Computer aided drug design is of two types: structure dependent drug design and ligand based drug design. Structure based drug design; main hypothesis is by this influence the potent molecule's capability to interact by hydrogen bond with special protein pulls a required biological impact which depends on its capability to favorably interact with a specific binding site on that molecular protein. And other ligand based computer aided drug design depends on ligand and involve the analysis of ligand molecule known/unknown to interact by hydrogen bond with target ligand and active molecule. Compounds found by ligand based virtual screening method are again and again more potent molecule (Klebe, 2000). The latest development is human immunodeficiency virus (HIV) potent inhibitor which has convincingly demonstrated the impact and the relevance of structure-based approaches to the discovery of new drugs (Lipkowitz & Boyed, 1996).

ADMET Properties

The pharmacological activity in our body or tissue, pharmaceutical compound has to pass through physiological barriers such as the BBB (blood brain barrier), gastrointestinal barrier, microcirculatory barrier and plasma member barrier before passing to blood circulatory system. Pharmaceutical compound are subsequently transported to effective receptor site for distribution into organs and tissue by specific pocket site and other wastage material out of the body this process is called excretion. ADMET

(Absorption, Distribution, Metabolism, Excretion and toxicity) properties check out biological activity of pharmaceutical compound (Song, Lim, & Tong, 2009). Drug development for novel pharmaceutical agent is filtering out one compound out of several screened compounds, and this reduces long time and cost for research and development. Today pharmaceutical industry and biotechnology laboratory develops several potential ligands and checks out ADEMT properties at every stage of drug development (Veselovsky & Ivanov, 2003).

Pre-Filtering

Initial step in ligand virtual screening is screening the generated library by the Lipinski's Rule of Five (Lipinski, Lombardo, Dominy, & Feeny, 2001; Kerns, & Carte, 2009). Lipinski's rule work depends on the analysis of profiling the calculated physical property-

- Maximum five hydrogen bond donor nature
- Molecular mass less than 500Da
- Octanol water partition coefficient less than five
- More than 10 Oxygen and Nitrogen atom accepter
- No. of rooted bond less than ten

Molecule chemical structure characteristic eligible of optimization and designed by combinatorial ligand and medicinal chemistry-

- ADME properties is good
- No toxic substructures

Thus lead molecule chemical structures are the starting point for drug development. The meaning of leads molecule structure requires at least one marketed preparation drug design based on this particular lead molecule structure (Clark, & Pickett, 2000).

Design of Combinatorial Natural Compound Library

Virtual high through screening use used in high performers computational to virtual screening large ligand molecule data base compound for most potent inhibiter screen. The performers a how ever virtual combinatorial library must be possible for natural library screening. Virtual screening can be earned in variation of molecule size and drug design inclusive of general virtual screening library that can be used to screen data base against proposed protein, selected library this are designed structure for a data base of related proposed target. And proposed target data base libraries that are specific structure designed for a single potent target. At last finally proposed data base methods is called generated data base (Sliwoski, Kothiwale, Meiler & Lowe, 2014).

Virtual Screening

Virtual screening is a standard process in drug discovery and selection of most potent chemical molecule structure this process involved in computer aided drug design. VS basically meninges data base library

Figure 3. Virtual screening method application in drug development.

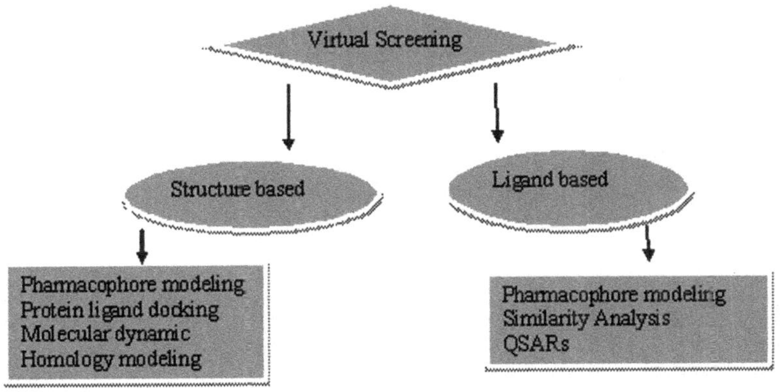

screen again proposed target protein molecule high energy scoring function in selection of data base library. This time Meany drug rejected in clinical trial phase because the drug is not potent for receptor. And pharmacokinetic including absorption, distribution metabolism, excretion and toxicology based blamed and reject clinical trial phase. The term virtual screening has been define in process computational based large data base chemical compound analysis and best compound selected. Virtual screening following the principal of Lipinski rules used in drug deployment. The selection of an applicable virtual screening process depends on much point e.g. on the availability of structure based biological information of the proposed target protein molecule and other selected ligand molecule the size of data base used for virtual screening and computation based resources. Virtual screening method can be categorized in two parts first part is ligand based and second part is protein structure based (Clark & Pickett, 2000) (Figure 3).

Ligand-Based

Ligand based drug development ligands bind to specific biological target. Mainly ligand based virtual screening procedure are QSARs, pharmacophore based modeling and similarity analysis.

Ligand Base Pharmacophore Modeling

Pharmacophore modeling introduced by Paul Ehrlich time duration the late 1800s (Schueler, 1960). The word pharmacophore coined by Schueler introduced in his book Drug design and Chemo biodynamics, a molecular structure that carry the essential features responsible for drug pharmacological activity (Schueler, 1960).International Union of Pure and Applied Chemistry (IUPAC) introduced the term pharmacophore in 1997, Pharmacophore is the ensemble of electronic and steric features that is necessary to ensure the optimal supramolecular interactions with a specific pharmacological target and to block its pharmacological activity. Computational pharmacophore structure is generally involved to generate novel initials point for drug development research center (Wermuth, Ganellin, Lindberg, & Mitscher, 1998). Many category of pharmacophore modeling based ligand development, such as Discovery of studio/Catalyst, phase (Leach, Gillet, Lewis, & Taylor, 2010). Ligand Scout and MOE (Dixon et al., 2006). These chemical ligand based can be labeled hydrogen bond accepter or donor, cation, anionic, hydrophobic or aromatic and any probity aggregate (Wolber, & Langer, 2005) (Figure 4).

Figure 4. Pharmacophore mapping of ligand and compound predicted by molecular docking.
[Source-Pharmacophore Modeling and Virtual screening for the Discovery of New type 4 cAMP Phosphodiesterase (PDE4) Inhibitors]

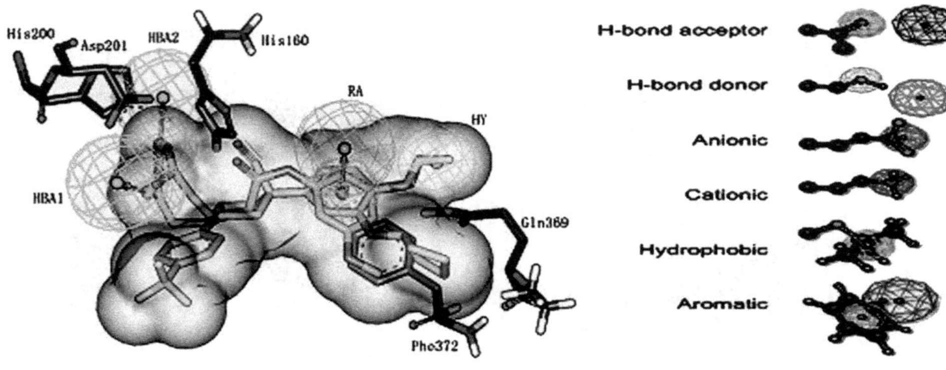

Similarity Analysis

Similarity search based algorithms use full techniques are finger print similarity analysis (2D finger print) or Electrostatic similarity analysis (3d shape) to find out similarity of a pharmacological activity query ligand with a biological data base. Fundamental developed for ligand chemical structure search, finger print similarity analysis very popular technique for conclusion of chemical molecular similarity between ligand based chemical compound (Gund, 2000). Finger print of data molecule similarity performed used in a coefficient score (Leach & Gillet, 2003).most popular finger print similarity analysis algorithms include ECFPs (Scitegic Extended Connectivity Fingerprints), 2D mol print and daylight finger print (Duan, Dixon, Lowrie, & Sherman, 2010).

Quantitative Structure Activity Relationship (QSAR)

Quantitative Structure Activity Relationship (QSAR) defined the mathematical correlation between structure characteristic and pharmaceutical target properties of ligand database (Perkins, Fang, Tong, & Welsh, 2003; Verma, Khedkar, & Coutinho, 2010) (Table 3).

Table 3. QSAR software and source of information link.

QSAR Software	Software Source
Topological index software (MolconnZ)	http://www.edusoft-lc.com
CODESSA descriptor software	http://www.semichem.com/codessa.html
Dragon descriptor software	http://www.disat.unimib.it/chm/Dragon.htm
Pomona College QSAR site	http://clogp.pomona.edu/medchem/chem/qsar-db
CoMFA 3-D QSAR method	http://www.tripos.com/software/qsar.html
QSAR and Modelling Society	http://www.ndsu.nodak.edu/qsar_soc/index.htm
Summaries of QSAR studies in literature	Journal-Quantitative Structure-Activity Relationship

Hence in contrast to hit drug development technique such as pharmacophore based modeling, QSAR are commonly used in the optimization phase of drug development (Fischer, 2008). QSAR technique 1st time introduced Corwin Herman Hansch (father of QSAR concept) in 1860 (Hansch, 1969) and this technique improved by two scientists Crum Brown and Fraser in 1865 expressed the idea chemical structure and relationship activity(Crum –Brown & Fraser,1969; Richet, 1893; Meyer, 1899; Overton, 1901).

Different type molecule structure like one dimension, two dimension, three dimensions and multidimensional Quantitative Structure Activity Relationship (QSAR) based have been design time period the past separate decades (Lill, 2007).one dimensional QSAR defined biological activity by correlation of the pharmaceutical ligand physicochemical properties eg.log P value. And two dimensional QSAR structure character of pharmaceutical ligand compound relation between structures based eg.2D-Pharmacophore (Lill, 2007).In three dimensional Quantitative structure activity relationship (QSAR) congeniality is correlated with the three dimensional structure of pharmaceutical ligand eg- CoMFA. CoMFA (Comparative molecular field analysis) is defined the 3Dimenstional visualization of electrostatic field and steric of pharmaceutical ligand molecule bioactive conformation and protein ligand binding (Cramer, Patterso, & Bunce, 1989). Three dimensional Quantitative Structure Activity Relationship used tool CoMSIA (comparative molecular similarity indices analysis) procedure calculation pharmaceutical ligand field characters like hydrogen bond accepter, hydrogen bond donor and hydrophobicity to created 3-dimenstional Quantitative structure activity relationship models (Klebe & Abraham, 1999) (Figure 5).

QSAR Modeling Process

Quantitative structure activity relationship modeling process mainly five phases (Figure 6).

Structure Based Virtual Screening

Structure based Virtual screening applied for drug development process pharmacological ligand target is available for three dimension ligand structure data. Structure based virtual screening interaction on ligand and protein and tool for optimization and hit drug development (Waszkowycz, 2008).

Molecular Dynamics Simulation

Molecular dynamic simulation is docking complex computational simulation method. Molecular dynamic come up of the first simulation method form the search function to the molecular dynamic of liquid phase introduced by Alder, Rahman and Wainwright in the later 1950s and early 1960s. There are two main category of molecular dynamics simulation process. In the classical working output to molecular

Figure 5. 1D, 2D, 3D structure

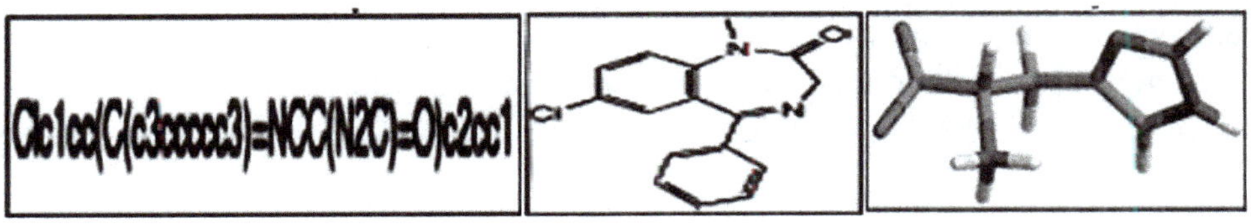

Figure 6. Flow chart of QSAR modeling process.

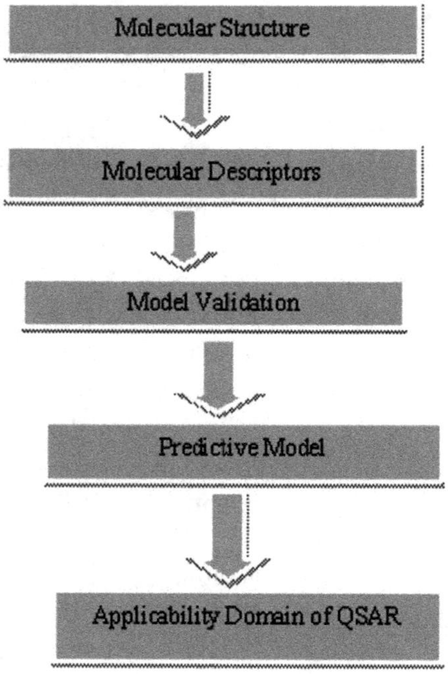

dynamics simulation partials are treated as classical object, homologues much the ball and stick model. Molecule atom approach to soft ball and elastic stick corresponding to bond (Sandeep, Priyadarshini, Pradhan, Munikumar, & Umamaheswari, 2012). The rule of classical work defines the dynamic of the method. The first principal of molecular dynamic simulation started in 1980 with the seminal work of car and Parinello accepted finally in to account the quantum nature of the chemical bond. Quantum molecular dynamics simulation performs an important correction over the access and they are used in given information on a number of biological problem. Computer molecular dynamic simulation act as a pool between microscopic distance and time parameter and microscopic earth sphere of the laboratory we provide a conjecture at the interaction between molecule particles and receive correct prediction of high amount characteristic. A molecular dynamic simulation is illustrated with figure (Figure 7).

Protein Ligand Docking

The Docking method is calculation of energy in complex including ligand and protein molecule. There are two role of docking research first is protein structure modeling and second is prediction information of biologically activity of ligand molecule. Docking is selection of scoring faction energy interact between ligand and protein ranking. Molecular characteristic such as hydrophilic nature, hydrogen bonding and electro static force as well as weight combination have been obtain a completely automated arrangement of molecule. Docking is basically work for accurate proposed structural modelling and correct prediction of the biological activity (Virtanen, 2013). The protein ligand docking development manly divided in two phase first know pocket site of pharmaceutical ligand docking development process and other

Figure 7. A simplified description of molecular dynamics simulation.

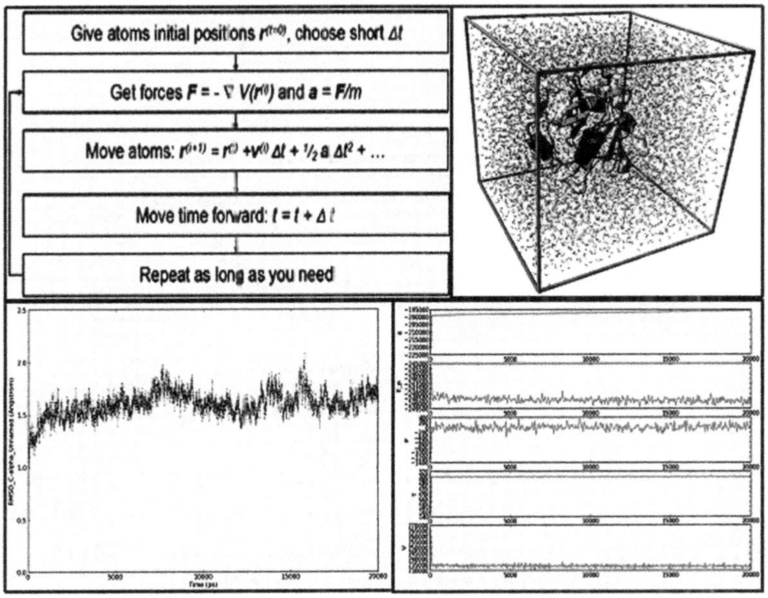

randomly pharmaceutical ligand binding and using scoring faction of ligand docking energy (Kirchmair, Markt, Distinto, Wolber, & Langer, 2008).

Structure Based Pharmacophore Modeling

Structure based Pharmacophore modeling used in the geographical information related to the pharmaceutical ligand protein target to create a topologically characterization of pharmaceutical ligand protein interaction (Leach, Gillet, Lewis, & Taylor, 2010).Three dimensional structure information on the pharmaceutical ligand protein is mainly got from multidimensional or X-ray crystallography spectroscopy and NMR. It is necessary to secure the credibility of the ligand bind site residues and pharmaceutical ligand co-ordinate by visually check out theirs degree of fitness to the corresponding electron density graph available for illustration at the Uppsala Electron Density Server (Kleywegt et al., 2004).Structure based pharmacophore models example for the optimization and generation found in literature (Markt, Schuster, Kirchmair, Laggner, & Langer, 2007 and Barreca, 2007). Salam et al. (2009) defined a different procedure for creating structure based pharmacophore using active analysis. Software programs that allow for the manual construction of pharmacophores from protein-ligand complexes include Schrodinger's Phase, Accelrys Discovery Studio, MOE by the Chemical Computing Group and Inte:Ligand's LigandScout (Table 4).

Homology Modeling

The large scale different between the number of possible sequence and number of laboratory procf protein molecular sequence, which is limitation by time, product cost and laboratory objection built-

Table 4. Structure based Pharmacophore modeling using various software.

Source	Software	Recent Published Use Cases
Accelrys	Catalyst (Discovery Studio)	http://dx.doi.org/10.1007/s00894-011-1105-5 http://dx.doi.org/10.1016/j.bmcl.2010.12.131
Schrödinger	Phase	http://10.1111/j.1747-0285.2011.01130.x http://cstest.ias.ac.in/cs/Volumes/100/12/1847.pd
Tripos	GASP	http://dx.doi.org/10.1016/j.jmgm.2010.02.004
Tripos	GALAHAD	http://dx.doi.org/10.1016/j.bmc.2011.09.016 http://dx.doi.org/10.1016/j.ejmech.2010.09.012
Inte:ligand	Ligandscout	http://dx.doi.org/10.1016/j.eplepsyres.2011.08.016
Chemical Computing Group	MOE	http://dx.doi.org/10.1007/s10822-011-9442-0 http://dx.doi.org/10.1016/j.ejmech.2010.07.020

in to the development of ligand structure determination could likely may be decide using homology modeling(Eswar, Eramian, Webb, Shen, & Sali, 2008). In non-attendance of laboratory proof structure homology modeling play important role of structure based drug development process .homology modeling is performed in seven phases (Krieger, Nabuurs, & Vriend, 2003).

1. Template recognition and initial alignment
2. Alignment correction
3. Backbone generation
4. Loop modeling
5. Side-chain modeling
6. Model optimization
7. Model validation

These phase may be continue until a good model is assembled (Cavasotto & Phatak, 2009). Although homology structure model are description of the known three dimension protein ligand structure, their property for virtual screening moment has been proved (Miguet, Zhang, Barbier, & Grigorov, 2006) (Figure 8).

Drug Discovery Process (Drug Cycle)

Approach for computer aided drug design deployment depend on the molecular structure and other biologically data information helpful regarding the propose target (Receptor/Enzyme) and screen ligand. Present time used in drug design deployment process two approach modeling design of drug directly and indirect design. In the direct strategies drug design based on relative analysis of the stretcher based characteristic know active and passive molecular compound. In direct drug design the three dimensional characteristic by the propose target (inhibiter) are directly consider (Frenking et al., 1996).

Figure 8. Steps of homology modeling
(Source- HOMOLOGY MODELING. Structural Bioinformatics)

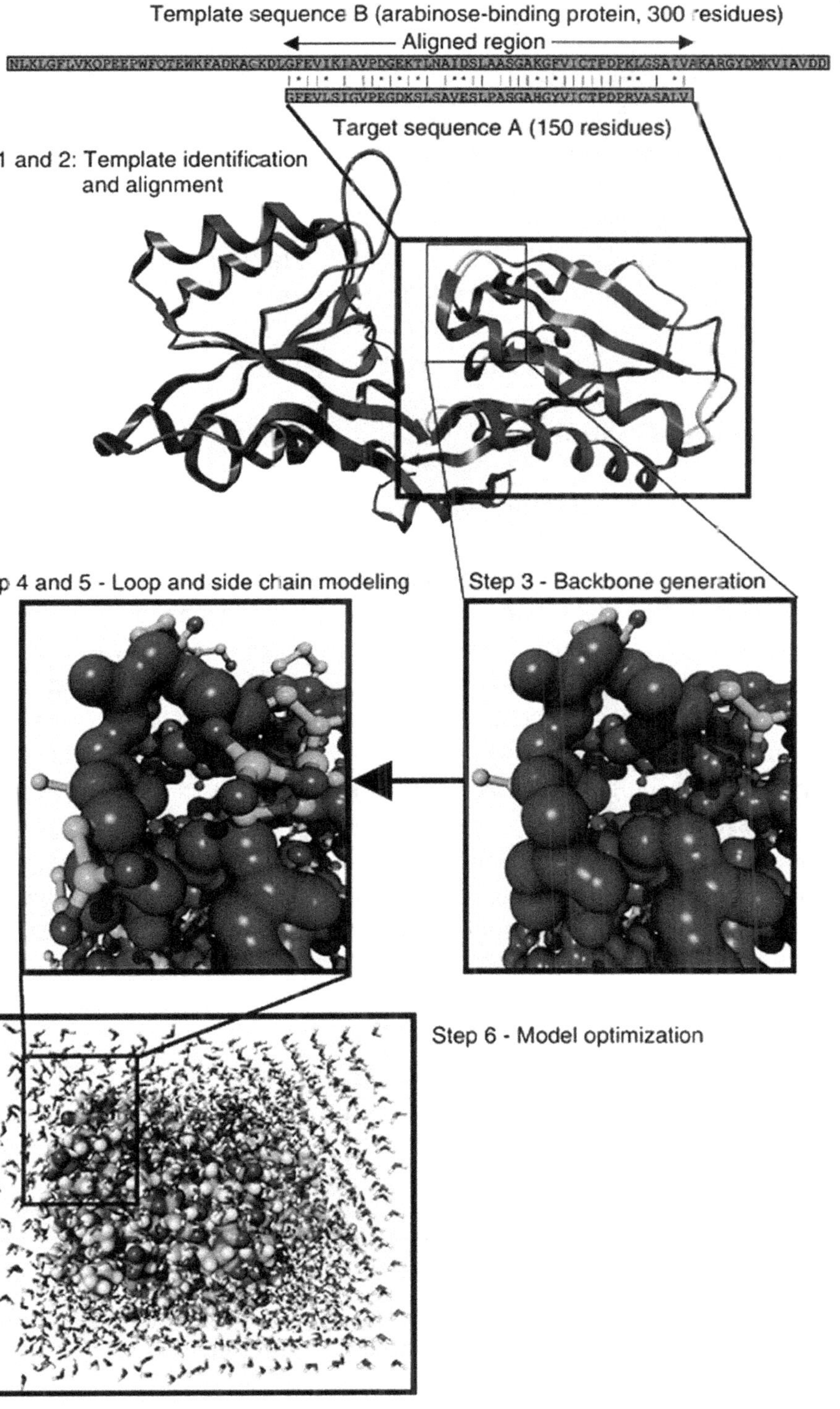

The strategy of drug discovery process has remained evasive despite important analysis. Like the biological approach bioinformatics on which the drug designs discovery process is based (Cavagnaro & Lewis, 1987). Discovery process strategies for drug development depend on following factors-

- Corporate sector, research, and marketing department cultures
- Individual scientists working within a company
- Synergies among various research disciplines
- Good quality of research management R&D leadership
- Individual and corporate experience
- Extent to which the management of a company is accustomed to risk Serendipity
- A particular company's market franchise (the therapeutic areas in which it markets drugs)

These processes are completed in 12-15 years (Figure 9)

Transmembrane Ion Channels

Voltage gated ion channel are a class of transmembrane ion channels that are activated by changes in electric potential difference. Sodium channels are integral membrane proteins that form ion channels which conducting sodium ions (Na^+) through a cell's plasma membrane (Jessell & Sanes, 2000).Voltage Gated Sodium channels (VGSCs) are members of the ion channel protein superfamily consisting of a large core protein, the α-subunit (220–260 kDa, ≈2000 amino acids), associated with one or more smaller regulatory β-subunits (22–36 kDa). VGSCs are transmembrane complexes play an essential role in neuronal and non-neuronal function, being responsible for the initiation and propagation of action potentials in excitable cells by allowing the influx of sodium ions. The α-subunit is sufficient for functional expression, forming the pore, determining the biophysical properties of the channel, and containing the ion selectivity filter. B-Subunits can modify the kinetic and voltage dependence properties of the channel and are involved in channel localization and interaction with cell adhesion molecules, extracellular matrix, and intracellular cytoskeleton. Voltage-dependent calcium channels (VDCC) are a group of voltage-gated ion channels found in excitable cells (e.g., muscle, glial cell, neurons etc.) with

Figure 9. Functional organization graph

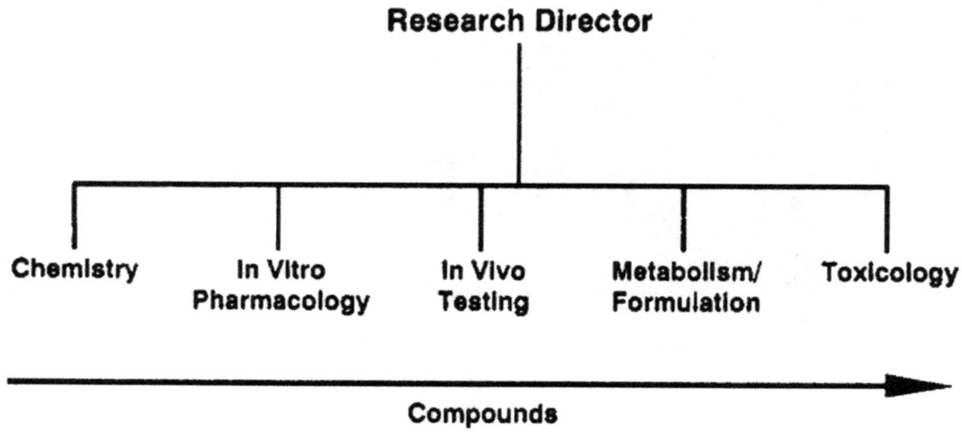

a permeability to the ion Ca^{2+}(William, Goldin, & Stephen, 2005). These channels are slightly permeable to sodium ions so they are also called Ca^{2-}-Na^{+} channels, but their permeability to calcium is about 1000-fold greater than to sodium under normal physiological conditions(Yamakaqe & Namiki, 2002). A physiological or resting membrane potential VDCCs are normally closed. They are activated (i.e., opened) at depolarized membrane potentials and this is the source of the "voltage-dependent" epithet Activation of particular VDCCs allows Ca^{2+} entry into the cell, which, depending on the cell type, results in activation of calcium-sensitive potassium channels, muscular contraction (Michael & Walsh, 1982),excitation of neurons, up-regulation of gene expression or release hormones or neurotransmitters. On the other hand, K+ channels are membrane proteins that allow rapid and selective flow of K+ ions across the cell membrane, and thus generate electrical signals in cells. Voltage-gated K+ channels (Kv channels), present in all animal cells, open and close upon changes in the transmembrane potential. Kv channels are one of the key components in generation and propagation of electrical impulses in nervous system. Voltage-gated K^{+} channels are selective for K^{+} over other cations such as Na^{+}. Sodium channels are integral membrane protein that form ion channels which conducting sodium ions Na^{+}through a cell's plasma membrane. In excitable cells such as neurons, myocytes and certain types of glia, sodium channels are responsible for the rising phase of action potentials. Sodium channels can be of two types: voltage-gated called VGSCs and the other ones that respond upon binding by a ligand and thus are called as ligand-gated sodium channel. The sequence set of DNAs for VGSC, VGKc, VGCC and its Docking sites with various neurotoxins can help us to understand the structure and function of these ion channels. Further, neurotoxins that bind can be a potent Analgesics, Also this can be useful in knowing the molecular basis of the diseases which are the result of disfunctioning or the alteration in their normal rhythmicity of the ion channels.

Calcium Channel Sub Unit

Calcium channel biochemical properties are ligand protein complex composed of near about four or five separate encoded subunit by multiple genes (William, 2000) (Figure 10).

Sodium channel are tetrodotoxin resistant degree due to changes in amino acid protein sequence a indusial position of domain and more expressed in root ganglion neurons and heart pace maker(Fozzard & Hanck, 1996) (Table 5).

BIOINFORMATICS AND MEDICAL SCIENCES (CLINICAL SCIENCES)

Bioinformatics has a deep effect in Medical sciences (Clinical Application). The molecular biological data base is very helpful for physicians to diagnose the disease and research strategies for therapy. Consider a situation where a patient with a genetic disease meets physicians. The physicians is not classified symptom casing disease physicians go to web information resource available at http://www.ncbi.gov. in which available detail gens related information on symptom. The information on the protein crystal structure can be acquired by following the link to web-protein data bank given in swiss port database. Following the other link to the DNA molecule sequence in the molecular genetic database also called gene bank the nucleotide sequencing of the gene is accrued along with data of gene asymmetry. Thus the Doctor/Physicians used in the biological database to collection of biological information about the

Figure 10. Transmembrane organization of sodium channel subunits. The primary structures of the subunits of the voltage-gated ion channels are illustrated as transmembrane-folding diagrams. Cylinders represent probable α-helical segments. Bold lines represent the polypeptide chains of each subunit, with length approximately proportional to the number of amino acid residues in the brain sodium channel subtypes. The extracellular domains of theβ1 and β2 subunits are shown as immunoglobulin-like folds. ψ, sites of probable N-linked glycosylation; P, sites of demonstrated protein phosphorylation by protein kinase A (circles) and protein kinase C (diamonds); shaded, pore-lining S5-P-S6 segments; white circles, the outer (EEDD) and inner (DEKA) rings of amino residues that form the ion selectivity filter and tetrodotoxin binding site; + +, S4 voltage sensors; h in shaded circle, inactivation particle in the inactivation gate loop; open shaded circles, sites implicated in forming the inactivation gate receptor. Sites of binding of α- and β- scorpion toxins and a site of interaction between αand β1 subunits are also shown.

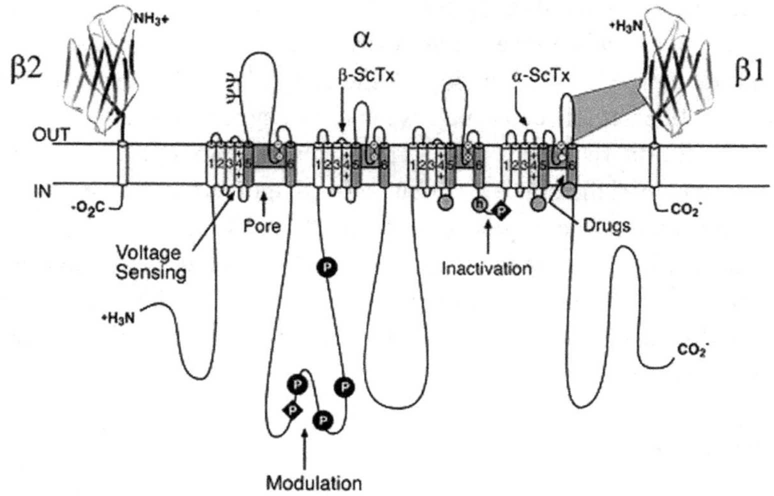

Table 5. Receptor site target on sodium channels.

Drug	Receptor Site	Domains
Tetrodotoxin, Saxitoxin, μ-Conotoxin	Neurotoxin receptor site-I	IS2–S6, IIS2–S6 IIIS2–S6, IVS2–S6
Veratridine, Batrachotoxin Grayanotoxin	Neurotoxin receptor site-II	IS6, IVS6
α-Scorpion toxins, Sea anemone toxins	Neurotoxin receptor site-III	IS5–IS6, IVS3–S4, IVS5–S6
β-Scorpion toxins	Neurotoxin receptor site-IV	IIS1–S2, IIS3–S4
Brevetoxins, Ciguatoxins	Neurotoxin receptor site-V	IS6, IVS5
δ-Conotoxins	Neurotoxin receptor site-VI	IVS3–S4
Local anesthetic drugs Antiarrhythmic drugs Antiepileptic drugs	Local anesthetic receptor site	IS6, IIIS6, IVS6

symptom which disease diagnose and device approach for therapy (Cote & Robboy, 1980; Slee, 1978 and Current procedural terminology, 1970).

The human genome project policy to complete the human gene sequencing process a gene database of all the dissimilarity in gene sequencing. And other bioinformatics tool is already acquired in certain clinical problem in diagnoses and treatment plan like PubMed etc (Markowitz & Ritter, 1995).

Most important of EMR (Electronic Medical Record) in medical science the information can be very easily acquired and shared in comparison to Conventional medical record. The EMR data expected for a study can be obtained directly from the electronic medical record thus producing research biological data collection for medical analysis a side effect of generally clinical data record keeping. The electronic medical record helpful for research protocol, point out to a physician when a eligible for a study, or when the protocol for a study calls for a specific management plan given the currently available data about that patient (Figure 11).

GENE THERAPY

Gene therapy is the therapeutic delivery of nucleic acid polymers into a patient's cells as a drug to treat disease. Gene therapy is a way to fix a genetic problem at its source level. The polymers are either expressed as proteins, interfere with protein expression, or correct genetic mutations. Biomedical helps to build up a therapeutic method to treat genetic diseases. The most common form uses DNA that encodes a functional, therapeutic gene to replace a mutated gene. The polymer molecule is caged within a carrier or vector, which carries the molecule inside affected cells.

Figure 11. Heterogeneity of Information in EMR and its advantages in designing better treatment procedures.
(source-www.mrc-lmb.cam.ac.uk/genomes/madanm)

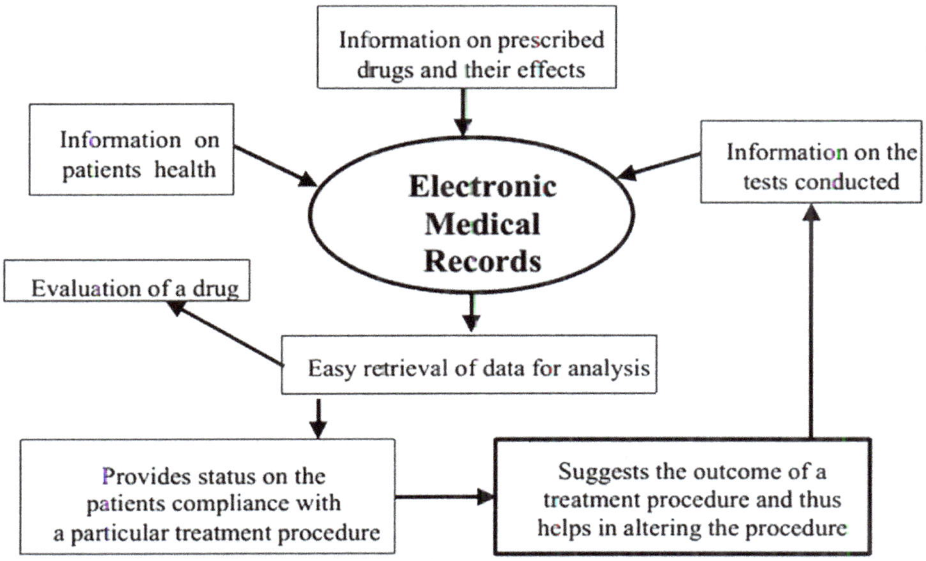

Gene therapy was conceptualized in 1972, by authors who urged caution before commencing human gene therapy studies. The first gene therapy experiment approved by the US Food and Drug Administration (FDA) occurred in 1990, when Ashanti DeSilva was treated for ADA – SCID. (Sheridan, 2011), Bioinformatics has led to identification of several genes and development of databases where large data is stored which can be seen for conducting gene therapy.

MICROBIAL GENOME APPLICATION

Microbial genome is ubiquitous and microorganisms are found in every place and any time. They have been found living and growing in crown of heat, cold emaciation, mineral acid, basicity and pressure. They are present in atmosphere, in human body and water, air and food. Generally use has been built of a different of microbial characters in the fermentation, bakery and food Technology Company. The coming of the whole genome sequence and their atmosphere, energy, healthy and food technology application. Introduced in 1994 department of energy (DOE) US proposed the microbial genome project (MGP) to sequencing gene of bacteria produced in energy formation, clean atmosphere, company processed food and harmful waste material.

Disease Causing Microorganisms

- Bacillus anthracis
- Brodetella pertusis
- Chlamydia trachomatis
- Clostridium botulinum
- Clostridium perfringens
- Clostridium tetani
- Corynebacterium diphtheriae
- Escherichia coli
- Gardinerella vaginalis
- Helicobacter pylori
- Haemophilus influenzae
- Klebsiella pneumoniae
- Legionella spp.
- Listeria monocytogenes
- Borrelia burgdorferi
- Anthrax
- Lyme disease
- Trachomas (blindness), etc.
- Botulism
- Gas gangrene & food poisoning
- Tetanus
- Diphtheria
- Typhoid fever
- Vaginitis

- Stomach ulcer
- Lung, ear infection, meningitis
- Atypical pneumoniae
- Legionnaire's disease
- Damage to fetus
- Whooping cough (pertusis)

Understanding of specialized organism system used on microbial host to live in climate environment with other host. (http://microbialgenomics.energy.gov/) (Figure 12)

MOLECULAR MEDICINE

The human genome study has profound effect on the area of modern clinical research and bio medical science. This may be due to genetic response to environmental pressure which results in change in genome like-Diabetes, cancer, cardiac disease etc. The new knowledge of the molecular mechanism properties of causing disease will offer potentially best treatment and develop specific tool for disease diagnosis, treatment and prevention (Muniba, 2010) (Figure 13).

PERSONALIZED MEDICINE

Personalized medicine is a medical system which points out the systematic use in information technology about clinical medicine and patient information is collected and this has created a new area i.e. pharma-

Figure 12. Bacteria Morphological Diversity: fm http://ag.arizona.edu/plp/courses/plp329/Micd invitro

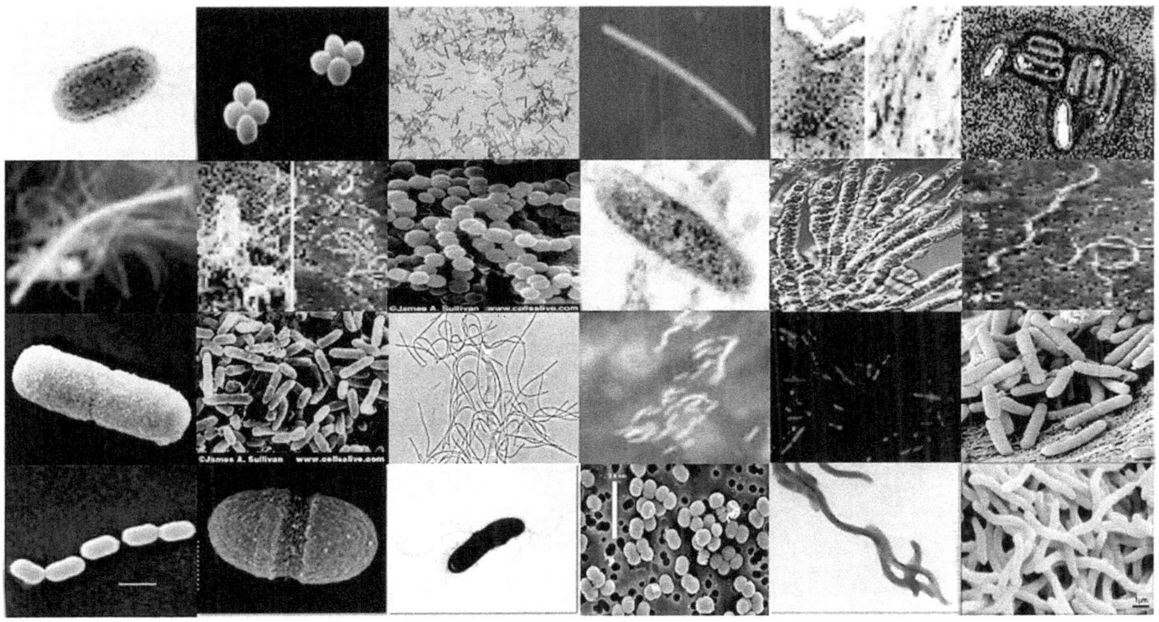

Figure 13. Integration of these disciplines molecular medicine.

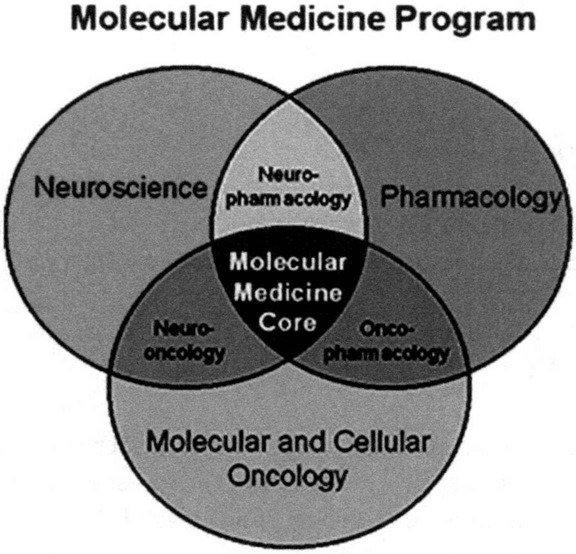

cogenomics (Indiana University Division of Clinical Pharmacology, 2010). This field studies affected body genetic character response to medicine. Some medicine have been rejected in market (development phase) because of a less presence of the personalized medicine patient population, displays advance effect to a medicine due to gene sequencing variant in their DNA molecule. Personalized medicine can be defined by this field and nature of human physiology change that permit the targeting of medical medicine treatment which may include cell or tissue therapeutics (Muniba, 2010) (Figure 14).

Figure 14. Different people respond differently to the same therapy.

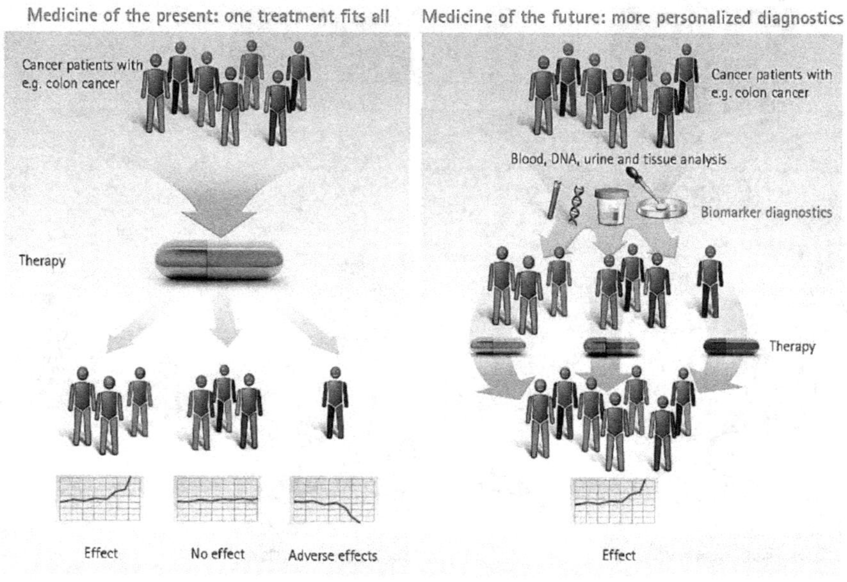

To date, the labeling of more than 100 approved drugs contain information on genomic biomarkers (including gene variants, functional deficiencies, expression changes, chromosomal abnormalities, and others). Some, but not all, of the labeling include specific actions to be taken based on genetic information. Pharmacogenomic information can appear in different sections of the labeling (e.g., Therapeutic Indications, Warnings and Precautions) (Table 6).

Medical product (drug) characteristic must be arranged with adequate information about the drug molecule and its application. Food and drug administration (FDA) desire medical product arranged to be adequately (U.S. Food and Drug Administration., 2013). Scientifically accurate, tricky and finally information must be communicated to health care practitioner for drug prescription (Margaret & Hamburg, 2013).

Table 6. Selected drugs with specific actionable guidance in labeling (arrange).

Biomarker	Therapeutic Range	Medicine (Drug)	Approval Time
PML/R ARα	Oncology	Arsenic Trioxide Tretinoin	2000 1995
CD30	Oncology	Brentuximab Vedotin	2011
DPD	Oncology	Capecitabine Fluorouracil	1998
EGFR; KR AS	Oncology	Cetuximab Panitumumab	2004 2006
ALK	Oncology	Crizotinib	2011
CD25/IL2	Oncology	Denileukin Diftitox	1999
ER/PR	Oncology	Letrozole Exemestane Fulvestrant	1997 1999 2002
C-Kit, PDGFR, FIP1L1	Oncology	Imatinib Lapatinib	2003 2007
HER 2	Oncology	Trastuzumab Everolimus Pertuzumab	1998 2009 2012
Ph Chromosome	Oncology	Imatanib Dasatanib Nilotinib	2003 2006 2007
G6PD	Oncology	Rasburicase	2002
CD20 antigen	Oncology	Tositumomab	2003
BRAF	Oncology	Vemurafenib	2011
UCD	Psychiatry	Valproic Acid	1978
CY P2C19	Psychiatry	Citalopram	1998
CYP2D6	Psychiatry, Neurology	Thioridazine Pimozide Aripiprazole Tetrabenazine Iloperidone	1962 1984 2002 2008 2009
CFTR	Pulmonary	Ivacaftor	2012
CYP2C9	Analgesics	Celecoxib	1998
CCR5	Antiviral	Maraviroc	2007
Chromosome 5qdeletion	Hematology	Lenalidomide	2005

BIOINFORMATICS IN AGRICULTURE

Application of bioinformatics in agriculture plays most important role in fast generation society, world economy and environment. Mainly crop is important part of agriculture. Today crop percentage yield has increased since last century. And will continue to increase as agronomy relies on new breeding technology and biotechnological approach (Xue, Zhao, Liang, Hou, and Wang, 2008).

FUTURE RESEARCH DIRECTIONS

Today large scale of commercial and academic enterprise such as pharmaceutical industry research & development and Quality control employ bioinformaticians to work, perform and analyse. There is large scale and complete bioinformatics demand from the academia and industry. Today increasing demand of Bioinformatics expert has arisen from most of the pharmaceutical laboratory and biomedical department. Bioinformatics growth has been global due to developed computer network allowed for easy access to molecular biological data and development of various type of software program for easy analysis.

CONCLUSION

Rapid advances in the field of computers coupled with increasing computer literacy among professionals favor the implementation of computer applications in medical practice. Further, the availability of numerous databases on the Internet has revolutionized the way by which a physician devices a strategy for treatment. Projects like the Human Proteomics Initiative is a classic example to show the necessity of integrating Bioinformatics to predict structures and functions of proteins, Medical Sciences - to identify proteins that are important in metabolic or other disorders and Pharmacology (drug discovery) - to identify novel drugs against the predicted targets. Thus it is apt to conclude that all the three areas must work in concert to achieve the ultimate goal of understanding the basis of life process and apply it for the betterment of human lives.

REFERENCES

P450 Drug interaction Table. (2010). *Indiana University Division of Clinical Pharmacology*. Retrieved from http://medicine.iupui.edu/clinpharm/ddis/table.asp

Altman, R. B. (1998). Bioinformatics in support of molecular medicine. In *Proceedings of American Medical Informatics Association Symposium (AMIA'98)* (pp. 53-61).

Barreca, M. L., De Luca, L., Iraci, N., Rao, A., Ferro, S., Maga, G., & Chimirri, A. (2007). Structure-based pharmacophore identification of new chemical scaffolds as non-nucleoside reverse transcriptase inhibitors. *Journal of Chemical Information and Modeling*, *47*(2), 557–562. doi:10.1021/ci600320q PMID:17274611

Bayat, A. (2002). Science, medicine and the future: Bioinformatics. *British Medical Journal, 324*(7344), 1018–1022. doi:10.1136/bmj.324.7344.1018 PMID:11976246

Cavagnaro, J., & Lewis, R. M. (1987). Toxicological evaluation of drugs. In M. Williams & J. B. Malick (Eds.), *Drug Discovery and Development* (pp. 259–298). Clifton, NJ: Humana Press. doi:10.1007/978-1-4612-4828-6_10

Cavasotto, C. N., & Phatak, S. S. (2009). Homology modeling in drug discovery: Current trends and applications. *Drug Discovery Today, 14*(13-14), 676–683. doi:10.1016/j.drudis.2009.04.006 PMID:19422931

Chung, S. Y., & Subbiah, S. (1996). A structural explanationfor the twilight zone of protein sequence homology. *Structure (London, England), 4*(10), 1123–1127. doi:10.1016/S0969-2126(96)00119-0 PMID:8939745

Clark, D. E., & Pickett, S. D. (2000). Computational Methods for the Prediction of Drug-Likeness. *Drug Discovery Today, 5*(2), 49–58. doi:10.1016/S1359-6446(99)01451-8 PMID:10652455

Cohen, J. (2004). Bioinformatics an Introduction for Computer Scientists: Brandeis University. *ACM Computing Surveys, 36*(2), 122–158. doi:10.1145/1031120.1031122

Cote, R. A., & Robboy, S. (1980). Progress in medical information management. Systematized nomenclature of medicine. *Journal of the American Medical Association, 243*(8), 756–762. doi:10.1001/jama.1980.03300340032015 PMID:6986000

Cramer, R. D., Patterso, D. E., & Bunce, J. D. (1989). Recent advances incomparative molecular field analysis (CoMFA). *Progress in Clinical and Biological Research, 291*, 161–165. PMID:2726839

Crum -Brown, A., & Fraser, T.R. (1969). On the connection between chemical constitution and physiological action. Part 1. On the physiological action of the ammonium bases, derived from Strychia, Brucia, Thebaia, Codeia, Morphia and Nicotia. *Transactions of the Royal Society of Edinburgh, 25*, 257–274.

Current Procedural Terminology (CPT). (1970). Current Procedural Terminology (CPT). *Journal of the American Medical Association, 212*(5), 873–874. doi:10.1001/jama.1970.03170180149024

Dixon, S. L., Smondyrev, A. M., Knoll, E. H., Rac, S., Shaw, D. E., & Friesner, R. A. (2006). PHASE: A new engine for pharmacophore perception, 3D QSAR model development, and 3D database screening: 1. Methodology and preliminary results. *Journal of Computer-Aided Molecular Design, 20*(10-11), 647–671. doi:10.1007/s10822-006-9087-6 PMID:17124629

Duan, J., Dixon, S. L., Lowrie, J. F., & Sherman, W. (2010). Analysis and comparison of 2D fingerprints: Insights into database screening performance using eight fingerprints Methods. *Journal of Molecular Graphics & Modelling, 29*(2), 157–170. doi:10.1016/j.jmgm.2010.05.008 PMID:20579912

Durbin, R., Eddy, S., Krogh, A., & Mitchison, G. (1998). *Biological Sequence Analysis*. Cambridge, UK: Cambridge University Press. doi:10.1017/CBO9780511790492

Eswar, N., Eramian, D., Webb, B., Shen, M., & Sali, A. (2008). Protein structure modeling with MODELLER. *Methods in Molecular Biology (Clifton, N.J.), 426*, 145–159. doi:10.1007/978-1-60327-058-8_8 PMID:18542861

Fischer, P. M. (2008). Computational chemistry approaches to drug discovery in signal transduction. *Biotechnology Journal*, *3*(4), 452–470. doi:10.1002/biot.200700259 PMID:18412174

Fitch, W. M. (1970). Distinguishing homologous from analogous proteins. *Systematic Zoology*, *19*(2), 99–110. doi:10.2307/2412448 PMID:5449325

Fozzard, H.A., & Hanck, D.A. (1996). Structure and function of voltage-dependent sodium channels: comparison of brain II and cardiac isoforms. *American Physiological Society, 76*(3), 887-926.

Frenking, G., Antes, I., Böhme, M., Dapprich, S., Ehlers, A. W., Jonas, V., ... Vyboishchikov, S.F. (1996). Reviews in Computational Chemistry. New York: VCH.

Gerstein, M., & Hegyi, H. (1998). Comparing genomes in terms of protein structure: Surveys of a finite parts list. *FEMS Microbiology Reviews*, *22*(4), 277–304. doi:10.1111/j.1574-6976.1998.tb00371.x PMID:10357579

Gund, P. (2000). Evolution of the pharmacophore Concept in Pharmaceutical Research. In O. F. Güner (Ed.), *Pharmacophore Perception, Development, and Use in Drug Design*. La Jolla, CA: International University Line.

Hansch, C. (1969). A quantitative approach to biochemical structure-activity relationships. *Accounts of Chemical Research*, *2*(8), 232–239. doi:10.1021/ar50020a002

Holstege, F. C., Wyrick, J. E., Lee, T. I., Hengartner, C. J., Green, M. R., Golub, T. R., & Young, R. A. et al. (1998). Dissecting the regulatory circuitry of a eukaryotic genome. *Cell*, *95*(5), 717–728. doi:10.1016/S0092-8674(00)81641-4 PMID:9845373

Jessell, T. M., & Sanes, J. R. (2000). The generation and survival of new cell. In E. R. Kandel, J. Schwartz, & T. M. Jessell (Eds.), *In principal of neural science* (pp. 41–62). New York, NY: McGraw-Hill.

Kerns, E. H., & Carte, G. T. (2009). Drug-like property concepts in Pharmaceutical design. *Current Pharmaceutical Design*, *15*(19), 2184–2194. doi:10.2174/138161209788682479 PMID:19601822

Kirchmair, J., Markt, P., Distinto, S., Wolber, G., & Langer, T. (2008). Evaluation of the performance of 3D virtual screening protocols: RMSD comparisons, enrichment assessments, and decoy selection--what can we learn from earlier mistakes. *Journal of Computer-Aided Molecular Design*, *22*(3-4), 213–228. doi:10.1007/s10822-007-9163-6 PMID:18196462

Klebe, G. (2000). Recent developments in structure-based drug design. *Journal of Molecular Medicine*, *78*(5), 269–281. doi:10.1007/s001090000084 PMID:10954199

Klebe, G., & Abraham, U. (1999). Comparative molecular similarity index analysis (CoMSIA) to study hydrogen-bonding properties and to score combinatorial libraries. *Journal of Computer-Aided Molecular Design*, *13*(1), 1–10. doi:10.1023/A:1008047919606 PMID:10087495

Kleywegt, G. J., Harris, M. R., Zou, J. Y., Taylor, T. C., Wahlby, A., & Jones, T. A. (2004). The uppsala electron-density server. *Acta Crystallographica. Section D, Biological Crystallography*, *60*(12), 2240–2249. doi:10.1107/S0907444904013253 PMID:15572777

Krieger, E., Nabuurs, S. B., & Vriend, G. (2003). Homology modeling. *Structural Bioinformatics*, *5*, 507–521. PMID:12647402

Langridge, R. (1974). Interactive three-dimensional computer graphics in molecular biology. *Federation Proceedings*, *33*(12), 2332–2335. PMID:4435233

Leach, A. R., & Gillet, V. J. (2003). An introduction to chemoinformatics. Springer.

Leach, A. R., Gillet, V. J., Lewis, R. A., & Taylor, R. (2010). Three-dimensional pharmacophore methods in drug discovery. *Journal of Medicinal Chemistry*, *53*(2), 539–558. doi:10.1021/jm900817u PMID:19831387

Lesk, A. M., & Chothia, C. (1980). How different amino acid sequences determine similar protein structures: The structure and evolutionary dynamics of the globins. *Journal of Molecular Biology*, *136*(3), 225–270. doi:10.1016/0022-2836(80)90373-3 PMID:7373651

Lill, M. A. (2007). Multi-dimensional QSAR in drug discovery. *Drug Discovery Today*, *12*(23-24), 1013–1017. doi:10.1016/j.drudis.2007.08.004 PMID:18061879

Lipinski, C. A., Lombardo, F., Dominy, B. W., & Feeny, P. J. (2001). Experimental and computational approaches to estimate solubility and permeability in drug discovery and development settings. *Advanced Drug Delivery Reviews*, *46*(1-3), 3–26. doi:10.1016/S0169-409X(00)00129-0 PMID:11259830

Lipkowitz, K. B., & Boyed, D. B. (1996). Reviews in Computational Chemistry. New York, NY: VCH Publishers.

Luscombe, N. M., Greenbaum, D., & Gerstein, M. (2001). What is Bioinformatics? An Introduction and Overview. *Yearbook of Medical Informatics*, 83–99. Retrieved from http://www.ebi.ac.uk/luscombe/publications.html

Margaret, A., & Hamburg, M. D. (2013). *Paving the Way for Personalized Medicine*. U.S. Food and Drug Administration.

Markowitz, V. M., & Ritter, O. (1995). Characterizing heterogeneous molecular biology database systems. *Journal of Computational Biology*, *2*(4), 547–556. doi:10.1089/cmb.1995.2.547 PMID:8634907

Markt, P., Schuster, D., Kirchmair, J., Laggner, C., & Langer, T. (2007). Pharmacophore modeling and parallel screening for PPAR ligands. *Journal of Computer-Aided Molecular Design*, *21*(10-11), 575–590. doi:10.1007/s10822-007-9140-0 PMID:17960326

Meyer, H. (1899). Zur Theorie der Alkoholnarkose. *Arch. Exp Pathol. Pharmakol*, *42*(2-4), 109–118. doi:10.1007/BF01834479

Miguet, L., Zhang, Z., Barbier, M., & Grigorov, M. G. (2006). Comparison of a homology model and the crystallographic structure of human 11beta-hydroxysteroid dehydrogenase type 1 (11betaHSD1) in a structure-based identification of inhibitors. *Journal of Computer-Aided Molecular Design*, *20*(2), 67–81. doi:10.1007/s10822-006-9037-3 PMID:16783599

Muniba, S. (2010). *Application of Bioinformatics in medicine*. Retrieved from http://www.biotecharticles.com/Bioinformatics-Article/Application-of-Bioinformatics-in-Medicine-222.html

NCBI (National Center for Biotechnology Information). Retrieved from http://www.ncbi.nlm.nih.gov

Overton, E. (1901). *Studien uber die Narkose, zugleich ein Beitrag zur allgemeiner Pharmakologie*. Jena, Switzerland: Gustav Fischer.

Pedersen, A. G., Jensen, L. J., Brunak, S., Staerfeldt, H. H., & Ussery, D. W. (2000). A DNA structural atlas for Escherichia coli. *Journal of Molecular Biology*, *299*(4), 907–930. doi:10.1006/jmbi.2000.3787 PMID:10843847

Perkins, R., Fang, H., Tong, W., & Welsh, W. J. (2003). Quantitative structure-activity relationship methods: Perspectives on drug discovery and toxicology. *Environmental Toxicology and Chemistry*, *22*(8), 1666–1679. doi:10.1897/01-171 PMID:12924569

Richards, W. G. (1994). Computer-Aided Drug Design. *Pure and Applied Chemistry*, *66*(8), 1589–1596. doi:10.1351/pac199466081589

Richet, M. C. (1893). Compt. *Rend. Soc. Biol.*, *45*, 775–776.

Russell, R. B., Saqi, M. A., Bates, P. A., Sayle, R. A., & Sternberg, M. J. (1998). Recognition of analogous and homologous protein folds—assessment of prediction success and associated alignment accuracy using empirical substitution matrices. *Protein Engineering*, *11*(1), 1–9. doi:10.1093/protein/11.1.1 PMID:9579654

Russell, R. B., Saqi, M. A., Sayle, R. A., Bates, P. A., & Sternberg, M. J. (1997). Recognition of analogous and homologous protein folds: Analysis of sequence and structure conservation. *Journal of Molecular Biology*, *269*(3), 423–439. doi:10.1006/jmbi.1997.1019 PMID:9199410

Russo, E. (2000). Proteomics Factories. *Scientist (Philadelphia, Pa.)*, *14*(3), 1.

Salam, N. K., Nuti, R., & Sherman, W. (2009). Novel method for generating structure based pharmacophores using energetic analysis. *Journal of Chemical Information and Modeling*, *49*(10), 2356–2368. doi:10.1021/ci900212v PMID:19761201

Sandeep, S., Priyadarshini, V., Pradhan, D., Munikumar, M., & Umamaheswari, A. (2012). Docking and molecular dynamics simulations studies of human protein kinase catalytic subunit alpha with antagonist. *Journal of Clinical & Scientific Research*, *1*, 15–23.

Schueler, F. W. (1960). *Chemobiodynamics and Drug Design*. New York, NY: McGraw-Hill.

Sheridan, C. (2011). Gene therapy finds its niche. *Nature Biotechnology*, *29*(2), 121–128. doi:10.1038/nbt.1769 PMID:21301435

Shortliffe, E. H., & Blois, M. S. (2000). The Computer meets medicine and biology: Emergence of a discipline. In E. H. Shortliffe & L. E. Perreault (Eds.), *Medical Informatics: Computer Applications in Health Care and Biomedicine* (2nd ed.; pp. 3–40). New York, NY: Springer Verlag.

Skolnick, J., & Fetrow, J. S. (2000). From genes to protein structure and function: Novel applications of computational approaches in the genomic era. *Trends in Biotechnology*, *18*(1), 34–39. doi:10.1016/S0167-7799(99)01398-0 PMID:10631780

Slee, V. N. (1978). The International Classification of Diseases: Ninth revision (ICD-9). *Annals of Internal Medicine*, *88*(3), 424–426. doi:10.7326/0003-4819-88-3-424 PMID:629506

Sliwoski, G., Kothiwale, S., Meiler, J., & Lowe, E. W. (2014). Computational Methods in Drug Discovery. *Pharmacological Reviews*, *66*(1), 334–395. doi:10.1124/pr.112.007336 PMID:24381236

Song, C. M., Lim, S. J., & Tong, J. C. (2009). Recent advances in computer-aided drug Design. *Briefings in Bioinformatics*, *10*(5), 579–591. doi:10.1093/bib/bbp023 PMID:19433475

Tatusov, R. L., Koonin, E. V., & Lipman, D. J. (1997). A genomic perspective on protein families. *Science*, *278*(5338), 631–637. doi:10.1126/science.278.5338.631 PMID:9381173

U.S. Food and Drug Administration. (2013). *Table of Pharmacogenomic Biomarkers in Drug Labels*. Retrieved from http://www.fda.gov/drugs/scienceresearch/researchareas/ph

Verma, J., Khedkar, V. M., & Coutinho, E. C. (2010). 3D-QSAR in drug design--a review. *Current Topics in Medicinal Chemistry*, *10*(1), 95–115. doi:10.2174/156802610790232260 PMID:19929826

Veselovsky, A. V., & Ivanov, A. S. (2003). Strategy of computer-aided drug design. *Current Drug Targets. Infectious Disorders*, *3*(1), 33–40. doi:10.2174/1568005033342145 PMID:12570731

Virtanen, S. (2013). *Virtual Screening Development of a Novel Structure-Based Method.* Jyvaskyla.

Walsh. (1982). *Calcium and Cell Function.* New York, NY: Academic Press,

Waszkowycz, B. (2008). Towards improving compound selection in structure based virtual screening. *Drug Discovery Today*, *13*(5-6), 219–226. doi:10.1016/j.drudis.2007.12.002 PMID:18342797

Wermuth, C. G., Ganellin, C. R., Lindberg, P., & Mitscher, L. A. (1998). Glossary of terms used in medicinal chemistry. *Pure and Applied Chemistry*, *70*(5), 1129–1143. doi:10.1351/pac199870051129

William, A. C. (2000). Structure and regulation of voltage –gated Ca channels. *Annual Review of Cell and Developmental Biology*, *16*(1), 521–555. doi:10.1146/annurev.cellbio.16.1.521 PMID:11031246

William, A. C., Goldin, A. L., & Stephen, G. W. (2005). International Union of Pharmacology. XLVII. Nomenclature and Structure-Function Relationships of Voltage-Gated Sodium Channels. *Pharmacological Reviews*, *57*(4), 397–409. doi:10.1124/pr.57.4.4 PMID:16382098

Wolber, G., & Langer, T. (2005). Ligand Scout: 3-D pharmacophores derived from protein-bound ligands and their use as virtual screening filters. *Journal of Chemical Information and Modeling*, *45*(1), 160–169. doi:10.1021/ci049885e PMID:15667141

Wooley, J. C. (1999). Trends in Computational Biology: A Summary based on a RECOMB Plenary lecture. *Journal of Computational Biology*, *6*(3/4), 459–474. doi:10.1089/106652799318391 PMID:10582579

Xue, J., Zhao, S., Liang, Y., Hou, C., & Wang, J. (2008). IFIP International Federation for Information Processing. In Computer and Computing Technologies in Agriculture (vol. 2, pp. 977–982). Boston: Springer.

Yamakaqe, M. & Namiki, A. (2002). Calcium channels--basic aspects of their structure, function and gene encoding; anesthetic action on the channels--a review. *Canadian Journal of Anesthesia/Journal canadien d'anesthésie, 49*, 151-164.

Zeng, J. (2000). Mini-Review: Computational Structure-Based Design of Inhibitors that Target Protein Surfaces. *Combinatorial Chemistry & High Throughput Screening, 3*(5), 355–362. doi:10.2174/1386207003331490 PMID:11032953

KEY TERMS AND DEFINITIONS

Bioinformatics: As an interdisciplinary field of science, bioinformatics combines computer science, statistics, mathematics, and engineering to analyze and interpret biological data.

Biomedical: Is the application of engineering principles and design concepts to medicine and biology for healthcare purposes (e.g. diagnostic or therapeutic).

Cheminformatics: Use of computer and informational techniques applied to a range of problems in the field of chemistry.

Database: A database is an organized collection of data.

Genomics: Is a discipline in genetics that applies recombinant DNA, DNA sequencing methods, and bioinformatics to sequence, assemble, and analyze the function and structure of genomes.

Pharmaceutical: Is a drug used to diagnose, cure, treat, or prevent disease.

Pharmacoinformatics: Drug discovery and development requires the integration of chemistry, biology, pharmacology, pharmaceutical technology and extensive use of information technology.

Proteomics: Is the large-scale study of proteins, particularly their structures and functions.

Section 5

Nutraceuticals and Phytopharmaceuticals

Chapter 6
An Overview and Therapeutic Applications of Nutraceutical and Functional Foods

Raj K. Keservani
Rajiv Gandhi Proudyogiki Vishwavidhyalaya, India

Anil K. Sharma
Delhi Institute of Pharmaceutical Sciences and Research, India

Rajesh K. Kesharwani
National Institute of Technology Warangal, India

ABSTRACT

Healthy nutrition is important for human beings for good health provided by global industry. Nutraceutical and functional food provide a prospect to reduce health care costs and improve the human health. Researchers carried out plenty of work for the preparation of nutraceutical and functional food product. This article also focused on recent advances on the nutraceutical and functional foods product on health benefits and their application in prevention of disease. Here we discussed about the health benefit of recently introduced nutraceutical and functional food products. With the modernised, competitive lifestyle and ever increasing stressful conditions this product is the need of the day.

INTRODUCTION

The nutraceutical is a portmanteau of nutrition and pharmaceutical. Reportedly, S. Defelice (1989), founder and chairperson of foundation for innovation in medicine, defined "any substance that may be food or part of a food and provides medical or health benefits, including the prevention and treatment of disease. Such products may achieved from isolated nutrients, dietary supplements and diets to genetically engineered 'designer' foods, herbal products, and processed foods such as cereals, soups, and beverages. According to the International Food Information Council (IFIC), a functional food provides a health benefit beyond basic nutrition (Biesalski, 2001; Keservani et al., 2010a). Any food can be consider as functional, on demonstration it can be produce beneficial effect to one or more target functions in the body or reduce disease risk besides basic nutrition (Sarkar, 2007). The nutraceutically and functionally used food products are Vitamins, minerals, trace elements, lipids, amino acid, carbohydrate, flavonoids,

DOI: 10.4018/978-1-5225-0754-3.ch006

plant extracts, and milk etc (Keservani et al., 2010b). The terminology functional foods was first came into light in Japan in the mid-1980s and deal with processed foods having ingredients that help specific bodily functions besides being nutritious. By latest, Japan is the lone nation that has prepared a particular regulatory approval procedure for functional foods. Called as Foods for Specified Health Use (FOSHU), these foods are apt candidates to have a seal of approval from the Japanese Ministry of Health and Welfare (Arai, 1996). The Institute of Medicine's Food and Nutrition Board (IOM/FNB, 1994) defined functional foods as "any food or food ingredient that may provide a health benefit beyond the traditional nutrients it contains" (Meyer, 1998; Keservani et al., 2010a).

Dietary plant flavonoids plays major role in cancer prevention, neuroprotection, and cardiovascular health through their anti-oxidant, anti-inflammatory, pro-apoptotic, and antiproliferative activities (Nordeen et al., 2013). The phytochemicals present in these foods (like phenylpropanoids, isoprenoids, polyphenols, anthocynidins, flavonoids, terpenoids, carotenoids, phytoestrogens and alkaloids etc) have therapeutic effects against a number of diseases like diabetes, heart disease, common cold, arthritis, cancer, hypertension, dyslipidemia, inflammatory bowel disease, depression etc (Iriti & Faoro, 2006). Pomegranate fruit extract (PFE), which contains anti-inflammatory via inhibiting the eicosanoid generating enzymes activity and Nitrous oxide (NO) production (Shukla et al., 2008).

PUFAs (Poly unsaturated fatty acids) and ω-3 fish oils in the diet or taken orally. Investigators have shown that the topical administration of PUFAs has also been effective for dry eye on the basis of preliminary human studies and animal data results (Cortina & Bazan, 2011). It was demonstrated in a randomized clinical trial that lycopene is used as therapeutic agent for prostate cancer (Kucuk et al., 2002). There are various nutraceutical components presents in plant extracts such as γ-linolenic acid, β-carotene, flavonoids etc with potential to reduce blood glucose and A1C levels in diabetics (Kagan et al., 1990; Davies et al., 1997; Sotaniemi et al., 1995; Huseini et al., 2006). Over the last century, researchers reported findings of the first huge level, across the nation investigation of fatty acids in U.S. organic and custom milk and concluded that the consumption of omega-6 fatty acids in western diets have enhanced, whereas omega-3 consumption have reduced, yielding omega-6 to omega-3 consumption ratios have raised to nutritionally unwanted amounts, usually 10 to 15, in comparison with a feasible optimal ratio of 2 to 3 (http://www.nutraceuticalsworld.com/).

Berislav Zlokovic studied how the brain's vascular system can assist in the progression of Alzheimer's disease and devised that, this is owing to elevated beta-amyloid accumulation on pericytes in old blood vessels, resulting into disturbing the integrity of the blood-brain barrier and a decrease capability to eliminate amyloid from the brain. Alzheimer's disease is the principal cause of dementia. It is an age-related disease that eventually diminishes a person's memory, thinking, and capability to carry out routine tasks. Brains from Alzheimer's patients generally have abnormally enhanced levels of plaques composed of depositions of beta-amyloid protein juxtaposed to brain cells, tau protein that aggregates together to make neurofibrillary tangles inside neurons, and extensive neuron loss. The European Food Safety Authority (EFSA) summarized in its prime full risk determination of the sweetener like aspartame and its metabolites (phenylalanine, methanol and aspartic acid) are safe for human consumptions at current levels. As per the report of Centers for Disease Control and Prevention (CDC), 75% of total healthcare expenses were spent on caring for people with preventable diseases, with only 3% spent on prevention (http://www.nutraceuticalsworld.com/).

According to Innova Market Insights, about 3% of global food and drink introductions in last one year by the end of September were branded as a protein rich or source-of-protein. Considering at latest new product events in yogurt, but data signal that more than 10% of launches across the globe utilised protein, nevertheless this was twisted by the Unites State, where over one-third of launches were branded employing this positioning. This data further go down to approximately 6% in Western Europe, United Kingdom begins resembling patterns as in the United State. The launching of Greek and Greek-style strained yogurts contain more amount of protein than that of standard line, which provides nice foundation for protein rich yogurts (as per Lu Ann Williams, Director of Innovation at Innova Market Insights). Majority of them are probiotics too. Men who are interested in good fitness demands more brogurt (subcategory of yogurt). Powerful yogurt introduces the first cycle of Greek yogurts for men in 2013, featuring 8-ounce cup with 25 g of natural protein per pot, launched by United State. Another progress pertains to the introduction of frozen yogurt with protein rich like Pro Yo in the United State and high protein strained yogurt (but not Greek or Greek-style) (http://www.nutraceuticalsworld.com/). The main aim of this chapter is to provide scattered information of dietary supplements, nutraceutical and functional food in management and prevention of disease and its health benefits in the gathered form.

Prebiotics

Prebiotics is a common term, which means substances that trigger the development and/or functions of friendly microflora (i.e. bacteria and fungi) that aids in the good health of their host. The most popular instance is inside the gastrointestinal tract, where prebiotics may modify the spread of microorganisms wthin gut microbiome. Nevertheless, hypothetically it is a much common nomenclature that may deal with other regions of the body too. For instance, few hand moisturizers are suggested to behave like prebiotics to enhance the funtionality and/or make up of the skin microbiota (Schloss, 2014).

Probiotics

Probiotics are microorganisms, which are trusted to yield health advantages upon consumption (Rijkers et al, 2011). The terminolgy probiotic is nowadays applied to tag intaked microorganism linked with favorable impact on humans and other animals (FAO-UN-WHO 2002). This group includes molecules or elements, probiotic microorganism. This group covers hugely bacteria. Criteria for selection are its survival in acid environment of stomach, bile and digestive enzymes generally present inside human gastrointestinal tract; capability to invade the human intestine; innocuous and useful for human uses. Probiotics administration is reported to be related with a reduced risk of allergy, asthma, cancer, infection of ear and urinary tract (Dahiya, 2013).

Dietary Supplements

Supplements as often apprehanded encompass vitamins, minerals, fiber, fatty acids, or amino acids, among other materials. A dietary supplement is purported to give nutrients that can or else not be taken in ample amounts (Park, 2013, Grace, 2013).

Superfood

Superfood is a commercial name applied to discus foods with associted health merits. The superfood terminology is not in parlance by dieticians and nutrition researchers, a number of whom raise quetions that specific foods possess the health advantages usually claimed by certain superfoods pro people (di Noia, 2014).

Medical Foods

The Orphan Drug Amendment to the FDCA of 1988 defines "medical food", as a food which is prepared to be ingested or administered orally under the supervision of a physician and which is purported for the particular dietary management of a disease or condition for which special nutritional needs, on the basis of proven scientific doctrines, are established by medical assessment (http://www.deplin.com/what-is-a-medical-food; Morgan et al, 2006).

NUTRACEUTICAL CONCEPTS

The nutraceutical products are recognized and produce health benefits like alleviating the threat of cancer and heart disease and also for prevention or treatment of hypertension, high cholesterol, excess weight, diabetes, osteoporosis, arthritis, macular degeneration (resulting in irreversible blindness), cataracts, menopausal manifestations, insomnia, memory and concentration loss, digestive upsets and constipation and other disease (Whitman, 2001; Heyland, 2001; Elizabeth, 2002).

Concept of nutraceutical (Figure 1) totally based on the nutrition and pharmaceutical, in the past years there was no verification method for food but in last few decades but, as food make up has been logically validated to lead towards life habit-associated diseases, and has turned a public concern. The notion of nutraceuticals has begun to be recognized as one of the approaches for prevention of such diseases (Brower, 1998; Kalra, 2003).

COMPARISON BETWEEN FUNCTIONAL FOODS, MEDICAL FOODS AND DRUGS

There are two main reasons which differentiate the functional food to medical foods and drug ie its distribution and regulation, functional food distributed and regulated differently than the medical food and

Figure 1. Nutraceutical concepts

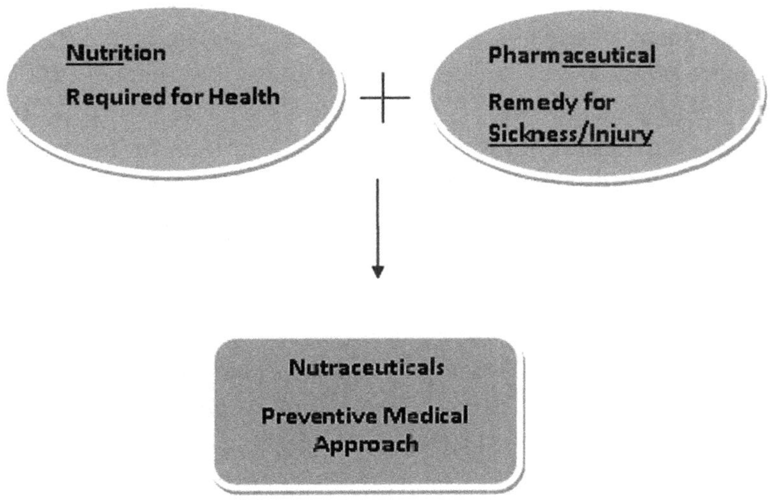

Table 1. Comparison between functional foods, medical foods and drugs

Difference	Functional Foods	Medical Foods	Prescription Drugs
Uses	Energy enhances; manage weight; boosts gut, bone or heart health; reduce threat of disease; improve memory	A disease or condition with specific nutritional requirements	In case of disease symptoms/ condition
Method of Procurement	Consumer selects, no prescription or supervision required	Used only under medical supervision	Health provider prescription
Channels of Distribution	Supermarkets, drug stores, online, principal retailers	Hospitals, pharmacy, drug stores, online	Pharmacy, hospitals
Regulatory Body	No specific body, but is known as food and is so subject to FDA regulation (FDA regulates any particular health claims that might be made)	No additional FDA review/approval required, but must adhere to controls with respect to foods, e.g., labeling (FDA control any perticular health claims that might be made)	FDA approval warranted, a multiyear, multistage review procedure
Amount Consumed	As needed	As desired	As per prescription by doctor

Source:www.pwc.com

drug (Table 1). The primary difference is that functional foods can be taken up without any prescription as part of daily life whereas medical foods and drugs are utlised during treatment or management of a condition under medical supervision (www.pwc.com).

PROTEIN, PEPTIDE, AND AMINO ACIDS AS NUTRACEUTICAL

Amino acids are physiologically vital organic compounds made up of amine (-NH2) and carboxylic acid (-COOH) functional groups, having a side-chain particular to every amino acid (Wagner and Musso, 1983). Amino acids are basic ingredient for human diet and have nutritional value. Several types of protein made up off varying amount of amino acids, which play role of foundation blocks of protein. There are approximately 20 amino acids that may be exploited to make protein. There are 8 essential amino acids that ought to be received by diet since the body cannot synthesize these amino acids (Table 2). There are about 6 provisionally essential amino acids also that the body faces difficulty in synthesizing, and so individuals are primarily based on dietary source for these amino acids. The body may readily synthesize the rest amino acids, so they are known as nonessential (Campbell, 2008). Other significant zone of the application of nutrition in recovery and relapse check is the incorporation of adequate amino acids that work as the foundation stone for strong substances in the brain termed neurotransmitters. These neurotransmitters, covering epinephrine and norepinephrine, GABA, serotonin and dopamine, are intimately associated with addiction habits. With the utilization of different amino acids, brain chemistry can be altered to assist normalize and restore deficiencies in the neurotransmitters that cause cravings that may contribute to addiction and relapse (Blum et al., 2001). The protein, peptide amino acid with their health benefits represented in Table 3.

This class possess the promise to cover integral protein (ie. soy protein), polypeptides, amino acids, and nitrogenous and sulphur amino acid derivative. Nowadays, some amino acids are being studied for their nutraceutical ability too. Arginine (Nittynen et al, 1999) and folic acid (Wildman and Medeiros 2000) have cardioprotective role. Arginine may also reduce atherogenesis (Nittynen et al, 1999).

Table 2. List of amino acids

Essential Amino Acids	Nonessential Amino Acids	Conditionally Essential Amino Acids
Isoleucine	Alanine	Arginine
Leucine	Asparagine	Cysteine
Lysine	Aspartic acid	Glutamine
Methionine	Glutamic acid	Histidine
Phenylalanine	Glycine	Proline
Threonine	Serine	Tyrosine
Tryptophan		
Valine		

(Young, 1994; Imura and Okada, 1998; Lourenço and Camilo, 2002; Holtcamp, 2012)

Table 3. Protein, peptide and amino acids with potential health benefits

Nutraceutical	Source	Health Benefits	References
Milk proteins, peptides Lactoferrin and immunoglobulin G.	Milk and derived products	Antihypertensive, antimicrobial, antiinflammatory and Inmunostimulating activities Important source of amino acids	(Lacomba et al., 2010 Campanella et al., 2009; Meltretter et al., 2008; De Simone et al., 2009)
Amino acids Sprouts	alga and sport drinks and tablets	Eeffect on the nervous system, antioxidant, anti-cancer and source of muscle energy	(Kim et al., 2006; Herrero et al., 2007; Ueno et al., 2008)
Immunomodulatoryproteins	Garlic (Allium sativum)	Immunomodulation activity	(Clement et al., 2010)
Total proteins	Ganoderma lucidum (fungi)	Prevention and treatment of hypertension, diabetes, hepatitis,cancers and AIDS	(Saltarelli et al., 2009)
Lysozyme-derived peptides	Hen's egg	Antimicrobial activity	(You et al., 2010)
Cyclopeptides	Cow cockle seed	Estrogen like activity in vivo	(Guclu-Ustundag et al., 2008)
Selenopeptides	Nuts	Antioxidant, anti-cancer, anti-heart disease	(Dernovics et al., 2007)

CARBOHYDRATE, GLYCOSIDE, AND FIBER AS NUTRACEUTICAL AND FUNCTIONAL FOODS

As the term defines, carbohydrates are based on the elements carbon, hydrogen, and oxygen. Nevertheless, carbohydrates in foods embrace a great diversity of structures, which in turn decide a broad range of physiological influences in the human body (Gray, 2003). Glycosides are compounds possessing a carbohydrate molecule (sugar) assocaited with a non- carbohydrate species. These compounds are generally present in plants, and they may be transformed, by hydrolytic break down, into a sugar and a non-sugar domain (aglycone). Particularly the sort of sugar identifies them that they have, as glucosides (glucose), pentosides (pentose), fructosides (fructose), etc. Many plant glycosides have exhibited action for cancer prevention, antidiabetic, anti-obese, antibacterial or antineoplastic activity (Erkucuk et al., 2009; D'Antuono et al., 2008; Baek et al., 2008; Dall'Acqua et al., 2007). Fiber also termed as non-starch carbohydrate comes from the cell wall of plants like cellulose, hemicelluloses and pectin. Like other carbohydrates, its prime role is to avail energy (Havrlentova et al., 2011). Carbohydrates acquire form of sugars, oligosaccharides, starches and fibers and are one of the three main macro nutrients that provide the body with energy (fat and protein are the others). There is now nice proof that minimum of 55% of per day calories should be obtained from carbohydrates. While it is essential to keep an adequate balance between calorie intake and expenditure, scientific investigations have proposed that a diet having an balanced level of carbohydrates can help to check body fat deposition; starch and sugars avail easily accessible fuel for physical activity; dietary fibers which are carbohydrates, facilitate the bowel working in right fashion (Wolever & Jenkins, 1986).

Carbohydrates are important source of energy in our diet, but certain structural characteristics enable their use beyond basic nutrition. The most important structural feature of bioactive carbohydrate is resistant to digestion in the upper gastrointestinal (GI) tract, primary because of the presence of glycosidic bonds that are different from the digestive enzyme-susceptible α-1,4 and α-1,6 linkages. Carbohydrates that are not digested in the upper GI tract will reach the colon and become food for the microflora that converts them into bioactive compounds. Dietary fibres were used in prevention and promotion of human health like bowel health, heart health, cancer, healthy weight and fetal developments (Rotimi, 2012). Fructose oligosaccharide and galactose oligosaccharide enriched infant products are present in the market; these are purported to augment the growing immune systems of neonates (DeVrese & Schrezenmeir, 2008). Zoetendal et al, suggested that fast uptake and fermentation of available carbohydrates leads to keeping up the micro biota in the human small intestine (Zoetendal et al., 2008). Dietary fiber is present in plant foods (fruit, vegetables and whole grains) and is indispensible for maintaining a healthy digestive system. Fiber can not be entirely digested and is usually known as bulk or roughage. The 2 types of fiber present in food are soluble and insoluble (Sivam et al., 2011). The glycoside with potential health benefits represented in Table 4.

The glucose derrived ascorbic acid (Vitamin C) is possibly one of the most familiar nutraceutical materials and is quite famous supplements. Ascorbic acid serves as a nutraceutical substance in general as antioxidants (Wildman et al, 1999).

Table 4. Glycoside with potential health benefits

Nutraceutical	Source	Health Benefits	References
Saponins	Vegetables	Trigger muscle growth and elevate testosterone levels. Antidiabetic or anti-obese effects, antibacterial and antineoplastic actions	(Brady et al., 2007)
Chondroitin sulfate	Raw materials, preparations and dietary supplements.	Treatment of osteoarthritis and few ophthalmologic diseases.	(Malavaki et al., 2008; Sim et al., 2007; Volpi et al., 2008)
Polysaccharide (1,3-α-galactan)	Poria cocos (fungus)	Anti-inflammatory activity	(Lu et al., 2010)
Glucosamine	Nutraceutical formulations and tablets	Treatment of osteoarthritis	(Volpi, 2009; Chen et al., 2006)
Glycosides (glucosinolates, glycyrrhetic acid, glycyrrzhin, liquiritin, steroidal glycosides)	Plants	Choleretic, anti inflammatory, anti-cancer, antioxidant, anorexant and diuretic	(Erkucuk et al., 2009)

LIPID AND FATTY ACIDS AS NUTRACEUTICAL AND FUNCTIONAL FOODS

Fat and oil structures correspond to triglycerol, in which three fatty acids are incorporated in one glycerol molecule through an ester union. The distribution of fatty acids in the three positions has great importance from the physiological and technological point of view, such as digestion, absorbption and physical properties such as melting point, solid content and spread properties (Henry, 2009). Numerous epidemiological and experimental investigations have documented the favorable influences of perilla oil on health (Li et al., 1998). Dietary sources of ALA, like perilla seed oil can possess the capability to stall the production of leucocytes in patients with asthma (Okamoto et al., 2000). The role of dietary fats and oils in health is a matter of permanent attention and it continues to be in the first line of biological research (Burlingame et al., 2009).

Fatty acids are carboxylic acids having an altering unbranched aliphatic tail (chain), which may be saturated or unsaturated. They are essential as nutritional materials in living organisms. Long- chain polyunsaturated fatty acids (PUFAs), particularly those of the ω-3 series, like α-linolenic (18:3 n-3), are indispensable for human metabolism and possess several favorable effects covering the prevention of numerous diseases, like coronary heart diseases, inflammation, autoimmune disorders, hypertension, hypotriglyceridemic effect, etc (Benatti et al., 2004; Schacky, 2003). The famous instances of polyunsaturated fatty acids (PUFAs) are the long chain ω-3-fatty acids, which are deemed important, as they can not be effectively synthesized by the body owing to the low action of the rate limiting enzyme Δ 6-desaturase. Various sorts of fish such as anchovies, salmon, mackerel, hearing, sardines, tuna and trout and marine mammals are especially great sources of PUFAs (Strobel et al., 2012). The lipid and their potential health benefits are presented in Table 5.

There are various fatty acids and their derivatives, which have drawn the attention of research groups because of their functional abilities. Like omega-3-Polyunsaturated fatty acids (ω-3-PUFA) present in greater amounts in plants, fish and other marine animals and conjugated linoleic acid (CLA) synthesized by bacteria inside rumen of gazing animals like cattle (Babayan 1987).

Table 5. Lipids with their potential health benefits

Nutraceutical	Source	Health Benefits	References
Plant sterols (Phytosterols)	Vegetable oils (olive, sunflower, rice bran, seeds,	Phytosterols reduce cholesterol linked with LDL, possess anti-cancer activity and modify the immune function and inflammation.	(Anwar et al., 2008)
Glycerolipids	Microalga	Antimicrobial and anti-inflammatory actions	(Mendiola et al., 2007; Herrero et al., 2007)
Sterols	Italian walnut	Lowers cholesterol and minimizes the danger of coronary heart disease	(Verardo et al., 2009)
Phytosterols and phytostanols	Milk and yoghurt	Decrease cholesterol levels	(Santos et al., 2007)
Squalene	Vegetable oil	Decrease cholesterol and anti-cancer activity	(Vazquez et al., 2007)
Milk lipids (triglycerides, diacylglycerides, saturated fatty acids and PUFAs).	Milk	Immuno-suppressive, anti-inflammatory, andantimicrobial features.	(Casado et al., 2009)
Terpenes and terpenoids	Essential oils	Antiseptic, carminative, antimicrobial, and antioxidative activities.	(Golmakani et al., 2008; Prieto et al., 2007; Perez-Fons et al., 2006)

MUSHROOM AS NUTRACEUTICAL AND FUNCTIONAL FOODS

Mushroom is a common name refered to the fruiting body of macrofungi (Ascomycota and Basidiomycota) and displays exclusively a squat reproductive phase of their life cycle (Das, 2010). Mushroom can be epigeous or hypogeous, sufficiently large to be visualized with the naked eyes and can be chosen by hand (Chang & Miles, 1992). From the taxonomic point of view, mainly basidiomycetes but few species of ascomycetes are mushroom producing fungi too. Total mushrooms on the earth are projected to be 140,000 species in which 10% (14,000 approximately) are recognized. Considering that the fraction of beneficial mushrooms amid the undiscovered and untested mushrooms will be only 5%, indicates that there are 7,000 undiscovered species still, which if discovered will be supplied with the feasible gain to humanity (Hawksworth, 2001). Human has been in search for the wild mushrooms since age old (Cooke, 1977). Several hundreds years ago, the fruiting body of higher fungi has been employed as a source of food (Mattila et al., 2001) because of their chemical make up which is fascinating from the nutrition aspects. Meanwhile the near the beginning days of culture, mushrooms were consumed primarily for their deliciousness and unparallelled flavors. Gruen and Wong suggested that edible mushrooms were profoundly nutritional and compared equally with meat, egg and milk food sources (Gruen & Wong, 1982). Crisan and Sands found that mushrooms commonly have 90% water,10% dry matter with the protein content changing between 27 and 48% and carbohydrates are less than 60% and lipids are between 2 to 8% (Crisan & sands, 1978).

Mushrooms are good sources of energy. They are poor suppliers of starch and lipids but with high proteins. Mushrooms have been observed promising to combat cancer, cholesterol lowering, stress, insomnia, asthma, allergies and diabetes (Bahl, 1983). Because of greater content of proteins, they may be exploited to fill the protein malnutrition void. The mushrooms are employed as functional foods since they are consumed as nutritional supplements and to boost immunity in the form of tablets. Overall, the world production of mushrooms is dominated by those mushrooms which are both edible and have medicinal properties. Oyster mushrooms are a assorted class of saprotrophic fungi from the genus Pleurotus (Kong, 2004). As per Croan, these mushrooms are a rich source of non-starchy carbohydrates, with great amount of dietary fiber and fair contents of proteins, like majority of amino acids, minerals and vitamins (Croan, 2004).

Medical mycology is contemporary of conventional applications of mushrooms. They have been exploited in medicine from the Neolithic and Paleolithic ages (Samorini, 2001). Though mushrooms as drug have been utilized in China since 100 A.D. (Gunde-Cimmerman, 1999), but it was barely in 1960 that researchers studied the core active contituents of mushrooms which are health modulating. Several Indian mushroom sources and its potential application are depicted in Table 6.

VITAMINS AS NUTRACEUTICAL AND FUNCTIONAL FOODS

Organic compounds which are needed in small quantities to maintain life known as vitamin. Various vitamins like vitamin A, D, E, K, B and vitamin C used as a nutraceutical and functional foods. Vitamin A is fat-soluble and a class of unsaturated nutritional organic substances, that comprise retinol, retinal, retinoic acid, and many provitamin A carotenoids, among which beta-carotene is the most outstanding (Fennema, 2008)._Vitamin A is essential for escalation, progress, vision and protection of the immune

Table 6. Mushroom sources with their potential health benefits

Source	Medicinal Effects	References
Lycoperdon perlatum	Antioxidant activity, antimicrobial activity	(Ramesh and Pattar, 2010)
Marasmius oreades	Antioxidant activity, antimicrobial activity	(Ramesh and Pattar, 2010)
Phellinus rimosus	Antioxidant activity and antitumor activity	(Ajith and Janardhanan, 2007)
Agaricus bisporus	Antioxidant activity, antimicrobial activity, antiproliferative activity	(Jagdish et al., 2009)
Astraeus hygrometricus	Immunoanhancing activity	(Chakraborty et al., 2004)
Cantharellus cibarius	Antioxidant activity, antimicrobial activity	(Ramesh and Pattar, 2010)
Volvariella bombycina	Antibacterial activity	(Jagadeesh et al., 2010)
Ganoderma lucidum	Antioxidant activity, antimutagenic activity	(Jones and Janardhanan 2000; Lakshmi et al., 2003)
Lentinus squarrosulus	Immunoanhancing activity	(Bhunia et al., 2010)
Lentinus tuberregium	Antibacterial activity	Manjunathan and Kaviyarasan (2010)
Pleurotus florida	Antioxidant activity, antiinflammatory, immmunoanhancing activity	(Jose and Janardhanan 2000; Jose et al., 2002; Roy et al., 2009; Dey et al., 2010)
Pleurotus ostreatus	Immunoenhancing activity	(Maity et al., 2011)
Pleurotus pulmonarius	Antioxidant activity, antimicrobial activity	(Ramesh and Pattar, 2010)
Pleurotus pulmonarius	Antitumor activity	(Jose et al., 2002)
Pleurotus sajor-caju	Antibacterial activity	(Tambekar et al., 2006)
Ramaria formosa	Antioxidant activity, antimicrobial activity	(Ramesh and Pattar, 2010)

system (Tanumihardjo, 2011). Vitamin A may be present in two main types in foods, retinol and carotenes (β-carotene, α-carotene) (DeMan, 1999).

Vitamin A is present in nature in various foods like dandelion greens, sweet potato, carrot, broccoli leaf, butter, kale, spinach, pumpkin, collardgreens, cheddar, cheese, cantaloupe, melon, egg, apricot, papaya, mango, pea, broccoli, milk, tomatoes, seaweed.

Vitamin D is fat-soluble, present in nature in very few foods, in addition to others, and obtainable as a dietary supplement. Vitamin D is synthesized endogenously upon smacking of ultraviolet rays from sunlight to the skin. Vitamin D accelerates calcium absorption in the gut and keeps sufficient serum calcium and phosphate amounts to permit usual mineralization of bone and to avert hypocalcemic tetany. In osteoblasts and osteoclasts conditions vitamin D is needed for bone remodeling and bone growth (Fennema, 2008; Tanumihardjo, 2011). Food source of vitamin D is fatty fish (like tuna, salmon, and mackerel), beef liver, cheese, egg yolks, mushrooms, milk, soy beverages, orange juice, yogurt, and margarine.

Vitamin E is fat-soluble material possessing unique antioxidant functions. In nature, vitamin E is found in 8 chemical states (α, β, γ, and λ-tocopherol and α, β, γ, and λ -tocotrienol) that exert changing levels of biological action. Alpha- (or α-) tocopherol is the lone subtype that is recognized to gather human needs (Traber, 2006). Vitamin E found in foods like spinach, turnip greens, chard, mustard greens, cayenne pepper, sunflower seeds, almonds, bell peppers, asparagus, collard greens, kale, tomatoes, broccoli, brussels sprouts, papaya, cranberries, raspberries, and carrots (Traber, 2006).

Vitamin K is known as the clotting factor. Vitamin K maintains strong bones during elderly condition researchers reported in some studies. Vitamin K may be obtained from the foods such as Green leafy vegetables, like kale, spinach, turnip greens, collards, swiss chard, mustard greens, parsley, romaine, green leaf lettuce, brussels sprouts, broccoli, cauliflower, and cabbage, fish, liver, meat, eggs, and cereals (Escott-Stump, 2008; Mason, 2011). Vitamin B (B1, B2, B3, B5, B6 and B12) are used as nutraceutical and functional foods. Food source and description of vitamin B1, B2, B3, B5, B6 are depicted in Table 7.

Vitamin C (also k/a L-ascorbic acid), soluble in water, generally occuring in few foods, in addition to others, and existing as a dietary supplement. Humans, distinct from majority of animals, are not capable to produce vitamin C endogenously; therefore, it is an indispensible dietary constituent (Li et al., 2007). For biosynthesis of collagen, L-carnitine, and certain neurotransmitters, vitamin C is required and implicated in protein metabolism too (Li et al., 2007; Carr & Frei, 1999). Vitamin C is also a vital physiological antioxidant (Frei et al., 1989) and has been exhibited to restore other antioxidants inside body, encompassing alpha-tocopherol (vitamin E) (Jacob & Sotoudeh, 2002). All fruits (like cantaloupe, citrus fruits and juices (like orange and grapefruit), Kiwi fruit, mango, papaya, pineapple, strawberries, raspberries, blueberries, cranberries, watermelon) and vegetables (like broccoli, brussels sprouts, cauliflower, Green and red peppers, Spinach, cabbage, turnip greens, and other leafy greens, Sweet and white potatoes, Tomatoes and tomato juice, Winter squash) contain vitamin C. List of various vitamins with their related health advantages is provided in table 3 (Keservani et al., 2010b). The list of fat and water soluble vitamins and their linked health advantages are depicted in Table 8.

Table 7. Description and food source of Vitamin B1, B2, B3, B5, B6 and B12

Type	Description	Food Source
Vitamin B1	Thiamine is water soluble and helps in energy production in the body.	Whole grain, unriched grains pork, dried beans, nuts, seeds (IM, 1998).
Vitamin B2	Riboflavin is a type of B vitamin. It is water soluble, which means it is not stored in the body.	Dairy products, eggs, green leafy vegetables, lean meats, legumes, milk, nuts, breads and cereals (Escott-Stump, 2008; IM, 1998).
Vitamin B3	Vitamin B_3 is a water-soluble vitamin - meaning that it dissolves in water - with pellagra-curative, antilipemic, and vasodilating properties,	Anchovies, beef, bread (whole wheat), beans, cheese, cereals, chicken, eggs, fish - tuna, salmon, lamb, leaf vegetables, legumes, liver, heart and kidney, milk, mushrooms, nuts, pasta (enriched), sunflower seeds, yeast extract (NCM, 2013).
Vitamin B5	Vitamin B5 (called pantothenic acid), is a member of the B-complex family of vitamins. It is an essential vitamin required by the body for cellular processes and optimal maintenance of fat.	Cucumber, avocado, asparagus, broccoli, celery, grapefruit, turnip greens, tomato, yogurt, eggs, sweet potato, collard greens, chard, bell peppers, and corn (Bender, 1992; Fox, 1984).
Vitamin B6	Vitamin B6 is a water-soluble vitamin. Water-soluble vitamins dissolve in water. The body cannot store them. Leftover amounts of the vitamin leave the body through the urine. That means you need a continuous supply of such vitamins in your diet.	Avocado, banana, legumes (dried beans), meat, nuts, poultry, whole grains (Escott-Stump, 2008; IM, 1998; Hamrick & Counts, 2008).
Vitamin B12	Vitamin B12 is a water-soluble vitamin. Water-soluble vitamins dissolve in water. After the body uses these vitamins, leftover amounts leave the body through the urine.	Organ meats (beef liver), shell fish (clams), meat, poultry, eggs,milk and other dairy foods, some breakfast cereals and nutritional yeasts (Escott-Stump, 2008; IM, 1998).

Table 8. List of fat and water soluble vitamins and their linked health benefits

Nutrients	Health Benefits of Vitamins
	Fat Soluble Vitamins
Vitamin A	Antioxidant, required for growth and development, keeps healthy vision, skin and mucous membranes can help in the prevention and treatment of some cancers and in the treatment of few skin disorders.
Vitamin D	Necessary for development of bones and teeth, aids the body absorb and utilise calcium
Vitamin E	Antioxidant, assists in maturity of blood cells, muscles, lung and nerve tissue, improves the immune system
Vitamin K	Needed for blood clotting
	Water Soluble Vitamins
Vitamin C	Antioxidant, essential for healthy bones, gums, teeth and skin, facilitates wound healing, can check common cold and minimizes its symptoms
Vitamin B1	Aids to transform food into energy, required in neurologic activities
Vitamin B2	Assists in energy generation and other chemical processes in the body, aids to keep healthy eyes, skin and nerve function
Vitamin B3	Aids to transform food into energy and keep proper brain function
Vitamin B6	Facilitates to synthesize indispensible proteins and Aids to transform protein into energy
Vitamin B12	Aids to produce the genetic material of cells, assists in formation of red blood cells, maintenance of central nervous system and synthesize amino acids and is part and parcel of metabolism of fats, protein and carbohydrates
Folic acid	Essential for production of the genetic materials of cells, required in first three months of pregnancy for checking birth defects, helps in red blood cell formation, protection against heart disease
Pantothenic acid	Facilitates synthesis of cholesterol, steroids and fatty acids, vital for intraneuronal synthesis of acetylcholine

PHYTOCHEMICAL (FLAVONOIDS) AS NUTRACEUTICAL AND FUNCTIONAL FOODS

Flavonoids are a group of plant secondary metabolites. Flavonoids were also known as Vitamin P as it influences the vascular capillaries permeability (Mobh, 1938). According to the IUPAC system, it can be grouped as flavonoids or bioflavonoids, isoflavonoids and neoflavonoids (McNaught & Wilkinson, 1997). Flavonoids exist as aglycones, glycosides and methylated derivatives. In plants, flavonoids aglycones (flavonoids without sugar residue) crop up in a number of structural types (Tapas et al., 2008).

Flavonoids are low molecular weight, polyphenolic compound existing in all dietary plants. Flavonoids are the most important plant pigments for flower colorations, producing yellow or red/blue pigmentations. By now more than 4000 molecule have been recognized in plants. The common character of such substances is phenyl benzopyrone framework (C6-C3-C6). Based on saturation level and patency pattern of the central ring flavonoid are further classified as flavanols, flavonols, flavononols, flavanones, flavones and isoflavones. Source (Figure 2) and example of these chemical with dietary source and their example mentioned table 9 (Ren et al., 2003; Harborne & Williams, 2000; Cook & Samman, 1996).

The principal active nutraceutical components in plants are flavonoids (Keservani & Sharma, 2014). Phenolic compounds (flavonols, flavones, flavonones, isoflavone, catechin, anthocyanin & chalcones) liable for the functional properties such as antioxidant capacity (Kerem et al., 2006; Almaraz et al., 2007), antibacterial capacity (Theodori et al., 2006), antiviral capacity (Evers et al., 2005), anti-inflammatory effect (Harris et al., 2006; Wu et al., 2006), cardio-protective ability (Moon et al., 2003; Celle et al., 2004), and the prevention of enzymatic browning (Chen et al., 2000). Important phytochemicals (nutraceuticals), with plant sources and medicinal characteristics are presented in Table 9 (Keservani et al., 2010b).

Figure 2. Structure of some dietary sources of flavonoids

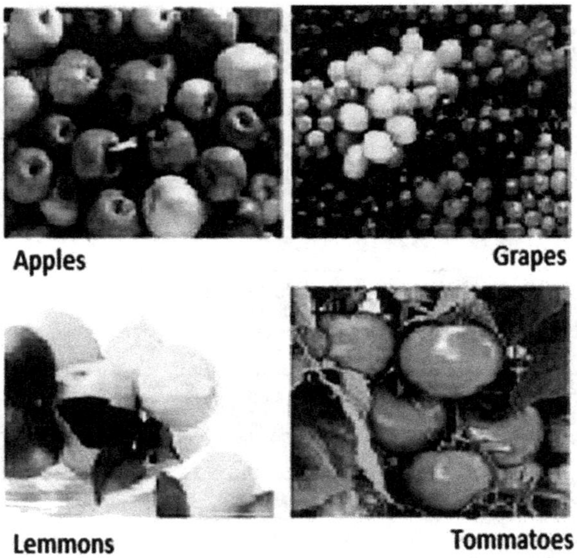

Table 9. Major phytochemicals (nutraceuticals), with plant sources and medicinal characteristics

Phytochemicals: Chemical Group	Plant Sources	Medicinal Property
	Alkaloids	
Quinine	Cinchona	Anti malarial
Tropane alkaloids	Solanaceous members: Deadly night shade, Datura	In treatment of heart ailments
Morphine	Opium poppy	Antidepressant, pain killer
Ergot alkaloids	Fungus: *Claviceps purpurea*	Abortificient
Vincristine	Periwinkle	Antineoplastic
Vinblastine	Periwinkle	Antineoplastic
Coumarin,	Fenugreek	Hypoglycaemic
Scopoletin	Fenugreek	Hypoglycaemic
Fenugreekine	Fenugreek	Hypoglycaemic
Trigonelliine	Fenugreek	Hypoglycaemic
	Carotenoid Terpenoids/ Isoprenoids	
α-carotene	Carrots	Antioxidants, anticarcinogenic
β-carotene	Fruits & vegetables	Antioxidants
β-cryptoxanthin	Oranges & tangerines	Antioxidants, anticancer
Lutein	Vegetables (kale, spinach, watercress, parsley)	Reduce risk of macular degeneration, protect against colon cancer
Zeaxanthin	Corn, avocado	Protects eye from macular degeneration and cataracts
Lycopene	Tomatoes, pink grapefruit, watermelon, guava, papaya	Reduces risk of prostate cancer in males

continued on following page

Table 9. Continued

Phytochemicals: Chemical Group	Plant Sources	Medicinal Property
Non-Carotenoid Terpenoids		
Perillyl alcohol	Cherries & mints	Anticancer
Saponins	Legumes (Chicks, peas, fenugreek, all pulse crops)	Reduces cholesterol levels in blood
Terpenol	Carrots	Anticancer
Terpene	limonoids Peels and membranes of citrus fruits	Anticarcinogenic
Flavonoid Polyphenolics		
Anthocyanins	Stawberries, raspberries, cherries, cranberries, pomegranate, apples, red grapes	Antioxidants
Betacyanins	Beet root	Antioxidant
Catechins	Tea	Antioxidant
Flavonones	Citrus fruits	Antioxidant
Flavones	Fruits & vegetables	Anticancer
Isoflavones	Soybean	Anticancer
Hesperetin	Citrus fruits	Antioxidant
Naringin	Grapefruit	Reduces cholesterol
Rutin	Asparagus, buckwheat & citrus fruits	Protects against cardio vascular ailments
Quercitin	Red onions, buckwheat, red grapes, green tea, apple skins	Anti-histaminic, antioxidant
Silymarin	Artichoke & milk thistle	Anti-atherosclerotic
Tangeretin	Tangerines	Anticancer
Tannins	Cranberries, pomegranate, cocoa & tea	Reduces blood cholesterol
Phenolic Acids		
Ellagic acids	Strawberries & raspberries	Prevents colon cancer
Chlorogenic acids	Blueberries, tomatoes, grapes & bell peppers	Antioxidant
p-coumaric acids	Red and green bell peppers, legumes	Antioxidant, anticancer
Phytic acids	Legumes and whole seed grains	Lowers blood glucose
Ferulic acids	Seeds of brown rice, whole wheat and oats, apple, artichoke, orange, peanut & pine apple	Antioxidant, anticancer
Vanillin	Vanilla bean	Antioxidant, anticancer
Cinnamic acid	Cinnamon, balsam tree resins	Antibacterial, antifungal
Hydroxycinnamic acid	Grapes, blueberries & blackberries	Antioxidant, anticancer
Non-Flavonoid Polyphenolics		
Curcumin	Curcuma	Anti-microbial, anticancer, antioxidant
Resveratrol	Grapes	Anti-inflammatory, anticancer
Lignans	Plant cell walls	Reduces skin cancer
Glucosinolates		
Isothiocyanates	Horseradish, radish & mustard	Anticancer
Phenethyl isothiocyanate	Watercress	Anticancer
Sulforaphene	Broccoli	Anticancer
Indoles	Broccoli	Anticancer

continued on following page

Table 9. Continued

Phytochemicals: Chemical Group	Plant Sources	Medicinal Property
Thiosulfonates	Garlic & onions	reduces blood pressure Anticancer, antimicrobial, and blood cholesterol
	Anthraquinones	
Senna	Legumes and pulses	Purgative,
Barbaloin	Aloe	Laxative, anti-helminthic
Hypericin	St. John's wort	Analgesic
Capsicum (hot peppers) Capsaicin Anticancer,	antiinflammatory,	antiapoptotic
Piperine	Black peppers, jalapeno peppers	Helps in digestion
	Terpenes	
Menthol (Monoterpene)	Plants of mint family	Topical pain reliever & anti-pyretic
Borneol (Monoterpene)	Pine oil	Disinfectant
Santonin (Sesquiterpene)	Wormwood	Photosensitizer
Gossypol (Sesquiterpene)	Cotton	Contraceptive

(Keservani et al., 2010b).

MINERALS AND TRACE ELEMENTS USED AS NUTRACEUTICAL AND FUNCTIONAL FOODS

Minerals are inorganic materials needed by the body in trace concentration for a number of activities, besides the 4 elements carbon, hydrogen, nitrogen, and oxygen existing in general organic molecules (Nelson & Cox, 2000). These cover the development of bones and teeth; as vital principles of body fluids and tissues; as parts of enzyme systems and for routine nerve activity. Few minerals are essential in higher concentrations than others, like calcium, phosphorus, magnesium, sodium, potassium and chloride. Rest are needed in trace amounts and are occasionally known as trace minerals, e.g. iron, zinc, iodine, fluoride, selenium and copper. Although needed in smaller concentrations, trace minerals are no less crucial than other minerals (http://www.nutrition.org.uk/nutritionscience/nutrients/minerals-and-trace-elements).The mineral and trace elements with potential health benefits depicted in Table 10 and Table 11 respectively.

REAGENTS DERIVED FROM OTHER SOURCES

Dehydroepiandrosterone (DHEA)

DHEA (Keservani et al., 2010b) can be produced from substances of natural origin, like soy and wild yam, by the transformation of components like diosgenin into DHEA (Whelan, 2006). DHEA supplementation has not been observed to be favorable for memory role in general middle aged or older adults (Grimley et al., 2006). Dehydroepiandrosterone (DHEA) is formed in the adrenal glands in the liver. The

Table 10. Minerals used as nutraceutical and functional foods

Minerals	Dietary Source	Health Benefits
Calcium	Dairy products, eggs, canned fish with bones (salmon, sardines), green leafy vegetables, nuts, seeds, tofu, thyme, oregano, dill, cinnamon (Drewnowski, 2010).	Necessary in formation of bones and teeth and sustaining bone strength, significant in nerve, muscle and glandular activities.
Iron	Red meat, fish (tuna, salmon), grains, dry beans, eggs, spinach, chard, turmeric, cumin, parsley, lentils, tofu, asparagus, leafy green vegetables, soybeans, shrimp, beans, tomatoes, olives, and dried fruit (Drewnowski, 2010; Human Nutrition: Iron 2009).	Assist in energy production, aids to carry and transfer oxygen to tissues.
Magnesium	Raw nuts, soybeans, cocoa mass, spinach, chard, sea vegetables, tomatoes, halibut, beans, ginger, cumin, cloves (Human Nutrition: Magnesium, 2009).	Necessary for healthy nerve and muscle function and bone formation, can aid to check premenstrual syndrome (PMS).
Phosphorous	Red meat, dairy foods, fish, poultry, bread, rice, oats (NHS Choices, 2011; Corbridge, 1995).	Required for building strong bones and teeth, helps in formation of genetic material, energy production and storage.

(Keservani et al., 2010b)

Table 11. List of trace elements use as nutraceutical

Trace Elements	Dietary Source	Health Benefits
Chromium	whole-grain products, processed meats, high-bran breakfast cereals, coffee, nuts, green beans, broccoli, spices (Lukaski, 1999)	Alongwith insulin assists in conversion of carbohydrates and fats into energy.
Cobalt	-	Vital component of vitamin B12, but ingested cobalt is metabolized *in vivo* to form the B12 coenzymes
Copper	Mushrooms, spinach, greens, seeds, raw cashews, raw walnuts, tempeh, barley (Nelson & Cox, 2000).	Crucial for haemoglobin and collagen production, healthy functioning of the heart, energy production, absorption of iron from digestive tract
Iodine	Sea vegetables, iodized salt, eggs. Alternate but inconsistent sources of iodine: strawberries, mozzarella cheese, yogurt, milk, fish, and shellfish (Human Nutrition: Iodine, 2009).	Required for proper functioning of the thyroid
Selenium	Brazil nuts, cold water wild fish (cod, halibut, salmon), tuna, lamb, turkey, calf liver, mustard, mushrooms, barley, cheese, garlic, tofu, seeds (Human Nutrition: Selenium, 2009).	Antioxidant, needed for healthy functioning of the heart muscle
Zinc	Calf liver, eggs, dry beans, mushrooms, spinach, asparagus, scallops, red meat, green peas, yogurt, oats, seeds, miso (Drewnowski, 2010; Human Nutrition: Zinc, 2009)	Necessary for cell reproduction, normal growth and development in children, wound healing, production of sperm and testosterone

(Keservani et al., 2010b)

testes produce it. DHEA amounts hit the highest point in the adults during their early 20s and then commence to reduce after age 25. This tapering has been linked with many diseases, embracing osteoporosis. So use of DHEA has been suggested to check or cure osteoporosis (Whelan et al., 2006; Jellin, 2009).

A review in 2003 observed the then existing proofs enough to propose that small serum concentrations of DHEAS can be related with coronary heart disease in men, but inadequate to assess whether DHEA supplementation would have any cardiovascular advantage (Thijs et al., 2003). Few in vitro investigations have found DHEA to possess antiproliferative as well as apoptotic impact on cancer cell lines at levels over 50 μM (Yang et al., 2002; Schulz et al., 1992; Loria, 2002).

Melatonin

Melatonin (Keservani et al., 2010b) is a material present in animals, plants, fungi and bacteria. In majority of these organisms, except for animals, its role is somewhat other than routine organization. In animals it is a hormone that forecasts the daily onset of darkness (Hardeland et al., 2006). It is produced in animal cells straightway from the essential amino acid tryptophan, whereas in other organisms via the Shikimic acid pathway (Tan et al., 2014; Acuna-Castroviejo et al., 2006). In animals, melatonin is part of the entrainment (synchronization) of the circadian rhythms of physiological activities covering sleep duration, blood pressure control, seasonal reproduction and several others (Altun & Ugur-Altun, 2007).

Melatonin is present in variety of plants covering feverfew (Tanacetum parthenium), St John's wort (Hypericum perforatum) (Paredes et al., 2009), rice, corn, tomato, grape (Iriti and Faoro, 2009) and other edible fruits (Tan et al., 2012). The physiological functions in plants cover control of their reaction to photoperiod, protection in opposition to tough milieus, and the role of an antioxidant (Tan et al., 2010). It controls plant progress by its capability to retard root development too, while boosting above-ground growth (Arnao and Hernández-Ruiz, 2006). Melatonin has been observed in foods such as cherries to approximately 0.17–13.46 ng/g (Burkhardt et al., 2001), bananas and grapes, rice and cereals, herbs, olive oil, wine and beer (Lamont et al., 2011). When birds intake high melatonin plant feed, like rice, the melatonin attaches to melatonin receptors in their brains (Hattori et al., 1995). When humans take foods high in melatonin like banana, pineapple and orange the blood levels of melatonin effectively rise (Sae-Teaw et al., 2012).

Melatonin biosynthesis in humans and few other organisms has 4 enzymatic stages beginning from the essential dietary amino acid tryptophan, followed by a serotonin passage. In the first two steps, L-tryptophan is first transformed to 5-hydroxy-L-tryptophan (5-HTP) by an enzyme, tryptophan 5-hydroxylase. 5-HTP is afterwards decarboxylated (CO_2 elimination) by 5-hydroxytryptophan decarboxylase to yield serotonin. This juncture is the rate limiting state like that now reaction is governed by light-dark situations (Norman and Henry, 2012).In addition to its role as synchronizer of the circadian rhythm, melatonin is a strong free-radical forager and broad-spectrum antioxidant as discovered in 1993 (Tan et al., 1993).

Numerous clinical investigations suggest that augmentation with melatonin is an impactful protective cure for migraines and cluster headaches (Dodic, and Capobianco, 2001). Few supplemental melatonin consumers claim a rise in flamboyant dreaming. Heavy doses of melatonin (50 mg) surprisingly prolonged REM sleep duration and dream function in people with as well as devoid of narcolepsy (Lewis, 1999). In exploratory investigations, sustained-release melatonin has exhibited sleep virtue refinement in patients having chronic schizophrenia (Shamir et al., 2000) and in patients with main depressive disorder as well(Dolberg et al., 1998; Dalton et al., 2000) and curing sleep-awake cycle disorders in children with neurodevelopment problems (Jan et al., 2000; De Leersnyder et al., 2003). Besides, as appended to antihypertensive therapy, sustained-release melatonin enhanced blood pressure regulation in patients with nocturnal hypertension as observed in a randomized double-blind placebo regulated investigation (Grossman et al., 2011).

MARKETED PRODUCTS OF NUTRACEUTICAL AND FUNCTIONAL FOODS

Till date plenty of nutraceutical and functional food products were formulated and marketed by various industries. Some of them were listed in Table 12 with their applications worldwide. These products provide medical benefit to human health by reducing or preventing the disease (http://www.nutraceuticalsworld.com/).

SUPPLIERS OF NUTRACEUTICAL AND FUNCTIONAL FOODS

Various industries and academic researcher were worked for formulation of nutritional and dietary supplements with the natural or artificial ingredients. List of ingredients with their suppliers are presented in Table 13 for medical benefit to human health (http://www.nutraceuticalsworld.com/).

Table 12. Nutraceutical and functional foods marketed product of with their application

Products	Company	Applications
100 Greek Yogurt	Chobani, New Berlin, NY	Tremendous source of protein and fiber and fine source of calcium.
Brain Shield	Life Extension	Supports normal, healthy levels of brain blood flow in both animals and in humans and etc.
Omega 3s	Klean Athlete, Pittsburgh, PA	Sports Nutrition.
Nutricosmetic and Bone & Joint Sips	Nippi Collagen, Vancouver, BC, and Singapore-based Unistraw Holdings	Promoting beauty, bone and joint health.
Quoquos Coconut Oil Lecithin Cocoa	Aecetia Foods, Ltd., NY	Dietary supplement aims to boost energy and stamina while reducing fatigue and recovery time after exercise or strenuous physical activity.
Patient One GastroOne	MediNutritionals Research LLC, Farmingdale, NY	Beneficial effects on GI tract health.
Patient One C-Cleanse	MediNutritionals Research LLC, Farmingdale, NY	Cleansing and colon health.
Lutemax	San Clemente, CA	Maintenance of healthy eye structure and function.
Sweet Kale	Brighteore Nutrition, Tampa/St. Petersburg, FL	Nutraceutical supplement.
AndroFlavone (for men) and FemFlavone (for women)	NeuroScience, Inc., Osceola, WI	Provide support for healthy reproductive hormone levels.
Kavinace Flash-Ease	NeuroScience, Inc., Osceola, WI	Women experiencing night sweats, hot flashes, sleep difficulties, and other common symptoms of menopause.
Magnesium-powered	Redd Remedies, Bradley IL	Cognitive function, memory, and overall brain health.
MenaQ7 Crystals	Norway-based NattoPharma's	Vitamin supplements for bone and cardiovascular health.
Mega 10	Metagenics, Inc., Aliso Viejo, CA	Blood lipid health and cardiovascular health.
Nordic Probiotic	Nordic Naturals, Watsonville, CA	Digestive issues or food sensitivities.
Liquid Melatonin	Life Extension, Fort Lauderdale, FL	Regulate the body's internal clock.
Baobab Fruit Powder	Kaibae, Santa Barbara, CA	Increase energy and relieve fatigue, sugar metabolism and lower cholesterol etc.

continued on following page

Table 12. Continued

Products	Company	Applications
GlycemicProTransglucosidase	Life Extension, Fort Lauderdale, FL	Maintain healthy blood glucose, cholesterol and insulin levels.
Intelligent probiotics	IQBiotix, Orange County, CA	Health benefits.
Coral Joint & Collagen Support	Coral LLC, Carson City, NV	Maintain healthy bones and joint flexibility.
GarciniaCambogia Extract	New Orleans, LA	Weight Loss.
Rootology	RedTreeNutraceuticals, Inc., Poughkeepsie, NY	Allergy Relief.
PQQ (pyrroloquinolinequinone) product	Jarrow Formulas, Los Angeles, CA	Support heart health and cognitive function.
Kellogg's Breakfast To Go	Kellogg Company, Battle Creek, MI	Nutritional suuplements.
AspregaProPac	ScimeraBioScience	Antibiotic-associated diarrhea.
Cod Liver Oil	Standard Process Inc., Palmyra, WI	Bone health, eye health, liver function, as well as cardiovascular and immune health.
Reishi Extract Mushroom Complex	Life Extension, Fort Lauderdale, FL,	Immune support.
NuControl	NuSirt Sciences, Inc., Nashville, TN	Ability to maintain a healthy weight and the management of overweight and obesity.
Ensure Complete.	Abbott Park, IL	Muscle, heart, immune system and bone support.
BelVita Breakfast Biscuits	Kraft Foods, East Hanover, NJ	Good source of fiber.
PRE3 MAX,	Tampa, FL's Re-Body	Pre-exercise energy optimizer.
Nutrilite	Amway, Ada, MI	Build, preserve and strengthen bones.
VitaGreens	VitalMax Vitamins, Delray Beach, FL	Improve overall health throughout the body.
The Stress and Anxiety Essence	Journey To Botanicals, Canton, OH	Stress and anxiety.
Fluxome resveratrol	Fluxome, Stenløse, Denmark,	Heart Strong Gum.
Algae Omega	Nordic Naturals, Watsonville, CA	Normal vision, heart health, immunity, positive mood and natural anti-inflammatory response.
NutriVeruspowder	Mannatech, Incorporated, Coppell, TX	Nutritional supplement.
Mr. Pink Ginseng Drinks	Mr. Pink Beverages, Los Angeles, CA	Energy drink.
Rodex Forte	LegerePharmaceuticals, Scottsdale, AZ	Heart disease, fatigue, weight loss and arthritis.
Alginex	ArkisBiotec, New York, NY	Weight loss.
Olive Leaf Olive Leaf Vascular Support	Life Extension, Fort Lauderdale, FL	Vascular Support.
Cardia 7	Basic Organics, Columbus, OH	Heart health.
B-Nexa	Upsher-Smith Laboratories, Inc., Maple Grove, MN	Nausea and vomiting of pregnancy.
ALPHA Brain	Onnit Labs, Austin, TX	Mental, physical and emotional balance.
Slender GR	Enzymedica, Port Charlotte, FL	Healthy weight management.
CocoGevity Plus	Youngevity Essential Life Sciences, San Diego, CA,	Dietary supplement.
Fertinatal	Fertility Nutraceuticals, LLC, New York, NY	Female fertility.
Airborne Chewables	Airborne, Inc., Minneapolis, MN	Immune support.
Nutra Rinse Mouthwash	Vitamin Mineral Shop LLC, Clinton Township, MI	Cleansing, Antiseptic properties, soothening and moisturizing action, support healthy gums and teeth .
D-Sorb	Cardium Therapeutics, San Diego, CA	Vitamin D supplement.

(http://www.nutraceuticalsworld.com/)

Table 13. Nutraceutical and functional foods supplier list with their uses

Products/Ingredients	Suppliers	Uses
Protein M+	Copalis	Anti-aging activity.
Lyc-O-Pro	LycoRed Ltd.	Prostate health.
OMEGA 60	DSM	
Glucevia	Naturex	Blood sugar control
Cluster Dextrin	Glico Nutrition	Advantage in building muscle, burning fat and delivering constant energy is dramatic
NeoFilm	Neogen Corporation	Simple microbial tests.
(D) ETAS (enzyme-treated asparagus extract) (E) Bluenesse (F) Venetron	Maypro Industries	Stress and sleep. Mental clarity. Mood support.
Synapsa	P.L. Thomas & Co., Inc.	Mental performance.
Flax protein powder	Glanbia Nutritionals	Protein fortification.
Orisett	NutraGenesis, LLC, Brattleboro and VT	Glucose management category.
BioEcolians prebiotic	Solabia	Which inhibits the hydrolytic action of the gastro-intestinal enzymes?
Nectevia	Steviva Ingredients	Organic Plant-Based Sweetener.
AppleActiv	AppleActives and Leahy Orchards	Joint health, cardiovascular health, cognitive function, immune health, and healthy stress response.
Fēnol organic polyphenol fiber	FutureCeuticals	Antioxidant activity.
Curcumin C3 Reduct	Sabinsa Corporation	Antioxidant activity.
EmulsiGel	Rousselot, Son, Netherlands	Stabilize emulsion.
PrefixPro	Deerland Enzymes	Digestive tract.
Prenulin	Pharmachem Laboratories Inc. Kearney, NJ,	Healthy blood glucose levels.
FIBERline	DuPont Nutrition & Health	Add fiber to whole meal bread.
Probiotic Lozenges	BLIS Technologies	Protection for the gums and teeth.
Guardian Chelox L	DuPont Nutrition & Health, New Century, KS	Antioxidant activity.
POMx	POM Wonderful	Antioxidant activity.
Vegeceuticals	WILD Flavors, Inc.	Applied to a variety of foods and beverages.
Benolea (EFLA943)	Frutarom USA	Cardiovascular health.
Actazin	Stratum Nutrition	Digestive health.

(http://www.nutraceuticalsworld.com/)

APPLICATION OF NUTRACEUTICAL AND FUNCTIONAL FOODS IN HEALTH BENEFITS AND PREVENTION OF DISEASES

Nutraceutical and functional foods are revolutionary products, which are applicable in the prophylaxis and treatment of diseases. Disease like cardiovascular disease (CVD), immune related disease, mental disorder, gastric disease, blood flow, joint pain, bone pain, obesity and others prevented and treated by nutraceutical and functional foods. For example fish, diet rich food and vegetables, grains, nuts & legumes, soy protein, carbohydrates, protein, amino acids, lipid and fatty acids, carotenoids, vitamin C, phytochemicals, coffee, tea and others dietary, nutraceutical and functional foods reduce the risk of various diseases like cardio vascular disease (CVD), sleep, mental disorder, immune response, anti-inflammatory, diabetes, pulmonary disease, anaemia, hair loss/hair growth, arthritis, brain function, ocular health, obesity, male fertility and others.

Cardio Vascular Disease (CVD)

Nutraceutical play important role in prevention and treatment of CVD reported by Rama CS and coworkers. Recent research finding on garlic, soy product, omega-3-fatty acids, dietary fibres, antioxidants, vitamins, prebiotics, probiotics, plant sterols, flavonoids have beneficial effect on hearts (Ramaa et al., 2006). Corn's impact on health of heart is inherent to not merely in its fiber, but in the appreciable concentrations of folate that corn provides. Corn maintains the homocysteine, an intermediate product of a significant metabolic process termed the methylation cycle. Homocysteine is the main culprit for damage of blood vessel during heart attack, stroke, or peripheral vascular disease. It has been predicted that intakes of 100% of the daily value (DV) of folate would, by itself, decrease the occurrences of heart attacks by 10%. (Bazzano et al., 2002).

Immune Response

Several investigations have raised concern that micronutrients like selenium, vitamins A, C and E may affect a number of constituents of the immune system (Erickson et al., 2000). Tsuchihashi and his colleagues (Tsuchihashi et al., 1987) exhibited an appreaciable rise of the bacteria Lactobacillus in rats subsequent to Spirulina amendments in their diet; which if happened in humans would perk up digestion, food absorption, and trigger the immune system to aid combat infections (Archer et al., 1985). The author recorded increased lymphocyte count and raised neutrophil phagocytosis in natural honey-fed rats as compared to control. This associated with past studies that prebiotics may improve immune function and natural honey is believed to have the prebiotics, oligosaccharides reported by Ajibola and coworkers (Ajibola et al., 2012). Keservani and co-workers reported that ditary supplements, nutraceuticals and functional foods like dietary fibre, probiotics, antioxidants, mushrooms, vitamins, folic acid, polysaccharides and phytochemicals were used as immunomodulators (Keservani et al., 2015d).

Mental Disorder

There are limited medications of natural origin that have been investigated for anxiety and insomnia. These covers kava, valerian and melatonin. Valerian and melatonin have a comparatively numerous clinical trials to validate their effect, however there is limited resaerch on kava, regarding which there have been growing issues pertaining to liver toxicity in the previous few years. Ginkgo biloba too has numerous clinical trials as evidences regarding its efficacy in regulating symptoms of early dementia (Mischoulon et al., 2009). Consumption of a diet high in omega-3 fatty acids has been linked with a decreased occurrences of a variety of psychiatric disorders such as depression and schizophrenia (Peet., 2004; Reis et al., 2006). One study suggested that Sam-e was better than a placebo and was active as a standard triclyclic antidepressant for the treatment of depression (Fetrow & Avila, 2001). Keservani et al., reported and briefly described nutraceuticals and functional foods like carbohydrate, protein, fat, vitamins, folic acids, caffeine, minerals and other plant and fruit-derived nutraceutical and functional foods part in the avoidance of mental disorder (Keservani et al., 2015b).

Brain Health

Shriharsh et al., studied the influence of nutraceutical and psychological interventions on cognitive activities of healthy human subjects and reported the nutraceutical and psychological interventions are likely to have positive influence on the cognitive function of healthy human subjects. However, better results were obtained when used in combination (Shriharsh et al., 2014). Ginkgo biloba is a herb that has been utilized from ancient times as a memory booster. All six of the brands that were tested (NeuroLogic, Deep Thought, Brain Pep, Mental Edge, Mind Balance, and Ginkgold), had ginkgo biloba. All the products, excluding Ginkgold, were found to have other materials too. Sales figure for ginkgo biloba, which is a part of several formula in famous herbal brands, make up over a billion dollars per year. (Solomon et al., 2002). Keservani and his coworkers noted role of dietary supplements in stress, parkinson's, and alzheimer's disease (Keservani et al., 2015a). Bastianetto and Quirion observed that daily consumption of red wine and ginkgo biloba can be favorable in the stabilization or improvement of memory activities in the aging brain (Bastianetto & Quirion 2002).

Liver Toxicity

Liver toxicity may be prevented by nutraceutical materials. Lee et al, studied the influences of the fruit extract from *Hovenia dulcis* (HD) on liver fibrosis in rats and concluded the extracts from HD fruit can control liver fibrosis and therefore could be used as a therapy to inhibit liver fibrosis (Lee et al., 2014). Carbon tetrachloride (CCl_4) when used as a xenobiotic resulted in oxidative stress, and may cause injury to hepatic cells (Kanter et al., 2005). Tarek et al., studied Z. officinale serves as a nutraceutical agent against liver fibrosis and concluded ginger has the capability to down-regulate free radicals rise, perk up liver and cholestatic biomarkers, improve hepatic marker enzymes, decrease collagen accumulation, fibrosis intensity and stabilize the hepatic cells architecture. Ginger ethanolic extract yielded the most potent impact in fine-tuning the chosen parameters (Tarek et al., 2011).

Diabetes

Berberine is the principal active constituent of the age old Chinese herb Coptis chinensis Franch, which has been employed to treat diabetes for several hundred years. Berberine is an over-the-counter drug, which is aimed to treat gastrointestinal infections in China (Affuso et al., 2012). Rajasekar et al., have shown that L-carnitine could enhance insulin activity in the fructose-fed rat model of insulin resistance. Skeletal muscle is an insulin-sensitive tissue, which is a domain of insulin resistance in the fructose-fed rat too and it is prone to oxidative destruction (Rajasekar et al., 2007).

Hypertension

α-linolenic acid (ALA), eicosapentaenoic acid and doosahexanoic acid (DHA) comprise the primary members of the omega-3 PUFA family. Omega 3- fatty acids are present in cold water fish, fish oil, flax,

flax seed and nuts (Mori et al., 1999). Omega-3 PUFA superbly lowered BP in observational, epidemiologic and in some small prospective clinical trial (Mori et al., 1999). Green tea, black tea and extract of active constituents in both have shown reductions in BP (Hodgson et al., 1999). High dose of vitamin B6 can lower the blood pressure studied by Aybak et al. (Aybak et al., 1995).

Respiratory and Pulmonary

Yeum et al., reported carotenoids may function as antioxidants and promote oxidative stress resistance (Yeum et al., 2009). Engelen's studies achieved some interesting conclusions, demonstrating an increased anabolic response to milk proteins (Engelen et al., 2012), in particular casein (oral and intravenous) was linked with lowered splanchnic extraction of essential amino acids in normal-weight COPD patients during and after exercise (Engelen et al., 2012). Tulsi is commonly used for its medicinal effects on respiratory tract infections, cardiac dysfunction and spasmodic problems (Ghosh & Bhattacharjee, 2014). Keservani and his colleagues reported role of antioxidants and nutraceuticals in pulmonary and respiratory health and disease prevention (Keservani et al., 2015c). Several flavonoids like catechins, flavonols and flavones are favorably attached with force expiratory volume in one second (FEV1) improvement and reciprocal to signs like chronic cough, shortness of breath (not chronic) and phlegm, proposing an advantageous impact of consuming catechins in patients with COPD. Research has demonstrated positive outcmes of flavonoids, like quercetin, on COPD and in the prophylaxis of the development of pulmonary emphysema in animal models (Lago et al., 2014).

Obesity

The intake of dietary fibers (fruits, vegetables, whole grains, legumes) is an important step in obesity check, dietary fiber supplements usually offer a beneficial add-on, as lifestyle alterations are tough to comply after a while and elevated cholesterol levels can be challenging to these modifications (Cicero & Ertek, 2008). Original plant of the resveratrol-enriched rice DJ-526, *Oryza sativa* japonica variety Dongjin grown by the Rural Development Administration of Korea, has features of having grains high in fiber and polyphenols possessing anti-obesity effect (Choi et al., 2012).

Sleep

A crucial part of keeping best health and well-being is having a fine sleep during night. Sleep permits the body to relax and recuperate from the previous day's functions, embracing physical patch up and mental boost, so as to get prepared for the next day's activities. Standardized extract of Ashwagandha (Withania somnifera), a plant grown in India that is honored for its capability to poise, strengthen, revivify, and refresh documented by Bruce (Bruce, 2008). Rong et al., also observed dietary supplements employed in management and prevention of insomnia.

Bone Health

The serum concentartions of Dehydroepiandrosteron (DHEA) have been associated to bone loss and levels of bone resorption (Wang et al., 2012; Ghebre et al., 2011), Nair et al., recorded benefit of DHEA to bone may be limited to elderly individuals with low serum DHEAS (Nair et al., 2006). β-cryptoxanthin is a type of carotenoid that has a promising impact in keeping bone health and in checking osteoporosis (Yamaguchi, 2008). The mechanism by which this is conferred probably implaicates symbiotic augmentation of each vitamin's effects on the manufacture and activation of osteocalcin (Koshihara et al., 1996). In light of the proof, vitamins D and K should be employed in combination to make the most of the likely valuable effects of each on bone health. Vitamin D promotes normal mineralization of bones and is needed for bone growth. Insufficient Vitamin D may lead to thinning of bones. Adequate Vitamin D and calcium intake protects adults from osteoporosis. Vitamin D is found in very few foods. Exposure to UV rays causes your body to synthesize Vitamin D (Cranney et al., 2007). A seed of grain amaranth terrific source of minerals like calcium, magnesium, and copper, a nice source of zinc, potassium, and phosphorus. It helps to build strong bones and a muscle, aid hydration, boost energy, and is vital in thousands of processes. The genus Amaranth (L.) includes more than 60 species (Kalac et al., 2000).

Ocular Health

The Lutein and Zeaxanthin used in eye health (Lockwood, 2007). Pinazo-Duran studied effects of a nutraceutical preparation having the mixture of antioxidants and ω-3 essential fatty acids in the expression of inflammation and immune response intermediates in tears from patients with dry eye disorders. They devised that inflammation and immune response (IIR) mediators exhibited varying expression styles in DED patients and these styles altered upon consuming combined preparation of antioxidant and EPUFAs supplementation. Our results can be considered for future protocols combining clinical/ biochemical data to assist in treatment of dry eye disorder (DED) patients (Pinazo-Duran et al., 2013). Kador investigated topical nutraceutical Optixcare EH reduces experimental ocular oxidative stress in rats and observed that topical application of 3% concentration of the ingredients in Optixcare EH decreases experimentally induced reactive oxygen moieties in rats exposed to many sources of ocular oxidative stress. Besides, Optixcare EH keeps tear volume in scopolamine-induced dry eye (Kador et al., 2014).

Arthritis

Arthritis, a chronic and growing incapacitating disease, influencess quality of life of humans and animals alike. Presently, as per the Arthritis Foundation, about 20% of the dog population (78.2 million) in the United States has arthritis. Fleck and coworker investigated anti-arthritic efficacy and safety of crominex® 3+ (Trivalent chromium, phyllanthus emblica extract, and shilajit) in moderately arthritic dogs and resulted that crominex® 3+ improved arthritic pain and enhanced quality of life devoid of any unwanted effects in fairly arthritic dogs.

Anaemia

Sickle cell disorder (SCD) is a class of genetic diseases having impact on the red cell hemoglobin (Bunn, 1997). Ciklavit is a plant extract formulation for the treatment of the sickle cell anemia. It possesses in general extracts of the plant Cajanus Cajan, proteins (essential amino acids), vitamins like vitamin C (ascorbic acid), and minerals like zinc. Ciklavit (Cajanus cajan extract) has been shown to possess antisickling features and to enhance good health of sicklers. The investigation also deciphered that the antisickling upshot of Ciklavit may not possibly be via nitric oxide production or arginase inhibition, as there were no significant deviations in such values. Initial findings of the antisickling component of Cajanus cajan proposed cajaminose (Iwu et al., 1988).

Hair Growth

Beer et al., studied and resulted that individuals consuming Cynatine HNS exhibited statistically outstanding improvements in their hair and nails versus placebo. Finally concluded Cynatine HNS is an influential supplement for fine tuning hair and nails in 90 days or less (Beer et al., 2014). *C. reflexa* collected from *Azadiracta indica* and *Zizyphus jujuba* were promising in the encouragement of hair growth, dandruff control, and decrease in hair fall activity reported by Anjum et al., (Anjum et al., 2014).

Anti-Inflammatory Action

Crataegi Fructus has a broad spectrum of pharmacological activities like enhancing digestion, cardiotonic effect, and hypolipodemic action. Oh et al. investigated blocking of inducible nitric oxide synthase and cyclooxygenase-2 by methanolic extract of *Crataegi Fructus* and summarized that the 70% methanolic extract of Crataegi Fructus causes important antioxidant and anti-inflammatory effects, probably through inhibiting iNOS and COX-2 induction (Oh et al., 2014).

Sexual Disorder

Lycopene, a lipid soluble carotenoid found in tomato-rich diets, is a powerful scavenger of free radicals preventing lipid peroxidation (Raj et al., 2014). To study differences in the nutrient intake of men with normal semen parameters and those with low sperm numbers, motility or morphology, Mendiola et al. examined specific nutrient intake of men attending infertility clinics in Spain. The authors demonstrated a positive relation between lycopene consumption and semen quality. The present data linking lycopene to an improvement in semen parameters is primarily observational, with small sample sizes under investigation (Mendiola et al., 2010).

CONCLUSION

Nutraceuticals are of immense significance in current system of Medical and Healthcare. A nutraceutical is defined as a material isolated or purified from food that is commonly marketed in medical preparations and possess a biological advantage or afford safeguard against chronic disease. Nutraceutical and Functional foods products will be providing good health in the future; it has been convincingly demonstrated as bebeneficial for their intended purposes when ingested as ingredient of a generally well-balanced and healthful diet. Also more information and evidences must be available toassist consumer for the correct choosing and using thefunctional foods and / or nutraceuticals to achieve the promised health benefits. All the species of mushrooms screened showed positive results for antioxidant activity. This indicates the medicinal importance of these mushrooms. The research strategies towards the nutraceuticals should improve the human health life and life quality in the future.

CONFLICT OF INTEREST

The authors declare no conflict of interest.

REFERENCES

Acuna-Castroviejo, D., Escames, G., Tapias, V., & Rivas, I. (2006). Melatonin, mitochondria and neuroprotection. In *Montilla, Pedro; Túnez, Isaac. Melatonin: Present and Future* (pp. 1–33). New York: Nova Science Publishers.

Affuso, F., Mercurio, V., & Ruvolo, A. (2012). A nutraceutical combination improves insulin sensitivity in patients with metabolic syndrome. *World J Cardiol*, *4*(3), 77–83. doi:10.4330/wjc.v4.i3.77 PMID:22451856

Ajibola, A., Chamunorwa, J. P., & Erlwanger, K. H. (2012). Nutraceutical values of natural honey and its contribution to human health and wealth. *Nutrition and Metabolism*, *9*(61), 1–12. PMID:22716101

Ajith, T. A., & Janardhanan, K. K. (2007). Indian medicinal mushrooms as a source of antioxidant and antitumor agents. *Journal of Clinical Biochemistry and Nutrition*, *40*(3), 157–162. doi:10.3164/jcbn.40.157 PMID:18398492

Almaraz, N., Campos, M. G., Avila, J. A., Naranjo, N., Herrera, J., & Gonzalez, L. S. (2007). Antioxidant activity of polyphenolic extract of monofloral honeybee collected pollen from mesquite (Prosopisjuliflora, Leguminosae). *Journal of Food Composition and Analysis*, *20*(2), 119–124. doi:10.1016/j.jfca.2006.08.001

Altun, A., & Ugur-Altun, B. (2007). Melatonin: Therapeutic and clinical utilization. *International Journal of Clinical Practice*, *61*(5), 835–845. doi:10.1111/j.1742-1241.2006.01191.x PMID:17298593

Anjum, F., Bukhari, S. A., Shahid, M., Bokhari, T. H., & Talpur, M. M. A. (2014). Exploration of Nutraceutical Potential of Herbal Oil Formulated from Parasitic Plant. *African Journal of Traditional, Complementary, and Alternative Medicines*, *11*(1), 78–86. PMID:24653557

Theodori, R., Karioti, A., Rancic, A., & Skaltsa, H. (2006). Linear sesquiterpene lactones from. Anthemis auriculata and their antibacterial activity. *Journal of Natural Products*, *69*(4), 662–664. doi:10.1021/np058084i PMID:16643047

Anwar, F., Przybylski, R., Rudzinska, M., Gruczynska, E., & Bain, J. (2008). Fatty acid, tocopherol and sterol compositions of Canadian prairie fruit seed lipids. *Journal of the American Oil Chemists' Society*, *85*(10), 953–959. doi:10.1007/s11746-008-1276-0

Arai, S. (1996). Studies on functional foods in Japan–State of the art. *Bioscience, Biotechnology, and Biochemistry*, *60*(1), 9–15. doi:10.1271/bbb.60.9 PMID:8824819

Archer, D. L., & Glinsmann, W. H. (1985). Intestinal infection and malnutrition initiate Acquired Immune Deficiency Syndrome (AIDS). *Nutrition Research (New York, N.Y.)*, *5*(1), 9–19. doi:10.1016/S0271-5317(85)80014-2

Arnao, M. B., & Hernández-Ruiz, J. (2006). The physiological function of melatonin in plants. *Plant Signaling & Behavior, 1*(3), 89–95. doi:10.4161/psb.1.3.2640 PMID:19521488

Aybak, M., & Sermet, A. (1995). Effect of oral pyridoxine hydrochloride supplementation on arterial blood pressure in patients with essential hypertension. *Arzneimittel-Forschung, 45*, 1271–1273. PMID:8595083

Babayan, V. K. (1987). Medium chain triglycerides and structural lipids. *Lipids, 22*(6), 417–420. doi:10.1007/BF02537271 PMID:3112486

Baek, J. Y., Lee, J. M., & Lee, S. C. (2008). Extraction of nutraceutical compounds from licorice roots with subcritical water. *Separation and Purification Technology, 63*(3), 661–664. doi:10.1016/j.seppur.2008.07.005

Bahl, N. (1983). Medicinal value of edible fungi. In *Proceeding of the International Conference on Science and Cultivation Technology of Edible Fungi*. Indian Mushroom Science.

Bastianetto, S., & Quirion, R. (2002). Natural extracts as possible protective agents of brain aging. *Neurobiological Aging, 23*(5), 891–897. doi:10.1016/S0197-4580(02)00024-6 PMID:12392793

Bazzano, L. A., He, J., Ogden, L. G., Loria, C., Vupputuri, S., Myers, L., & Whelton, P. K. (2002). Dietary intake of folate and risk of stroke in US men and women: NHANES I Epidemiologic Follow-up Study. National Health and Nutrition Examination Survey. *Stroke, 33*(5), 1183–1188. doi:10.1161/01.STR.0000014607.90464.88 PMID:11988588

Beer, C., Wood, S., & Veghte, R. H. (2014). A Clinical Trial to Investigate the Effect of Cynatine HNS on Hair and Nail Parameters. *TheScientificWorldJournal, 2014*, 1–6. doi:10.1155/2014/641723 PMID:25386609

Benatti, P., Peluso, G., Nicolai, R., & Calvani, M. (2004). Polyunsaturated fatty acids: Biochemical, nutritional and epigenetic properties. *Journal of the American College of Nutrition, 23*(4), 281–302. doi:10.1080/07315724.2004.10719371 PMID:15310732

Bender, D. A. (1992). *Nutritional biochemistry of the vitamins*. New York: Cambridge University Press.

Bhunia, S. K., Dey, B., Maity, K. K., Patra, S., Mandal, S., Maiti, S., & Islam, S. S. et al. (2010). Structural characterization of an immunoenhancing heteroglycan isolated from an aqueous extract of an edible mushroom, *Lentinus squarrosulus* (Mont.) Singer. *Carbohydrate Research, 345*(17), 2542–2549. doi:10.1016/j.carres.2010.09.015 PMID:20934687

Biesalski, H. K. (2001). Nutraceuticals: the link between nutrition and medicine. In K. Kramer, P. P. Hoppe, & L. Packer (Eds.), *Nutraceuticals in health and disease prevention* (pp. 1–26). New York: Marcel Dekker. doi:10.1201/9780203908174.ch1

Blum, K., Ross, J., Reuben, C., Gastelu, D., & Miller, D. K. (2001). *Nutritional gene therapy: Natural Healing in Recovery*. Counselor Magazine.

Brady, K., Ho, C. T., Rosen, R. T., Sang, S., & Karwe, M. V. (2007). Effects of processing on the nutraceutical profile of quinoa. *Food Chemistry, 100*(3), 1209–1216. doi:10.1016/j.foodchem.2005.12.001

Brain, L. (2007). *Nutraceuticals* (2nd ed.). London: Pharmaceutical press.

Brower, V. (1998). Nutraceuticals: Poised for a healthy slice of the healthcare market. *Nature Biotechnology, 16*(8), 728–731. doi:10.1038/nbt0898-728 PMID:9702769

Bruce, A. (2008). Essentra® - A Patented Extract that Reduces Stress and Enhances Sleep. *NutraGenesis, LLC*, 1–4.

Bunn, H. F. (1997). Pathogenesis and treatment of sickle cell disease. *The New England Journal of Medicine, 337*(11), 762–769. doi:10.1056/NEJM199709113371107 PMID:9287233

Burkhardt, S., Tan, D. X., Manchester, L. C., Hardeland, R., & Reiter, R. J. (2001). Detection and quantification of the antioxidant melatonin in Montmorency and Balaton tart cherries (Prunus cerasus). *Journal of Agricultural and Food Chemistry, 49*(10), 4898–4902. doi:10.1021/jf010321+ PMID:11600041

Burlingame, B. et al.. (2009). Fats and fatty acids in human nutrition. JointFAO/WHO. Expert Consultation. *Annals of Nutrition & Metabolism, 55*, 1–3. doi:10.1159/000228993 PMID:20104000

Campanella, L., Martini, E., Pintore, M., & Tomassetti, M. (2009). Determination of lactoferrin and immunoglobulin G in animal milks by new immunosensors. *Sensors (Basel, Switzerland), 9*(3), 2202–2221. doi:10.3390/s90302202 PMID:22574009

Campbell, B. (2008). *Nutritional Supplements in Sports and Exercise*. J. Humana Press. LLC.

Carr, A. C., & Frei, B. (1999). Toward a new recommended dietary allowance for vitamin C based on antioxidant and health effects in humans. *The American Journal of Clinical Nutrition, 69*, 1086–1107. PMID:10357726

Casado, B., Affolter, M., & Kussmann, M. (2009). OMICS-rooted studies of milk proteins, oligosaccharides and lipids. *Journal of Proteomics, 73*(2), 196–208. doi:10.1016/j.jprot.2009.09.018 PMID:19793547

Celle, T., Heeringa, P., Strzelecka, A. E., Bast, A., Smits, J. F., & Janssen, B. J. (2004). Sustained protective effects of 7-monohydroxyethylrutoside in an in vivo model of cardiac ischemia perfusion. *European Journal of Pharmacology, 494*(2-3), 205–212. doi:10.1016/j.ejphar.2004.05.017 PMID:15212976

Chakraborty, I., Mondal, S., Pramanik, M., Rout, D., & Islam, S. S. (2004). Structural investigation of a water-soluble glucan from an edible mushroom, *Astraeus hygrometricus. Carbohydrate Research, 339*(13), 2249–2254. doi:10.1016/j.carres.2004.07.013 PMID:15337453

Chang, S. T., & Miles, P. G. (1992). Mushroom biology-A new decipline. *The Mycologist, 6*(2), 64–65. doi:10.1016/S0269-915X(09)80449-7

Chen, J. J., Lee, Y. C., Cheng, T. J., Hsiao, H. Y., & Chen, R. L. C. (2006). Determination of glucosamine content in nutraceuticals by capillary electrophoresis using in-capillary OPA labeling techniques. *J. Food Drug Anal, 14*(2), 203–206.

Chen, L., Mehta, A., Berenvaum, M., Zangerl, A. R., & Engeseth, J. (2000). Honeys from different floral sources as inhibitors of enzymatic browning in fruit and vegetable homogenates. *Journal of Agricultural and Food Chemistry, 48*(10), 4997–5000. doi:10.1021/jf000373j PMID:11052768

Choi, H. et al.. (2012). Comparative nutritional analysis for genetically modified rice, Iksan483 and Milyang204, and nontransgenic counterparts. *J. Korean soc. Appl. Biol. Chem., 55*, 19–26.

Cicero, A. F. G., & Ertek, S. (2008). Natural Sources of Antidyslipidaemic Agents: Is There an Evidence-Based Approach for Their Prescription. *Medit. J. Nutri. Metab.*, *1*(2), 85–93. doi:10.1007/s12349-008-0011-6

Clement, F., Pramod, S. N., & Venkatesh, Y. P. (2010). Identity of the immunomodulatory proteins from garlic (*Allium sativum*) with themajor garlic lectins or agglutinins. *International Immunopharmacology*, *10*(3), 316–324. doi:10.1016/j.intimp.2009.12.002 PMID:20004743

Cook, N. C., & Samman, S. (1996). Flavonoids-Chemistry, metabolism, cardioprotective effects, and dietary sources. *The Journal of Nutritional Biochemistry*, *7*(2), 66–76. doi:10.1016/0955-2863(95)00168-9

Cooke, R. C. (1977). *Fungi, man and his environment*. London: Largman.

Corbridge, D. E. C. (1995). Phosphorus: An outline of its chemistry, biochemistry, and technology (5th ed.). Amsterdam: Elsevier Science Pub Co.

Cortina, M. S., & Bazan, H. E. (2011). Docosahexaenoic acid, Protectins, and Dry Eye. *Current Opinion in Clinical Nutrition and Metabolic Care*, *14*(2), 132–137. doi:10.1097/MCO.0b013e328342bb1a PMID:21157308

Cranney, A., Horsley, T., & O'Donnell, S. (2007). Effectiveness and Safety of Vitamin D in Relation to Bone Health. *Evid. Rep. Technol. Assess*, *158*, 1–235. PMID:18088161

Crisan, E. W. S. (1978). A nutritional value. In The biology and cultivation of edible mushrooms. Academic Press.

Croan, S. C. (2004). Conversion of conifer wastes into edible and medicinal mushrooms. *Forest Products Journal*, *54*, 68–76.

D'Antuono, L. F., Elementi, S., & Neri, R. (2008). Glucosinolates in Diplotaxis and Eruca leaves: Diversity, taxonomic relations and applied aspects. *Phytochemistry*, *69*(1), 187–199. doi:10.1016/j.phytochem.2007.06.019 PMID:17669448

Dahiya, K. (2013). Nutraceuticals and Their Impact on Human Health. *J Plant Biochem Physiol*, *1*, 4.

Dall'Acqua, S., & Innocenti, G. (2007). Steroidal glycosides from Hoodia gordonii. *Steroids*, *72*(6-7), 559–568. doi:10.1016/j.steroids.2007.03.008 PMID:17485103

Dalton, E. J., Rotondi, D., Levitan, R. D., Kennedy, S. H., & Brown, G. M. (2000). Use of slow-release melatonin in treatment-resistant depression. *Journal of Psychiatry & Neuroscience*, *25*(1), 48–52. PMID:10721684

Das, K. (2010). Diversity and conservation of wild mushrooms in Sikkim with special reference to Barsey Rhododendron Sanctuary. *NeBIO*, *1*(2), 1–13.

Davies, S., Howard, J. M., Hunnisett, A., & Howard, M. (1997). Age-related decreases in chromium levels in 51,665 hair, sweat, and serum samples from 40,872 patients – implications for the prevention of cardiovascular disease and type II diabetes. *Metabolism: Clinical and Experimental*, *46*(5), 469–473. doi:10.1016/S0026-0495(97)90179-7 PMID:9160809

De Leersnyder, H., Bresson, J. L., de Blois, M. C., Souberbielle, J. C., Mogenet, A., Delhotal-Landes, B., & Munnich, A. et al. (2003). Beta 1-adrenergic antagonists and melatonin reset the clock and restore sleep in a circadian disorder, Smith-Magenis syndrome. *Journal of Medical Genetics*, *40*(1), 74–78. doi:10.1136/jmg.40.1.74 PMID:12525548

De Simone, C., Picariello, G., Mamone, G., Stiuso, P., Dicitore, A., Vanacore, D., & Ferranti, P. et al. (2009). Characterisation and cytomodulatory properties of peptides from Mozzarella di Bufala Campana cheese whey. *Journal of Peptide Science*, *15*(3), 251–258. doi:10.1002/psc.1093 PMID:19035578

DeMan, J. (1999). *Principles of Food chemistry* (3rd ed.). Aspen Publication Inc. doi:10.1007/978-1-4614-6390-0_1

Dernovics, M., Giusti, P., Lobinski, R. (2007). *ICP-MS-assisted nanoHPLC-electrospray Q/time*. Academic Press.

Dernovics, M., Giusti, P., & Lobinski, R. (2007). of-flight MS/MS selenopeptide mapping in Brazil nuts. *Journal of Analytical Atomic Spectrometry*, *22*(1), 41–50. doi:10.1039/B608041C

DeVrese, M., & Schrezenmeir, J. (2008). Probiotics, prebiotics and synbiotics. *Advances in Biochemical Engineering/Biotechnology*, *111*, 1–66. doi:10.1007/10_2008_097 PMID:18461293

Dey, B., Bhunia, S. K., Maity, K. K., Patra, S., Mandal, S., Maiti, S., & Islam, S. S. et al. (2010). Chemical analysis of an immunoenhancing water-soluble polysaccharide of an edible mushroom, *Pleurotus florida* blue variant. *Carbohydrate Research*, *345*(18), 2736–2741. doi:10.1016/j.carres.2010.09.032 PMID:20971448

di Noia, J. (2014). *Defining powerhouse fruits and vegetables: a nutrient density approach. Preventing chronic disease*. National Center for Chronic Disease Prevention and Health Promotion.

Dodick, D. W., & Capobianco, D. J. (2001). Treatment and management of cluster headache. *Current Pain and Headache Reports*, *5*(1), 83–91. doi:10.1007/s11916-001-0015-0 PMID:11252143

Dolberg, O. T., Hirschmann, S., & Grunhaus, L. (1998). Melatonin for the treatment of sleep disturbances in major depressive disorder. *The American Journal of Psychiatry*, *155*(8), 1119–1121. doi:10.1176/ajp.155.8.1119 PMID:9699707

Drewnowski, A. (2010). The Nutrient Rich Foods Index helps to identify healthy, affordable foods. *The American Journal of Clinical Nutrition*, *91*(4), 1095S–1101S. doi:10.3945/ajcn.2010.28450D PMID:20181811

Elizabeth, A. C. (2002). Over the counter products: Nonprescription medications, nutraceuticals, and herbal agents. *Clinical Obstetrics and Gynecology*, *45*(1), 89–98. doi:10.1097/00003081-200203000-00010 PMID:11862061

Engelen, M. P., De De Castro, C. L., Rutten, E. P., Wouters, E. F., Schols, A. M., & Deutz, N. E. (2012). Enhanced anabolic response to milk protein sip feeding in elderly subjects with COPD is associated with a reduced splanchnic extraction of multiple amino acids. *Clinical Nutrition (Edinburgh, Lothian)*, *31*(5), 616–624. doi:10.1016/j.clnu.2012.04.006 PMID:22682082

Engelen, M.P., Rutten, E.P., De Castro, C.L., Wouters, E.F., Schols, A.M., & Deutz, N.E. (2012) Casein protein results in higher prandial and exercise induced whole body protein anabolism than whey protein in chronic obstructive pulmonary disease. *Metabolism, 61*(9), 1289–1300.

Erickson, K. L., Medina, E. A., & Hubbard, N. E. (2000). Micronutrients and innate immunity. *The Journal of Infectious Diseases, 182*(s1), S5–S10. doi:10.1086/315922 PMID:10944478

Erkucuk, A., Akgun, I. H., & Yesil-Celiktas, O. (2009). Supercritical CO2 extraction of glycosides from Stevia rebaudiana leaves: Identification and optimization. *The Journal of Supercritical Fluids, 51*(1), 29–35. doi:10.1016/j.supflu.2009.07.002

Erkucuk, A., Akgun, I. H., & Yesil-Celiktas, O. (2009). Supercritical CO2 extraction of glycosides from *Stevia rebaudiana* leaves: Identification and optimization. *The Journal of Supercritical Fluids, 51*(1), 29–35. doi:10.1016/j.supflu.2009.07.002

Escott-Stump, S. (2008). Nutrition and Diagnosis-Related Care (8th ed.). Lippincott Williams & Wilkins.

Evers, D. L., Chao, C. F., Wang, X., Zhang, Z. G., Huong, S. M., & Huang, E. S. (2005). Human cytomegalo virus-inhibitory flavonoids: Studies on antiviral activity and mechanism of action. *Antiviral Research, 68*(3), 124–134. doi:10.1016/j.antiviral.2005.08.002 PMID:16188329

Fennema, O. (2008). Fennema's Food Chemistry. CRC Press.

Fetrow, C. W., & Avila, K. R. (2001). Efficacy of the dietary supplement S-adenosyl-L-methionine. *The Annals of Pharmacotherapy, 35*(11), 1414–1425. doi:10.1345/aph.1Z443 PMID:11724095

Fleck, A., Gupta, R. C., Goad, J. T., Lasher, M. A., Canerdy, T. D., & Kalidindi, S. R. (2014). Anti-arthritic efficacy and safety of crominex® 3+ (Trivalent chromium, phyllanthus emblica extract, and shilajit) in moderately arthritic dogs. *Journal of Veterinary Science & Animal Husbandry., 1*(4), 1–8.

Fox, H. M. (1984). Pantothenic acid. In L. J. Machlin (Ed.), *Handbook of Vitamins* (Vol. 437). New York: Marcel Dekker.

Frei, B., England, L., & Ames, B. N. (1989). Ascorbate is an outstanding antioxidant in human blood plasma. *Proceedings of the National Academy of Sciences of the United States of America, 86*(16), 6377–6381. doi:10.1073/pnas.86.16.6377 PMID:2762330

Ghebre, M. A., Hart, D. J., Hakim, A. J., Kato, B. S., Thompson, V., Arden, N. K., & Zhai, G. et al. (2011). Association between DHEAS and bone loss in postmenopausal women: A 15-year longitudinal population-based study. *Calcified Tissue International, 89*(4), 295–302. doi:10.1007/s00223-011-9518-9 PMID:21789637

Ghosh, S., & Bhattacharjee, P. (2014). Supercritical carbon dioxide extract of *Ocimum sanctum* improves nutraceutical properties of ice cream. *Nutrafood., 13*(2), 69–78. doi:10.1007/s13749-014-0004-7

Golmakani, M. T., & Rezaei, K. (2008). Comparison of microwave-assisted hydrodistillation with the traditional hydrodistillation method in the extraction of essential oils from *Thymus vulgaris* L. *Food Chemistry, 109*(4), 925–930. doi:10.1016/j.foodchem.2007.12.084 PMID:26050009

Grace, E. (2013). *How to choose the best supplement*. Health Beacon.

Gray, J. (2003). *Carbohydrates: Nutritional and Health Aspects*. Washington, DC: ILSI Press.

Grimley, E. J., Malouf, R., Huppert, F., & van Niekerk, J. K. (2006). Malouf, Reem, ed. Dehydroepiandrosterone (DHEA) supplementation for cognitive function in healthy elderly people. Cochrane Database of Systematic Reviews, 4.

Grossman, E., Laudon, M., & Zisapel, N. (2011). Effect of melatonin on nocturnal blood pressure: Meta-analysis of randomized controlled trials. *Vascular Health and Risk Management*, *7*, 577–584. PMID:21966222

Gruen, V. E. C., & Wong, H. X. (1982). Immunomodulatory and antitumour activities of a polysaccharide-peptide complex from a mycelial culture of Trichoderma sp. *The Sciences*, *57*, 269–281.

Guclu-Ustundag, O., & Mazza, G. (2008). Extraction of saponins and cyclopeptides from cow cockle seed with pressurized low polarity water. *Food Science and Technology (Campinas.)*, *41*, 1600–1606.

Hamrick, I., & Counts, S. H. (2008). Vitamin and mineral supplements. *Wellness Prevent*, *35*(4), 729–747. PMID:18928827

Harborne, J. B., & Williams, C. A. (2000). Advances in flavonoid research since 1992. *Phytochemistry*, *55*(6), 481–504. doi:10.1016/S0031-9422(00)00235-1 PMID:11130659

Hardeland, R., Pandi-Perumal, S. R., & Cardinali, D. P. (2006). Melatonin. *The International Journal of Biochemistry & Cell Biology*, *38*(3), 313–316. doi:10.1016/j.biocel.2005.08.020 PMID:16219483

Harris, G. K., Qian, Y., Leonard, S. S., Sbarra, D. C., & Shi, X. L. (2006). Luteolin and chrysin differentially inhibit cyclooxygenase-2 expression and scavenge reactive oxygen species but similarly inhibit prostaglandin-E2 formation in RAW 264.7 cells. *The Journal of Nutrition*, *136*(6), 1517–1521. PMID:16702314

Hattori, A., Migitaka, H., Iigo, M., Itoh, M., Yamamoto, K., Ohtani-Kaneko, R., & Reiter, R. J. et al. (1995). Identification of melatonin in plants and its effects on plasma melatonin levels and binding to melatonin receptors in vertebrates. *Biochemistry and Molecular Biology International*, *35*(3), 627–634. PMID:7773197

Havrlentova, et al.. (2011). Cereal β-glucans and their significance for the preparation of functional foods-a review. *Czech Journal of Food Science*, *29*(1), 1–14.

Hawksworth, D. L. (2001). Mushrooms: The extent of the unexplored potential. *Int. J. Med. Mushr*, *3*(4), 333–337. doi:10.1615/IntJMedMushr.v3.i4.50

Henry, J. (2009). Processing, manufacturing, uses and labeling of fat in the food supply. *Annals of Nutrition & Metabolism*, *55*(1-3), 273–300. doi:10.1159/000229006 PMID:19752546

Herrero, M., Ibáñez, E., Fanali, S., & Cifuentes, A. (2007). Quantitation of chiral amino acids from microalgae by MEKC and LIF detection. *Electrophoresis*, *28*(15), 2701–2709. doi:10.1002/elps.200600599 PMID:17592610

Herrero, M., Vicente, M. J., Cifuentes, A., & Ibanez, E. (2007). Characterization by high performance liquid chromatography/electrospray ionization quadrupole time-of-flight mass spectrometry of the lipid fraction of *Spirulina platensis* pressurized ethanol extract. *Rapid Communications in Mass Spectrometry*, *21*(11), 1729–1738. doi:10.1002/rcm.3017 PMID:17487827

Heyland, D. K. (2001). In search of the magic nutraceuticals: Problems with current approaches. *The Journal of Nutrition*, *131*(9), 2591–2595. PMID:11533319

Hodgson, J. M., Puddey, I. B., Burke, V., Beilin, L. J., & Jordan, N. (1999). Effect of blood pressure of drinking green and black tea. *Journal of Hypertension*, *17*(4), 457–463. doi:10.1097/00004872-199917040-00002 PMID:10404946

Holtcamp, W. (2012). The emerging science of BMAA: Do cyanobacteria contribute to neurodegenerative disease? *Environmental Health Perspectives*, *120*(3), a110–a116. doi:10.1289/ehp.120-a110 PMID:22382274

Huseini, H. F., Larijani, B., Heshmat, R., Fakhrzadeh, H., Radjabipour, B., Toliat, T., & Raza, M. (2006). The efficacy of silybum marianum (L.) Gaertn. (silymarin) in the treatment of type II diabetes: A randomized, double-blind, placebo-controlled, clinical trial. *Phytotherapy Research*, *20*(12), 1036–1039. doi:10.1002/ptr.1988 PMID:17072885

Imura, K., & Okada, A. (1998). Amino acid metabolism in pediatric patients. *Nutrition (Burbank, Los Angeles County, Calif.)*, *14*(1), 143–148. doi:10.1016/S0899-9007(97)00230-X PMID:9437700

Institute of Medicine (IM). (1998). *Food and Nutrition Board. Dietary Reference Intakes for Thiamin, Riboflavin, Niacin, Vitamin B6, Folate, Vitamin B12, Pantothenic Acid, Biotin, and Choline*. Washington, DC: National Academy Press.

Iriti, M., Faoro, F. (2006). Grape phytochemicals: A bouquet of old and new nutraceuticals for human health. *Med Hypoth*, 833-838.

Iriti, M., & Faoro, F. (2009). Bioactivity of grape chemicals for human health. *Nat. Prod. Commun.*, *4*(5), 611–634. PMID:19445314

Iwu, M. M., Igboko, A. O., Onwubiko, H., & Ndu, U. E. (1988). Effect of cajaminose from Cajanus cajan on gelation and oxygen affinity of sickle cell haemoglobin. *Journal of Ethnopharmacology*, *23*(1), 99–104. doi:10.1016/0378-8741(88)90118-3 PMID:3419206

Jacob, R. A., & Sotoudeh, G. (2002). Vitamin C function and status in chronic disease. *Nutrition in Clinical Care*, *5*(2), 66–74. doi:10.1046/j.1523-5408.2002.00005.x PMID:12134712

Jagadeesh, R., Raaman, N., Periyasamy, K., Hariprasath, L., Thangaraj, R., Srikumar, R., & Ayyappan, S. R. (2010). Proximate analysis and antibacterial activity of edible mushroom *Volvariella Bombycina. Int. J. Microbiol. Res*, *1*(3), 110–113.

Jagadish, L. K., Krishnan, V. V., Shenbhagaraman, R., & Kaviyarasan, V. (2009). Comparative study on the antioxidant, anticancer and antimicrobial property of *Agaricus bisporus* (J. E. Lange) Imbach before and after boiling. *African Journal of Biotechnology*, *8*, 654–661.

Jan, J. E., Hamilton, D., Seward, N., Fast, D. K., Freeman, R. D., & Laudon, M. (2000). Clinical trials of controlled-release melatonin in children with sleep-wake cycle disorders. *Journal of Pineal Research*, *29*(1), 34–39. doi:10.1034/j.1600-079X.2000.290105.x PMID:10949538

Jellin, J. M. (2009). *Natural medicines comprehensive database*. Retrieved from http://www.naturaldatabase.com

Jones, S., & Janardhanan, K. K. (2000). Antioxidant and antitumor activity of *Ganoderma lucidum* (curt ex Fr.). P. Karst-Reshi (Aphyllophoromycetieae) from south India. *Int. J. Med. Mushr*, *2*(3), 195–200. doi:10.1615/IntJMedMushr.v2.i3.20

Jose, N., Ajith, T. A., & Janardhanan, K. K. (2002). Antioxidant, anti-inflammatory and antitumor activities of culinarymedicinal mushroom *Pleurotus pulmonarius* (Fr.) Quel. (Agaricomycetideae). *Int. J. Med. Mushr*, *4*(4), 329–335. doi:10.1615/IntJMedMushr.v4.i4.60

Jose, N., & Janardhanan, K. K. (2000). Antioxidant and antitumor activity of *Pleurotus florida*. *Current Science*, *79*, 941–943.

Kador, P. F., Guo, C., Kawada, H., Randazzo, J., & Blessing, K. (2014). Topical Nutraceutical Optixcare EH Ameliorates Experimental Ocular Oxidative Stress in Rats. *Journal of Ocular Pharmacology and Therapeutics*, *30*(7), 593–602. doi:10.1089/jop.2014.0016 PMID:25188009

Kagan, V., Khan, S., Swanson, C., Shvedova, A., Serbinova, E., & Packer, L. (1990). Antioxidant action of thioctic acid and dihydrolipoic acid. *Free Radical Biology & Medicine*, *9S*, 15. doi:10.1016/0891-5849(90)90220-D

Kalac, P., & Moudry, J. (2000). Chemical composition and nutritional value of amaranth grains[in Czech]. *Czech Food Scienc*, *18*, 201–206.

Kalra, E. K. (2003). Nutraceutical Definition and Introduction. *AAPS PharmSci*, *5*(3), 25. doi:10.1208/ps050325 PMID:14621960

Kanter, M., Coskun, O., & Budancamanak, M. (2005). Hepatoprotective effects of Nigella sativa L. and Urtica dioica L. on lipid peroxidation, antioxidant enzyme systems and liver enzymes in carbon tetrachloride-treated rats. *World Journal of Gastroenterology*, *11*(42), 6684–6688. doi:10.3748/wjg.v11.i42.6684 PMID:16425366

Kerem, Z., Chetrit, D., Shoseyov, O., & Regev-Shoshani, G. (2006). Protection of lipids from oxidation by epicatechin, trans-resveratrol, and gallic and caffeic acids in intestinal model systems. *Journal of Agricultural and Food Chemistry*, *54*(26), 10288–10293. doi:10.1021/jf0621828 PMID:17177572

Keservani, R. K., Singh, S., Singh, V., Kesharwani, R.K., & Sharma, A. K. (2015b). Nutraceuticals and Functional Foods in the Prevention of Mental Disorder. CRC Press, Taylor and Francis.

Keservani, R. K., Kesharwani, R. K., & Sharma, A. K. (2015c). *Pulmonary and Respiratory Health: Antioxidants and Nutraceuticals*. CRC Press, Taylor and Francis.

Keservani, R. K., Kesharwani, R. K., Sharma, A. K., & Jarouliya, U. (2015d). Dietary Supplements, Nutraceutical and Functional Foods in Immune Response (Immunomodulators). CRC Press, Taylor and Francis.

Keservani, R. K., Kesharwani, R. K., Sharma, A. K., & Ahmad, M. F. (2015a). *Stress, Parkinson's,Alzemer's disease: Role of Dietary Supplements*. CRC Press, Taylor and Francis.

Keservani, R. K., Kesharwani, R. K., Sharma, A. K., Vyas, N., & Chadoker, A. (2010b). Nutritional Supplements: An Overview.[IJCPR]. *Int. J. Curr. Pharm. Rev. Res.*, *1*, 59–75.

Keservani, R. K., Kesharwani, R. K., Vyas, N., Jain, S., Raghuvanshi, R., & Sharma, A. K. (2010a). Nutraceutical and functional food as future food: A Review. *Der Pharmacia. Lett*, *2*, 106–116.

Keservani, R. K., & Sharma, A. K. (2014). Flavonoids: Emerging trends and potential health benefits. *J Chin. Pharm. Sci.*, *23*(12), 815–822.

Kim, S. J., Kawaharada, C., Suzuki, T., Saito, K., Hashimoto, N., Takigawa, S., & Yamauchi, H. et al. (2006). Effect of natural light periods on rutin, free amino acid and vitamin C contents in the sprouts of common (Fagopyrum esculentum Moench) and tartary (F. tataricum Gaertn.) buckwheats. *Food Science and Technology Research*, *12*(3), 199–205. doi:10.3136/fstr.12.199

Kong, W. S. (2004). Descriptions of commercially important Pleurotus species. In Oyster mushroom cultivation. Part II. Oyster mushrooms. Seoul: Heineart Incorporation.

Koshihara, Y., & Hoshi, K. (1996). Vitamin K2 promotes 1α,25(oh)2 vitamin D3-induced mineralization in human periosteal osteoblasts. *Calcified Tissue International*, *59*, 466–473. PMID:8939773

Kucuk, O., Sarkar, F. H., Sak, W., Djuric, Z., Pollak, M. N., & Khachik, F. (2002). Phase II randomized clinical trial of lycopene supplementation before radical prostatectomy. *Cancer Epidemiology, Biomarkers & Prevention*, *10*, 861–868. PMID:11489752

Lacomba, R., Salcedo, J., Alegria, A., & Lagarda, M. J. (2010). Determination of sialic acid and gangliosides in biological samples and dairy products: A review. *J. Pharmaceut. Biomed*, *51*(2), 346–357. doi:10.1016/j.jpba.2009.04.023 PMID:19481897

Lago, J. H. G., Toledo-Arruda, A. C., Mernak, M., Barrosa, K., Martins, M., Tibério, I., & Prado, C. (2014). Structure-Activity Association of Flavonoids in Lung Diseases. *Molecules (Basel, Switzerland)*, *19*(3), 3570–3595. doi:10.3390/molecules19033570 PMID:24662074

Lakshmi, B., Ajith, T.A., & Sheena, M., NidhI, G., & Janardhanan, K.K. (2003). Antiperoxidative, anti-inflammatory and antimutagenic activities of ethanol extract of the mycelium of *Ganoderma lucidum* occurring in South India. *Teratogenesis, Carcinogenesis, and Mutagenesis*, *22*, 1–13. PMID:12616600

Lamont, K. T., Somers, S., Lacerda, L., Opie, L. H., & Lecour, S. (2011). Is red wine a SAFE sip away from cardioprotection? Mechanisms involved in resveratrol- and melatonin-induced cardioprotection. *Journal of Pineal Research*, *50*(4), 374–380. doi:10.1111/j.1600-079X.2010.00853.x PMID:21342247

Lee, J. J., Yang, S. Y., Kim, D. H., Hur, S. J., Lee, J. D., Yum, M. J., & Song, M. D. (2014). Liver fibrosis protective effect of hovenia dulcis fruit. *Current Topics in Nutraceutical Research*, *12*(1/2), 43–50.

Lewis, A. (1999). *Melatonin and the Biological Clock*. McGraw-Hill.

Li, D., Ng, A., Mann, N., & Sinclair, A. J. (1998). Meat fat can make a significant contribution to dietary arachidonic acid. *Lipids*, *33*, 437–440. doi:10.1007/s11745-998-0225-7 PMID:9590632

Li, Y., & Schellhorn, H. E. (2007). New developments and novel therapeutic perspectives for vitamin C. *The Journal of Nutrition*, *137*, 2171–2184. PMID:17884994

Loria, R. M. (2002). Immune up-regulation and tumor apoptosis by androstene steroids. *Steroids*, *67*(12), 953–966. doi:10.1016/S0039-128X(02)00043-0 PMID:12398992

Lourenço, R., & Camilo, M. E. (2002). Taurine: A conditionally essential amino acid in humans? An overview in health and disease. *Nutricion Hospitalaria*, *17*(6), 262–270. PMID:12514918

Lu, M.-K., Cheng, J.-J., Lin, C.-Y., & Chang, C.-C. (2010, January). anti-inflammatory effect of a water-soluble 1,6-branched 1,3-α-D-galactan from cultured mycelia of *Poria cocos*. *Food Chemistry*, *118*(2), 349–356. doi:10.1016/j.foodchem.2009.04.126

Lu, M. K., Cheng, J. J., Lin, C.-Y., & Chang, C. C. (2010). Purification, structural elucidation, and Lukaski, H.C. (1999). Chromium as a supplement. *Annual Review of Nutrition*, *19*(1), 279–302.

Maity, K. K., Patra, S., Dey, B., Bhunia, S. K., Mandal, S., Das, D., & Islam, S. S. et al. (2011). A heteropolysaccharide from aqueous extract of an edible mushroom, *Pleurotus ostreatus* cultivar: Structural and biological studies. *Carbohydrate Research*, *346*(2), 366–372. doi:10.1016/j.carres.2010.10.026 PMID:21129732

Malavaki, C. J., Asimakopoulou, A. P., Lamari, F. N., Theocharis, A. D., Tzanakakis, G. N., & Karamanos, N. K. (2008). Capillary electrophoresis for the quality control of chondroitin sulfates in raw materials and formulations. *Analytical Biochemistry*, *374*(1), 213–220. doi:10.1016/j.ab.2007.11.006 PMID:18054774

Mason, J. B. (2011). Vitamins, trace minerals, and other micronutrients. In L. Goldman & D. Ausiello (Eds.), *Cecil Medicine. Saunders* (p. 225). Philadelphia, Pa.: Elsevier.

Mattila, P., Konko, K., Eurola, M., Pihlawa, J. M., & Astola, J. (2001). Contents of vitamins, mineral elements, and some phenolic compounds in cultivated mushrooms. *Journal of Agricultural and Food Chemistry*, *49*(5), 2343–2348. doi:10.1021/jf001525d PMID:11368601

McNaught, A. D., & Wilkinson, A. (1997). *IUPAC Flavonoids (isoflavonoids and neoflavonoids) IUPAC Compendium of Chemical Terminology* (2nd ed.). Oxford, UK: Blackwell Scientific.

Meltretter, J., Schmidt, A., Humeny, A., Becker, C. M., & Pischetsrieder, M. (2008). Analysis of the peptide profile of milk and its changes during thermal treatment and storage. *Journal of Agricultural and Food Chemistry*, *56*(9), 2899–2906. doi:10.1021/jf073479o PMID:18419126

Mendiola, J., Torres-Cantero, A. M., Vioque, J., Moreno-Grau, J. M., Ten, J., Roca, M., & Bernabeu, R. et al. (2010). A low intake of antioxidant nutrients is associated with poor semen quality in patients attending fertility clinics. *Fertility and Sterility*, *93*(4), 1128–1133. doi:10.1016/j.fertnstert.2008.10.075 PMID:19147135

Mendiola, J. A., Torres, C. F., Martín-Álvarez, P. J., & Santoyo, S. (2007). Use of supercritical CO2 to obtain extracts with antimicrobial activity from *Chaetoceros muelleri* microalga. A correlation with their lipidic content. *European Food Research and Technology*, *224*(4), 505–510. doi:10.1007/s00217-006-0353-6

Meyer, A. (1998). The 1998 top 100® R&D survey. *Food Processing.*, *58*(8), 32–40.

Mischoulon, D., Fava, M., & Stahl, S. (2009). Folate Supplementation. *The Journal of Clinical Psychiatry, 70*(5), 767–769. doi:10.4088/JCP.08lr04824a PMID:19552872

Mobh, S. (1938). Research for Vitamin P. *Journal of Biochemistry, 29*(3), 487–501.

Moon, S., Cho, G., Jung, S., Gal, S., Kwon, T. K., Lee, Y.-C., & Kim, C.-H. et al. (2003). Quercetin exerts multiple inhibitory effects on vascular smooth muscle cells: Roleof ERK1/2, cell-cycle regulation, and matrix metalloproteinase-9. *Biochemical and Biophysical Research Communications, 301*(4), 1069–1078. doi:10.1016/S0006-291X(03)00091-3 PMID:12589822

Morgan, S. L., & Baggott, J. E. (2006). Medical foods: Products for the management of chronic diseases. *Nutrition Reviews, 64*(11), 495–501. doi:10.1111/j.1753-4887.2006.tb00182.x PMID:17131945

Mori, T. A., Bao, D. Q., Burke, V., Puddey, I. B., & Beilin, L. J. (1999). Docohexanoic acid but not eicasapentanoic acid lowers ambulatory blood pressure and heart rate in humans. *Hypertension, 34*(2), 253–260. doi:10.1161/01.HYP.34.2.253 PMID:10454450

Nair, K. S., Rizza, R. A., O'Brien, P., Dhatariya, K., Short, K. R., Nehra, A., & Jensen, M. D. et al. (2006). DHEA in elderly women and DHEA or testosterone in elderly men. *The New England Journal of Medicine, 355*(16), 1647–1659. doi:10.1056/NEJMoa054629 PMID:17050889

Nelson, D. L., & Cox, M. M. (2000). Lehninger Principles of Biochemistry (3rd ed.). W. H. Freeman.

Niacin Compound Summary (NCS). (n.d.). PubChem, National Center for Biotechnology Information, U.S. National Library of Medicine.

Nittynen, L., Nurminen, M. L., Korpela, I., & Vapaatalo, H. (1999). Role of arginine, taurine and homocysteine in cardiovascular disease. *Annals of Medicine, 31*(5), 318–326. doi:10.3109/07853899908995898 PMID:10574504

Nordeen, S. K., Bona, B. J., Jones, D. N., Lambert, J. R., & Jackson, T. A. (2013). Endocrine disrupting activities of the flavonoid nutraceuticals luteolin and quercetin. *Horm. Canc., 4*(5), 293–300. doi:10.1007/s12672-013-0150-1 PMID:23836117

Norman, A. W., & Henry, H. L. (2012). *Hormones* (3rd ed.). Oxford, UK: Academic Press.

Nutraceutical World. (n.d.). Retrieved from http://www.nutraceuticalsworld.com/

Nutrition, H. (2009). *Iodine*. George Mateljan Foundation.

Nutrition, H. (2009). *Iron*. George Mateljan Foundation.

Nutrition, H. (2009). *Magnesium*. George Mateljan Foundation.

Nutrition, H. (2009). *Selenium*. George Mateljan Foundation.

Nutrition, H. (2009). *Zinc*. George Mateljan Foundation.

Oh, J. U., Jang, H., & Kim, S. J. (2014). Inhibition of inducible nitric oxide synthase and cyclooxygenase-2 by methanolic extract of *Crataegi Fructus*. *Current Topics in Nutraceutical Research., 12*(1/2), 35–42.

Okanoto, M. et al.. (2000). Effects of perilla seed oil supplementation on leukotriene generation by leucocytes in patients with asthma associated with lipometabolism. *International Archives of Allergy and Immunology*, *122*(2), 137–142. doi:10.1159/000024369 PMID:10878492

Paredes, S. D., Korkmaz, A., Manchester, L. C., Tan, D. X., & Reiter, R. J. (2009). Phytomelatonin: A review. *Journal of Experimental Botany*, *60*(1), 57–69. doi:10.1093/jxb/ern284 PMID:19033551

Park, M. (2013). *Half of Americans use supplements*. CNN.

Peet, M. (2004). International variations in the outcome of schizophrenia and the prevalence of depression in relation to national dietary practices: An ecological analysis. *The British Journal of Psychiatry*, *184*(5), 404–408. doi:10.1192/bjp.184.5.404 PMID:15123503

Perez-Fons, L., Aranda, F. J., Guillén, J., Villalaín, J., & Micol, V. (2006). Rosemary (*Rosmarinus officinalis*) diterpenes affect lipid polymorphism and fluidity in phospholipid membranes. *Archives of Biochemistry and Biophysics*, *453*(2), 224–236. doi:10.1016/j.abb.2006.07.004 PMID:16949545

Pinazo-Duran, M. D., Galbis-Estrada, C., Pons-Vázquez, , Cantu-Dibildox, J., Marco-Ramirez, C., & Benitez-del-castillo, F. (2013). Effects of a nutraceutical formulation based on the combination of antioxidants and ω-3 essential fatty acids in the expression of inflammation and immune response mediators in tears from patients with dry eye disorders. *Clinical Interventions in Aging*, *8*, 139–148. doi:10.2147/CIA.S40640 PMID:23430672

Prieto, J. M., Iacopini, P., Cioni, P., & Chericoni, S. (2007). In vitro activity of the essential oils of *Origanum vulgare, Satureja montana* and their main constituents in peroxynitrite-induced oxidative processes. *Food Chemistry*, *104*(3), 889–895. doi:10.1016/j.foodchem.2006.10.064

Probiotics in food: health and nutritional properties and guidelines for evaluation. (2002). Food and Agricultural Organization of the United Nations and World Health Organization (FAO-UN-WHO).

Raj, M. V., Selvakumar, K., Krishnamoorthy, G., Revathy, S., Elumalai, P., & Arunakaran, J. (2014). Impact of lycopene on epididymal androgen and estrogen receptors' expression in polychlorinated biphenyls-exposed rat. *Reproductive Sciences (Thousand Oaks, Calif.)*, *21*(1), 89–101. doi:10.1177/1933719113492213 PMID:23749762

Rajasekar, P., & Anuradha, C. V. (2007). Effect of L-carnitine on skeletal muscle lipids and oxidative stress in rats fed high-fructose diet. *Experimental Diabetes Research*, *2007*, 72741. doi:10.1155/2007/72741 PMID:17641743

Ramaa, C. S., Shirode, A. R., Mundada, A. S., & Kadam, V. J. (2006). Nutraceuticals--an emerging era in the treatment and prevention of cardiovascular diseases. *Current Pharmaceutical Biotechnology*, *7*(1), 15–23. doi:10.2174/138920106775789647 PMID:16472130

Ramesh, C., & Pattar, M. G. (2010). Antimicrobial properties, antioxidant activity and bioactive compounds from six wild edible mushrooms of Western Ghats of Karnataka, India. *Pharmacognosy Res*, *2*(2), 107–112. doi:10.4103/0974-8490.62953 PMID:21808550

Reis, L. C., & Hibbeln, J. R. (2006). Cultural symbolism of fish and the psychotropic properties of omega-3 fatty acids. *Prostaglandins, Leukotrienes, and Essential Fatty Acids*, *75*(4-5), 227–236. doi:10.1016/j.plefa.2006.07.014 PMID:16962306

Ren, W., Qiao, Z., Wang, H., Zhu, L., & Zhang, L. (2003). Flavonoids: Promising anti-cancer agents. *Medicinal Research Reviews*, *23*(4), 519–534. doi:10.1002/med.10033 PMID:12710022

Rijkers, G. T., de Vos, W. M., Brummer, R. J., Morelli, L., Corthier, G., & Marteau, P. et al.. (2011). Health benefits and health claims of probiotics: Bridging science and marketing. *The British Journal of Nutrition*, *106*(9), 1291–1296. doi:10.1017/S000711451100287X PMID:21861940

Rong, X. Y., Xiang, L. M., & Gui, G. J. (2014). Dietary supplements and insomnia. *Current Topics in Nutraceutical Research*, *12*(1/2), 51–56.

Rotimi, E. A. (2012). Functional foods and nutraceuticals. Springer.

Roy, S. K., Das, D., Mondal, S., Maiti, D., Bhunia, B., Maiti, T. K., & Islam, S. S. (2009). Structural studies of an immunoenhancing water-soluble glucan isolated from hot water extract of an edible mushroom, *Pleurotus florida*, cultivar Assam Florida. *Carbohydrate Research*, *344*(18), 2596–2601. doi:10.1016/j.carres.2009.09.010 PMID:19836727

Sae-Teaw, M., Johns, J., Johns, N. P., & Subongkot, S. (2012). Serum melatonin levels and antioxidant capacities after consumption of pineapple, orange, or banana by healthy male volunteers. *Journal of Pineal Research*, *55*(1), 58–64. doi:10.1111/jpi.12025 PMID:23137025

Saltarelli, R., Ceccaroli, P., Iotti, M., Zambonelli, A., Buffalini, M., Casadei, L., & Stocchi, V. et al. (2009). Biochemical characterisation and antioxidant activity of mycelium of *Ganoderma lucidum* from Central Italy. *Food Chemistry*, *116*(1), 143–151. doi:10.1016/j.foodchem.2009.02.023

Samorini, G. (2001). *Fungi Hallucinogeni. Studi etnomicologici*. Bologna, Italy: Telesterion. Dozza.

Santos, R., Limas, E., Sousa, M., da Conceição Castilho, M., Ramos, F., & da Silveira, M. I. N. (2007). Optimization of analytical procedures for GC-MS determination of phytosterols and phytostanols in enriched milk and yoghurt. *Food Chemistry*, *102*(1), 113–117. doi:10.1016/j.foodchem.2006.05.001

Sarkar, S. (2007). Functional foods as self-care and complementary medicine. *Nutrition & Food Science*, *37*(3), 160–167. doi:10.1108/00346650710749053

Schacky, C. V. (2003). The role of Omega-3 fatty acids in cardiovascular disease. *Current Atherosclerosis Reports*, *5*(2), 139–145. doi:10.1007/s11883-003-0086-y PMID:12573200

Schloss, P. D. (2014). Microbiology: An integrated view of the skin microbiome. *Nature*, *514*(7520), 44–45. doi:10.1038/514044a PMID:25279916

Schulz, S., Klann, R. C., Schönfeld, S., & Nyce, J. W. (1992). Mechanisms of cell growth inhibition and cell cycle arrest in human colonic adenocarcinoma cells by dehydroepiandrosterone: Role of isoprenoid biosynthesis. *Cancer Research*, *52*(5), 1372–1376. PMID:1531325

Shamir, E., Laudon, M., Barak, Y., Anis, Y., Rotenberg, V., Elizur, A., & Zisapel, N. (2000). Melatonin improves sleep quality of patients with chronic schizophrenia. *The Journal of Clinical Psychiatry*, *61*(5), 373–377. doi:10.4088/JCP.v61n0509 PMID:10847313

Shriharsh, V. et al.. (2014). Effect of nutraceutical and psychological interventions on cognitive functions of healthy human subjects. *Indian Journal of Traditional Knowledge.*, *13*(1), 95–102.

Shukla, M., Gupta, K., Rasheed, Z., Khan, K. A., & Haqqi, T. M. (2008). Bioavailable constituents/metabolites of pomegranate (*Punicagranatum* L) preferentially inhibit COX2 activity *ex vivo* and IL-1beta-induced PGE_2 production in human chondrocytes in vitro. *Journal of Inflammation*, *5*(9), 1–10. PMID:18261214

Sim, J. S., Im, A. R., Cho, S. M., Jang, H. J., Jo, J. H., & Kim, Y. S. (2007). Evaluation of chondroitin sulfate in shark cartilage powder as a dietary supplement: Raw materials and finished products. *Food Chemistry*, *101*(2), 532–539. doi:10.1016/j.foodchem.2006.02.011

Sivam, A. S., Sun-Waterhouse, G. I., Waterhouse, S., Quek, S. Y., & Perera, C. O. (2011). Physicochemical properties of bread dough and finished bread with added pectin fiber and phenolic antioxidants. *Journal of Food Science*, *76*(3), 97–107. doi:10.1111/j.1750-3841.2011.02086.x PMID:21535837

Solomon, P. R., Adams, F., Silver, A., Zimmer, J., & DeVeaux, R. (2002). Ginkgo for memory enhancement: A randomized controlled trial. *Journal of the American Medical Association*, *288*(7), 835–840. doi:10.1001/jama.288.7.835 PMID:12186600

Sotaniemi, E. A., Haapakoski, E., & Rautio, A. (1995). Ginseng therapy in non-insulin dependent diabetic patients. *Diabetes Care*, *18*(10), 1373–1375. doi:10.2337/diacare.18.10.1373 PMID:8721940

Strobel, C., Jahreis, G., & Kuhnt, K. (2012). Survey of n-3 and n-6 polyunsaturated fatty acids in fish and fish products. *Lipids in Health and Disease*, *11*(1), 144. doi:10.1186/1476-511X-11-144 PMID:23110317

Tambeker, D. H., Sonar, T. P., Khodke, M. V., & Khante, B. S. (2006). The novel antimicrobials from two edible mushrooms: *Agaricus bisporus* and *Pleurotus sajor caju. Int. J. Pharmacol*, *2*(5), 584–587. doi:10.3923/ijp.2006.584.587

Tan, D. X., Chen, L. D., Poeggeler, B., Manchester, L. C., & Reiter, R. J. (1993). Melatonin: A potent, endogenous hydroxyl radical scavenger. *Endocrine Journal*, *1*, 57–60.

Tan, D. X., Hardeland, R., Manchester, L. C., Korkmaz, A., Ma, S., Rosales-Corral, S., & Reiter, R. J. (2012). Functional roles of melatonin in plants, and perspectives in nutritional and agricultural science. *Journal of Experimental Botany*, *63*(2), 577–597. doi:10.1093/jxb/err256 PMID:22016420

Tan, D. X., Hardeland, R., Manchester, L. C., Paredes, S. D., Korkmaz, A., Sainz, R. M., & Reiter, R. J. et al. (2010). The changing biological roles of melatonin during evolution: From an antioxidant to signals of darkness, sexual selection and fitness. *Biological Reviews of the Cambridge Philosophical Society*, *85*(3), 607–623. PMID:20039865

Tan, D. X., Zheng, X., Kong, J., Manchester, L., Hardeland, R., Kim, S., & Reiter, R. et al. (2014). Fundamental Issues Related to the Origin of Melatonin and Melatonin Isomers during Evolution: Relation to Their Biological Functions. *International Journal of Molecular Sciences*, *15*(9), 15858–15890. doi:10.3390/ijms150915858 PMID:25207599

Tanumihardjo, S. A. (2011). Vitamin A: Biomarkers of nutrition for development. *The American Journal of Clinical Nutrition*, *94*(2), 658S–665S. doi:10.3945/ajcn.110.005777 PMID:21715511

Tapas, A. R., Sakarkar, D. M., & Kakde, R. B. (2008). Flavonoids as Nutraceuticals: A Review. *Tropical Journal of Pharmaceutical Research*, *7*(3), 1089–1099. doi:10.4314/tjpr.v7i3.14693

Tarek, K. M., Manal, A. H., Manal, H. S., Reem, M. H., & Asmaa, F. A. N. (2011). Zingiber officinale acts as a nutraceutical agent against liver fibrosis. *Nutrition and Metabolism*, *8*(40), 1–11. PMID:21241467

Theodori, R., Karioti, A., Racnic, A., & Skaltsa, H. (2006). Linear sesquiterpene lactones from Thijs, L., Fagard, R., Forette, F., Nawrot, T., Staessen, J.A. (2003). Are low dehydroepiandrosterone sulphate levels predictive for cardiovascular diseases? A review of prospective and retrospective studies. *Acta Cardiologica*, *58*(5), 403–410.

Traber, M. G. (2006). Vitamin E. In M. E. Shils, M. Shike, A. C. Ross, B. Caballero, & R. Cousins (Eds.), *Modern Nutrition in Health and Disease* (10th ed.). MD: Lippincott Williams & Wilkins, Baltimore.

Tsuchihashi, N., Watanabe, T., & Takai, Y. (1987). Effect of Spirulina platensis on caecum content in rats. *Bull Chiba Hygiene Coll*, *5*, 27–30.

Ueno, H., Wang, J., Kaji, N., Tokeshi, M., & Baba, Y. (2008). Quantitative determination of amino acids in functional foods by microchip electrophoresis. *Journal of Separation Science*, *31*(5), 898–903. doi:10.1002/jssc.200700517 PMID:18266297

Vazquez, L., Torres, C. F., Fornari, T., Senorans, F. J., & Reglero, G. (2007). Recovery of squalene from vegetable oil sources using countercurrent supercritical carbon dioxide extraction. *The Journal of Supercritical Fluids*, *40*(1), 59–66. doi:10.1016/j.supflu.2006.04.012

Verardo, V., Bendini, A., Cerretani, L., Malaguti, D., Cozzolino, E., & Caboni, M. F. (2009). Capillary gas chromatography analysis of lipid composition and evaluation of phenolic compounds by micellar electrokinetic chromatography in Italian walnut (*Juglans Regia l.*): Irrigation and fertilization influence. *Journal of Food Quality*, *32*(2), 262–281. doi:10.1111/j.1745-4557.2009.00249.x

Volpi, N. (2009). Capillary electrophoresis determination of glucosamine in nutraceutical formulations after labeling with anthranilic acid and UV detection. *Journal of Pharmaceutical and Biomedical Analysis*, *49*(3), 868–871. doi:10.1016/j.jpba.2009.01.006 PMID:19200685

Volpi, N., & Maccari, F. (2008). Quantitative and qualitative evaluation of chondroitin sulfate in dietary supplements. *Food Anal. Methods*, *1*(3), 195–204. doi:10.1007/s12161-008-9020-9

Wagner, I., & Musso, H. (1983). New naturally occurring amino acids. *Angewandte Chemie International Edition in English*, *22*(22), 816–828. doi:10.1002/anie.198308161

Wang, Y. D., Tao, M. F., Cheng, W. W., Liu, X. H., Wan, X. P., & Cui, K. (2012). Dehydroepiandrosterone indirectly inhibits human osteoclastic resorption via activating osteoblastic viability by the MAPK pathway. *Chinese Medical Journal*, *125*, 1230–1235. PMID:22613593

Whelan, A. M., Jurgens, T. M., & Bowles, S. K. (2006). Natural health products in the prevention and treatment of osteoporosis: Systemic review of randomized controlled trials. *The Annals of Pharmacotherapy*, *40*(5), 836–849. doi:10.1345/aph.1G226 PMID:16670364

Whitman, M. (2001). Understanding the perceived need for complementary and alternative nutraceuticals: Lifestyle issues. *Clinical Journal of Oncology Nursing*, *5*, 190–194. PMID:11899764

Wildman, R. E. C., & Medeiros, D. M. (2000). Food in relation to the human body. In Advance Human Nutrition. CRC Press.

Wolever, T. M. S., & Jenkins, D. J. A. (1986). The use of the glycemic index in predicting the blood glucose response to mixed meals. *The American Journal of Clinical Nutrition*, *43*, 167–172. PMID:3942088

Wu, Y. H., Zhou, C. X., Li, X. P., Song, L., Wu, X., Lin, W., & Zhao, Y. et al. (2006). Evaluation of antiinflammatory activity of the total flavonoids of aggerapterodonta on acute and chronic inflammation models. *Phytotherapy Research*, *20*(7), 585–590. doi:10.1002/ptr.1918 PMID:16673449

Yamaguchi, M. (2008). β-cryptoxanthin and Bone Metabolism: The Preventive Role in Osteoporosis. *Journal of Health Science*, *54*(4), 356–369. doi:10.1248/jhs.54.356

Yang, N. C., Jeng, K. C., Ho, W. M., & Hu, M. L. (2002). ATP depletion is an important factor in DHEA-induced growth inhibition and apoptosis in BV-2 cells. *Life Sciences*, *70*(17), 1979–1988. doi:10.1016/S0024-3205(01)01542-9 PMID:12148690

Yeum, K. J., Aldini, G., Russell, R. M., & Krinsky, N. I. (2009). Antioxidant/Prooxidant Actions of Carotenoids. In Carotenoids: Nutrition and Health. Birkhauser Verlag Basel.

You, S. J., Udenigwe, C. C., Aluko, R. E., & Wu, J. (2010). Multifunctional peptides from egg white lysozyme. *Food Research International*, *43*(3), 848–855. doi:10.1016/j.foodres.2009.12.004

Young, V. R. (1994). Adult amino acid requirements: The case for a major revision in current recommendations. *The Journal of Nutrition*, *124*(8), 1517S–1523S. PMID:8064412

Zoetendal, E. G., Raes, J., van den Bogert, B., Arumugam, M., Booijink, C. C., Troost, F. J., & Kleerebezem, M. et al. (2012). The human small intestinal microbiota is driven by rapid uptake and conversion of simplecarbohydrates. *The ISME Journal*, *6*(7), 1415–1426. doi:10.1038/ismej.2011.212 PMID:22258098

Chapter 7
Phytoparmaceuticals and Its Applications in Therapy

Alejandra Hernández-Ceruelos
Cuerpo Académico de Salud Pública, Área Académica de Medicina, Universidad Autónoma del Estado de Hidalgo, Mexico

Sergio Muñoz-Juarez
Cuerpo Académico de Salud Pública, Área Académica de Medicina, Universidad Autónoma del Estado de Hidalgo, Mexico

Patricia Vázquez-Alvarado
Cuerpo Académico de Salud Pública, Área Académica de Odontología, Universidad Autónoma del Estado de Hidalgo, Mexico

ABSTRACT

Medicinal plants have been used to treat illnesses since medicine began. Nowadays, 80% of the population in the planet uses drugs directly or indirectly derived from plants. In the past, natural products were used empirically; people experimented with them as helpful for their well-being and learned to treat ailments with specific plants. Henri Leclerc introduced the terminology of phytotherapy into medical science and this concept refers to study of the use of extracts of natural origin as medicines or health-promoting agents. Usually pharmacology isolates an active compound from a given plant, phytotherapy aims to reserve the complexity of constituents from a plant with moderately less processing. Phytopharmaceuticals (PP) are composed by one plant species or by complex mixtures of plants, presented in a natural or in a pharmaceutical form. The tendency is to use standardized plant extracts in the formulation, obtained by a patented extraction process. PP need to fulfill the same requirements as other medical products: safety, efficacy and consistent quality.

CONCEPTS

Medicinal plants are the source of raw materials for traditional medicine such as, Ayurvedic, Chinese, Unani, Homeopathy, and Siddha but also for modern medicine base in natural products. These days, plant materials are used in industrial scale as home remedies, over-the-counter drugs, and ingredients

DOI: 10.4018/978-1-5225-0754-3.ch007

for the pharmaceutical industry. They represent a substantial proportion of the market around the world, especially in developing countries (*Bardaranayake, 2006).*

The concept phytopharmaceutical is derived from the Greek root *Phyton* which means plant and *Pharmakon* which means medicine. The literal translation is a drug based on a plant. Phytotopharmaceuticals must be considered as drugs, whose active compounds are exclusively plant based, and they are constituted of plant parts, extracts, juices or distillates. The conception is that a plants or parts of them are therapeutic entities in phytotherapy (Wichyl, 2004).

The term phytomedicine was first introduced by Henry Le Clerc (1870-1955) and it is related to the therapeutic application of medicinal plants. Today phytomedicine is defined as the science or the art to use of botanical medicine to prevent or treat illnesses (Braun, 2010).

The term "herbal medicine" is full of misconceptions, related to the diversity of its approaches. Herbal medicine can be categorized into three general groups: phytotherapy over-the-counter, herbal medicine and traditional herbalism. Among these, phytotherapy is the one that follows scientific methodology and generates results related to the effects of the phytopharmaceutical. Based on the general principles of phytotherapy, plant material contains a number of pharmacologically active compounds, and they should be seen as a single unit. For example, an extract can be standardized, in order to contain a well characterized concentration of active compounds and then could be tested for a clinical condition (Mohamed, Shuid, Borhanuddin & Fozi 2012).

In 2002 the botanical trade of herbs and medicinal plants, in the U.S.A. was estimated, a retail of approximately US$ 1.6 billion. China with exports of over 120,000 tons and India with some 32,000 tons per year, both dominated the international markets. It was estimated that Europe, annually imported about 40,000 tons of medicinal plants with a market value of US$ 1 billion form Africa and Asia. For foreign-exchange reserves the medicinal plants are a new contributor beginning to emerge. To satisfy the demands on this growing market, some analyses are being conducted to unearth new plant sources of herbal remedies and medicines (Dasture 2002).

Medicinal plants are a major resource base for the traditional medicine and pharmaceutical industry; they also provide health security and livelihood to a huge part of Indian population. In 2015, there is a new renaissance in traditional and alternative health care systems, resulting in world herbal trade which stands at US a $ 120 billion marked. It is expected to reach US$ 7 trillion by 2050. The National Medicinal Plants Board (NMPB) set-up in November 2000 by the Government of India has the primary mandate of coordinating all matters relating to medicinal plants and support policies and programs for growth of trade, export, conservation and cultivation. The Board is located in the Department of Ayurveda, Yoga & Naturopathy, Unani, Siddha & Homeopathy (AYUSH) of the Ministry of Health & Family Welfare (National Medicinal Plants Board, 2015).

PP are multicomponent mixtures of natural origin either in the crude state or as pharmaceutical formulation and their use increases due to the advantages in the therapy of several diseases such as good tolerability. They need to fulfill the same requirements as other medicinal products safety, efficacy and consistent quality. Usually, standard pharmacology separates and purifies a single active compound from a specific plant; on the other hand phytotherapy aims to preserve the complex mix of active compounds from it, avoiding the necessity of more processes (Schweim & Schwewim 2014).

Standardized PP must have a specific content and concentration of diverse active metabolites well characterized that will act as the active drug Substances with exogenous origin have to be quantified and they have to be under the limits recommended by the regulatory agencies of every country (Zuin & Vilegas, 2000).

HISTORY

Since ancient times the plant kingdom has supplied mankind not only with food and raw materials but also with potent medications. Plants are natural chemical factories producing thousands of different metabolites which exhibit a multitude of biological activities (Rischer & Oksman- Caldentey, 2005). Nowadays, around the world 80% of the global population uses medicines, derived directly or indirectly from plants. Worldwide, such medicines are equivalent to the 25% of the pharmaceutical battery. The use of medicinal plants is particularly important in the Chineses health system. Other regions of the planet with a wide use of natural products for therapy are Africa, South and Central America, India, Tibet, Indonesia and Pacific Islands. (Bhattaram et al., 2002).

Traditionally, people through history have experienced with natural products and they had discovered which plant was useful for their health, in that way they learned empirically to treat specific illnesses (Ciuman 2012). The first evidence about the use of ancient medicinal plants were discovered in prehistoric graves with an antiquity of 60,000 years (Bhattaram et al., 2002). The oldest records for the usage of medicinal plants date back to 5000 B.C. in clay tablets form Mesopotamia. Sheng-Nongs Herbal Book, document the use of herbs in China, dated back to 3000 B.C. and included use of 365 plants, animals and minerals useful as medication. In Egypt Ebers papyrus was written in 1534 B.C. describe medicinal uses for plants as, it presents a group of 8000 prescriptions referring to the use of 700 plants like pomegranate, castor oil plant, aloe, garlic, onion among others (Petrovska, 2012).

The Ayurvedic and Chinese Traditional Medicine systems date back to ancient time, with an ever-expanding knowledge of plant properties and their medicinal qualities that were preserved in ancient texts. This body of knowledge has been constantly updated and passed down to newer generations in revised versions, while preserving its originality and values. Currently, only China has a frequently updated inventory of traditional medicines used, with India starting to initiate similar efforts. The Chinese government is one of the most active governments in the world in promoting the use of traditional medicine and integrating it with allopathic, conventional medicine (Mohamed et al., 2012).

In ancient Greece the works of Hippocrates enclosed 300 therapeutic plants with some physiological effect. In Rome, Pliny the elder and Galen documented the use many plants. During the middle ages the expertise for therapeutic procedures, cultivation of medicinal plants and preparation of medicines were monopolized on monasteries. While in old times the medicinal plants were primarily used as infusions, decoctions and macerations, during the 16th and 18th centuries, the necessity of plants or their compounds as drugs increased. During the 19th century the discovery, organic compounds and isolations of alkaloids and glycosides marked the turning point for the beginning of scientific pharmacy, including the discovery of tannins, saponosides, etheric oils, vitamins and hormones (Petrovska, 2012).

In several parts of the world there have been continued uses of plats in the folklore medicine. The chemical scrutiny during the 19th century and preference was given to plants which gave pharmacologically active compounds. Paul Erhlich at the Institute for Experimental Therapy in Frankfurt Germany was a pioneer to propound his theories on drug action and plants as an important source of drugs (Amuka 2013).

Seidler defined for the first time the term Pharmacognosy as a discipline of the pharmaceutical sciences in 1815. His definition was: ‘‘With the name Pharmacognosy we mean the science which has the task to learn everything about drugs originating from plants or animals in all aspects, except under the physiological effect, to describe them correctly and under a general vision connect this knowledge’’ (Gurib-Fakim 2006).

Chemical synthesis lifted the focus of drug discovery efforts from looking at natural sources to the laboratory synthesis in the late 1980s. Of the 1,135 new drugs approved from 1981 to 2010, 50% were natural derivatives and analogues (Cragg and Newman 2013). Harshberger in 1896 defined the term Ethnobotany as “a study of plants used by primitive and aboriginal people”. In 1916, the concept was extended by Robbins, Harrington and Freire-Marreco, and they suggested that Ethnobotany should include the research and evaluation of the effects of the vegetal environment upon the life customs and all phases of life amongst not only in primitive societies, as well as beliefs and history of these tribal peoples knowledge'' (Gurib-Fakim, 2006).

At the beginning of the twenty first century there has been a tendency in the pharmaceutical industry and it is to return to natural sources as possible new drugs. Various nature-origin phytochemicals such as essential oils, alkaloids, stilbenoids, polysaccharides, polyphenols have renewed the attention on them as therapeutic drugs for their biological activities (Xiao, 2015).

Historically, apothecaries and then pharmaceutical corporations to produce relatively crude therapeutic formulations have used plant extracts. In the last half of the twentieth century, drug preparations of partly purified natural products became typical prior to single molecule medicines (David et al., 2014).

PP contain a mainly constituent responsible its mechanism of action, It also has auxiliary components, supporting and structure stabilizing compounds or they are made of different herbs that will increase therapeutic effect (Ciuman, 2012).

PHYTOPHARMACEUTICAL PRODUCTION

Natural products or secondary metabolites are the result of millions of years of evolutions of terrestrial and marine organism adapting to various abiotic and biotic stresses. They are therefore encoded to be bioactive (Lamottke, Ripoll & Walzack, 2011). Plants are natural chemical factories producing thousands of different metabolites with a multitude of biological activities to support their sessile lifestyle; only a minimal percentage of the total known herbal species have been studied chemically to some extent (Rischer & Oksman- Caldentey, 2005).

Plants, similar to all life species, are affected by the interaction with the environment where they grow and live. Therefore, secondary metabolites are produced for the adaptation of the plants to particular conditions. The concentration of secondary metabolites can also vary from one part of the plant to another depending on the stimulus that triggers their production (Harborne & Williams, 2000).

Considering quality as one of the main factors related to consumer acceptance and sustainability in the market, it is important to strictly control and standardize all the stages involved in the production of PP preparations, such as the selection of the starting plant material, the extraction conditions, and the quantification of secondary metabolites or bioactive compounds in the final product (Cortés-Rojas et al., 2012).

Plants that are used as fresh ingredients for the industry are provided through direct collection or by cultivation, with their own disadvantages and advantages. For the industry, the method of farming a plant is the chosen one, as it is better for the control the entire supply chain and the chemical variation will decrease. The use of cultivated medicinal plants eliminates adulteration or misidentification of plant material. One weaknesses of the cultivation method is that the product is much more expensive than the one harvested in the wild. Another disadvantage is that many of the medicinal plants are difficult to cultivate, they grow slow and the farmers must invest a money before they can have any economical profit. (Lubbe & Verpoorte, 2011).

Quality and safety of the fresh herbal material depend on many factors, some intrinsic as plant´s genetic and other external such as environment, the way they are harvested or collected from the wild, the post-harvest transportation, storage and process., Unintentional pollution by microscopic species or chemical compounds through any manufacture phases can also lead to deterioration in the quality of the herbal product. When medicinal plants are harvested from the wild population, they might be mixed with other type or plant parts through misidentification of the species, an accidental contamination or deliberated adulteration. All of this will have hazardous consequences (WHO 2003).

Uncontrolled production conditions may lead to an increasing risk of microbial contamination. Thus microbial spoilage of the raw herbal material is one of the factors governing the global market of herbs. Although a large range of microorganisms can be found in herbs, including bacteria, yeasts and moulds. Despite the beneficial effects of herbs, some microorganisms and their metabolites can be found which could lead to serious health problems. Among the microorganisms that may be present, moulds are the most relevant, mainly due to their mycotoxins production capacity (Santos et al., 2013).

Regulation and sustainable methods for wild harvesting must be implemented in order to protect the species of medicinal. A long-term alternative solution would be to promote the domestic cultivation of medicinal plants. Farming also unlocks the opportunity of applying biotechnology in order to resolve complications that are characteristic to the production of herbal medicines. Farming offers the occasion to improve yield and accomplish a uniform, high quality product. (Canter, Thomas & Ernts 2005).

The use of controlled environment system for the production of medicinal plants has a potential to provide mass quantities of consistent standardized and optimized plant material free of biotic and abiotic contamination. Selection, breeding and cloning of higher specific genotypes and the chemical characterization of medicinally active constituents can be achieved and thus the applications of this technology has a significant potential (Zobayed, Afreen & Kozai, 2005)

Farming of certain herbs has showed to be problematic since they have low germination or particular environmental necessities. There might just be a lack of information about the detailed requirements for pollination, seed germination and development. Low growth rates often are the result of mycological infection or mechanical injury to seeds. The improvement on germination can be achieve by seed treatments or by warranting the optimum storing conditions. Stratification, as well as, artificial imitation of the environment is needed for seed germination, for example, it may be necessary to soak or chill them in order to have a successful sprout. (Canter et al., 2005).

The metabolic composition of plants is the result of enzymatic activity, which in turn is ultimately controlled by genes regulating the biosynthetic pathways at different levels. Controlled growth systems can also make possible to contemplate the manipulation of phenotypic difference in the concentration of medicinally important metabolites. This controlled production increases the potency of the plant, it reduce toxin levels and provide a standardized extracts. The objective compounds are virtually always secondary metabolites, which may vary in concentration depending on temperature and light conditions like with the antioxidants, stress can alter the concentration of proline, infection decreases the rate of flavonoids and herbivore fauna affects the concentration of alkaloids. (Mc Chesney 1999).

When plants are cultivated in a controlled environment, where climatic aspects and disturbance could be observed at as uniform, the quality of secondary metabolites of a specific plant would be established with some grade of predictability (Ncube et al., 2012).

The ideal time to harvest medicinal plants should be during the period to ensure the fabrication of finished herbal products of the finest likely quality. The best period for harvest must be determined according to the quality and amount of biologically active constituents rather than the by the total vegetative harvested, considering the quality top season and the time of day for the targeted medicinal plant parts. During harvest, precautions should be taken to avoid foreign matter, wild plant material or toxic plants are mixed with the collected therapeutic plant of interest (WHO 2003).

Before processing for quality control, there must be taken final samples, dividing the average into four. Every portion most be representative of the raw material. The final samples are tested for the following characteristics (WHO 1998):

- Grade of fragmentation measure with the sieve test
- Determination and quantification of impurities
- Moistness degree and ash content
- Concentration of active metabolites

For standardization there are two classifications. The first category correspond to the "true" standardization, where a certain phytochemical or group of metabolites that are known to be the responsible of the therapeutic activity. For example, *Ginkgo biloba* contains 26% of ginkgo flavones and 6% terpenes. These metabolites are very much concentrated and no longer denote the whole herb, therefore it is considered as PP. However the industrial process may result in the loss of effectiveness and potentiate the adverse side-effects or increase the herb–drug interactions. The second kind of standardization, based itself on manufacturers assuring the presence of an specific percentage of some compounds as markers of therapeutic capacity or quality of the herbal product (Bandaranayake, 2006)

Harvest, drying, and storage conditions can also influence the value of the fresh material. Therefore, these techniques need to be seriously standardized as well. Moreover, processing of the raw material to the finished product can influence the constituents and, consequently, the quality of the final product. Dissimilar polarity of the solvent and a different method of extraction lead to obtain an extract preparation with considerably different concentrations of the active compounds. Besides, external pollutants like heavy metals, pesticides or aflatoxins have to be considered (Bauer, 1998).

Post-harvest modification of plant metabolites must be concern, as it can lead to significant variations due to plant internal enzymes like hydrolases (glycosidases), peroxidases or polyphenol oxidases (Bucar, Wube & Schmid,2013). Moreover, processing of the raw product to the finished material should influence the concentration and kind of constituents and consequently the quality of the formulation (Bauer 1998).

PHYTOPHARMACEUTICAL FORMS

Either the dried plant of the extract derived from the plant is considered by definition the active substance. The use of special extracts has several advantages like the concentration of active substances can be raised and smaller amounts of the substance are needed to achieve the effect. Undesirable byproducts can be removed by the process of extraction, so that the PP will be better tolerated (Schweim & Schweim, 2014).

The part of the herb to be employed and its presentation depend on the intended use for the herb. In its natural state (fresh or dried) herbs are mainly marketed in herbal stores, but transformed into essential oils, aromas or extracts which are often used in the pharmaceutical, perfume, cosmetic, decor and food industries (Santos et al., 2013).

According to WHO (1996) Plant preparations consist of comminuted or pulverized plant parts, as well as, extracts, tinctures, fatty or essential oils, expressed juices and preparations whose production involves fractionation, purification or concentration. The manufacturing process must be described in fully detail. If any other materials are added during manufacture for adjusting the plant preparation to assured the level of active compound or the characteristic constituents or for any other reason, the additional ingredients should be declared in the manufacturing procedures. A technique for identification of the plant preparation should be added. If a proof of identity of an active principle is not possible, it must be adequate to pinpoint a characteristic constituent or mixture of substances, for example, the chromatographic fingerprint ensures reliability on the quality of the preparation.

Apart from the many advantages which cultivation can offer, the development of modern methods of processing and preserving the raw material of medicinal plants dehydration through drying in vacuum packs, liyophilisation, etc. helps to maintain their quality for a longer time (Capasso et al., 2000). For fresh plants, pharmaceutical forms include, fruit pulps, juices, press juices, gums, resin and balsams (List and Smith, 1989).

Herbal infusions are prepared by immersing the herb material with hot water or alcohol (ethanol) or a mixture of both. A decoction consists on rudely bruised herb material boiled in water for a definite period. Tinctures are solutions of the active principles of the plant in high concentration on alcohol and water as vehicle. These extraction procedures lead to the manufacture of the herbal preparations that go form of fresh juice, cold and hot infusions, decoctions, tinctures, gums, pastes and powders. The resulting remedies come in numerous forms, including oral tablets, capsules, gel caps, extracts, and infusions. Solid or powdered extracts are prepared by vaporization of the diluents used in the method of extraction of the raw material (Bandaranayake, 2006).

Extracting the compounds of importance from the non-soluble medium in which they are inserted needs more than a few issues to be taken into account. These include the polarity and stability of the extractives and the solvent, the purity of the solvent selected for the extraction, as well as, its toxicity, volatility and viscosity, besides the probability of artifact creation during the extraction method, and the total of bulk material. Secondary metabolites usually are inside the plant cells, thus crushing of the raw material and breaking tissue and cell integrity before extraction increases its output (Bucar et al., 2012). The solvents more frequently used for extraction in order of polarity are hexane, light petroleum, chloroform, ethyl acetate, alcohol and methanol (Van Beek & Montoro 2009)

For seeds, it is nearly impossible to extract oil from uncracked seeds using scCO2 or any organic solvent. Consequently, different milling procedures have been proposed in order to increase the interfacial surface and facilitate oil release from the seed. Flaking, chopping, and crushing were informed as the most effective pretreatments regarding to oil yield after. The pretreatment of canola seeds include to be heated at 55 °C and 36 MPa. For amaranth seeds, the method of flouring in a Tema mill resulted more effective than only crushing and blending in complete breaking of the rind making possible to achieve the highest rate and yield (Ivanovic et al., 2014).

The majority of separation and purification methods still use simple extraction procedures with solvents of different polarity, water and their mixtures. The methods include maceration, percolation, Soxhlet extraction, ultrasound-assisted extraction and turbo-extraction (Bucar et al., 2012). The standardization of herbal preparations industrial process is the basic necessity for the establishment of reproducible and consistent quality of herbal preparations. Since different manufacturing processes can lead to different extract quality, it cannot be transferred into a product by applying analytical methods, if the extract was not produced under the same standarized conditions. (Bauer 1998).

Extraction method may change the concentration of metabolites. For example, in *Hypericum perforatum* (St. John´s Wort), aqueous preparations made from tea bags, contain the complete flavone glycoside spectrum as well as hypericine, but biapigenin and hyperforin however, are not soluble in water, then it can be extracted in an infusion. Ethanol and methanol extract a good quality of flavonoids. On the other hand hypericin and pseudohypericin have not been confirmed in hypericum oils (Meier, 2001).

Although dry herbal extracts are more stable in comparison to their aqueous form, they have a complex conformation and hold a number of active molecules and hydrophilic compounds with a tendency to absorb moisture leading to microbial growth and hydrolysis The incorporation of dry extracts into granulated dosage forms is a suitable alternative to overcome such issues. Pellets are a multiparticulate drug delivery system; they provide several technological and therapeutic benefits since they consist of a "multiple unit" dosage form with a well-defined diameter of 0.5-2 mm and minimum surface/volume ratio, which ensures a good drug dissolution ratio, fewer irritation of the intestinal tract and lower risk of side effects (Beringhs et al., 2013)

Maceration is performed at room temperature by immersing the plant material in a solvent with eventual stirring. The advantage of this method is that offers modest extraction conditions but implies high solvent consumption, long period of and small extraction yields. Extraction efficiency is upgraded by percolation, for example, packing the pre-soaked plant material in a container that allows the constantly controlled subtraction of the extract via a valve at the bottom and adding fresh solvent from the top. Other method is Soxhlet extraction a popular method due to its reduced solvent consumption; however, thermo-labile compounds can be despoiled during the process. For liquid samples, the extraction with organic solvents or mixtures of then can be done, either simply in a separating funnel or similar to a Soxhlet apparatus in a perforator (Bucar 2012).

Essential oils are used primarily as natural preservatives, flavourants and fragrances in cosmetic products. In addition, studies related to biological properties of oils have been intensified, indicating ectoparasitic, insect repellent, anticholinesterase anti- diarrheal, antimicrobial and cytotoxic activities. Several pharmacopeias possess monographs of plants which are good sources of essential oils. Since these complex mixtures are also used as raw material for different approaches, some of them have specific essential oils monographs with parameters of quality such as density, refractive index and optical rotation (Fernandes et al., 2013)

For the preparation of solid or powdered extracts, there must be evaporation of the solvents used in the process of extraction of the raw plant. Phytotherapeutic agents are significantly concentrated in order to improve their beneficial efficacy. During the manufacturing process, it is possible to remove some secondary compounds present in the plants, which may provoke unwanted side effects. By definition the extracts must also contain marker compounds which are, chemically well-defined constituents that are of interest for control purposes, and not necessary related to any therapeutic activity (Bandaranayake, 2006).

Spray drying is a technique commonly employed for the micro-encapsulation of herbal-extract-based compositions using several wall materials, such as carbohydrates, gums and proteins. Nevertheless, spray dried powders might present some disadvantages, such as small particle sizes and low densities, leading to inadequate flow and reconstitution properties, which are responsible for difficulties in further product handling. Fluidization is a promising alternative technology, which allows for the simultaneous drying, encapsulation and agglomeration of herbal compositions in a single step, reducing operation costs, saving time and generating a coarse product with improved physicochemical properties adequate for further processing in pharmaceutical, food and agricultural sectors (Benelli et al., 2015). Spray dried extracts have high stability, are easier to handle, standardize, transport and store that liquid forms (Couto et al., 2013).

QUALITY CONTROL

For propose of performing quality control of PP there are three important definitions:

Identity: confirming the herb is the herb the one that should be
Purity: Is free of contaminants
Content or Assay: The active compounds are within the defined limits

From a regulatory perspective the formulation of herbal pharmacopoeia and monographs is gaining increasing priority worldwide to standardize natural medicines. The American herbal pharmacopoeia, British herbal pharmacopoeia and European Scientific Cooperative on Phytotherapy (ESCOP) monographs have already established a trend of formulating referred texts on plant medicines (Dahami, 2013).

Published monographs in a pharmacopeia are the most practical approach for quality control of herbal drugs and there are many available. When pharmacopeial monographs are unavailable, development and validation of analytical procedures have to be carried out by the manufacturer. The best strategy is to follow closely the pharmacopeial definitions of identity, purity, and content or assay. Valuable sources for general analytical procedures are included in the pharmacopeias, in guidelines published by the WHO (Bandaranayake, 2006).

Monographs contain the a description of the herb, including all the botanical data, the methods for laboratory analysis, therapeutic indications, and if the plant may interact with some drugs Monographs, talk about the traditional and standardized therapeutic uses of herbs, therefore, they provide a foundation for clinical practice. (Lee, 1999).

For a thoughtful quality management, the definition of individual quality criteria and specifications are a must for every PP form. The specific criteria have to be contained in a monograph or a master file in a similar way to the specified in a monograph of a National Pharmacopea, but according to Bauer (1998) every monograph most include for quality:

1. Proof of identity
2. Sensoric features
3. Fingerprint-chromatograms
4. Purity
5. Moisture
6. Ash
7. Physical constants
8. Solvent residues
9. Content of active principle or lead compound
10. Biological activity description

And for safety the methods to determine:

1. Microbiological contamination
2. Foreign materials
3. Heavy metals
4. Pesticide residues
5. Aflatoxins
6. Radioactivity
7. Adulterations

The quality control of PP is closely linked to the concentrations of their chemical constituents. Their major components are slightly different according to their growing conditions, which such as topographical origin; therefore, there must be a selection of only several specific components as essential quality criteria. That is the reason why characteristic chromatographic fingerprint is developed (Yi et al., 2008).

Methods of standardization have to take into consideration the very complete aspects that contribute to the quality of the herbal drugs, that is the correct identity of the sample, organoleptic evaluation, pharmacognostic evaluation, volatile matter, quantitative evaluation like ash residues or extractive values, as well as, phytochemical evaluation, and tests for quantify the presence of xenobiotics, microbial load, toxicity, and biological activity. The phytochemical profile is of special significance since it is directly associated to the activity of the herbal drugs (Rajani & Kanaki 2008).

For the past years, the chromatographic fingerprints is a well-known method that is based on high-performance liquid chromatography (HPLC), capillary electrophoresis fingerprint (CEFP), gas chromatography (GC), Capillary electrophoresis (CE) and ultra- performance liquid (UPLC). Those methods have been accepted as rapid and reliable means for identification and qualification of herbal drugs (Wei-Jun, et al. 2009). UPLC system using high linear velocities with columns packed with porous 1.7 miliparticles improves radically the peak resolution, sensitivity and speed of analysis (Wei-Jung et al., 2009)

Thin layer chromatography fingerprinting is a very useful tool for PP made up of essential oils, resins, and gums, since they are complex mixtures of compounds that no longer have any organic structure. It is a dominant and fairly rapid solution to distinguish between chemical classes, where macroscopy and microscopy will fail. Chromatograms of essential oils, are broadly published in the scientific literature, making easier the identification. HPLC is the preferred method for quantitative analysis of more complex mixtures. Yet the separation of volatile components such as essential and fatty oils can be achieved with HPLC, it is best accomplished by GC or GC/MS. Founded on the concept of photoequivalence, the chromatographic fingerprints of PP can be used to make a statement the matter of quality control. Systems based on information theory, similarity estimation, chemical pattern recognition, spectral correlative chromatograms, multivariate resolution, the combination of chromatographic fingerprints and chemometric evaluation for evaluating fingerprints are all potent tools for quality control of PP. (Bandaranayake, 2006).

Metabolomics is a systematic study of the unique chemical fingerprints that specific cellular processes leave behind, specifically the study of small molecule metabolite profiles. Nuclear magnetic resonance and mass sprectrometry, are analytical tools that along with diverse types of chromatography system are employed in metabolomics fingerprinting for the detection of metabolites, giving a pattern recognition for quality control (Van der Kooy, et al., 2009).

Stability and consistency of processed and manufactured products are issues often neglected in the herbal arena with relatively few studies published on these topics. Modern analytical techniques in conjunction with the above information should enable the development of meaningful criteria for the shelf-life of herbal products and ensure processing techniques retain herbal efficacy in endproducts (Wills, Bone & Morgan, 2000).

The United States Pharmacopeia (USP) and National Formulary together with the FDA and they have published authoritative standards for many botanical supplements. Doctors should advise their patients to only purchase products carrying NF or USP logotypes on their labels. Consecutively, patients can be advised to select producers from their own countries or those in Europe as well as Japan and Australia, since their herbal medicines by law must be made according the code of pharmaceutical Good Manufacturing Practice (Pribitkin, 2005).

Unlike pharmaceuticals, the literature regarding stability of herbal remedies is scant, which may be due to inadequate analytical methods and standards or scarce reporting. Since the quantification of constituents in herbal products is difficult, assumptions are often made in a way that the purity and potency is retained as long as appearance of a product remains unchanged, which is un-scientific. Therefore, it is imperative to carry out proper stability studies on extracts as well as herbal products. Stability of a product is affected by a number of physical factors such as temperature, moisture and light, and chemical factors such as hydrolysis, oxidation, polymerization and isomerisation. Temperature allows the rate of degradation of active components due to promote an increase in their kinetic energy resulting in the fraction of colliding molecules. Moisture contents increase the rate of decomposition and make the product susceptible to hydrolysis. In case of herbal crude powders or extracts, it facilitates the growth of microbes which not only deteriorate the constituents but may also produce toxic substances. Decomposition of pharmaceutical preparation because of the oxidation is nearly as probable as that with hydrolysis and the rate of oxidation is also temperature related. For example, the rate of fatty acids peroxidation accelerates as the temperature exceeds 50°C. Polymerizations, addition of similar molecules, isomerisation, and the variation of isomeric forms, are the additional factors affecting the stability. Sunlight as a form of energy also facilitates the degradation and affects the stability of pharmaceuticals. The temperature and sunlight are particularly important for extracts containing volatile and photo-labile constituents. Increase in temperature and exposure to sunlight decreases the activation energy and helps molecules to cross the energy barrier to start a reaction (Khalid et al., 2011).

Most herbal extracts exhibit a fair degree of hygroscopicity although the opposite phenomenon "efflorescence" is not uncommon. Hygroscopicity information and extent of the same are very important in formulation of solid dosage forms, as it will have serious implications of the manufacture steps, environmental controls on the manufacturing, design of packs and packaging, and most importantly on the stability and microbial qualities of the material and formulations (Anantha- Narayana, 2013).

Lipid-based drug delivery systems have been explored in various researches and have revealed their capacity for controlled and targeted drug delivery. Pharmacosomes are amphophilic phospholipid complexes of drugs bearing active hydrogen that bind to phospholipids. They improve the biopharmaceutical properties to the drug, resulting in better bioavailability. Phytosomes are new mixtures comprising of lipophilic complexes of components of plant origin like *Silybum Marianum, Ginkgo Biloba,* Ginseng. They are also called as phytolipids delivery system. They have an extraordinary lipophilicity, which improves bioavailability and therapeutic properties. These are advanced form of PP have improved pharmacokinetic and pharmacological parameter, whose end result can valuably be used in treatment of acute liver diseases, either metabolic or infective origin. Phytosomes are manufactured by a patent process in which individual constituent of herbal extract like flavonolignans and terpenoids are united on a molecular level to the phospholipids like phosphatidylcholine through a polar end. Phytosomes that are used as a medicament have also a wide scope in cosmetology. Phytosomes forms are a bridge between the convectional delivery system and novel delivery system. As herbal novel drug delivery systems have lot of possible applications, several researchers are working to develop a novel drug delivery systems like mouth dissolving tablets, sustained and extended release formulations, mucoadhesive systems, transdermal dosage forms, microparticles, microcapsules, nanoparticles, implants etc. (Devy, Jain & Valli, 2010).

Ma and colleagues investigated the effect and mechanism of Shuanghua aerosol on upper respiratory tract infections in children aged from 3 to 14 years. Shuanghua aerosol consists of *Flos Chrysanthemum Indicum, Flos Lonicera, Herba Houttuynia, Radix Bupleurum* and menthene. The control treatment was Shuanghuanglian aerosol which consists of *Flos Lonicera, Fructus Forsythia* and *Radix Scutellaria*. The authors conclude that the aerosol has obvious anti-inflammatory and antiviral effects and has a good healing effect in treating infantile upper respiratory tract infections (Ma, Duan & Wang, 2000).

Another pharmaceutical form used in PP are the microcapsules that entrapped herbal water-soluble extracts, for example, *Calendula officinalis* L. was set by layer-by-layer adsorption of carrageenan and oligochitosan onto calcium carbonate microparticles with their subsequent dissolving after the treatment of EDTA. The entrapment was performed by using adsorption and co-precipitation techniques. The co-precipitation provided better entrapment of the calendula into the carbonate matrix compared to adsorption. *In vitro* release kinetics was studied using artificial gastric juice. Using the model of acetate ulcer in rats, it has been demonstrated that the extract of calendula released from the microcapsules speeded up gastric tissue repair (Borodina et al., 2008).

Nanoparticles and nanoemulsions are colloidal systems with particles varying in size from 10 nm to 1000 nm. In nanoparticle systems particle size is well determined, above the 100 nm is the standardized measure, but they have also been reported in literature even higher than 200 nm. Nanoparticles might also be defined as submicronic colloidal systems. The nanospheres have a matrix type structure in which the active ingredient is dispersed throughout while the nanocapsules have a polymeric membrane and an active ingredient core. Nanonization holds many advantages, such as increasing compound solubility, reducing medicinal doses, and improving the absorbency of herbal medicines compared with the respective crude drugs preparations (Saraf, 2010).

Nanoparticles of traditional Chinese herbs are helpful to increase their absorption and distribution and effects in the body. Chinese herbs, including peach seed, safflower, angelica root, *Szechwan lovage rhizome, Rehmannia root,* red peony root, leech, gadfly, earth worm and ground beetle, were mixed and set through drying, mincing, extracting, crushing into liquid particles with ultrasonic wave, filtering and nanometerizing into nanoparticles with nanometer collider. Nanoparticles of the herbs showed significant thrombolytic effects, consequentialy there was a quick recovery from arterial embolism and diminution of thrombi. The thrombolytic effects of nanoparticles were much intensified than their non-nanoparticle form (Shen et al., 2008).

Administration of medication via micro particulate systems is beneficial because microspheres can be ingested or injected and they can be design for a desired release rate and be used for site-specific delivery of drugs. They also can offer organ-targeted release.A series of plant active ingredients, such as rutin, camptothecin, zedoary oil, tetrandrine, quercetine and *Cynara scolymus* extract has been prepared into microspheres (Saraf, 2010).

A study on palatal mucoadhesive tablet holding an herbal formulation showed the constant release abilities. The ingredients of the herbal formulation i.e. sage, Echinacea, Lavender and Mastic gum have previously demonstrated antimicrobial activity. In the study, the herbal formulation included these four herbal medicinal incorporated into a slow dissolving mucoadhesive tablet, designed to fit the palate. Results indicated that the adhesive tablet containing the herbal formulations were effective in reducing oral malodor and volatile sulfur compounds levels responsible of the bad breath (Devy et al., 2010).

Furthermost of the PP formulation is administered orally since it is very convenient for the patient and also for their manufacturing advantages compared with other dosage forms. For the oral drug, there are two critical slower rate-determining steps in absorption. If the drug is hydrophilic by high aqueous solubility, then dissolution is going to be rapid and the absorption of such drugs will have a degree of permeation from side to side of the biomembrane (Gunasekaran 2014).

The absence of technical-practical training related to phytotherapy during professional development is considered the main obstacle on prescribing phytotherapy in primary services. Integration of PP and medicinal plant could improve access to therapeutic options in the first level of attention (Antonio, Tesser & Moretti-Pires, 2014).

Beyond actions of several compounds on more than a only target, it is suggested to also stand up from mutual interactions of related chemical moieties at both the pharmacokinetic and pharmacodynamic level (Zadoyan & Fuhr, 2012). PP are metabolized by phase I/II enzymes, including cytochrome P450 enzymes (CYP) and glucuronosyltransferases (UGTs) and also processed by phase II transporters such as P-glycoprotein (Pgp), increasing the likelihood of hepatotoxicity. While cytochrome P450-mediated herb-drug interactions have been widely analyzed, the effects of herbal extracts and constituents on UDP-glucuronosyl transferase (UGT) enzymes have been less studied. *In vitro* and *in vivo* studies showed that noni, St. John's wort, grape seed, milk thistle, hawthorn, green tea, *Ginkgo biloba*, soy, cranberry, and valerian are rich in phytochemicals that modify UGT enzymes. However, the *in vivo* consequences of these interactions are not well understood (Eichhorn, Greten & Efferth, 2011).

CLINICAL TRIALS

Clinical trials must be performed according to a protocol that has been written and approved by the Research and Ethics Committees before the study begins. The acceptable protocols are those that are the ones designed with a multidisciplinary team of experts of various disciplines. The trial protocol ought to include a justification for the trial and a very clear defined the question of research that the trial will answer. The population under study must also be well-defined, demonstrating both inclusion and exclusion criteria and the techniques to be used for enrolling participants into the study (WHO1990).

Pharmacological studies about synergistic effects must be confirmed in clinical trials. Particularly in comparison with synthetic standard drugs, the trials must use the same indication and equivalent dosages. Two hundred comparative, doble-blind, placebo controlled trials have been done using standardized mono- and multi extracts mixtures in contrast to standard drugs, indicating that synergistic effects of the compounds in the plant are the reason of this therapeutic equality (Wangner 2011).

Conditions for which consumers use phytomedicines in Germany, a country where herbal drugs are widely used, include: common cold (66%), flu 38%, digestive and or intestinal diseases (25%) stocmach ulcer (34%), nervousness (21%, circulatory disorders (15%), skin diseases (15%), fatigue and (exhaustion 12%). (Calixto, 2000).

Here are some examples of preclinical and clinical studies that scientifically support the use of PP.

Aloe vera

Aloe vera (family: Liliaceae) is one of the most familiar herbs in the world and the use in traditional medicine includes the succulent leaves. The gel of the leaf fresh or dry is obtained by cutting or slicing a leaf. A topical application of the gel offers great healing effect for the skin. *Aloe vera* contains many important nutrients, including B vitamins, amino acids and other nutrients good for health. Its pharmacological properties also include antioxidant capacity, wound healing, antibacterial, antifungal, and immunomodulating effects. Traditionally burn wound healing is one of major indications of *Aloe vera* gel, and this propertiy has been studied in several animal and clinical studies. Few studies have compared the efficacy of this gel with silver sulfadiazine in the treatment of burns in patients The findings of this clinical study showed that Aloe cream promoted burn wound healing more effectively tan silver sulfadiazine cream with smaller lesions and shorter healing times. The reepithelialization process was more rapidly in the skin of patients treated with aloe than in those treated with the silver compound. The mechanism of the remarkable efficacy of aloe cream in the healing of burn injuries may be elucidated by its antimicrobial, cell proliferation, and anti-inflammatory effects (Khorasani et al. 2009)

Reports have shown that polysaccharides isolated from *Aloe vera* demonstrated various pharmacological effects, such as antiinflammatory, wound healing, antihepatitis, antigastric ulcer, and antitumorigenicity in animals, although some side effects of Aloe have been found in humans. Hence, some experimental studies have been performed to confirm the upper dose of *Aloe vera* gel without any side effects to establish the maximal allowable daily intake of active Aloe (Radha & Laxmipriya 2015).

Loranthus ferrugineus

Loranthus ferrugineus (L. ferrugineus) from *Loranthaceae*, a mistletoe, is a medicinal herb used for a variety of human ailments. The results showed that mistletoe possesses a remarkable effect in concentration dependently inhibiting norepinephrine induced vasoconstriction. In addition, further examination showed that LFME can modulate norepinephrine induced aortic ring contraction through a reversible noncompetitive antagonism mechanism. *L. ferrugineus* antioxidant properties and effects on cholinergic pathways are of particular interest, because cholinergic abnormalities may affect memory or play a role in Alzheimer's disease: perhaps *L. ferrugineus* action on cholinergic pathways may explain its memory enhancement and gerontological effects that have been observed in elderly people. Extracts of mistletoe were tested on the isolated guinea pig ilium preparation *in vitro*, to test for gut contractility actions. Indeed, this work showed that crude extract retained the ability to dose dependently increase intestinal smooth muscle contractility. Importantly, these effects were significantly reduced upon pre-incubation with atropine, enhanced in the presence of neostigmine, and unchanged in the presence of hexamethonium, suggesting a direct cholinomimetic action via muscarinic receptor activation, and that bioactive constituents within *L. ferrugineus* serve as a substrate for intestinal AChE (Ameer et al., 2015).

Hypericum perforatum

Multiple clinical studies have shown St. John's Wort (*Hypericum perforatum*) to be effective and safe in the management of mild to moderate depression. Some studies, however, has reported interactions with various drugs. St John´s Wort is not indicated for severe depression Efficacy at least 80% of that of the synthetic drug offers a rationale for the preferred use of the studied *Hypericum* preparation mild to moderate depression (Behnke et al., 2002).

Bidens pilosa L.

Bidens pilosa L., Asteraceae, is a medicinal plant native of South America that nowadays is disseminated all over the world, mainly in tropical and subtropical regions. Flavonoids and other phenolic compounds of *Bidens pilosa* L., asteraceae, have been linked to its biological activities reported for this plant include antidiabetic, antitumoral, antimicrobial, hepatoprotective, and antioxidant. (Cortés-Rojas et al., 2012).

Isatis tinctoria L.

Isatis tinctoria L. (woad, Brassicaceae) has a long and well documented history as an indigo dye plant in temperate climates, and as a medicinal herb. *Isatis* extracts and selected constituents have been screened for antiviral, antifungal, antibacterial and cytoinhibitory activities. Tryptanthrin was originally isolated by Honda et al. (1980) as an antidermatophytic. The antimycobacterial activity of the compound against *Mycobacterium smegmatis* prompted a synthetic programme on indoloquinazoline derivatives. Tryptanthrin had been isolated from *Isatis tinctoria.* Tryptanthrin strongly inhibited COX-2 catalyzed eicosanoid synthesis in LPS-stimulated Mono Mac 6 cells (Hamburger, 2002).

Vitex agnus-castus

Most women (70–90%) experience premenstrual symptoms. A collection of these symptoms, that occurs regularly during the 2 weeks prior to menses and vanishes after the menstrual flow starts (and sufficiently severe to interfere with some aspects of life), is named premenstrual syndrome (PMS). Most frequent PMS signs are acne, breast swelling and tenderness, food cravings, swelling and weight gain, headache or joint pain, and psychological and emotional features. Headache, with undefined clinical characteristics, is regarded as a symptom of PMS. In fact, in migrainous women there is a close relationship between female sex hormone fluctuation and migraine. In the Middle Ages, Vitex agnus-castus is a hytopharmaceutical compound, considered worldwide to be a valid tool to treat PMS.VAC was used in Europe to suppress sexual urges and became a symbol of chastity (from this indication, popular names of ''Chaste Tree'' and ''Chasteberry''. Traditionally Vitex agnus-castus is a phytopharmaceutical compound, considered worldwide to be a valid tool to treat PMS. Vitex agnus-castus has been used to treat depression, sleep disorders, gynecological complaints (e.g. dysmenorrhoea, endometriosis, PMS, menopausal disorders), lactation disorders, anxiety, acne, flatulence, and to suppress appetite. Mainly this phytopharmaceutical have pharmacological activities that work on the reproductive steroid, dopaminergic, and opiatergic systems and modulate inflammation and it seems to be safe and well tolerated and could improve preventative management of both menstrual related and non-menstrual-related migraine headaches (Ambrosini, et al., 2013).

Pinus pinaster

In vitro, French maritime pine bark extract (*Pinus pinaster)* showed good antioxidant power, especially in the human low-density lipoprotein model. A study evaluated the effect of long term supplementation with the extract on rats and Syrian hamsters, especially on plasma antioxidant activity and atherosclerosis prevention Effective skin bleaching, firming and anti-wrinkle effects were observed after 28 days of 100 mg of extract intake per day, with a high level of safety. It represents an interesting alternative to topical products and supports the skin from the inside out (Piriou et al., 2014).

Ginko biloba l.

Ginkgo is broadly prescribed in Europe, particularly in France and Germany, for the management of intermittent claudication and cerebral insufficiency. The last concept is an unclear term that covers a range of complications such as absentmindedness, confusion, tiredness, lack of energy, lack of concentration, forgetfulness, and depression. Resulting of a review of 40 studies, Ginkgo was beneficial in cerebral insufficiency, because it improved mental function. It is not unexpected that researchers should try the use of Ginkgo towards degenerative conditions, some studies have showed and effect to some degree in improving cognitive functioning in patients with Alzheimer's disease (Wesnes, 2000).

Today, the evidence for the efficacy of EGb 761® an extract of Ginko, in the treatment of dementia syndromes has accumulated from a series of randomized, placebo-controlled, double-blind studies. EGb 761® not only improves memory and concentration but also enables patients with dementia to cope better with the demands of everyday life and alleviates neuropsychiatric symptoms. EGb 761® improved cognitive function, including attention and memory, in patients with mild cognitive impairment, with benefits visible even in those with very mild impairment. EGb 761® treatment was found effective in vestibular as well as in non-vestibular vertigo. The extract not only alleviated the severity of vertigo symptoms but also decreased the lateral sway amplitude in tests of equilibrium control. Likewise, EGb 761® attenuated the severity of dizziness associated with neurodegeneration in dementia disorders (Lang et al., 2013)

Panax ginseng

The roots of *Panax ginseng* C.A. Meyer have several triterpene glycosides named ginsenosides (or panaxosides), which contribute to the adaptogenic and physical performance augmenting properties of the ginseng extracts. They are used in old-style Chinese medicine to heal a large number of illnesses, ranging from dyspepsia, gastritis, insomnia, anaemia, abnormal blood pressure, *Diabetes mellitus*, and neurasthenia, overstrain and fatigue (Wesnes, 2000).

It had been demonstrated by clinical trials and animal experiments that Ginseng and its extract ginsenoside could alleviate cardiomyocyte ischemia, restrict myocardial infarction size, and exertmarked protection effect on myocardial reperfusion injury. More recent research revealed that cardiomyocyte apoptosis that is a key part in myocardial ischemia-reperfusion injury, and ginsenoside exerted an inhibitory effect upon cardiomyocyte apoptosis in ischemia-reperfusion injury (Li, Weizhen & Zhengxiang 2002).

Matricaria recutita

Native Western Asia, Southern and Eastern Europe chamomile flowers have been used as medications, they can be drunk as infusion, consumed in tablets, or applied as oils for relaxation and for helping to sleep. German chamomile (*Matricaria recutita*) is also very popular as a single ingredient in herbal teas and is the most broadly used herbal merchandise for sleep. Although chamomile reputed mechanism of action is not completely identified, preclinical studies suggest that the flavonoid component apigenin produces sedative effects through modulation of y-aminobutryic acid (GABA) receptors. Chamomile is generally well accepted; only a narrow number of event reports have documented allergic responses (Zick et al., 2011).

Hypoglycemic and hypocholestrolemic effects of chamomile extract and the protective effects of this herb against complications of hyperglycemia associatedwith diabetes have been demonstrated in experimental studies on animals and clinical trials on humans. Such effects have been attributed to two classes of compounds: sesquiterpenic and the phenolic compounds. Such flavonoid compounds include apigenin, quercetin, patuletin and luteolin, and their glucosides (Rafraf, Zemestani & Asghari-Jifaaradi, 2015).

Oral mucositis manifests as usually painful, erythematous, erosive, and/or ulcerative lesions of the oral mucosa related to toxicity and myelosuppression stemming from cancer treatment, such as chemotherapy and head and neck radiotherapy. An immunohistochemical study reveals an increase in pro-inflammatory cytokines with the development of mucositis. Topical treatment with chamomile extract (Ad-Muc^{R}) leads to a decline in IL-1b and TNF-a levels, associated with lesser oral mucositis severity (Curra et al., 2013).

Triticum aestivum

Wheatgrass is prepared from the cotyledons of common wheat plant. Its juice is the extract from the pulp and it has been used for the treatment of intestitnal diseases and thalassemia. By radical scavenging correlation with phenolic and flavonoid contents inside, it exhibits an antioxidant activity. Clinical usage of wheat grass juice for ulcerative colitis, showing a significant reduction in disease activity index, reverity and rectal bleeding (Wan, et al., 2014).

Melastoma malabathricum

Locally known as Senduduk, it is abundant in India, Southeast and South of Asia, Its leaves have reported pharmacological activities, mainly as antiulcer agents. A methanolic standardized extract of leaves showed a gastroprotective activity, due to tis antioxidant activity, as well as antisecretory and cytoprotective mechanism, The modulation of No and SH compounds contributed to the gastroprotection mechanism (Zakaria, et al., 2015).

Nigella sativa

A plant commonly used in the Middle Eastern and North African traditional medicine was validated for its multi-factorial anti-diabetic actions. The crude aqueous extract tested in experimental rats was able to restore glucose homeostasis and to improve glucose tolerance as efficiently as metformin. It enhance insulin sensitivity in liver cells, and to possess an insulinotropic and insulin-like activities in cultured pancreatic β-cells, skeletal muscle cells and adipocytes. A crude aqueous extract of *Nigella sativa* seeds directly inhibits the electrogenic intestinal absorption of glucose *in vitro* (El-Abhar & Schaalan, 2014).

Zingiber officinale

Commonly known as Ginger; its rhizome possesses pharmacological effects. Ginger essential oil could prevent postoperative nausea. It is also anti-inflammatory, analgesic and antibacterial. Fresh and soft pound plaster of ginger is beneficial to alopecia, lyses of gaseousness, swelling and pain. Eating ground cooked and dusted ginger on broth could help to relieve joint pain. Mixture of fresh ginger with salt and lemon juice after meals causes digestion reinforcement and changes the taste of mouth (Khodaie & Sadeghpoor, 2015).

Citrus spp.

Ethanolic extracts of *Citrus reticulate* (orange) and *Citrus aurantifolia* (lime) peels, both rich in phenolic flavonoids compounds, showed anticarcinogenic antiproliferative, co- cgenitherapeutic and estrogenic effects. Particularly orange peel ethanolic extract was a potential phytoestrogen with proliferatve effect on WiDr cells., and increased bone density, improved blood cholesterol profile in ovariectomized rats (Meiyanto, Hermawan & Anindyajati, 2012).

Allium sativum

A study made in the USA to determine if garlic could control dyslipidemia. The predominant type of garlic preparation used was dried garlic powders and in some cases aged garlic extract.

Three randomized clinical trials have evaluated the effect of garlic intake on gastric cancer risk. In one study, which involved over 5,000 Chinese men and women at high risk for stomach cancer, researchers compared the effects of taking a combination of 200 mg synthetic allitridum (an extract of garlic used as a medicine in China) daily and 100 micrograms selenium every other day with taking a placebo for 5 years. In the group that received allitridum and selenium, the risk for all tumors combined was reduced by 33 percent and the risk for stomach cancer was reduced by 52 percent in comparison with the group that received only the placebo (Li et al., 2004).

A study in Japan compared the effects of daily high-dose 2.4 mL and low-dose 0.16 mL intake of aged-garlic extract after 6 and 12 months of use on individuals with colorectal adenomas (noncancerous tumors). At the end of 12 months, 67 percent of the low-intake group developed new adenomas compared with 47 percent in the high-intake group (Tanaka et al., 2004).

Vitis vinifera

A study of healthy volunteers found that taking grape seed extract did substantially increase levels of antioxidants in their blood. Antioxidants are substances that destroy free radicals -- harmful compounds in the body that damage DNA (genetic material) and even cause cell death. Free radicals are believed to contribute to aging, as well as the development of a number of health problems, including heart disease and cancer. Other uses include chronic venous insufficiency, edema, high cholesterol and blood pressure; it improves blood sugar control in diabetic patients, improves night vision and protects elastin and collagen in skin (University of Maryland Medical Center, 2015).

Camellia sinensis

Traditional tea infusion is characterized by a high content of flavonoids. Enhanced plasma levels of catechins have consistently been found following the consumption of green and black tea, ranging from 0.63–1.8 µmol/L for green and 0.2–0.34 µmol/L for black tea. The plasma levels peaked after 1.5–2.6 h and were back to baseline within 24 h (Rietvel & Wiseman, 2015).

Significant reduction of DNA damage after consumption of green and black tea has been reported in population studies. Recently conducted intervention trials also indicate that tea consumption may lead to protection of DNA against oxidation (Xue et al., 1992; Shim et al 1995).

Vaccinium oxicoccus

Cranberry is a rich source of proanthocyanidis, this compounds may inhibit P-fimbriated E. coli adherence to uroepithelial cells. Also, it can minimize the inflammatory component of urinary tract infection. People that consumed well-standardized cranberry extract decreased the number of infections, duration and the need of medical attention (Ledda et al., 2015).

Celendula officinalis

Commonly known as Marigold, presents some antioxidant action, anti-inflammatory, antibacterial, antifungal and antiviral properties. An ethanolic extract of calendula used as mouthwash was used to treat oropharyngeal mucositis, in patients with radiotherapy and chemotherapy, decreasing the intensity but it could not prevent the occurrence (Babaee et al., 2013).

Calendula ethanolic extracts has also showed hepatic chemoprotection against aflatoxin, inducing significant improvement biochemical and histological parameters *in vivo*. Anti-inflammatory activity of calendula extracts rich in carvacol, promote liver regeneration, inhibition of interleukin 6 and TNF-α and COX enzymes (Hamzawy et al., 2013).

Eucalyptus spp.

Essential oil of several Eucalyptus species have showed clinical efficacy for respiratory diseases in particular of the anti-obstructed efficacy in acute bronchitis and impact on lung function. The combination in the oil of 1,8-cineol,a-pinene and limonene showed efficacy against bronchitis in a placebo controlled clinical trial. (Bhattaram, 2002).

Hypoxis spp.

Hypoxis species extract of *H. hemerocallidea* sterols and sterloins, have the potential to enhance the immune system. They can also act as inhibitors of nuclear factor κB mediating the pathway in which the immune cells involved in the inflammatory response. It also exhibit antibacterial properties, having a better effect with a combination of *H. colchicifolia* and *H. hemerocallieda* (Ndhlala et al., 2013).

An extract fo *Hypoxis rooperi*, is used in Germany, with 70% of dry weight contains β-sitosterol. Patients treated for benign prostatic hyperplasia in a clinical trial. There was a symptomatic improvement in patients treated with the extract, and maintained the improvement for 12 months (Lowe et al., 1998).

Andrographis paniculata

Known as sabiloto, it is traditionally used as antimalarial agent. Methanol extract acted against Plasmodium falciparum with an IC_{50} of 7.2 µg/ml. A PP obtained from fractionated ethanol extracts using two fractions from ethanol extract, using ethyl acetate for purification. Formulation as granulated and solid dispersion tables were administered to mice. The PP inhibited parasite growth´s significantly (Widyawaruyanti, 2014).

Valeriana officinalis

Root extracts from valeriana, are popular supplements used for the treatment of sleep disorders, anxiety, epilepsy and neurodegenerative diseases. Its tinctures have antioxidant effects. Valeriana decreases levels of corticosterone and serotonin in brain and plasma, reducing stress in rats (Jung et al., 2014).

Most sleep studies have used 400 to 900 mg of aqueous or aqueous- alcoholic extracts; the main impact was the improvement on sleep latency and structure with a gradual onset of efficacy rather than to exert a general sedative effect, while sleep electroencephalogram changes were pronounced after several days of intake (Committee on Herbal Medicinal Products, 2007).

An aqueous extract of the aerial parts of *Melissa officinalis* showed antioxidant and neuroprotective properties induced neurotoxicity (oxidative stress), especially in the hippocampus and striatum, in mice at a dose corresponding to100 mg plant material/kg/day for 90 days. An ethanolic liquid extract was tested for its potential anti-ulcerogenic activity against indometacin-induced ulcers in rats at oral doses of 2.5 to 10 ml/kg. Acid output was reduced and mucin secretion increased. An increase in prostaglandin E2 release and a decrease in leukotrienes were observed. The anti- ulcerogenic effect was also confirmed histologically. 600 mg of a methanolic extract of Melisa was given to 18 healthy volunteers that were subjected to mil laboratory- induced psychological stress at 1 h after treatment, the effect on the mood and stress ameliorate the negative mood effects, significantly increased self-ratings of calmness and reduced self-ratings of alertness and increased the speed of mathematical processing (Claeson, 2013).

CONCLUSION

The industrial usage of dietary supplements and PP around the world is expanding continuously. New technologies for quality control, cost-risk ratio, and validation of positive benefits will allow the development of phytopharmaceutical industry.

REFERENCES

Ambrosini, A., Di Lorenzo, C., Coppola, G., & Pierelli, F. (2013). Use of *Vitex agnus-castus* in migrainous women with premenstrual syndrome: An open-label clinical observation. *Acta Neurologica Belgica*, *113*(1), 25–29. doi:10.1007/s13760-012-0111-4 PMID:22791378

Ameer, O., Salman, I., Quek, K., & Asmawi, M. (2015). Loranthus ferrugineus: A Mistletoe from Traditional Uses to Laboratory Bench. *Journal of Pharmacopuncture*, *18*(1), 7–18. doi:10.3831/KPI.2015.18.001 PMID:25830054

Amuka, O. (2013). An overview in support of continued research into phytomedicine: past, present and future. In A. Garib-Famkim & J. N. Eloff (Eds.), *Chemistry for Sustainable development in Africa* (pp. 3–15). Heidelberg, Germany: Springer- Verlag. doi:10.1007/978-3-642-29642-0_1

Anantha-Narayana, D. B. (2013). Approaches to pre-formulation R and D for PP emanating from herb based traditional Ayurvedic processes. *Journal of Ayurveda and Integrative Medicine*, *4*(1), 4–8. doi:10.4103/0975-9476.109542 PMID:23741154

Antonio, G., Tesser, C., & Moretti-Pires, R. (2014). Phytotherapy in primary health care. *Revista de Saude Publica*, *48*(3), 541–553. PMID:25119949

Babaee, N., Moslemi, D., Khalilpour, M., Vejdani, F., Monghadamnia, Y., Bijani, A., & Moghadamnia, A. et al. (2013). Antioxidant capacity of *calendula officinalis* flowers extract and prevention of radiation induced oropharyngeal mucositis in patients with head and neck cancers: A randomized controlled clinical study. *DARU Journal of Pharmaceutical Sciences.*, *21*(1), 18–24. PMID:23497687

Bandaranayake, W. M. (2006). Quality Control, Screening, Toxicity, and Regulation of Herbal Drugs. In Modern Phytomedicine: Turning Medicinal Plants into Drugs (pp. 25-57). Weinheim, Germany: Wiley-VCH Verlag GmbH & Co. KGaA.

Bauer, R. (1998). Quality criteria and standardization of PP: Can acceptable drug standards be achived. *Drug Information Journal*, *32*, 101–110.

Behnke, K., Jensen, G., Graubaum, H., & Gruenwald, J. (2002). *Hypericum perforatum* Versus Fluoxetine in the Treatment of Mild to Moderate Depression. *Advances in Natural Therapy.*, *19*(1), 43–52. doi:10.1007/BF02850017 PMID:12008860

Benelli, L., Cortés-Rojas, D., Souza, C., & Pereira-Oliveira, W. (2015). Fluid bed drying and agglomeration of phytopharmaceutical compositions. *Powder Technology*, *273*, 145–153. doi:10.1016/j.powtec.2014.12.022

Beringhs, A., Fagner, M., Souza, F., Angela, M., de Campo, A., Ferraz, H., & Sonaglio, D. (2012). Technological development of Cecropia glaziovi extract pellets by extrusion-spheronization. *Brazilian Journal of Pharmacognosy*, *23*(1), 160–168.

Bhattaram, V. A., Graefe, U., Kohlert, C., Veit, M., & Derendorf, H. (2002). Pharmacokinetics and bioavailability of herbal medicinal products. *Phytomedicine*, *9*, 1–33. doi:10.1078/1433-187X-00210 PMID:12222652

Borodina, N., Rumsh, D., Kunizhev, M., Sukhorukov, B., Vorozhtsov, N., Feldman, M., & Markvicheva, E. A. et al. (2008). Entrapment of herbal extracts into biodegradable microcapsules. *Biochemistry (Moscow) Supplement Series B. Biomedical Chemistry*, *2*(2), 176–182. doi:10.1134/S199075080802008X

Braun, L. (2010) Principles of herbal medicine. In General practice: the integrative approach. Sydney. Australia: Elsevier.

Bucar, F., Wube, A., & Schmid, M. (2013). Natural product isolation- how to get from biological material to pure compounds. *Natural Product Reports*, *30*(4), 525–545. doi:10.1039/c3np20106f PMID:23396532

Calixto, J. (2000). Efficacy, safety, quality control, marketing and regulatory guidelines for herbal medicines (phytotherapeutic agents). *Brazilian Journal of Medical and Biological Research*, *33*(2), 179–189. doi:10.1590/S0100-879X2000000200004 PMID:10657057

Canter, P., Thomas, H., & Ernst, E. (2005). Bringing medicinal plants into cultivation: Opportunities and challenges for biotechnology. *Trends in Biotechnology*, *23*(4), 180–185. doi:10.1016/j.tibtech.2005.02.002 PMID:15780709

Capasso, R., Izzo, A., Pinto, L., Bifulco, T., Vitobello, C., & Mascolo, N. (2002). Phytotherapy and quality of herbal medicines. *Fitoterapia*, *71*, 58–65. doi:10.1016/S0367-326X(00)00173-8 PMID:10930714

Ciunab, R. R. (2012). Phytotherapeutic and naturopathic adjuvant therapies in otorhinolaryngology. *European Archives of Oto-Rhino-Laryngology*, *269*(2), 389–397. doi:10.1007/s00405-011-1755-z PMID:21922427

Claeson, P. (n.d.). *Assessment report on Melissa officinalis L.* London: European Medicines Agency.

Committee on Herbal Medicinal Products. (2007). *Assessment report on Valeriana officinales L., Radix* (pp. 3–21). London, MD: European Medicines Agency.

Cortés-Rojas, D., Chagas-Paula, A., Da Costa, F., Souza, C., & Oliveira, W. (2013). *Bidens pilosa L.* populations: A key step in the standardization of phytopharmaceutical preparations. *Brazilian Journal of Pharmacognosy.*, *23*(1), 28–35.

Couto R., Martins F., Chaul L., Conceicao E., Alexandre L., Freitas P., Bara M., Paula J. (2013). Spray drying of *Eugenia dysenterica* extract: effects of in-process parameters on product quality. *Revista brasileira de Farmacognosia, 23*(1), 115-123.

Cragg, G. M., & Newman, D. J. (2013). Natural products: A continuing source of novel drug leads. *Biochimica et Biophysica Acta*, *1830*(6), 3670–3695. doi:10.1016/j.bbagen.2013.02.008 PMID:23428572

Curra, M., Martinis, M., Lauxen, I., Pellicioli, A., Filho, M., Pavesi, V., & Martinis, M. et al. (2013). Effect of topical chamomile on immunohistochemical levels of IL-1b and TNF-a in 5-fluorouracil-induced oral mucositis in hamsters. *Cancer Chemotherapy and Pharmacology*, *71*(2), 293–299. doi:10.1007/s00280-012-2013-9 PMID:23096219

Dasture, A. (2002). Global market potentials of ayuvedra drugs- some facts. *Ancient Science of Life*, *XXI*(4), 281–286. PMID:22557067

David, B., Woldenfer, J. L., & Dias, D. A. (2014). The pharmaceitucial industry and natural products: Historical status and new trends. *Phytochemistry Reviews*, *14*(2), 299–315. doi:10.1007/s11101-014-9367-z

Devi, V., Jain, N., & Vali, K. (2010). Importance of novel drug delivery systemps in herbal medicines. *Pharmagonogsy Review*, *4*(7), 27–31. PMID:22228938

Dhami, N. (2013). Trends in Pharmacognosy: A modern science of natural medicines. *Journal of Herbal Medicine.*, *3*(4), 123–131. doi:10.1016/j.hermed.2013.06.001

Eichhorn, T., Greten, H., & Efferth, T. (2011). Self-medication with nutritional supplements and herbal over-thecounter products. *Natural Products and Bioprospecting.*, *1*(2), 62–70. doi:10.1007/s13659-011-0029-1

El-Abhar, H., & Schaalan, M. (2014). Phytotherapy in diabetes: Review on potential mechanistic perspectives. *World Journal of Diabetes*, *5*(2), 176–197. PMID:24748931

Fernandes, C., Mascarenhas, M., Zibetti, F., Lima, G., Oliveira, R., Rocha, L., & Falcão, D. (2013). HLB value, an important parameter for the development of essential oil PP. *Brazilian Journal of Pharmacognosy*, *23*(1), 108–114.

Gunasekara, T., Haile, T., Nigusse, T., & Dhanaraju, M. (2014). Nanotechnology: An effective tool for enhancing bioavailability and bioactivity of phytomedicine. *Asian Pacific Journal of Tropical Biomedicine*, *4*(1), S1–S7. doi:10.12980/APJTB.4.2014C980 PMID:25183064

Gurib-Fakim, A. (2006). Medicinal plants: Traditions of yesterday and drugs of tomorrow. *Molecular Aspects of Medicine*, *27*(1), 1–93. doi:10.1016/j.mam.2005.07.008 PMID:16105678

Hamburger, M. (2002). *Isatis tinctoria* – From the rediscovery of an ancient medicinal plant towards a novel anti-inflammatory phytopharmaceutical. *Phytochemistry Reviews*, *1*(3), 333–344. doi:10.1023/A:1026095608691

Hamzawy, M., El-Denshary, E., Hassan, N., Mannaa, F., & Abdel-Wahhab, M. (2013). Dietary Supplementation of *Calendula officinalis* Counteracts the Oxidative Stress and Liver Damage Resulted from Aflatoxin. *ISRB Nutrition*, 538427-538436.

Harborne, J. B., & Williams, C. A. (2000). Advances in flavonoid research since 1992. *Phytochemistry*, *5*(6), 481–504. doi:10.1016/S0031-9422(00)00235-1 PMID:11130659

Ivanovic, J., Meyer, F., Stamenic, M., Jaeger, P., Zizovic, I., & Eggers, R. (2014). Pretreatment of natural materials used for supercritical fluid extraction of commercial phytopharmaceticals. *Chemical Engineering & Technology*, *9*(9), 1606–1611. doi:10.1002/ceat.201300715

Jung, H., Yoo, D., Kin, W., Nam, S., Kim, H., Choi, J., & Yoon, Y. et al. (2014). *Valeriana officinalis* root extract suppresses physical stress by electric shock and psychological stress by nociceptive stimulation-evoked responses by decreasing the ratio of monoamine neurotransmitters to their metabolites. *Complementary and Alternative Medicine.*, *14*(1), 476–483. doi:10.1186/1472-6882-14-476 PMID:25495725

Kahalid, H., Zhari, I., Amirin, S., & Pazilah, I. (2011). Accelerated stability and chemical kinetics of ethanol extracts of fruit of *Piper sarmestosum* using high performance liquid chromatography. *Iranian Journal of Pharmaceutical Research*, *10*(3), 403–413. PMID:24250372

Khodaie, L., & Sadeghpoor, O. (2015). Ginger form acient times to the new outlook. *Jundishapur Journal of Natural Pharmaceutical Products.*, *10*(1), 1–5. doi:10.17795/jjnpp-18402 PMID:25866718

Khorasani, G., Hosseinimerh, S., Azadbakht, M., Zamani, A., & Mahdavi, M. (2009). Aloe Versus Silver Sulfadiazine Creams for Second-Degree Burns: A Randomized Controlled Study. *Surgery Today*, *39*(7), 587–591. doi:10.1007/s00595-008-3944-y PMID:19562446

Lamottke, K., Ripoll, C., & Walzack, R. (2011). The roots of innovation. *European Biopharmaceutical Review*, *15*, 52–56.

Lang, F., Hoerr, R., Noeldner, M., & Koch, E. (2013). Ginkgo biloba Extract EGb 761®: From an Ancient Asian Plant to a Modern European Herbal Medicinal Product. In Evidence and Rational Based Research on Chinese Drugs (pp. 431-470). Wien, Austria: Wiley-VCH Verlag GmbH & Co. KGaA.

Ledda, A., Bottari, A., Luzzi, R., Belcaro, G., Hu, S., Dugall, M., & Togni, S. et al. (2015). Cranberry supplementation in the prevention of non-severe lower urinary tract infections: A pilot study. *European Review for Medical and Pharmacological Sciences*, *19*, 77–80. PMID:25635978

Lee, L. (1999). Introducing herbal medicine into conventional health care settings. *Journal of Nurse-Midwifery*, *44*(3), 253–266. doi:10.1016/S0091-2182(99)00042-7 PMID:10380444

Li, G., Weizhen, L., & Zhengxiang, L. (2002). Effect of Ginsenoside-Rb on cardiomyocyte Apoptosis after Ischemia and Reperfusion in Rats. *Journal of Huazjong Univerity of Science and Technology*, *22*(3), 212-215.

Li, H., Li, Q., Wang, Y., Xu, X., Fan, W., Wang, M., & Xie, X. et al. (2004). An intervention study to prevent gastric cancer by micro-selenium and large dose of allitridum. *Chinese Medical Journal*, *117*(8), 1155–1160. PMID:15361287

Lowe, F., Dreikorn, K., Borkowski, A., Braechman, J., Denis, L., Ferrari, P., & Senge, T. et al. (1998). Review of Recent Placebo-Controlled Trials Utilizing Phytotherapeutic Agents for Treatment of BPH. *The Prostate*, *37*(3), 187–193. doi:10.1002/(SICI)1097-0045(19981101)37:3<187::AID-PROS8>3.0.CO;2-T PMID:9792136

Lubbe, A., & Verpoorte, R. (2011). Cultivation of medicinal and aromatic plants for specialty industrial materials. *Industrial Crops and Products*, *34*(1), 785–801. doi:10.1016/j.indcrop.2011.01.019

Ma, B., Duan, X., & Wang, Z. (2000). Clinical and experimental study on Shuanghua aerosol in treating infantile upper respiratory tract infection. *Zhongguo Zhong Xi Yi Jie He Za Zhi.*, *20*, 653–655. PMID:11789167

McChesney, J. D. (1999). Quality of botanical preparations: environmental issues and methodology for detecting environmental contaminants. In M. A. Liebert (Ed.), *Botanical Medicine: Efficacy, quality assurance and regulation* (pp. 127–131). New Rochelle Inc. Publishers.

Meier, B. (2001). Comparing phytopharmaceuticlas: The example of St. John's wort. *Advances in Natural Therapy*, *18*(1), 35–46. doi:10.1007/BF02850249 PMID:11512531

Meiyanto, E., Hermawan, A., & Anindyajati, A. (2012). Natural products for cancer-targeted therapy: citrus flavonoids as potent chemopreventive agents. *Asian Pacific Journal of Cancer Prevention*, *13*(2), 427–436. doi:10.7314/APJCP.2012.13.2.427 PMID:22524801

Mohamed, I., Shuid, A., Borhanuddin, B., & Fozi, N. (2012). The Application of Phytomedicine in Modern Drug Development. *The Internet Journal of Herbal and Plant Medicine*, *1*(2), 16–22.

National Medicinal Plans Board, Government of India, Ministry of Ayush. (n.d.). Retrieved from http://www.nmpb.nic.in

Ncube, B., Finnie, J. F., & Van Staden, J. (2012). Quality from the field: The impact of environmental factors as quality determinants in medicinal plants. *South African Journal of Botany*, *82*, 11–20. doi:10.1016/j.sajb.2012.05.009

Petrovska B.B. (2012). Historical review of medicinal plants´s usage. *Pharmacognosy Review, 6*(11), 1-5.

Piriou, Y., Sirvent, A., Natalizio, A., & Girad-ory, F. (2014). Skin-lightening and anti-ageing effect of a food supplement containing *Pinus pinaster* extract. *Naturafood*, *13*(3), 123–131. doi:10.1007/s13749-014-0036-z

Pribitkin E. (2005). Herbal medicine and surgery. *Seminar in Integrative Medicine, 3*, 17-23.

Radha, M., & Laxmipriya, N. (2015). Evaluation of biological properties and clinical effectiveness of Aloe vera: A systematic review. *Journal of Traditional and Complementary Medicine*, *5*(1), 21–26. doi:10.1016/j.jtcme.2014.10.006 PMID:26151005

Rafraf, M., Zemestani, M., & Asghari-Jifaaradi, M. (2015). Effectiveness of *chamomile* tea on glycemic control and serum lipid profile in patients with type 2 diabetes. *Journal of Endocrinological Investigation*, *38*(2), 163–170. doi:10.1007/s40618-014-0170-x PMID:25194428

Rajani, M., & Kanaki, S. (2008). Phytochemical Standardization of Herbal Drugs and Polyherbal Formulations. In Bioactive Molecules and Medicinal Plants (pp 349-369). Berlin, Germany: Springer-Verlag Berlin Heidelberg. doi:doi:10.1007/978-3-540-74603-4_19 doi:10.1007/978-3-540-74603-4_19

Rietveld, A., & Wiseman, S. (2003). Antioxidant Effects of Tea: Evidence from Human Clinical Trials. *The Journal of Nutrition*, *133*(10), 3285S–3292S. PMID:14519827

Rischer, H., & Oksman-Caldentey, K. M. (2005). Biotechnological utilization of plant genetic resources for the production of PP. *Plant Genetic Resources*, *3*(2), 83–89. doi:10.1079/PGR200564

Santos, L., Marin, S., Sanchis, V., & Ramos, A. J. (2013). Mycotoxin in medicinal/aromatic herbs-a review. *Boletín Latinoamericanos y del Caribe de Plantas Medicinales y Aromáticas*, *12*(2), 119–142.

Saraf, A. (2010). Applications of novel drug delivery system for herbal formulations. *Fitoterapia*, *81*(7), 680–689. doi:10.1016/j.fitote.2010.05.001 PMID:20471457

Schweim, J., & Schweim, H. (2014). Status quo and future developments of combinations of medicinal products. *Synergy*, *1*(1), 70–75. doi:10.1016/j.synres.2014.07.007

Shen, Y. J., Zhang, Z. W., Luo, X. G., Wang, X. F., & Wang, H. L. (2008). Nanoparticles of traditional chinese herbs inhibit thrombosis in vivo. *Haematologica*, *93*, J1457.

Shim, J. S., Kang, M. H., Kim, Y. H., Roh, J. K., Roberts, C., & Lee, I. P. (1995). Chemopreventive effect of green tea (Camellia sinensis) among cigarette smokers. *Cancer Epidemiology, Biomarkers & Prevention*, *4*, 387–391. PMID:7655335

Tanaka, S., Haruma, K., Kunihiro, M., Nagata, S., Kitada, Y., Manabe, N., & Chayama, K. et al. (2004). Effects of aged garlic extract (AGE) on colorectal adenomas: A double-blinded study. *Hiroshima Journal of Medical Sciences*, *53*(3–4), 39–45. PMID:15726891

Van Beek, T., & Montoro, P. (2009). Chemical analysis and quality control of Ginkgo biloba leaves, extracts, and PP. *Journal of Chromatography. A*, *1216*, 2002–2032. doi:10.1016/j.chroma.2009.01.013 PMID:19195661

Wagner, H. (2011). Synergy research: Approaching a new generation of PP. *Fitoterapia*, *82*, 34–37. doi:10.1016/j.fitote.2010.11.016 PMID:21075177

Wan, P., Chen, H., Guo, Y., & Bai, A. (2014). Advances in treatment of ulcerative colitis with herbs: From bench to bedside. *World Journal of Gastroenterology*, *20*(39), 14099–14104. doi:10.3748/wjg.v20.i39.14099 PMID:25339799

Wei-Jun, K., Yan-Ling, Z., Xiao-He, X., Cheng, J., & Zu-Lun, L. (2009). Quantitative and chemical fingerprint analysis for quality control of Rhizoma Coptidischinensis based on UPLC-PAD combined with chemometrics methods. *Phytomedicine*, *16*(10), 950–959. doi:10.1016/j phymed.2009.03.016 PMID:19553096

Wei-Jun, K., Yan-Ling, Z., Xiao-He, X., Jia-Bo, W., Han-Bing, L., & Zu-Lun, L. (2009). Spectrum–effect relationships between ultra performance liquid chromatography fingerprints and anti-bacterial activities of *Rhizoma coptidis*. *Analytica Chimica Acta*, *634*(2), 279–285. doi:10.1016/j.aca.2009.01.005 PMID:19185133

Wesnes, K., Ward, T., McGinty, A., & Petrini, O. (2000). The memory enhancing effects of a Ginkgo biloba/Panax ginseng combination in healthy middle-aged volunteers. *Psychopharmacology*, *152*(4), 353–361. doi:10.1007/s002130000533 PMID:11140327

WHO. (1990) Global programme on aids and traditional medicine programme. Report of a WHO consultation on traditional medicine and AIDS: Clinical evaluation of traditional medicines and natural products.

WHO. (1996). Expert committee on specifications for pharmaceutical preparations-WHO technical report series, No. 863, Annex 11. In *WHO Guidelines for the Assessmet of Herbal Medicines, Thirty-fourth report* (pp. 1–8). Munich, Germany: World Health Organization.

WHO. (2003). *WHO guidelines on good agricultural and collection practices (GACP) for medicinal plants*. Geneva, Switzerland: World Health Organization.

Wichtl, M. (2004). *Herbal drugs and PP: A handbook for practice on a scientific basis*. Stuttgart, Germany: CRC Press.

Widyawaruyanti, A., Asrory, M., Wiwied, E., Setiawan, D., Radjaram, A., Tumewu, L., & Hafid, A. (2014) In vivo Antimalarial Activity of *Andrographis paniculata* Tablets. *Procedia Chemistry, 13*, 101-104.

Wills, R., Bone, K., & Morgan, M. (2000). Herbal products: Active constituents, modes of action and quality control. *Nutrition Research Reviews*, *13*(01), 47–77. doi:10.1079/095442200108729007 PMID:19087433

Xiao, J. (2015). Phytochemicals in medicine and food. *Phytochemistry Reviews*, *14*(3), 317–320. doi:10.1007/s11101-015-9407-3

Xue, K. X., Wang, S., Ma, G. J., Zhou, P., Wu, P. Q., Zhang, R. F., & Wang, Y. Q. et al. (1992). Micronucleus formation in peripheral-blood lymphocytes from smokers and the influence of alcohol- and tea-drinking habits. *International Journal of Cancer*, *50*(5), 702–705. doi:10.1002/ijc.2910500506 PMID:1544703

Yi, C., Shang-Bin, Z., Ming-Yong, X., Shao-Ping, N., Wei, L., Chang, L., & Yuan-Xing, W. et al. (2008). Quality control and original discrimination of Ganoderma lucidum based on high-performance liquid chromatographic fingerprints and combined chemometrics methods. *Analytica Chimica Acta*, *623*(2), 146–156. doi:10.1016/j.aca.2008.06.018 PMID:18620918

Zakaria, Z., Balan, T., Mamat, S., Mohtarrudin, N., Kek, T., & Salleh, M. (2015). Mechanisms of gastroprotection of methanol extract of *Melastoma malabathricum* leaves. *Complementary and Alternative Medicine.*, *15*(1), 135–150. doi:10.1186/s12906-015-0638-z PMID:25927982

Zobayed, S. A., Afreen, F., & Kozai, T. (2005). Necessity and production of medicinal plants under controlled environments. *Environment Control in Biology*, *43*(4), 243–252. doi:10.2525/ecb.43.243

Chapter 8
A Perspective on the Phytopharmaceuticals Responsible for the Therapeutic Applications

Rajesh K. Joshi
Regional Medical Research Centre (Indian Council of Medical Research), India

ABSTRACT

The word phytopharmaceutical deals with a complex mixture of compounds derived from the plant source that is used as a medicine or drug. Primitive human societies have been depending on plants and plant products for various remedies. Several plants in the different forms have been reported in traditional medicine and to find a rational for the treatment of various diseases than to isolated single compounds. Many of the single compounds isolated from the plant origin are effectively used in the medicine. The search of natural products in drug discovery has been greatly enhanced in the last few years. The impetus to use phytopharmaceutical agents for the treatment of disease, most of the plant based drugs are quite safe and have lesser adverse effects and are claimed that it works as synergistic effects.

INTRODUCTION

Primitive human societies have been depending on plants and plant products for various remedies. In certain areas, these folk medicinal prescriptions are endemic and have survived through ages from one generation to next through word of mouth. They do not exist as written knowledge. Generally, these systems of medicines depend on old people's experiences. The person, prescribing these medicines has so-called scientific knowledge about the diseases. Indigenous systems of medicine are specially conditioned by cultural heritage and myths. In India, the reference to the curative properties of some herbs in the Rig Veda seems to be the earliest records of use of plants in medicine. The identity of several plants referred to in Suktas of the Rig Veda can be fixed with reasonable certainty, e.g. of *Semal, Pithvan, Palash,* and *Pipal.* A more detailed account is available in the Atharva Veda. The period of Rig Veda is

DOI: 10.4018/978-1-5225-0754-3.ch008

estimated to be between 3500 and 1800 B.C. After the Vedas, there is no information on the development of this science in India for a period of about 1,000 years. Then appeared the two most important works on Indian system of medicine, the works of Charak and Susruta, namely the Charak-Samhita and Susruta-Samhita. The latter deals with about 700 drugs, some of these are not indigenous to India. In the modern era, the medicinal plants are being replaced more and more by synthetic drugs. But of late it is being realized that synthetics, though useful as life saving drugs, are responsible for many hazardous side effects. This has led to the revival of interest in herbal medicine with the reawakening of efforts to promote indigenous system of medicine.

Since antiquity, man has used plants to treat common infectious diseases and some of these traditional medicines are still included as part of the habitual treatment of various maladies. For example, the use of bearberry (*Arctostaphylos uva-ursi*) and cranberry juice (*Vaccinium macrocarpon*) to treat urinary tract infections have been reported in different manuals of phytotherapy, while species such as lemon balm (*Melissa officinalis*), garlic (*Allium sativum*) and tee tree (*Melaleuca alternifolia*) are described as broad-spectrum antimicrobial agents (Rios& Recio, 2005).

Variety of plant extracts, such as an extract of the root of *Sophora flavescens*, an extract of stem bark of *Magnolia obovata*, and oil of *Melaleuca alternifolia*, have been used as traditional medicines for microbial infections, strongly suggests that natural products are the major source of important antimicrobial agents (Sohn et al., 2004). Several essential oils and their isolates have been found to exhibit strong antibacterial and antifungal activity. According to Wan et al. (1998), the majority of the essential oils assayed for their antibacterial properties showed a more pronounced effect against the Gram positive bacteria. The resistance of Gram negative bacteria to essential oil has been ascribed to their hydrophilic outer membrane, which can block the penetration of hydrophobic compounds into target cell membrane (Wan et al. 1998). The essential oils of the medicinal and aromatic plants rather than their extracts that have had the greatest use in the treatment of infectious pathologies in the respiratory system, urinary tract, gastrointestinal and biliary systems, as well as on the skin (Rios & Recio, 2005).Various essential oils viz., *Plectranthus mollis* (Joshi, 2014a), *Ocimum basilicum* (Joshi, 2014b), *Artemisia absinthium* (Joshi, 2013a), *Ocimum gratissimum*, *Ocimum sanctum* (Joshi, 2013b),*Cyathocline purpurea* (Joshi, 2013c), *Senecio belgaumensis* (Joshi, 2012a), *Lantana camara* (Joshi, 2012b), *Tridax procumbens* (Joshi& Badakar, 2012), *Phlomis bracteosa* (Joshi et al., 2011), *Feronia elephantum* (Joshi et al., 2011), *Erigeron floribundus* (Joshi et al., 2011), *Craniotome furcata* (Joshi, 2010) and *Anaphalis nubigena* var. *monocephala* (Joshi et al., 2009) have been reported promising *in vitro* antimicrobial activity.

The essential oils seem to have no specific cellular targets. As typical lipophiles, they pass through the cell wall and cytoplasmic membrane, disrupt the structure of their different layers of polysaccharides, fatty acids and phospholipids and permeabilize them. Cytotoxicity appears to include such membrane damage. The cytotoxic property is a great importance in the applications of essential oils not only against certain human or animal pathogens or parasites but also for the preservation of agricultural or marine products (Bakkali et al., 2008). Cytotoxic activities of essential oils or their major components, sometimes activated by light, have also been demonstrated in the mammalian cells *in vitro* by short-term viability assays using specific cell staining or fluorescent dyes including NRU (Neutral Red Uptake) test, MTT (3-(4,5-dimethylthiazol-2-yl)-2,5-diphenyl-tetrazolium bromide) test, Alamar Blue (resazurin) test, Trypan Blue exclusion test or Hoechst 33342 and propidium iodide test (Bakkali et al., 2008).

Essential oils have a calming, stimulating, pain alleviating and mood enhancing effect. They improve the functioning of internal organs like heart, lungs etc. Till now they were on the periphery of pharmacological preparations, inflammatory and flavouring agents. This is because they have multiple beneficial effects than just being pain relievers (Shukla & Shukla, 1997). Aromatherapy by essential oils and their isolates have been studied as an emerging trend of treatment for some physiological disorder (Buchbauer & Jirovetz, 1994). Pharmacology, pharmaceutical botany, medical and clinical microbiology, phytopathology, and food preservation are some fields in which the essential oils can be applied (Daferera et al., 2000).

Terpenoids are also used as chemical messengers. In the communication between different parts of the same organism, the messenger is referred to as a hormone. Chemicals that carry signals from one organism to another are known as semiochemicals, and grouped into two main classes. If the signal is between two members of the same species, the messenger is called a pheromone. Chemicals which carry message between members of different species are known as allelochemicals (Devon& Scott, 1972).

The ancient medical literature reports that surgery was performed but that physicians also recommended the use of some natural, and especially plant products, which represent an interesting point of comparison with current knowledge (Nobili et al., 2009). Curcumin has been widely studied because of its antioxidant and anti-inflammatory properties. It inhibits growth and induces apoptosis in a range of different cell types. Curcumin has ability to inhibit signaling through NF-kB and reduce expression of COX-2, LOX, NOS, MMP-9, uPA, TNF-a, cyclin D1, downregulates growth factor receptors EGFR, HER2, inhibits Bcl-2, Bcl-XL, IAP, Inhibits activity of protein kinases (EGFR, HER2, ERK, JNK, PKB/Akt, PKC, CYPs, GSTP1-1 and Inhibits VEGF production (Manson et al., 2005). Epigallocatechin-3-gallate, a polyphenol found in green tea, also affects growth, inducing G0/G1 cell cycle arrest and apoptosis in many cell types, and appears to modulate a range of signalling pathways and target molecules. Epigallocatechin-3-gallate inhibits the activity of 5-cytosine-DNA methyltransferase, p38, TNF-α- release, urokinase, LOX, COX. angiogenesis and VEGFR phosphorylation and VEGF induction. It also downregulates signalling through Her2 neu, PDGFR, transcription factors AP-1 and NF-kB (Manson et al., 2005).

Podophyllotoxins have a long therapeutic history. Podophyllotoxins have been extracted from the root of the Indian podophyllum plant (*Podophyllum peltatum*). Podophyllotoxin was used as a remedy by the American Indians for its emetic, cathartic, and anthelmintic effects. From a wide program of chemical synthesis (about 600 derivatives from 1950s to 1960s), two active compounds, etoposide and teniposide, emerged. Unlike other podophyllotoxin derivatives, etoposide and teniposide have no effect on microtubular structure or function at concentrations used in the clinic (Nobili et al., 2009). Psoralen is a natural photodynamic compound belongs to the family of furocoumarins, whose chemical structure consists of a furan ring fused with coumarin. It is produced by a variety of plants as a natural defence against pest. It occurs in *Psoralea corylifolia*, from which the natural compound derives its name, as well as in the common fig, celery, parsley, and parsnips. Its extended π-electron system, psoralen displays UV light-induced photosensitizing activity, useful in photodynamic treatment of various diseases, including psoriasis, vitiligo and other skin conditions like cutaneous T-cell lymphoma (Nobili et al., 2009). Natural products play a relevant role in cancer therapy today with substantial numbers of anticancer agents used in the clinic being either natural or derived from natural products from various sources such as plants, animals and microorganisms (also of marine origin) (Nobili et al., 2009).

Use of plants as a source of medicine has been an ancient practice and is an important component of the health care system in India (Pandey et al., 2013). In India, about70 percent of rural population depends on the traditional Ayurvedic system of medicine. Most healers/practitioners of the traditional systems of medicine prepare formulations by their own recipes and dispense to the patients. In the Western countries, approximately 40 per cent of people are using the herbal medicine for the treatment of various diseases (Pandey et al., 2013).The results of the herbal treatments led to their increased acceptance by the local people of Thailand. In a recent scientific studies that supported treatment with herbal preparations at the Kabchoeng Hospital of Thailand, where the efficacy and safety of *Cinnamon stomachic* mixture has been reported. The research suggested that this preparation was suitable for the treatment of patients with functional dyspepsia, in clinical randomized controlled trials, compared with simethicone (Chotchoungchatchai et al., 2012). The folk healers maintained knowledge regarding the proper use of indigenous plants for healing diseases specific to that area. Various preparations have been derived from folk medicine knowledge that consisted of medicinal plants that were available in the local area and were used for symptoms that related to diseases of the local people of Thailand (Chotchoungchatchai et al., 2012). For implementation of herbal medicine into hospitals, some uncertainty exists about the safety, effectiveness, and cost-effectiveness of complementary and alternative medicine methods, expanding their use, where reasonable evidence of their effectiveness and good evidence of their safety exists, might yield health, social, and economic benefits (Pandey et al., 2013).

Nature has gifted varieties of plant species occurring from different regions of world, whereas some species are found in particular zones. The alpine flora has their own properties to produce secondary metabolites compared to temperate region plants and vice versa. A plant can be considered as a system where many biochemical reactions occur. The secondary metabolites of plant or phytopharmaceutical are the product of biosynthesis where several factors alter the synthesis route. These factors are soil, climate, rainfall, altitude, grazing frequency, sunshine length etc, where plant produced different metabolites. As per the geoclimatic distribution of the flora, botanicals are consumed by the people as their own localities to cure the diseases. Some plants are frequently used in the food preparation almost as their daily recipes. A single plant is used in the treatment of various diseases or as a food supplement can varies phytochemicals as per the geoclimatic distribution. As the development of technologies more efforts are utilized to search of new chemical entities for treatment of the diseases which are safe from adverse effects. Now a day's various bioactive compounds are investigated from those where the plants are traditionally used for treatment of particular disease.

The isolated compounds which are found to be potent biological activities have been synthesized in laboratories as a modern medicine to fulfill the requirements of patients. A multidisciplinary approach to drug discovery, involving the generation of truly novel molecular diversity from natural product sources, combined with total and combinatorial synthetic methodologies, and including the manipulation of biosynthetic pathways (so-called combinatorial biosynthesis), provides the best solution to the current productivity crisis facing the scientific community engaged in drug discovery and development (Newman & Cragg, 2007). The exploration of Nature as a source of novel active agents that may serve as the leads and scaffolds for elaboration into desperately needed efficacious drugs for a multitude of disease indications (Newman & Cragg, 2007). For this purpose plant cell can be cultured as an alternative potential renewable source for sustainable production of phytopharmaceuticals. Though several studies on such aspects have been published in peer reviewed journals of national and international repute, the amount of research transferred from laboratory to published papers are more as compared to apply research findings to field or real ground is very less (Hurakadle et al., 2010; Pai et al., 2008). The greatest discovery in this field was made by Haberlandt (1902), where he showed un-natural successful growing of plant tissue and further use of plant growth regulators to control the organogenesis phenomenon. Since then it come across many successes stories in using this technique to grow, multiply and transfer number of plant species belonging to above mentioned categories. The only success being in agriculture industry wherein, varieties of banana, sugarcane have been widely used commercially apart from floriculture crops frequently using this technique. Medicinal plant industry is a booming cell which has several branches such as nutraceuticals, cosmetics, health medicines and several others. Most of today's herbal industries rely on the natural plant population as it being easy and less cost bearing in comparison to the costlier technologies in biotechnology field.

The discovery of fungal endophytes that produce novel compound has significant biological and commercial implications. Commercially, the fungal culture can be scaled up to provide adequate production to satisfy new drug development and patient treatment needs. This production reduces the need to harvest wild populations of the source plants, preserving these species for the future (Eyberger et al., 2006). Endophytic fungi from herbs could the sources of new drugs for treatment of various diseases in humans, animals, and plants. Endophytes are microorganisms that live within plants for at least a part of their life cycle without causing any visible manifestation of disease (Bacon & White, 2000). The fungi in the plant appear to "peacefully coexist" with each other in the nutrient-rich tissues of the host plant. This coexistence may actually be more of a "chemical truce" (Rahman, 2000). Medicinal plants have been recognized as a repository of fungal endophytes with novel metabolites of pharmaceutical importance (Strobel et al., 2004). Distinctly from plants, endophytes can be cultured quickly and the biomass can be accumulated by large scale fermentation. Production of bioactive compounds can be increased by using biotechnology on endophytic fungi in order to meet demands while keeping biodiversity and sustainable ecosystem (Onifade, 2007).

A successful account of the necessity of other source like endophytes from *Taxus brevifolia* for production of taxol has been described by the Stierle and Strobel, (1995). According to Stierleand Strobel, (1995), the highly functionalized taxol a diterpene was isolated primarily from the inner bark of the relatively rare and slow growing Pacific yew tree, *Taxus brevifolia*, and a few related species, in extremely small quantities (<0.02% dry wt). The emergence of taxol as an effective anticancer agent created a difficulty viz., how to ensure an adequate supply of a natural compound of non-microbial origin. Although the pharmaceutical potential of taxol elevated the status of the yew from a nuisance weed to a precious commodity and natural resource, it did not alter the underlying problem; there were simply not enough trees to supply the growing demands for taxol. Advanced preclinical and phase I clinical development of taxol required several collections ranging in size from 5,000 to 15,000 pounds of dry bark. A mature Pacific yew (100 years old) yields approximately 10 pounds of dry bark, so each collection required the sacrifice of 500 to 1500 trees. As the efficacy of the compound became more apparent, the demand for additional taxol was increased. In 1987-1988 a 60,000-pound bark collection was undertaken with little controversy. The need for a second 60,000-pound bark collection in 1989, however, sparked concern about the impact such collection sizes may have on the continued existence of the species.

Even with this estimate, however, it was clear that additional sources of taxol would be necessary. In 1991-1993, a single course of clinical treatment was 125-300 mg of taxol, and typical treatments extended for ten or more courses. Treatment of the 12,000 women who die annually of ovarian cancer alone would consume as much as 36 kg of the drug. Isolation methods yielded 1 kg of taxol from 25,000 pounds of dried bark, or the bark of 2,500 yews. Simply treating ovarian cancer over a one-year period would consume 90,000 mature yews. The recent approval of taxol for the treatment of breast cancer will triple the projected demand. Should taxol prove as effective against other refractory cancers (head and neck and non-small cell lung cancers) as clinical trials have indicated, it is not unreasonable to assume that the demand for taxol may exceed 300 kg, or 750,000 trees per year. This represents an enormous demand on a limited resource. There are simply not enough yews growing in North America to satisfy projected needs of this drug over the next twenty years (Stierle & Strobel, 1995).

Several research groups have addressed the supply problem in a variety of ways. Total syntheses from simple precursors were published virtually simultaneously by Holton et al., (1994) and Nicolaou, et al., (1994) and their co-workers. Although these syntheses are chemical masterpieces, they will probably not answer the supply question (Stierle & Strobel, 1995). To fulfill the requirement of the taxol, a novel endophytic fungus isolated from the inner bark of the Northwest Pacific yew tree was able to synthesize taxol in de novo fashion (Stierle & Stierle, 2000).

The clinically-active agents, topotecan (Hycamtin) and irinotecan® (Camptosar®; CPT-11), are semi-synthetically derived from camptothecin, isolated from the Chinese ornamental tree *Camptotheca acuminata* Decne (Cragg & Newman, 2009). Camptothecin has also been reported to be produced by an endophytic fungus of the family Phycomycetes, subsequently identified as *Entrophospora infrequens*, isolated from the inner bark of *Nothapodytes foetida* (Cragg & Newman, 2009). Despite being dropped from clinical trials by NCI in the 1970s due to severe bladder toxicity, extensive research on the structural modification of camptothecin led to the development of the more effective derivatives, topotecan (Hycamtin®) and irinotecan (CPT-11; Camptosar®). Topotecan is used for the treatment of ovarian and small cell lung cancers, while irinotecan is used for the treatment of colorectal cancers. This class of agents acts through inhibition of topoisomerase I, another important enzyme involved in the replication pathway of DNA during cell cycle progression and, to date, remains by far the most important class of topoisomerase I inhibitors (Cragg & Newman, 2004).

Many endophytes have the potential to synthesize various bioactive metabolites that may directly or indirectly be used as therapeutic agents against numerous diseases (Strobel et al., 2004; Staniek et al., 2008). In recent years, substantial efforts to discover effective inhibitors of α-glucosidases from natural sources have been made (Miller et al., 2012; Rivera-Chavez et al., 2013). Endophytic fungi are thus a rich source of novel organic compounds with interesting biological activities and a high level of biodiversity (Hussain et al., 2009). Novel antibiotics, antimycotics, immunosuppressants, anticancer, anti-diabetic compounds are few natural products have been obtained from endophytic fungi (Dompeipen et al., 2009). A non-peptidal fungal metabolite (L-783,281) was isolated froman endophytic fungus *Pseudomassaria* sp. collected from an African rainforest near Kinshasa in the Democratic Republic of the Congo (Zhang et al., 1999). This compound acts as an insulin mimetic and unlike insulin, is not destroyed in the digestive tract and may be given orally. Oral administration of L-783,281 to two mouse models of diabetes resulted in significant lowering of blood glucose levels. These results may lead to new therapies for diabetes (Zhang et al., 1999). The compounds thielavins A, J and K have been isolated from an endophytic fungus from *Hintonia latiflora*. All these compounds showed in vitro α-glucosidase inhibitory action which was higher than that of acarbose. The a-glucosidase inhibitory properties of thielavin K were corroborated in vivo since it induced a noted anti-hyperglycemic action during an oral sucrose tolerance test (3.1, 10.0 and 31.6 mg/kg) in normal and nicotinamide–streptozotocin diabetic mice. In addition, at a dose of 10 mg/kg, it provoked a moderate hypoglycemic activity in diabetic mice (Rivera-Chavez et al., 2013). Fungal endophytes have begun to be recognized as a rich and diverse source of natural products. Podophyllotoxin, an aryltetralin lignan, is a valuable natural product as a precursor to three anticancer drugs, etoposide, teniposide, and etoposide phosphate. Destruction of wild populations of the primary source plant (*Podophyllum emodi* Wall. Ex Royle) and difficulties of total synthesis of the compound have led many laboratories to search for alternative sources. Endophyte fungi are widespread and perhaps ubiquitous in their occurrence in higher plants (Eyberger et al., 2006).

BACKGROUND

The word phytopharmaceutical deals with a complex mixture of compounds derived from the plant source that is used as a medicine or drug. Plants are the "Sleeping Giants of Drugs Development" as they form a reservoir of potential useful untapped source of drugs that have been serving mankind since the dawn of civilization.

The plant chemicals used for these latter purposes are largely the secondary metabolites, which are derived biosynthetically from plant primary metabolites (e.g., carbohydrates, amino acids, and lipids) and are not directly involved in the growth, development, or reproduction of plants. These secondary metabolites can be classified into several groups according to their chemical classes, such alkaloids, terpenoids, and phenolics. The functions of secondary metabolites in the plants are not understood, but it is believed that these compounds are utilized by the plants for self-defense against microbes or by other external predators. Moreover, the quantitative and qualitative divergence of secondary metabolites may be due to the geographical, climatic, and soil conditions, which in turn may affect the composition and/or synthesize new secondary metabolites\chemotypes from the same plant species (Joshi, 2013d; 2014c). It was observed that *Ritu* or season influences secondary metabolite concentration in the plants or its parts. The ability to synthesize and accumulate the compounds in plants varied greatly throughout the seasons. Consequently, to obtain optimum utility of the plant as a source of medicine, the screening for presence of the secondary metabolites during different season is useful (Ketkar et al., 2015). Several plants in the different forms have been reported in traditional medicine and to find a rational for the treatment of various diseases than to isolated single compounds. The phytopharmaceuticals or extracts are under pipeline in clinical trials for treatment of diseases. The efficacy of phytopharmaceutical agents used in different forms by the people for centuries was validated in many cases by pre-clinical and clinical studies. The impetus to use phytopharmaceutical agents for the treatment of disease, most of the plant based drugs are quite safe and have lesser adverse effects and are claimed that it works as synergistic effects. Synergy effects of the mixture of phytopharmaceuticals and their byproducts contained in plants are claimed to be responsible for improved effectiveness. The multi-drug theory is already being practiced worldwide in the treatment of AIDS and other infectious diseases, hypertension, numerous types of cancer and rheumatic diseases. However, many of the single compounds isolated from the plant origin are effectively used in the medicine.

MAIN FOCUS OF THE CHAPTER

The search of natural products in drug discovery has been greatly enhanced in the last few years. In recent years many of the natural products of medicinal value are the source of drugs, which have been used effectively for centuries in traditional medicine. All the chemical structures are depicted in Figures 1, 2 and 3 wherein the compounds are numbered in parenthesis. In 1805, morphine (1) became the first pharmacologically active compound to be isolated in pure form from a plant. Morphine is profusely found in dried latex of unripe seedpods of *Papaver somniferum* commonly known opium poppy. Morphine is belongs as a narcotic analgesic drug which directly acts on the central nervous system of the body to relieve pain. Codeine (2) or 3-methylmorphine is also found in *Papaver somniferum* in low quantity but it can be derived from morphine. Codeine is used mainly as an antitussive agent, but also as a non-narcotic analgesic. It has been said that it is useful in treating malaria patients. Its use in the treatment of diarrhoea, however, is out of date, because more effective substitutes are now available (Theuns et al., 1986).

Figure 1. Chemical structures of: (1) Morphine; (2) Codeine; (3) Ephedrine; (4) Atropine; (5) Caffeine; (6) Theobromine; (7) Theophylline; (8) Pilocarpine; (9) Quinine; (10) Artemisinin.

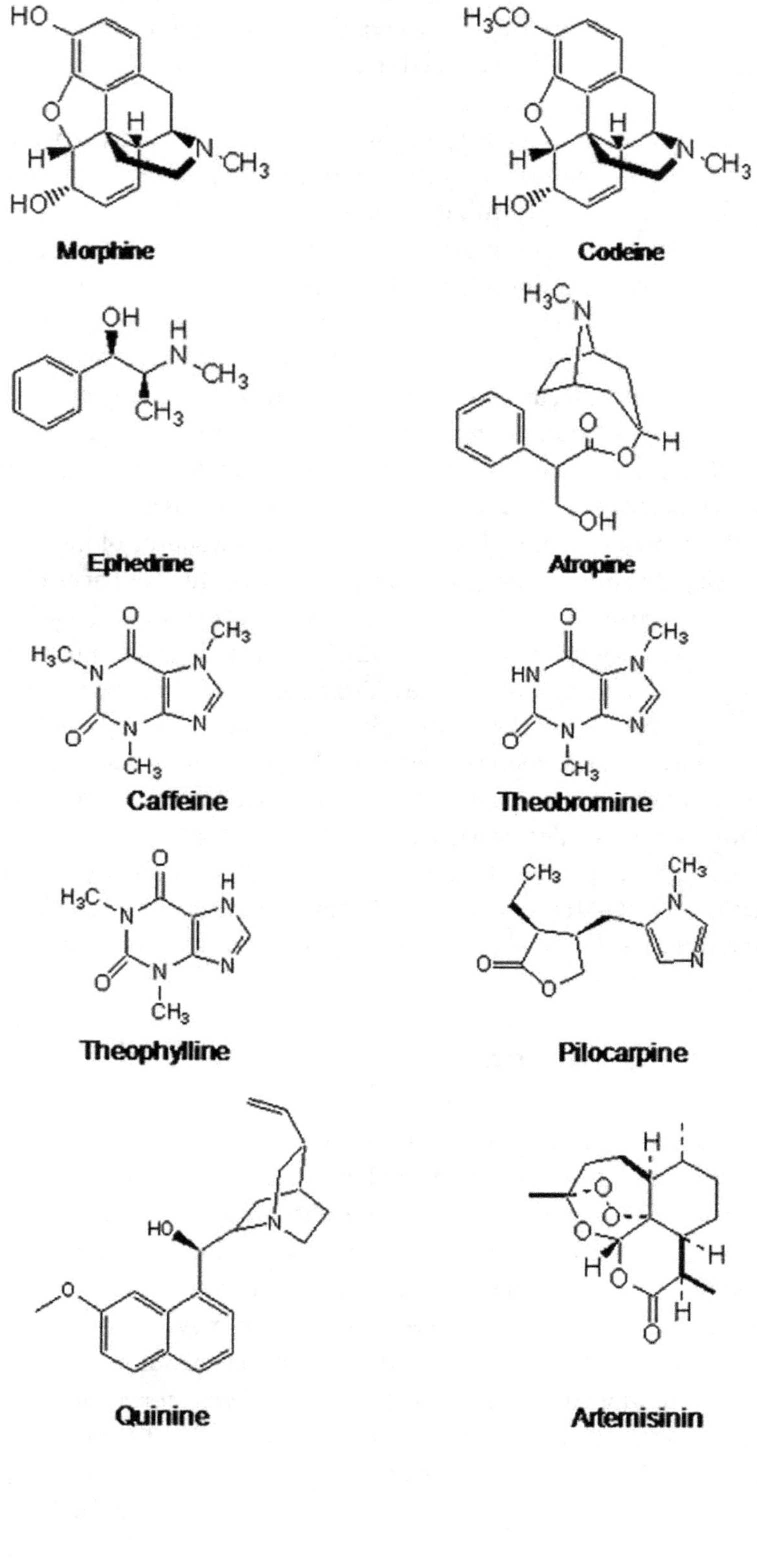

Figure 2. Chemical structures of: (11) Artesunate; (12) Paclitaxel; (13) Docetaxel; (14) camptothecin; (15) Topotecan; (16) Belotecan; (17) delta-9-Tetrahydrocannabinol; (18) Cannabidiol.

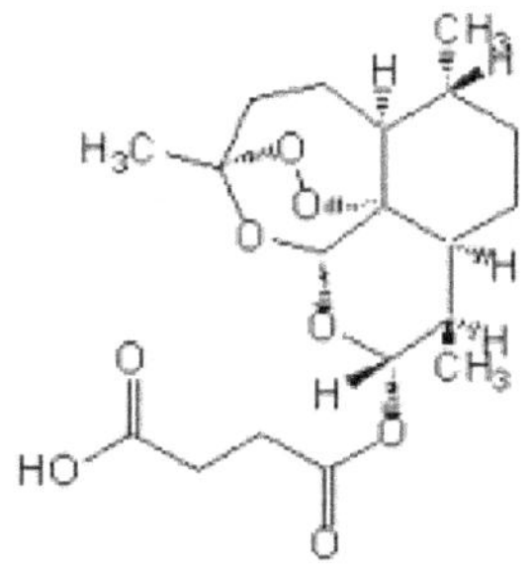

Artesunate

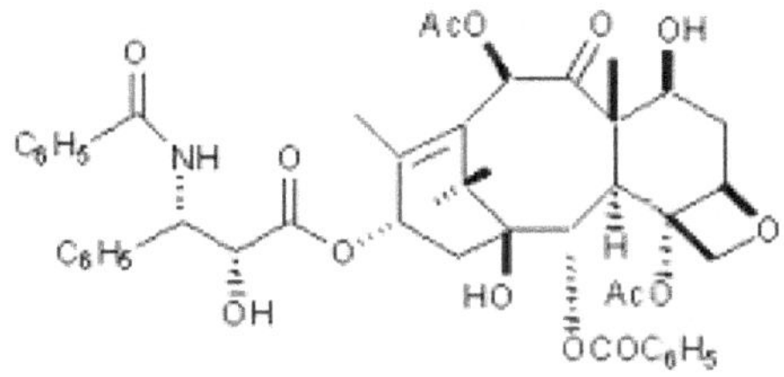

Paclitaxel

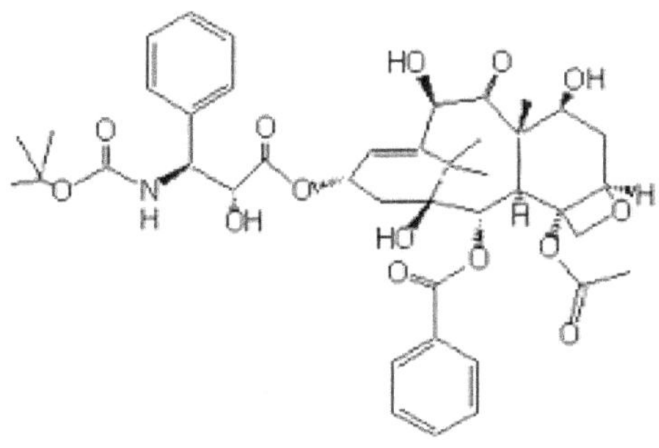

Docetaxel

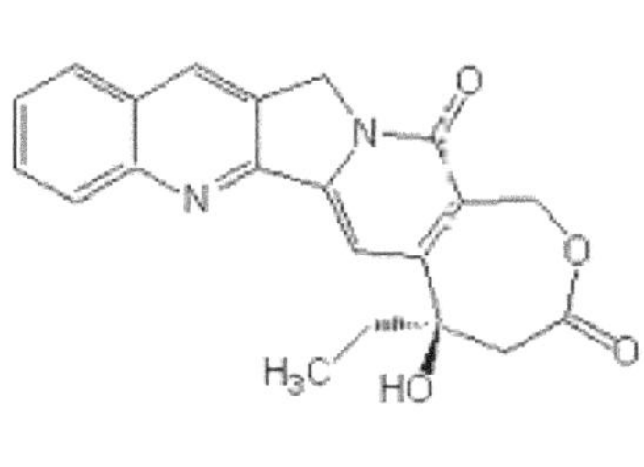

Camptothecin

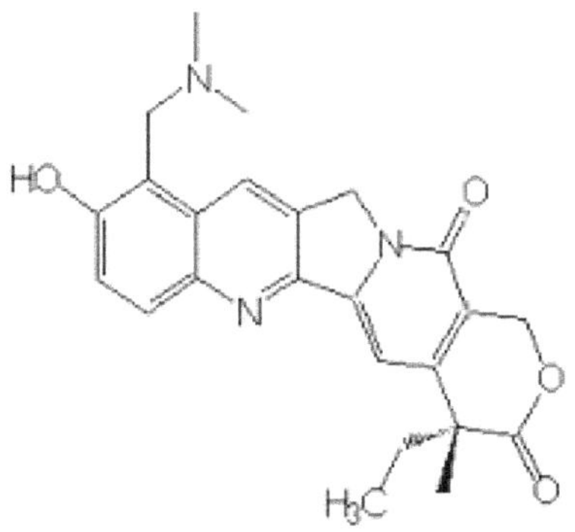

Topotecan

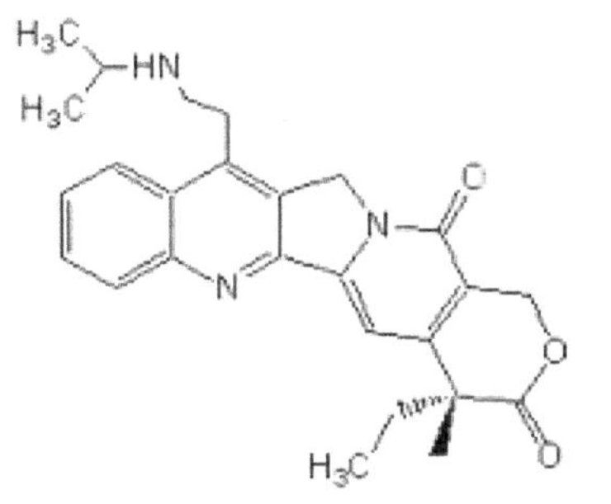

Belotecan

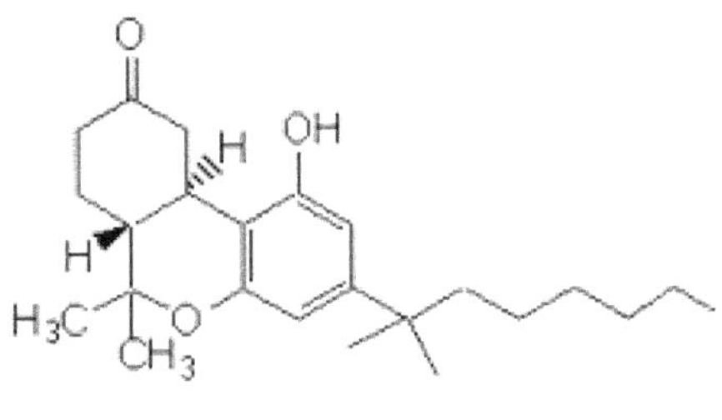

delta-9-Tetrahydrocannabinol

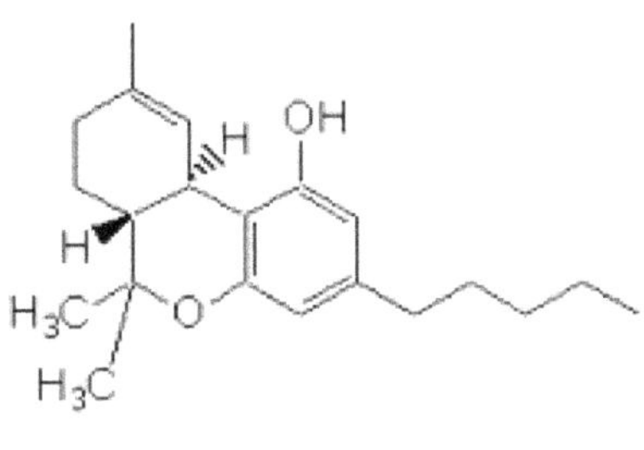

Cannabidiol

Figure 3. Chemical structures of: (19) Galanthamine; (20) Physostigmine; (21) Nitisinone; (22) Leptospermone; (23) Shikimic acid; (24) Oseltamivir phosphate

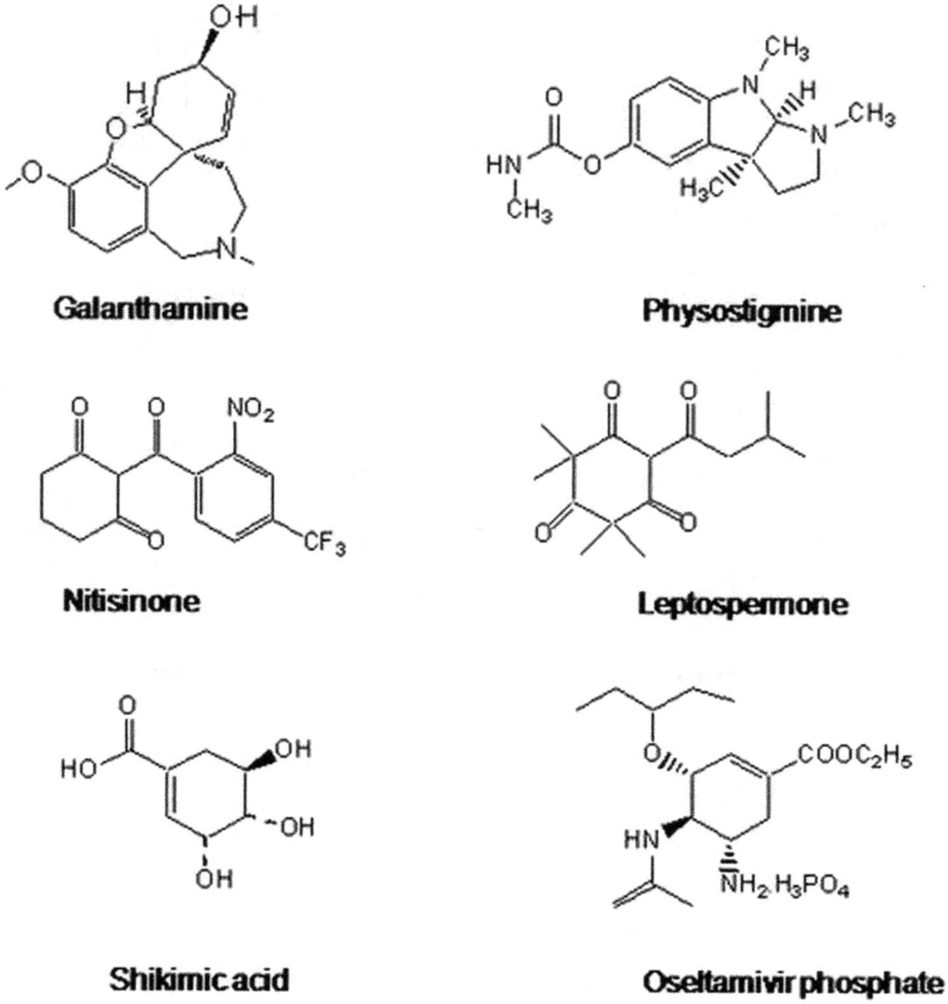

Ephedrine (3) is a sympathomimetic alkaloid, isolated from traditional Chinese herb *má huáng*known as *Ephedra sinica.* The ephedrine is used for therapeutic purpose, primarily as a bronchodilator and decongestant. Its pharmacological applications are related to its sympathomimetic properties, which in turn occur due to its stimulating action on α-, β1-, and β2-adrenergic receptors through direct and indirect effects. Nowadays, there is a concern about the indiscriminate use of ephedrine, since it started to be used to weight loss and enhance athletic performance (Limberger et al., 2013).

The drug atropine (4) is a tropane alkaloid isolated from the plants *Atropa belladonna* of the family Solanaceae. In general, atropine counters the "rest and digest" activity of glands regulated by the parasympathetic nervous system. This occurs because atropine is a competitive antagonist of the muscarinic acetylcholine receptors (acetylcholine being the main neurotransmitter used by the parasympathetic nervous system). Atropine dilates the pupils, increases heart rate, and reduces salivation and other secretions (http://en.wikipedia.org/wiki/Atropine) (see Figure 1).

Caffeine (5) (1,3,7-trimethylpurine-2,6-dione), is a bitter white crystalline central nervous system stimulant psychoactive (Nehlig et al., 1992) alkaloid and has mild diuretic property (FDA, 2010). The chief source of caffeine is a plant *Coffea arabica* of the family Rubiaceae commonly known as coffee. The beans, leaves, and fruit of more than 60 plants contain varying quantities of caffeine (Kovacs, 2008; Andrews et al. 2006). In those plants caffeine serves as a pesticide, killing or paralyzing insects that feed on the plants. Coffee, tea, and cocoa are the major plants containing caffeine that are cultivated. Guarana, kola nuts, and yerba maté are also cultivated for use as sources of caffeine in energy drinks and snacks. The FDA says that caffeine is both a drug and a food additive. Caffeine is used in both prescription and over-the-counter medicines to treat tiredness or drowsiness and to improve the effect of some pain relievers. People with heart problems shouldn't use caffeine because it makes their hearts work too hard, and people with anxiety problems or panic attacks may find that caffeine makes them feel worse (http://www.fda.gov/downloads/UCM200805.pdf). Caffeine is used for prevention and treatment of bronchopulmonary dysplasia which is a chronic pulmonary condition that usually evolves after premature birth and respiratory distress syndrome (Kugelman & Durand, 2011; Schmidt, 2005). Caffeine therapy for apnea of prematurity improves weight gain (Schmidt et al., 2007), neurodevelopmental disability in infants, with very low birth weight. Caffeine is an adenosine-receptor blocker that inhibits adenosine induced vasodilatation by blocking these receptors used to treat orthostatic hypotension due to autonomic failure (Schmidt et al., 2006).

Theobromine (6) (3,7 dehydro3,7 dimethyl-IH-purine-2,6-dione) also known as 3,7-dimethylxanthine is a purine alkaloids. It is widely distributed in nature in a variety of plants such as *Commelia thea* (tea leaves), *Theobroma cacao* (cocoa), *Cola acuminata* (cola), *Paullinia cupana*, *Ilex aquifolium* and other *Ilex* species including Theaceae, Sterculiaceae, Sapindaceae (Eteng et al., 1997). Theobromine is used as a diuretic, central nervous system stimulants (Leonard et al., 1987), myocardial stimulants, vasodilators and smooth muscle relaxants (Windholz, 1983).

Theophylline (7) is the typical alkaloid in mate´ and green tea. Only the slightest of traces has been established in cacao (Matissek, 1997). Theophylline has been used in the treatment of asthma for over 70 years, but its use has recently declined, as inhaled corticosteroids have become the mainstay of asthma control and inhaled β_2-agonists are more effective bronchodilators (Ito et al., 2002). Asthma is a chronic inflammatory disease of the airways characterized by reduced airway patency, which is regulated by bronchodilators such as β-agonists, and by the infiltration of inflammatory and immune cells, which is treated by corticosteroids (Ito et al., 2002). There is increasing evidence that theophylline has anti-inflammatory or immunomodulatory actions in asthma (Barnes & Pauwels, 1994).

Pilocarpine (8) is an imidazole alkaloid found large amount in the plant *Pilocarpus microphyllus* (Pinheiro, 1997). This plant is a shrub and found in the under storey of the pre-Amazonian rain forest and in the state of Maranhão (Sandhu et al., 2006). The pilocarpine is a cholinergic parasympathomimetic agent with predominantly muscarinic action, it may stimulate cholinergic receptors on the surfaces of the exocrine glands, causing a reduction of the symptoms of xerostomia, includes dry mouth, mucosal burning, and fissured lips and/or tongue, with difficulty in eating, swallowing, conversing, and wearing removable prosthetic devices such as dentures and even in patients with no measurable salivary flow at rest (Gornitsky et al., 2004). Xerostomia represents a frequent and significant radiation-induced side effect in the treatment of head and neck cancers. It leads to increased incidence of dental caries, oral mucositis, and impaired mastication (Gornitsky et al., 2004). Moreover, various studies reported that pilocarpine improves the overall condition of xerostomia when prescribed after radiotherapy (LeVeque et al., 1993; Johnson et al., 1993).

Quinine (9) is cinchona alkaloid isolated from the bark of several species of cinchonatrees. The high yield obtained from the plant *Cinchona ledgeriana* (Song, 2009). Quinine had a profound influence on modern colonial history and a number of historians have highlighted the importance of this single drug as one of the "tools of empire" (Meshnick & Dobson, 2001). Quinine was used as the antimalarial drug caused by *Plasmodium falciparum*. As per the recommendation of World Health Organization (WHO) quinine should be used when artemisinins are not available (WHO, 2006).

Artemisinin (10), having very strong potential as the non-conventional antimalarial drug, is a sesquiterpene lactone with endoperoxide bridge and has been isolated from *Artemisia annua*, a pervasive wormwood with a long history of use, known as 'Qinghao'. The Chinese scientist extracted a crystalline compound named "Qinghaosu" (QHS) from 'Qinghao', *Artemisia annua*(Kinghorn, 1987) and this stable peroxide emerged as a potent antimalarial (Luo & Shen, 1987).

Artesunate (11), a derivative of artemisinin isolated from *Artemisia annua* is recommended by the WHO in preference to quinidine for the treatment of severe malaria and has been used worldwide for many years (http://www.cdc.gov/malaria/diagnosis_treatment/artesunate.html). In laboratory models artesunate has demonstrated cytotoxic effects against a variety of cancer cells. However, there is little available information about the antitumor effects of artesunate on human gastric cancer cells (Zhang et al., 2015).

The taxane class agents (paclitaxel and docetaxel) are one of the most important cancer chemotherapeutics in the past several years. Both drugs are very similar in mechanism of action, preclinical and clinical activities. Paclitaxel (12) (Taxol), one of microtubule-stabilizing anticancer agent, was first obtained from the bark of Pacific yew (*Taxus brevifolia)* in 1971. The Pacific yew is a highly toxic plant but it was employed medicinally by several native of North American Indian tribes who used it to treat a variety of complaints (Moreman, 1988). Paclitaxel is used for the treatment of metastatic pancreatic cancer, non-small cell lung cancer and breast cancer (http://www.cancer.gov/about-cancer/treatment/drugs/fda-nanoparticle-paclitaxel) (see Figure 2).

Docetaxel (13) is semi-synthetically derived compound from 10-deacetylbaccatin III extracted from the needles of the European yew (*Taxus baccata)*. Docetaxel is used for treatment of various diseases viz., head and neck cancer, gastric cancer, breast cancer, prostate cancer, and non-small cell lung cancer (http://www.cancer.gov/about-cancer/treatment/drugs/fda-docetaxel). The laboratory studies showed that the paclitaxel a chemotherapy drug, can be used in the treatment of renal fibrotic diseases. Mechanistically, paclitaxel treatment blocks the STAT3 activity by disrupting the association of STAT3 with tubulin and STAT3 nucleus translocation (Zhang et al., 2015).

The compound camptothecin (14), a planar pentacyclic ring system containing a pyrrol (3,4-b) quinoline and α-hydroxy lactone was isolated from the plant *Camptotheca acuminata* Decne (Nyssaceae), a tree that is native to China, growing in relatively warm areas of southeastern provinces of Szechwan, Yunnan, and Kwangsi (Perdue et al., 1970). Topotecan(15) is a chemotherapeutic agent that is a topoisomerase inhibitor. It is a water-soluble derivative of camptothecin. It is used in form of the hydrochloride to treat ovarian cancer and lung cancer, as well as other cancer types (http://www.ebi.ac.uk/chebi/searchId.do?chebiId=CHEBI:63632. In addition, a semi-synthetic camptothecin derivative, belotecan (16), was launched in Korea for treatment of small-cell lung and cervical cancer (Butler, 2005).

Two FDA-approved drugs, dronabinol and nabilone, contain delta-9-tetrahydrocannabinol (THC) (17). They treat nausea caused by chemotherapy and increase appetite in patients with extreme weight loss caused by AIDS (NIDA, 2015). THC is the main ingredient of the plant marijuana, and is principally responsible for the psychoactive effects (Cooper & Haney, 2009). Marijuana is the crude drug derived from the plant *Cannabis sativa*, belongs to the family Cannabaceae that has only one genus *Cannabis* with only one species *sativa* that is highly variable (Elsohly & Slade, 2005). Cannabis has had a long history of use (over 5000 years) starting in Central and Northeast Asia with current use spreading worldwide as a recreational drug or as a medicine albeit unauthorized. The cannabis plant (*Cannabis sativa*) and products thereof (such as marijuana, hashish and hash oil) have a long history of use both as a medicinal agent and intoxicant. Over the last few years there have been an active debate regarding the medicinal aspects of cannabis. Currently cannabis products are classified as Schedule I drugs under the Drug Enforcement Administration (DEA) Controlled Substances act, which means that the drug is only available for human use as an investigational drug (Russo, 2001; 2002; Elsohly, 2002; Elsohly & Slade, 2005). Cannabidiol (18) (CBD) another compound of marijuana exhibited prominent anticancer activity (Scott et al., 2013).The United Kingdom, Canada, and several European countries have approved nabiximolssynthetic cannabinoids, a mouth spray containing THC and CBD. It treats muscle control problems. The United States is conducting clinical trials for its safe use in treating cancer pain (NIDA, 2015*).In vitro* studies of THC and CBD both alone and in combination with radiotherapy in a number of glioma cell lines (T98G, U87MG, and GL261) inhibit glioma growth as well as neutralize oncogenic processes such as angiogenesis. High-grade glioma is one of the most aggressive cancers in adult humans and long-term survival rates are very low as standard treatments for glioma remain largely unsuccessful. These studies suggested a potential clinical benefit for glioma patients by using these treatment modalities.

Alzheimer's disease (AD) was first described by the German psychiatrist, Alois Alzheimer, in 1907. Alzheimer's disease is a neurological disorder in which the death of brain cells causes memory loss and cognitive decline. It is a neurodegenerative disease, which means there is progressive brain cell death that happens over a course of time (National Institute of Neurological Disorders and Stroke (NINDS), 2013).The total brain size shrinks with Alzheimer's - the tissue has progressively fewer nerve cells and connections (NINDS 2013; Alzheimer's Association, 2013a). The most recent census has enabled researchers to give estimates that in 2010, 4.7 million people of 65 years of age and older were living with Alzheimer's disease in the US (Hebert et al., 2013). In 2013 statistical report from the Alzheimer's Association gives a proportion of the population affected - just over a tenth of people in the over-65 age group have the disease in the US. In the over-85s, the proportion goes up to about a third (Alzheimer's Association, 2013b). The development of galanthamine (galantamine) (19) a drug commonly used today in the treatment of AD. It is a natural product known from several members of the Amaryllidaceae and the idea for developing a natural product from these species seems to be based on ethnobotanical information. This alkaloid was first isolated from snowdrop (*Galanthus* spp., most notably *G. woronowii*), but today it is obtained from *Narcissus* spp. and *Leucojum* spp. (esp. *L. aestivum*) as well as synthetically (Heinrich & Teoh, 2004). Galantamine has a unique, dual mode of action. It is a reversible, competitive inhibitor of acetylcholinesterase, and proven activity as an allosteric modulator of nicotinic acetylcholine receptors (nAChRs). This latter activity is thought to be particularly important since decreases in the expression and activity of nAChRs make a large contribution to the reduction in central cholinergic neurotransmission in patients with AD (Lilienfeld, 2002). Physostigmine (20) or serine is a parasympathomimetic alkaloid, widely regarded as the antidote to anticholinergic toxicity, is a naturally occurring cholinesterase inhibitor found in the Calabar bean (Watkins et al., 2014) and short span of action has rendered it useless for treating Alzheimer's disease (Scheindlin, 2010).The Calabar bean or ordeal bean (*Physostigma venenosum* Balf. of the family Leguminosae) is the seed of a leguminous plant, a native of tropical Africa, poisonous to humans (Lloyd, 1897) (see Figure 3).

Tyrosinemia type 1 is a rare genetic metabolic disorder characterized by lack of the enzyme fumarylacetoacetate hydrolase (FAH), which is needed to break down the amino acid tyrosine. Failure to properly break down tyrosine leads to abnormal accumulation of tyrosine and its metabolites in the liver, resulting in severe liver disease. Tyrosine may also accumulate in the kidneys and central nervous system (McKiernan, 2006). Tyrosinemia type 1 affects males and females in equal numbers. It is estimated to occur in one of every 100,000-120,000 births in the United States. In one region of the Quebec province of Canada, the disorder is estimated to occur in approximately one in 1,850 births. The birth prevalence is also higher in Norway where it is estimated to be one in 60,000 (NORD, 2012). The triketones, an important new class of herbicides, are reported to be derivatives of the plant-produced phytotoxin leptospermone, derived from the bottlebrush plant (Callistemon spp.) (Duke et al., 2000). *Callistemon citrinus* commonly known as Bottlebrush belongs to a family Myrtaceae and comprises over 30 species that has a great medicinal importance (Mabberly, 1997). *Callistemon* spp. are also used as weed control (Wheeler, 2005) and as bioindicators for environmental management (Burchett et al., 2002). Nitisinone (21) is a derivative of leptospermone (22), a new class of herbicide isolated from the *Callistemon citrinus*. Both the compounds nitisinone and leptospermone inhibit 4-hydroxyphenyl pyruvate dioxygenase (HPPD), the enzyme involved in plastoquinone and tocopherol biosynthesis in plants (Duke et al., 2000). In humans, inhibition of HPPD prevents tyrosine catabolism, leading to the accumulation of tyrosine metabolites, 4-hydroxyphenyl pyruvic acid and 4-hydroxyphenyl lactic acid, which can be excreted through the urine (Hall et al., 2001). The drug nitisinone was approved by the FDA for the treatment of hereditary tyrosinemia type 1 diseases.

Shikimic acid (23) was first isolated in 1885 by Eijkman from the fruit of the Japanese plant *Illicium religiosum* Sieb. The elucidation of its structure nearly 50 years later, and the discovery of shikimic acid, the starting material in the commercial synthesis of the antiviral agent oseltamivir under the trade name Tamiflu (Enrich et al., 2008). Oseltamivir phosphate (24) (Tamiflu) is an orally active neuraminidase inhibitor developed for the treatment and prophylaxis of influenza viruses A and B. The starting material for the oseltamivir synthesis is (−)-shikimic acid, an important biochemical intermediate in plants and microorganisms.

One of the compound fulyzaq (crofelemer), the first anti-diarrheal drug for HIV/AIDS patients has been recently approved by U.S. Food and Drug Administration (FDA). The compound crofelemer is a proanthocyanidin oligomer, isolated from red latex of the plant *Croton lechleri* (Euphorbiaceae) found in the western Amazonian regions of South America (Orozco-Topete et al., 1997). Native populations of South America have used the sap of the plant for self-treatment of secretory diarrhea for many years (Crutchley et al., 2010). Crofelemer is a first-in-class agent that may be useful for different types of secretory diarrhea, since it prevents chloride and fluid secretion into the bowel by directly inhibiting 2 distinct intestinal chloride channels (Crutchley et al., 2010). Crofelemer possesses a unique mechanism of action through inhibition of both cyclic adenosine monophosphate (cAMP)–stimulated cystic fibrosis transmembrane conductance regulator (CFTR) and calcium stimulated (CaCC) chloride intestinal Channels (Crutchley et al., 2010). The drugcrofelemer has been investigated for the treatment of several types of secretory diarrhea, including traveler's diarrhea (DiCesare et al., 2002), AIDS-associated diarrhea (Holodniy et al., 1999) and infectious diarrhea such as cholera (Bardhan et al., 1999).

Some of the botanical compounds, which have been demonstrated to have positive effects in cancer therapy, have a long history behind them. It was recently demonstrated that the green tea antioxidant epigallocatechin-3-gallate significantly slowed breast cancer growth in female mice: its use is attested in ancient Japanese texts (Nobili et al., 2009). The juice, peel and oil of *Punica granatum* has also been shown to possess anticancer activity, including interference with tumour cell proliferation, cell cycle, invasion and angiogenesis (Lansky & Newman, 2007). Promising and selective anti-cancer effects have been observed with Saffron (stigmata of *Crocus sativus* L.) *in vitro* and *in vivo*, but not yet in clinical trials (Nobili et al., 2009). Homoharringtonine was isolated from the Chinese tree *Cephalotaxus harringtonia* var. *drupacea* (Sieb and Zucc.), and a racemic mixture of harringtonine and homoharringtonine has been used successfully in China for the treatment of acute myelogenous leukemia and chronic myelogenous leukemia. Purified homoharringtonine has shown efficacy against various leukemias, including some resistant to standard treatment and has been reported to produce complete hematologic remission in patients with late chronic phase myelogenous leukemia (Cragg & Newman, 2009). Vinca alkaloids are isolated from the periwinkle plant *Catharanthus roseus*, also known as *Vinca rosea*. The extracts of *Vinca rosea* possess many therapeutic effects including anti-tumour activity. The compounds vincristine, vinblastine and vindesine are the first Vinca alkaloids with anti-tumour activity to be identified from the plant *Vinca rosea* (Nobili et al., 2009).

The compound vinflunine, a bis-fluorinated vinorelbine derivative, has been synthesized by super-acid chemistry. Due to its favourable preclinical anti-tumour activities, including microtubule dynamics disruption, anti-angiogenesis and prolonged multidrug resistance development, vinflunine is now being widely studied in phase I–III clinical trials (Nobili et al., 2009).There are many flavonoids in the plant kingdom which may possess cancer chemopreventive efficacy. The isoflavone genistein from soya and the flavone quercetin a constituent of onions, are examples of flavonoids which prevent cancer in rodent models of carcinogenesis. The compound genistein is currently in clinical trial for the prevention of recurrent localized prostate cancer subsequent to radical prostatectomy (Manson et al., 2005). Rohitukine, isolated as the constituent responsible for anti-inflammatory and immunomodulatory activity from *Dysoxylum binectariferum* Hook. f. (Meliaceae) which is phylogenetically related to the Ayurvedic plant *D. malabaricum* Bedd.used for rheumatoid arthritis. It is currently in phase I and phase II clinical trials, either alone or in combination with other anticancer agents, against a broad range of tumors, including leukemias, lymphomas and solid tumors (Cragg& Newman, 2009).

The plants have provided humans with many of their essential needs, including life-saving pharmaceutical agents from the antiquity. A number of terrestrial as well as marine flora are available and many of them have not yet been screened for biological activities and it need to explore the active constituents in the search for new medicines, particularly with the development of highly sensitive and versatile analytical methods are available.

ISSUES, CONTROVERSIES, PROBLEMS

Plants have been the mainstay of the oldest known systems of medicine in the world and have survived the ravages of time spanning thousands of years. Existing biological resources can be exploited in the search for new molecules, because while there are many compounds already under investigation for their chemopreventive properties, we have only begun to scratch the surface in terms of the number of possible efficacious agents in the plant kingdom (Manson et al., 2005).

The advent of next generation sequencing technology has led to the discovery of rare private mutations which has revolutionized our understanding of the genetics of complex diseases, with major focus on Cancer. The development of high-throughput platforms like Roche-454, Illumina Hiseq, Ion Torrent PGM etc., has provided the geneticists with large chunks of genomic data like never before, and its relevant bioinformatics pipelines contributing to uncover myriad cancer biological complexity and heterogeneity. Thus, there is a growing trend of studies undertaking whole genome and exome-sequencing from individuals affected with different subtypes of cancer thereby identifying and validating specific driver events and novel target genes by integrative approaches to understand their oncogenic potential and intratumoral diversity. The recent developments in diverse study designs and approaches in cancer genomics globally, viz., whole-genome, exome sequencing, transcriptome, methylome analysis, genome wide association studies, gene regulation analysis, cytogenetic analysis, DNA- Protein interaction analysis (CHIP-Seq), small RNA discovery to name a few have been inclusively studied. The focus on the future perspective of these genomic and epigenomic studies in developing important therapeutic targets and their subsequent validation by effective clinical trials that leads to cancer drug discovery, personalized medicines, painless and costless treatment, patients management and lifespan. Moreover, importance of dietary and natural resources as the medicine particularly phytochemicals for cancer prevention are required.

One of the major issue, more than 70% of all cancer patients are very interested in herbal drugs. However, many of them do not inform their oncologist about their use (Kelberet a., 2014). As 19 to 75% of all cancer patients suffer from sleep disturbances. The cancer patients often have difficulties to sleep and are restless, so that they can use herbal drugs such as valerian in order to avoid chemically defined sedatives and hypnotics as they fear becoming addicted. However, they state that warnings that valerian (*Valeriana officinalis*) may stimulate CYP 3A4 (Kelberet a., 2014).

Nutraceuticals are emerged as potential cancer preventive natural sources from food (Baichwal, 1999). It was hypothesized that this observation is related to diet or more specifically to nutraceuticals present in fruits, vegetables, common beverages, grains, marine products, medicinal plants, and herbs (Jankun et al., 2006). The nutraceuticals are natural bioactive chemical compounds and have value in health promoting, disease preventing or semi-medicinal properties. The nutraceuticals are found as natural products from (a) the food industry (b) the herbal and dietary supplement (c) pharmaceutical industry and (d) the newly emerged bioengineered microorganisms, agro products or active biomolecules. It may range from isolated nutrients, herbal products, dietary supplements and diets to genetically engineered "custom" foods and processed products such as cereals, soups and beverages (Dureja et al., 2003). Many dietary agents have extremely promising modes of action when investigated in cultured cells, but *in vivo* are much less effective. One of the reasons is bioavailability. Many purified dietary compounds have limited solubility, making it difficult to attain plasma or tissue concentrations equivalent to those showing activity *in vitro*. On a cautionary note, there may be a very good reason why many of these compounds are poorly available to tissues, so any attempts to use them in humans at higher doses than are available from the diet should be assessed for possible toxic consequences (Manson et al.,2005). Chemically the nutraceuticals may be classified as isoprenoid derivatives (terpenoids, carotenoids, saponins, tocotrienols, tocopherols, terpenes), phenolic compounds (couramines, tannins, lignins, anthocyanins, isoflavones, flavanones, flavanoids), and carbohydrate derivatives (ascorbic acid, oligosaccharides, non-starch polysaccharides) etc. (Sharma, 2009). The validation of nutraceuticals against cancer is under progress. In recent reports on cancer protection by nutraceuticals were evidenced for lymphoma (Russell et al., 2007), skin cancer (Hercberg et al., 2007), pancreatic cancer (Larsson et al., 2006), while vitamins and minerals were validated in chemoprevention trial of different cancers (Sandler et al., 2001). Two prominent nutraceuticals (curcumin and EGCG from green tea) have been implicated in anti-cancer activity (Manson et al., 2005). Natural product based drug discovery is increasing based on new technologies, such as combinatorial synthesis and high-throughput screening and their associated approaches. The vincristine, irinotecan, etoposide and paclitaxel are classic examples of plant-derived compounds; actinomycin D, mitomycin C, bleomycin, doxorubicin and l-asparaginase are drugs coming from microbial sources, and cytarabine is the first drug originating from a marine source. To date, new generations of taxanes, anthracyclines, vinca alkaloids, camptothecins, as well as the novel class of epothilones have been developed. Some of these are in clinical use, others in clinical trials. Other agents originating from marine sources (both plants and animals) (e.g. trabectedin-ET-743, bryostatin-1, neovastat) have also entered clinical trials (Nobili et al., 2009). Most *in vitro* studies investigating a new dietary agent initially look for indications of growth inhibition, cell cycle arrest and induction of apoptosis in tumour cell lines (Manson et al., 2005).

There is concomitant increase in the prevalence of type1 diabetes, the major driver of the epidemic is the more common form of diabetes, namely type2 diabetes which accounts for more than 90% of all diabetes cases. Nowhere is the diabetes epidemic more pronounced than in India as estimated that 32 million people had diabetes in the year 2000 (Wild et al., 2004). The International Diabetes Federation (IDF) estimates the total number of diabetic subjects to be around 40.9 million in India and this is further set to rise to 69.9 million by the year 2025 (Sicree et al., 2006). The most disturbing trend is the shift in age of onset of diabetes to a younger age in the recent years. This could have long lasting adverse effects on nation's health and economy (Mohan et al., 2007). Several plants are used for the management of the diabetes. Some example of the plants viz.,*Acacia arabica or nilotica* (Singh, 2011), *Capparis sepiaria* (Selvamani et al., 2008), *Catharanthus roseus* (Rasineni et al., 2010; Singh et al., 2001), *Barleria prionitis* (Geetha and Wahi, 2001), *Barleria lupulina* (Suba et al., 2004), *Balanites aegypticea* (Baragob et al., 2014), *Aegle marmelos* (Seema et al., 1996; Das et al, 1996), *Allium cepa*(Augusti, 1973; Mathew & Augusti, 1975; Gupta et al.,1977), *Artemisia pallens*(Subramonium et al., 1996); *Areca catechu* (Chempakam, 1993), *Beta vulgaris* (Yoshikawa et al., 1996), *Biophytum sensitivum* (Puri & Baral, 1998), *Brassica juncea* (Khan et al., 1995), *Caesalpinia bonducella*(Sharma et al., 1997), *Cajanus cajan*(Amalraj & Ignachimuthu, 1998), *Citrullus colocynthis* (Abdel-Hassan et al., 2000), *Eugenia jambolana, Tinospora cordifolia* (Grover et al., 2000), *Feronia elephantum* (Joshi et al., 2009a), *Coccinia indica* (Mukherjee et al., 1972), *Eugenia uniflora*(Arai et al., 1999), *Bambusa arundinacea* (Joshi et al., 2009b), *Andrographis paniculata*(Nugroho et al. 2012), *Gymnema sylvestre* (Thakur et al., 2012) and may more plant possessing anti-diabetic activity in *in vivo* models. Several compounds viz., S-methyl cysteine sulphoxide (sulphur containing amino acid) (Kumari et al., 1995), allicin (Mathew & Augusti, 1973), S-allyl cysteine sulphoxide (sulphur containing amino acid) (Sheela & Augusti, 1992), C-flavonol glucoside called as shamimin (Saleem et al., 1999), andrographolide (Nugroho et al., 2012), gymnemic acid, gymnemagenin (Persaud et al., 1999; Porchezhian & Dobriyal, 2003)and many more compounds have been isolated from various plants containing anti-diabetic activity.

Parthenin (a sesquiterpene pseudoguaianolide) isolated from *Parthenium hysterophorus* exhibits significant anti-malarial activity against a multidrug resistant strain of *Plasmodium falciparum*. Molecular matching of the oxygen atoms of parthenin and the new anti-malarial drug qinghaosu (Artemisinin) show that both molecules to be amphipathic with common areas for their oxygen atoms and hydrogen framework (Hooper et al., 1990). Parthenin also shows antiamoebic (Sharma & Bhutani, 1988) and allelopathic properties (Kanchan, 1975; Patil &Hegde, 1988). Forskolin (also called Coleonol) is a labdane diterpene that is produced by the Indian Coleus plant (*Coleus forskohlii*). Forskolin is commonly used to raise levels of cyclic AMP (cAMP) in the study and research of cell physiology Forskolin activates the enzyme adenylyl cyclase and increases intracellular levels of cAMP. cAMP is an important second messenger necessary for the proper biological response of cells to hormones and other extracellular signals. It is required for cell communication in the hypothalamus/pituitary gland axis and for the feedback control of hormones (Mulhall et al., 1997). The flavonoids are known to exhibit several biological activities including anti-HIV activity (Vlietinck et al., 1998). The anti-HIV prenylated flavonoids as 6, 8-diprenylaromadendrin, 6, 8-diprenylkaempferol and lonchocarpol an isolated from the plant *Monotes africanus* exhibited HIV-inhibitory activity in the XTT-based, whole-cell screen. (Meragelman et al., 2001). *Ixeris chinensis* Nakai (Compositae) known as Siyekucai, is a perennial plant, and used as a folk medicine in China for the treatment of bronchitis, pneumonia, pharyngitis, dysentery and poisonous indigestion on the basis of its anti-febrile, antidotal and analgesic effects (Shiojima et al., 1996). Three new guaianolides, 10α-hydroxy-3-oxoguaia-4(15),11(13)-dieno-12,6α-lactone, 10α-hydroxy-3-oxo-4βH-guaia-11(13)-eno-12,6α-lactone, and 10α-hydroxy-3-oxoguaia-4,11(13)-dieno-12,6α-lactone have been isolated from the methanolic extract of the whole plant of *Ixeris chinensis* (Zhang et al., 2002). 3-Hydroxy-4-pyrone-3α-D-Glucopyranoside a novel glucoside has been isolated from aerial parts of *Erigeron karwinskyanus* DC (Mathela et al., 1984), and shows a strong biological activity against certain pathogens viz., *Aspergillus, Penicillium* and *Fusarium* species (Mathela et al., 1986).

The major issue for the plant based drug especially isolated compounds which are present in plant with low yield. It cannot execute the demand of pharmaceutical industries. For this reason biotechnology should be apply taking consideration into enhancement of the compound of interest. Plant tissue culture is an option to solve the purpose. Though this statement is controversial we must think over in the way to en-cash the amount of manpower and cost involved in such research. Here in this section it is attempting to highlight such issues in plant biotechnology especially related to tissue culture. Manipulation of DNA to alter its expression in medicinal plants is an area that is widely expanding, provided that the character of interest is present shelled to small number of genes. Although the primary target of trait for manipulation in medicinal plants is the content of active compounds, to which other traits such as development as crops, basic agronomic characters related to uniformity, stability, growth and development, and resistance to biotic and abiotic stresses, can serve as secondary also to be improved (Bajaj, 1998; Dubey & Guerra, 2002). The application of biotechnological approaches to medicinal plants does not start from a low baseline. There is already considerable interest in manipulating plant biosynthetic pathways to produce drug precursors, food components or pesticides; for example, through trichomes, specialized surface organs that manufacture, store and exude secondary metabolites (Stevenson, 2004).

In *Mentha* spp. (mints), biosynthetic pathways have been engineered to modify essential oil production in the trichomes and to enhance the resistance of the plant to fungal infection and abiotic stresses (Veronese et al., 2001). There is a long history of experimental and commercial production of high-value phytochemicals by tissue culture, an *in vitro* system for growing plant organs, explants, tissues and cells or protoplasts. Genetic transformation of cultures using bacterial vectors to transfer genes into the cultured plant DNA has been widely employed to improve product output in such systems. For example, hairy root cultures, transformed by infecting cells with the bacterium *Agrobacterium rhizogenes*, often sustain stable and high productivity in hormone-free culture conditions (Sevon & Oksman-Caldentey, 2002). An efficient transgene delivery system is thus already in place for several important medicinal plants, including *Papaver somniferum* (Park & Facchini, 2000), *Artemisia* spp. (wormwoods) (Chen et al., 1999), members of the family Solanaceae (Moyano et al., 1999) and *Taraxacum platycarpum* (Lee et al., 2004).

Tissue culture often promotes genetic disturbances, which result in somaclonal variation, greatly extending the range of useful variation available to the breeder (Kukreja & Dhawan, 2000). Tissue culture can also contribute to the conservation of valuable biodiversity (Augustine & D'Souza, 1997) and somatic embryogenesis. The micro-propagation of whole plants from cultured cells, has a potentially significant part to play in establishing breeding material from wild populations (Kintzios & Michaelakis, 1999) and in mass-producing material for selection or engineering (Lakshmanan et al., 2002).

The other option could be the plant endophytic fungi, where not only the possibilities to get plethora ofcompound of interest but also can be obtain new biologically active compounds in mass production. In this issue several plant endophytic fungi have been reported in the literature with varieties of the compounds which exhibited prominent biological activities. It must be considerable that genuine endophytic fungus producing the secondary metabolites likes signature constituent(s) or other compound(s) that produced by the plant itself, though in small quantity. Several research groups now a day are working in this area.

Herbs are natural products and their chemical composition varies depending on several factors, such as botanical species, used chemotypes, the anatomical part of the plant used (seed, flower, root, leaf, and so on) and also storage, sun, humidity, type of ground, time of harvest, geographic area; and merchandized products containing on the label the same product varying in their content and concentrations of chemical constituents from batch to batch; and even the same manufacturer can merchandize in different periods and products containing different substances although standardized to achieve a high pharmaceutical quality. This variability can result in significant differences in pharmacological activity involving both pharmacodynamic and pharmacokinetic issues (Firenzuoli& Gori, 2007).

Currently, the major pharmaceutical companies have demonstrated renewed interest in investigating higher plants as sources for new lead structures along with development of standardized phytotherapeutic agents with proven efficacy, safety, and quality. Herbal medicinal preparations are normally very popular in developing countries because of being economical, backed with a long history of traditional use and also in some developed countries such as Germany, France, Italy and United States where appropriate guidelines for registration of such medicines (Sharma et al., 2010).Chemicals known to have medicinal benefits are referred to as "active ingredients" or "active principles" and their presence depends on a number of factors including the plant species, the time and season of harvest, the type of soil, the way the herb is prepared.The impact of variability of the constituents in herbs or herbal preparations due to genetic, cultural and environmental factors is a major issue in herbal medicines.

Standardization of active chemical constituents of herbal drugs as a finished product must be carried out using standard available protocols. Now a day various sophisticated techniques viz., high performance thin layer chromatography (HPTLC), high performance liquid chromatography (HPLC),gas chromatography (GC), gas chromatography–mass spectrometry (GC-MS), liquid chromatography–mass spectrometry (LC-MS) are frequently used in identification of known phytochemicals. The qualitative and quantitative divergence of the compounds in herbal materials may be due to the climatic, which in turn may affect the composition and other secondary metabolites of the plants (Joshi, 2013d; 2014c) and can accumulate the compound at a particular period and environment. According to WHO (1996a and b, 1992), standardization and quality control of herbals is the process involved in the physicochemical evaluation of crude drug covering aspects, such as selection and handling of crude material, safety, efficacy and stability assessment of finished products, documentation of safety and risk based on experience, provision of product information to consumer and product promotion. Quality of herbal medicines indices such as: macro and microscopic examination, foreign organic matter, ash values, moisture content, extractive values, crude fibre, qualitative and quantitative chemical evaluation, chromatographic examination and toxicological studies. The name of marker constituent(s) along with percentage of each herb either single preparation or multidrug formulation should be mentioned in the final and market product and must be under the strict surveillance of drug regulatory authority.

Various problems appeared during the clinical trial of the crude raw herbmaterial viz., chemical variations as per geographicallocations, climatic conditions, environmental hazards, harvesting methods, collection protocols, etc. which makes it a difficult task to standardize the end product for are producible quality (Bauer& Tittel, 1996). Adverse and side effects is another open problem, because in citizens still prevail the respect for everything that is natural tout court, more as a cultural-fashion based choice than thinking that the patient is introducing in his/her body chemical substances of vegetal origin; not knowing that salicylic glucosides and lactonic sesquiterpenes of many Compositae are often responsible of allergic reactions. Some constituents of the plants are cancerogenic like safrole, bergapten and pyrrolizidines alkaloids. Not of minor importance especially for the old patient using contemporary more synthetic drugs is the problem of drug interferences. Some plants reduce or improve the bioavailability of some drugs due to induction or inhibition of cytochromes (Firenzuoli & Gori, 2007).

In the case of wild harvesting, continual selection of the largest wild-growing individuals or those with the traits considered desirable from a medicinal point of view, if it involves destruction of the whole plant or its reproductive organs, will inevitably lead to a degradation of the wild population. It cannot use medicinal plants on a large scale without modifying the characteristics of the plant populations available to us. If medicinal herbs are brought into cultivation, then we can at least attempt to do this in a controlled manner and at the same time can attempt to conserve wild populations. A particular challenge for medicinal plants is the degree to which synergistic effects can be not only conclusively demonstrated but also realistically defined for biotechnological intervention. Otherwise, increasing understanding of what the active components in herbs are and how they work will simply lead to their isolation as plant-derived drugs, and biotechnological interest in the plants and whole extracts from them will not be justifiable.

NOTE

In 2004, the FDA created a pathway for drug makers to get approval of drugs derived from plants. While it has received about 500 applications, it approved only one prescription botanical drug in the 8 years since, until today. There are lots of opportunities for developments of phytopharmaceuticals. Undoubtedly a very few molecules from plant origin have been characterized in detail as a drug candidates. One of the question arises taking into consideration of the yield of compound in the plant, if the compound showing prominent biological activity. Can it supply the demand of the drug based on the plant itself? The plant origin drug can only utilized for the research purpose and may not complete the demand of plant based drugs for disease like diabetes or other life style diseases. Otherwise alternate sources viz., plant tissue culture and endophytes can be the option for potential renewal sources for sustainable production of phytopharmaceuticals.

Quality control using modern analytical tools for testing the various qualitative parameters of herbal medicine as a final market product must be emphasized as per the allopathic medicine norms adopted by the various government agencies of the globe and WHO guidelines must be strictly implemented universally.

REFERENCES

Abdel-Hassan, I. A., Abdel-Barry, J. A., & Mohammeda, S. T. (2000). The hypoglycemic and antihyperglycemic effect of *Citrullus colocynthis* fruit aqueous extract in normal and alloxan induced diabetic rats. *Journal of Ethnopharmacology, 71*(1-2), 1–2. doi:10.1016/S0378-8741(99)00215-9 PMID:10904143

Alzheimer's Association. (2013a). *Alzheimer's disease facts and figures*. Author.

Alzheimer's Association. (2013b). *The role of plaques and tangles*. Author.

Amalraj, T., & Ignachimuthu, S. (1998). Hypoglycemic activity of *Cajanus cajan* (seeds) in mice. *Indian Journal of Experimental Biology, 36*, 1032–1033. PMID:10356965

Andrews, K. W., Schweitzer, A., Zhao, C., Holden, J., Roseland, J., Brandt, M., & Yetley, E. (2006). Caffeine, theobromine and theophylline content of commonly purchased weight loss and sport performance enhancing dietary supplements. *Experimental Biology*, 1–5.

Arai, I., Amagaya, S., Komatsu, Y., Okada, M., Hayashi, T., Kasai, M., & Momose, Y. et al. (1999). Improving effects of the extracts from *Eugenia uniflora* on hyperglycemia and hypertriglyceridemia in mice. *Journal of Ethnopharmacology, 68*(1-3), 307–314. doi:10.1016/S0378-8741(99)00066-5 PMID:10624893

Augusti, K. T. (1973). Studies on the effects of a hypoglycemic principle from *Allium cepa* Linn. *The Indian Journal of Medical Research, 61*, 1066–1071. PMID:4757998

Augustine, A. C., & D'Souza, L. (1997). Regeneration of an anticarcinogenic herb, *Curculigo orchioides* (Gaertn.). *In Vitro Cellular & Developmental Biology. Plant, 33*(2), 111–113. doi:10.1007/s11627-997-0006-x

Bacon, C. W., & White, J. F. (2000). *Microbial Endophytes*. New York: Marcel Deker Inc.

Baichwal, R. S. (1999). Developments in nutraceuticals. *Pharmacy Times, 1*, 19–20.

Bajaj, Y. P. S. (1998). Biotechnology for the improvement of medicinal plants. *Acta Horticulturae, 457*(457), 37–45. doi:10.17660/ActaHortic.1998.457.4

Bakkali, F., Averbeck, S., Averbeck, D., & Idaomar, M. (2008). Biological effects of essential oils-A review. *Food and Chemical Toxicology, 46*(2), 446–475. doi:10.1016/j.fct.2007.09.106 PMID:17996351

Baragob, A. A., AlMalki, W. H., Shahid, I., Bakhdhar, F. A., Bafhaid, H. S., & Eldeen, O. I. (2014). The hypoglycemic effect of the aqueous extract of the fruits of *Balanites aegypticea* in Alloxan-induced diabetic rats. *Pharmacognosy Research, 6*(1), 1–5. doi:10.4103/0974-8490.122909 PMID:24497735

Bardhan, P. K., Khan, W. A., Salam, A., Saha, D., Golman, D., Harris, M. S., & Chaturvedi, P. (2009). *Safety and efficacy of a novel anti-secretory anti-diarrheal agent Crofelemer (NP-303), in treatment of adult infectious diarrhea and cholera, with or without the use of antibiotics. 13th International Conference on Emerging Infectious Diseases in the Pacific Rim*, Kolkata, India.

Barnes, P. J., & Pauwels, R. A. (1994). Theophylline in the management of asthma: Time for reappraisal? *The European Respiratory Journal, 7*(3), 579–591. doi:10.1183/09031936.94.07030579 PMID:8013614

Bauer, R., & Tittel, G. (1996). Quality assessment of herbal preparations as a precondition of pharmacological and clinical studies. *Phytomedicine, 2*, 193-198.

Buchbauer, G., & Jirovetz, L. (1994). Aromatherapy-use of fragrances and essential oils as medicaments. *Flavour and Fragrance Journal*, *9*(5), 217–222. doi:10.1002/ffj.2730090503

Burchett, M., Mousine, R., &Tarran, J. (2002).Phytomonitoring for urban environmental management. *Air Pollution & Plant Biotechnology*, 61-91.

Butler, M. S. (2005). Natural products to drugs: Natural product derived compounds in clinical trials. *Natural Product Reports*, *22*(2), 162–195. doi:10.1039/b402985m PMID:15806196

Chempakam, B. (1993). Hypoglycemic activity of arecoline in betel nut*Areca catechu* L. *Indian Journal of Experimental Biology*, *31*, 474–475. PMID:8359856

Chen, D. H., Liu, C. J., Ye, H. C., Li, G. F., Liu, B. Y., Meng, Y. L., & Chen, X. Y. (1999). Ri-mediated transformation of *Artemisia annua* with a recombinant farnesyl diphosphate synthase gene for artemisinin production. *Plant Cell, Tissue and Organ Culture*, *57*(3), 157–162. doi:10.1023/A:1006326818509

Chotchoungchatchai, S., Saralamp, P., Jenjittikul, T., Pornsiripongse, S., & Prathanturarug, S. (2012). Medicinal plants used with Thai traditional medicine in modern healthcare services: A case study in Kabchoeng hospital, Surin Province, Thailand. *Journal of Ethnopharmacology*, *141*(1), 193–205. doi:10.1016/j.jep.2012.02.019 PMID:22366679

Cooper, Z. D., & Haney, M. (2009). Actions of delta-9-tetrahydrocannabinol in cannabis: Relation to use, abuse, dependence. *International Review of Psychiatry (Abingdon, England)*, *21*(2), 104–112. doi:10.1080/09540260902782752 PMID:19367504

Cragg, G. M., & Newman, D. J. (2004). A tale of two tumor targets: Topoisomerase I and tubulin. The Wall and Wani contribution to cancer chemotherapy. *Journal of Natural Products*, *67*(2), 232–244. doi:10.1021/np030420c PMID:14987065

Cragg, G. M., & Newman, D. J. (2009). Nature: A vital source of leads for anticancer drug development. *Phytochemistry Reviews*, *8*(2), 313–331. doi:10.1007/s11101-009-9123-y

Crutchley, R. D., Miller, J., & Garey, K. W. (2010). Crofelemer, a novel agent for treatment of secretory diarrhea. *The Annals of Pharmacotherapy*, *44*(5), 878–884. doi:10.1345/aph.1M658 PMID:20388859

Daferera, D. J., Ziogas, B. N., & Polissiou, M. G. (2000). GC-MS analysis of essential oils from some Greek aromatic plants and their fungi toxicity on *Penicillium digitatum. Journal of Agricultural and Food Chemistry*, *48*(6), 2576–2581. doi:10.1021/jf990835x PMID:10888587

Das, A. V., Padayatti, P. S., & Paulose, C. S. (1996). Effect of leaf extract of *Aegle marmelos* (L.) Correa ex Roxb.on histological and ultra structural changes in tissues of streptozotocin induced diabetic rats. *Indian Journal of Experimental Biology*, *34*, 341–345. PMID:8698423

Devon, T. K., & Scott, A. I. (1972). *Handbook of Naturally occurring Compounds: The Terpenes*. London: Academic Press.

DiCesare, D., DuPont, H. L., Mathewson, J. J., Ashley, D., Martinez-Sandoval, F., Pennington, J. E., & Porter, S. B. (2002). A double blind, randomized, placebo-controlled study of SP-303 (Provir) in the symptomatic treatment of acute diarrhea among travelers to Jamaica and Mexico. *The American Journal of Gastroenterology*, *97*(10), 2585–2588. doi:10.1111/j.1572-0241.2002.06027.x PMID:12385443

Dompeipen, E. J., Srikandace, Y., Suharso, W. P., Cahyana, H., & Simanjuntak, P. (2009). Potential endophytic microbes selection for antidiabetic bioactive compounds production. *Asian Journal of Biochemistry*, *6*(6), 465–471. doi:10.3923/ajb.2011.465.471

Dubey, T., & Guerra, D. J. (2002). Use of biotechnology for growing medicinal plants. *Recent Progress in Medicinal Plants*, *5*, 47–61.

Duke, S. O., Dayan, F. E., Romagni, J. G., & Rimando, A. M. (2000). Natural products as sources of herbicides: Current status and future trends. *Weed Research*, *40*(1), 99–111. doi:10.1046/j.1365-3180.2000.00161.x

Dureja, H., Kaushik, D., & Kumar, V. (2003). Developments in nutraceuticals. *Indian Journal of Pharmacology*, *35*, 363–372.

Elsohly, M. A. (2002). Chemical constituents of Cannabis. In F. Grotenhermen & E. Russo (Eds.), *Cannabis and cannabinoids. Pharmacology, toxicology, and therapeutic potential*. Binghamton, New York: The Haworth Press.

Elsohly, M. A., & Slade, D. (2005). Chemical constituents of marijuana: The complex mixture of natural cannabinoids. *Life Sciences*, *78*(5), 539–548. doi:10.1016/j.lfs.2005.09.011 PMID:16199061

Enrich, L. B., Scheuermann, M. L., Mohadjer, A., Matthias, K. R., Eller, C. F., Newman, M. S., & Poon, T. (2008). Liquidambar styraciflua: A renewable source of shikimic acid. *Tetrahedron Letters*, *49*(16), 2503–2505. doi:10.1016/j.tetlet.2008.02.140

Eteng, M. U., Eyong, E. U., Akpanyung, E. O., Agiang, M. A., & Aremu, C. Y. (1997). Recent advances in caffeine and theobromine toxicities: A review. *Plant Foods for Human Nutrition (Dordrecht, Netherlands)*, *51*(3), 231–243. doi:10.1023/A:1007976831684 PMID:9629863

Eyberger, A. L., Dondapati, R., & Porter, J. R. (2006). Endophyte fungal isolates from *Podophyllum peltatum* produce podophyllotoxin. *Journal of Natural Products*, *69*(8), 1121–1124. doi:10.1021/np060174f PMID:16933860

Firenzuoli, F., & Gori, L. (2007). Herbal medicine today: Clinical and research issues. *Evidence-Based Complementary and Alternative Medicine*, *4*(s1), 37–40. doi:10.1093/ecam/nem096 PMID:18227931

Food and Drug Administration. (2010). *Caffeine intake by the U.S. population*. Retrieved from (http://www.fda.gov/downloads/AboutFDA/CentersOffices/OfficeofFoods/CFSAN/CFSANFOIAElectronicReadingRoom/UCM333191.pdf)

Geetha, M., & Wahi, A. K. (2001). Antidiabetic activity of *Barleria prionitis* Linn. *Journal of Natural Remedies*, *1*, 64–66.

Gornitsky, M., Shenouda, G., Sultanem, K., Katz, H., Hier, M., Black, M., & Velly, A. M. (2004). Double-blind randomized, placebo-controlled study of pilocarpine to salvage salivary gland function during radiotherapy of patients with head and neck cancer. *Oral Radiology & Endodontology, 98*, 45–52.

Grover, J. K., Vats, V., & Rathi, S. S. (2000). Anti-hyperglycemic effect of *Eugeniajambolana*and *Tinosporacordifolia*in experimental diabetes and their effects on key metabolic enzymes involved in carbohydrate metabolism. *Journal of Ethnopharmacology, 73*(3), 461–470. doi:10.1016/S0378-8741(00)00319-6 PMID:11091000

Gupta, R. K., Gupta, S., & Samuel, K. C. (1977). Blood sugar lowering effects of various fractions of onion. *Indian Journal of Experimental Biology, 15*, 313–314. PMID:914348

Haberlandt, G. (1902). Kulturversuche mit isolierten Pflanzenzellen.*S. B. Weisen Wien Naturwissenschaften, 111*, 69–92.

Hall, M. G., Wilks, M. F., Provan, W. M., Eksborg, S., & Lumholtz, B. (2001). Pharmacokinetics and pharmacodynamics of NTBC (2-(2-nitro-4-fluoromethylbenzoyl)-1,3-cyclohexanedione) and mesotrione, inhibitors of 4-hydroxyphenyl pyruvate dioxygenase (HPPD) following a single dose to healthy male volunteers. *British Journal of Clinical Pharmacology, 52*(2), 169–177. doi:10.1046/j.0306-5251.2001.01421.x PMID:11488774

Hebert, L. E., Weuve, J., Scherr, P. A., & Evans, D. A. (2013). Alzheimer disease in the United States (2010-2050) estimated using the 2010 census. *Neurology, 80*(19), 1778–17783. doi:10.1212/WNL.0b013e31828726f5 PMID:23390181

Heinrich, M., & Teoh, H. L. (2004). Galanthamine from snowdrop-the development of a modern drug against Alzheimer's disease from local Caucasian knowledge. *Journal of Ethnopharmacology, 92*(2-3), 147–162. doi:10.1016/j.jep.2004.02.012 PMID:15137996

Hercberg, S., Ezzedine, K., Guinot, C., Preziosi, P., Galan, P., Bertrais, S., & Malvy, D. (2007). Antioxidant supplementation increases the risk of skin cancers in women but not in men. *The Journal of Nutrition, 137*, 2098–2105. PMID:17709449

Holodniy, M., Koch, J., Mistal, M., Schmidt, J. M., Khandwala, A., Pennington, J. E., & Porter, S. B. (1999). A double blind, randomized, placebo-controlled phase II study to assess the safety and efficacy of orally administered SP-303 for the symptomatic treatment of diarrhea in patients with AIDS. *The American Journal of Gastroenterology, 94*(11), 3267–3273. doi:10.1111/j.1572-0241.1999.01535.x PMID:10566728

Holton, R. A., Somoza, C., Kim, H. B., Liang, F., Biediger, R. J., Boatman, P. D., & Kim, S. (1994). First total synthesis of taxol. 1. Functionalization of the B ring. *Journal of the American Chemical Society, 116*(4), 1597–1598. doi:10.1021/ja00083a066

Hooper, M., Kirby, G. C., Kulkarni, M. M., Kulkarni, S. N., Nagasampagi, B. A., O'Neill, M. J., & Warhurst, D. C. (1990). Antimalarial activity of parthenin and its derivatives. *European Journal of Medicinal Chemistry, 25*(9), 717–723. doi:10.1016/0223-5234(90)90190-E

Hurakadle, P. J., Gadkar, S. S., & Pai, S. R. (2010). Callus culture studies on *Jasminum malabaricum*-An endemic medicinal plant. *Planta Medica, 77*.

Hussain, H., Krohn, K., Draeger, S., Meier, K., & Schulz, B. (2009). Bioactive chemical constituents of a sterile endophytic fungus from *Meliotus dentatus*. *Records of Natural Products*, *3*, 114–117.

Ito, K., Lim, S., Caramori, G., Cosio, B., Chung, K. F., Adcock, I. M., & Barnes, P. J. (2002). A molecular mechanism of action of theophylline: Induction of histone deacetylase activity to decrease inflammatory gene expression. *Proceedings of the National Academy of Sciences of the United States of America*, *99*(13), 8921–8926. doi:10.1073/pnas.132556899 PMID:12070353

Jankun, J., Selman, S. H., Aniola, J., & Skrzypczak-Jankun, E. (2006). Nutraceutical inhibitors of urokinase: Potential applications in prostate cancer prevention and treatment. *Oncology Reports*, *16*, 341–346. PMID:16820913

Johnson, J. T., Ferretti, G. A., Nethery, W. J., Valdez, I. H., Fox, P. C., Ng, D., & Gallagher, S. C. et al. (1993). Oral pilocarpine for post-irradiation xerostomia in patients with head and neck cancer. *The New England Journal of Medicine*, *329*(6), 390–305. doi:10.1056/NEJM199308053290603 PMID:8326972

Joshi, R. K. (2010). In vitro antimicrobial and antioxidant activity of the essential oil of *Craniotome furcata*. *Journal of Applied and Natural Science*, *2*, 57–62.

Joshi, R. K. (2012a). In vitro antimicrobial activity of the essential oil of the endemic plant *Senecio belgaumensis*. *Journal of Biologically Active Products from Nature*, *2*(6), 382–386. doi:10.1080/22311866.2012.10719147

Joshi, R. K. (2012b). Comparative analysis by GC-MS and *in vitro* antimicrobial activity of the essential oils of noxious weed (*Lantana camara* L.) from Western Ghats region of North West Karnataka, India. *Journal of Biologically Active Products from Nature*, *2*(3), 135–143. doi:10.1080/22311866.2012.10719120

Joshi, R. K. (2013a). Volatile composition and antimicrobial activity of the essential oil of *Artemisia absinthium* growing in Western Ghats region of North West Karnataka, India. *Pharmaceutical Biology*, *51*(7), 888–892. doi:10.3109/13880209.2013.768676 PMID:23570523

Joshi, R. K. (2013b). Chemical composition, *in vitro* antimicrobial and antioxidant activities of the essential oils of *Ocimum gratissimum, O. sanctum* and their major constituents. *Indian Journal of Pharmaceutical Sciences*, *75*(4), 457–462. doi:10.4103/0250-474X.119834 PMID:24302801

Joshi, R. K. (2013c). Chemical constituents and antibacterial property of the essential oil of the roots of *Cyathocline purpurea*. *Journal of Ethnopharmacology*, *145*(2), 621–625. doi:10.1016/j.jep.2012.11.045 PMID:23220198

Joshi, R. K. (2013d). Pulegone and menthone chemotypes of *Mentha spicata* Linn.from Western Ghats region of North West Karnataka, India. *National Academy Science Letters*, *36*(3), 349–352. doi:10.1007/s40009-013-0141-3

Joshi, R. K. (2014a). Chemical composition and antimicrobial activity of the essential oil of *Plectranthus mollis* (Lamiaceae) from Western Ghats region, Karnataka, India. *Revista de Biologia Tropical*, *62*, 423–431. doi:10.15517/rbt.v62i2.9396 PMID:25102628

Joshi, R. K. (2014b). Chemical composition and antimicrobial activity of the essential oil of *Ocimum basilicum* L. (sweet basil) from Western Ghats of North West Karnataka, India. *Ancient Science of Life*, *33*(3), 149–154. doi:10.4103/0257-7941.144618 PMID:25538349

Joshi, R. K. (2014c). 2,4,6-Trimethoxy-styrene new chemotype from the essential oil of *Zanthoxylum ovalifolium* Wight from India. *National Academy Science Letters*, *37*(4), 331–333. doi:10.1007/s40009-014-0243-6

Joshi, R. K., & Badakar, V. (2012). Chemical composition and *in vitro* antimicrobial activity of the essential oil of the flowers of *Tridax procumbens* L. *Natural Product Communications*, *7*, 941–942. PMID:22908588

Joshi, R. K., Badakar, V. M., Kholkute, S. D., & Khatib, N. (2011). Chemical composition and antimicrobial activity of the essential oil of the leaves of *Feronia elephantum* (Rutaceae) from North West Karnataka. *Natural Product Communications*, *6*, 141–143. PMID:21366066

Joshi, R. K., Mujawar, M. H. K., Badakar, V., & Khatib, N. A. (2011). *In vitro* antimicrobial activity of the essential oil of *Erigeron floribundus*. *International Journal of Research in Ayurveda and Pharmacy*, *2*, 236–238.

Joshi, R. K., Pande, C., Mujawar, M. H. K., & Kholkute, S. D. (2009). Chemical composition and antimicrobial activity of the essential oil of *Anaphalis nubigena* var. *monocephala*. *Natural Product Communications*, *4*, 993–996. PMID:19731610

Joshi, R. K., Pande, V., & Thakuri, B. C. (2011). Antimicrobial activity of the essential oil of *Phlomis bracteosa*. *Scientific World*, *9*(9), 63–65. doi:10.3126/sw.v9i9.5521

Joshi, R. K., Patil, P. A., Mujawar, M. H. K., Kumar, D., & Kholkute, S. D. (2009a). Hypoglycemic activity of aqueous leaf extract of *Feronia elephantum* in normal and streptozotocin- induced diabetic rats. *Pharmacologyonline*, *3*, 815–821.

Joshi, R. K., Patil, P. A., Mujawar, M. H. K., Kumar, D., & Kholkute, S. D. (2009b). Hypoglycemic activity of *Bambusa arundinacea* leaf aqueous extract in euglycemic and hyperglycemic Wistar rats. *Pharmacologyonline*, *3*, 789–795.

Kanchan, S. D. (1975). Growth inhibitors from *Parthenium hysterophorus* Linn. *Current Science*, *44*, 358–359.

Kelber, O., Nieber, K., & Kraft, K. (2014). Valerian: No evidence for clinically relevant interactions. *Evidence-Based Complementary and Alternative Medicine*, *2014*, 1–8. doi:10.1155/2014/879396 PMID:25093031

Ketkar, P. M., Nayak, S. U., Pai, S. R., & Joshi, R. K. (2015). Monitoring seasonal variation of epicatechin and gallic acid in the bark of *Saraca asoca* using reverse phase high performance liquid chromatography (RP-HPLC) method. *Journal of Ayurveda and Integrative Medicine*, *6*(1), 29–34. doi:10.4103/0975-9476.146568 PMID:25878461

Khan, B. A., Abraham, A., & Leelamma, S. (1995). Hypoglycemic action of *Murraya Koeingii* (curry leaf) and *Brassica juncea* (mustard): Mechanism of action. *Indian Journal of Biochemistry & Biophysics*, *32*, 106–108. PMID:7642200

Kinghorn, A. D. (1987). Biologically active compounds from plants with reputed medicinal and sweetening properties. *Journal of Natural Products*, *50*(6), 1009–1024. doi:10.1021/np50054a002 PMID:3327919

Kintzios, S., & Michaelakis, A. (1999). Induction of somatic embryogenesis and in vitro flowering from inflorescences of chamomile (*Chamomilla recutita* L.). *Plant Cell Reports*, *8*(7-8), 684–690. doi:10.1007/s002990050643

Kovacs, B. (2008). *Sources of caffeine*. Retrieved from http://www.Medicinenet.Com

Kugelman, A., & Durand, M. (2011). A comprehensive approach to the prevention of bronchopulmonary dysplasia. *Pediatric Pulmonology*, *46*(12), 1153–1165. doi:10.1002/ppul.21508 PMID:21815280

Kukreja, A. K., & Dhawan, O. P. (2000). Somaclonal breeding for improvement of herb and essential oil yield in mints: A case study. *Journal of Medicinal & Aromatic Plant Sciences*, *22*, 431–442.

Kumari, K., Mathew, B. C., & Augusti, K. T. (1995). Antidiabetic and hypolipidemic effects of S-methyl cysteine sulphoxide isolated from *Allium cepa* Linn. *Indian Journal of Biochemistry & Biophysics*, *32*, 49–54. PMID:7665195

Lakshmanan, P., Danesh, M., & Taji, A. (2002). Production of four commercially cultivated *Echinacea* species by different methods of *in vitro* regeneration. *The Journal of Horticultural Science & Biotechnology*, *77*(2), 158–163. doi:10.1080/14620316.2002.11511473

Lansky, E. P., & Newman, R. A. (2007). *Punica granatum* (pomegranate) and its potential for prevention and treatment of inflammation and cancer. *Journal of Ethnopharmacology*, *19*(2), 177–206. doi:10.1016/j.jep.2006.09.006 PMID:17157465

Larsson, S. C., Hakansson, N., Giovannucci, E., & Wolk, A. (2006). Folate intake and pancreatic cancer incidence: A prospective study of Swedish women and men. *Journal of the National Cancer Institute*, *98*(6), 407–413. doi:10.1093/jnci/djj094 PMID:16537833

Lee, M. H., Yoon, E. S., Jeong, J. H., & Choi, Y. E. (2004). *Agrobacterium rhizogenes*-mediated transformation of *Taraxacum platycarpum* and changes of morphological characters. *Plant Cell Reports*, *22*(11), 822–827. doi:10.1007/s00299-004-0763-5 PMID:14986056

Leonard, T. K., Waison, R. R., & Mohs, M. S. (1987). The effect of caffeine on various body systems: A review. *Journal of the American Dietetic Association*, *87*, 1048–1053. PMID:3301987

LeVeque, F. G., Montgomery, M., Potter, D., Zimmer, M. B., Rieke, J. W., Steiger, B. W., & Muscoplat, C. C. (1993). A multicenter, randomized, double-blind, placebo-controlled, dose-titration study of oral pilocarpine for treatment of radiation-induced xerostomia in head and neck cancer patients. *Journal of Clinical Oncology*, *11*, 1124–1131. PMID:8501499

Lilienfeld, S. (2002). Galantamine-a novel cholinergic drug with a unique dual mode of action for the treatment of patients with Alzheimer's disease. *CNS Drug Reviews*, *8*(2), 159–176. doi:10.1111/j.1527-3458.2002.tb00221.x PMID:12177686

Limberger, R. P., Jacques, A. L. B., Schmitt, G. C., & Arbo, M. D. (2013). Pharmacological effects of ephedrine. In K. G. Ramawar & J. M. Merillon (Eds.), *Natural Products*. Heidelberg, Germany: Springer-Verlag Berlin. doi:10.1007/978-3-642-22144-6_41

Lloyd, J. U. (1897). *Physostigma by venenosum (Calabar)*. Chicago: The Western Druggist.

Luo, X. D., & Shen, C. C. (1987). The chemistry, pharmacology, and clinical applications of qinghaosu (Artemisinin) and its derivatives. *Medicinal Research Reviews*, *7*(1), 29–52. doi:10.1002/med.2610070103 PMID:3550324

Mabberly, D. J. (1997). *A Portable Dictionary of the Vascular Plants* (2nd ed.). Cambridge, UK: Cambridge University Press.

Manson, M. M., Farmer, P. B., Gescher, A., & Steward, W. P. (2005). Innovative agents in cancer prevention. *Recent Results in Cancer Research. Fortschritte der Krebsforschung. Progres Dans les Recherches Sur le Cancer*, *166*, 257–275. doi:10.1007/3-540-26980-0_17 PMID:15648195

Mathela, D. K., Mathela, C. S., & Taskinen, J. (1986). Polyacetylenes and terpenoids from *Erigeron karwinskyanus*. *Journal of the Indian Chemical Society*, *63*, 603–604.

Mathela, D. K., Pant, A. K., & Mathela, C. S. (1984). A pyrone glycoside from *Erigeron karwinskyanus*. *Phytochemistry*, *23*(9), 2090–2091. doi:10.1016/S0031-9422(00)84988-2

Mathew, P., & Augusti, K. T. (1975). Hypoglycaemic effects of onion, *Allium cepa* Linn.on diabetes mellitus-a preliminary report. *Indian Journal of Physiology and Pharmacology*, *19*, 213–217. PMID:1223000

Mathew, P. T., & Augusti, K. T. (1973). Studies on the effect of allicin (diallyl disulphide-oxide) on alloxan diabetes.Hypoglycemic action and enhancement of serum insulin effect and glycogen synthesis. *Indian Journal of Biochemistry & Biophysics*, *10*, 209–212. PMID:4792931

Matissek, R. (1997). Evaluation of xanthine derivatives in chocolate-nutritional and chemical aspects. *Zeitschrift für Lebensmitteluntersuchung und -Forschung A*, *205*, 175-184.

McKiernan, P. J. (2006). Nitisinone in the treatment of hereditary tyrosinaemia type 1. *Drugs*, *66*(6), 743–750. doi:10.2165/00003495-200666060-00002 PMID:16706549

Meragelman, K. M., Mckee, T. C., & Boyd, M. R. (2001). Anti-HIV prenylated flavonoids from *Monotes africanus*. *Journal of Natural Products*, *64*(4), 546–548. doi:10.1021/np0005457 PMID:11325248

Meshnick, S. R., & Dobson, M. J. (2001). The history of antimalarial drugs. In P. J. Posenthal (Ed.), *Antimalarial chemotherapy mechanism of action, resistance and new drug directions in drug discovery*. Humana Press. doi:10.1385/1-59259-111-6:15

Miller, K. I., Qing, C., Sze, D. M., Roufogalis, B. D., & Neilan, B. A. (2012). Culturable endophytes of medicinal plants and the genetic basis for their bioactivity. *Microbial Ecology*, *64*(2), 431–449. doi:10.1007/s00248-012-0044-8 PMID:22430508

Moerman, D. (1988). *Native American Ethnobotany*. Timber Press.

Mohan, V., Sandeep, S., Deepa, R., Shah, B., & Varghese, C. (2007). Epidemiology of type 2 diabetes: Indian scenario. *The Indian Journal of Medical Research*, *125*, 217–230. PMID:17496352

Moyano, E., Fornale, S., Palazon, J., Cusido, R. M., Bonfill, M., Morales, C., & Pinol, M. T. (1999). Effect of *Agrobacterium rhizogenes* T-DNA on alkaloid production in Solanaceae plants. *Phytochemistry, 52*(7), 1287–1292. doi:10.1016/S0031-9422(99)00421-5

Mukherjee, K., Ghosh, N. C., & Datta, T. (1972). *Coccinia indica* Linn.As potential hypoglycemic agent. *Indian Journal of Experimental Biology, 10*, 347–349. PMID:4658184

Mulhall, J. P., Daller, M., Traish, A. M., Gupta, S., Park, K., Salimpour, P., & Goldstein, I. et al. (1997). Intracavernosal forskolin: Role in management of pharmacotherapy vasculogenic impotence resistant to standard 3-agent. *The Journal of Urology, 158*, 1752–1759. doi:10.1016/S0022-5347(01)64118-1 PMID:9334594

National Institute of Neurological Disorders and Stroke. (2013). *Dementia: hope through research.* Bethesda, MD: Office of Communications and Public Liaison, National Institute of Neurological Disorders and Stroke, US National Institutes of Health.

National Institute on Drug Abuse. (2015). *Is Marijuana Medicine?* National Institute on Drug Abuse, Drug Facts.

National Organization for Rare Disorders. (2012). *Physician's Guide to Tyrosinemia Type 1*. The National Organization for Rare Disorders.

Nehlig, A., Daval, J. L., & Debry, G. (1992). Caffeine and the central nervous system: Mechanisms of action, biochemical, metabolic and psychostimulant effects. *Brain Research. Brain Research Reviews, 17*(2), 139–170. doi:10.1016/0165-0173(92)90012-B PMID:1356551

Newman, D. J., & Cragg, G. M. (2007). Natural products as sources of new drugs over the last 25 Years. *Journal of Natural Products, 70*(3), 461–477. doi:10.1021/np068054v PMID:17309302

Nicolaou, K. C., Yang, Z., Liu, J. J., Ueno, H., Nantermet, P. G., Guy, R. K., & Sorensen, E. J. (1994). Total synthesis of taxol. *Nature, 367*(6464), 630–634. doi:10.1038/367630a0 PMID:7906395

Nobili, S., Lippi, D., Witort, E., Donnini, M., Bausi, L., Mini, E., & Capaccioli, S. (2009). Natural compounds for cancer treatment and prevention. *Pharmacological Research, 59*(6), 365–378. doi:10.1016/j.phrs.2009.01.017 PMID:19429468

Nugroho, A. E., Andrie, M., Warditiani, N. K., Siswanto, E., Pramono, S., & Lukitaningsih, E. (2012). Antidiabetic and antihiperlipidemic effect of Andrographis paniculata (Burm. f.) Nees and andrographolide in high-fructose-fat-fed rats. *Indian Journal of Pharmacology, 44*(3), 377–381. doi:10.4103/0253-7613.96343 PMID:22701250

Onifade, A. K. (2007). Research trends: Bioactive metabolites of fungal origin. *Research Journal of Biological Sciences, 2*, 81–84.

Orozco-Topete, R., Sierra-Madero, J., Cano-Dominguez, C., Kershenovich, J., Ortiz-Pedroza, G., Vazquez-Valls, E., & Rozhon, E. J. (1997). Safety and efficacy of Virend for topical treatment of genital and anal herpes simplex lesions in patients with AIDS. *Antiviral Research, 35*(2), 91–103. doi:10.1016/S0166-3542(97)00015-6 PMID:9217246

Pai, S. R., Nimbalkar, M. S., Pawar, N. V., Kedage, V. V., & Dixit, G. B. (2008). *In vitro* embryo culture and ex situ regeneration studies in *Ancistrocladus heyneanus* Wall. Ex Grah. *Plant Cell Biotechnology & Molecular Biology*, *9*, 95–100.

Pandey, M. M., Rastogi, S., & Rawat, A. K. S. (2013). Indian traditional Ayurvedic system of medicine and nutritional supplementation. *Evidence-Based Complementary and Alternative Medicine*, *2013*, 1–12. PMID:23864888

Park, S. U., & Facchini, P. J. (2000). *Agrobacterium rhizogenes* mediated transformation of opium poppy, *Papaver somniferum* L., and *California poppy, Eschscholzia californica*Cham., root cultures. *Journal of Experimental Botany*, *51*(347), 1005–1016. doi:10.1093/jexbot/51.347.1005 PMID:10948228

Patil, T. M., & Hegde, B. A. (1988). Isolation and purification of a sesquiterpene lactone from the leaves of *Parthenium hysterophorus*-Its allelopathic and cytotoxic effects. *Current Science*, *57*, 1178–1181.

Perdue, R. E., Smith, R. L., Wall, M. E., Hartwell, J. L., & Abbott, B. J. (1970). *Camptotheca acuminata Decaisne (Nyssaceae). Source of camptothecin, an antileukemic alkaloid.US department of agriculture agricultural research service*. Technical Bulletin No.1415.

Persaud, S. J., Al-Majed, H., Raman, A., & Jones, P. M. (1999). *Gymnema sylvestre* stimulates insulin release in vitro by increased membrane permeability. *The Journal of Endocrinology*, *163*(2), 207–212. doi:10.1677/joe.0.1630207 PMID:10556769

Pinheiro, C. U. B. (1997). Jaborandi (*Pilocarpus* sp., Tutaceae): A wild species and its rapid transformation into a crop. *Economic Botany*, *51*, 49–58. doi:10.1007/BF02910403

Porchezhian, E., & Dobriyal, R. M. (2003). An overview on the advances of *Gymnema sylvestre*: Chemistry, pharmacology and patents. *Die Pharmazie*, *58*, 5–12. PMID:12622244

Puri, D., & Baral, N. (1998). Hypoglycemic effect of *Biophytum sensitivum* in the alloxan diabetic rabbits. *Indian Journal of Physiology and Pharmacology*, *42*, 401–406. PMID:9741656

Rahman, A. (2000). *Studies in Natural Product Chemistry*. Elsevier Science B.V.

Rasineni, K., Bellamkonda, R., Singareddy, S. R., & Desireddy, S. (2010). Antihyperglycemic activity of *Catharanthus roseus* leaf powder in streptozotocin-induced diabetic rats. *Pharmacognosy Research*, *2*(3), 195–201. doi:10.4103/0974-8490.65523 PMID:21808566

Rios, J. L., & Recio, M. C. (2005). Medicinal plants and antimicrobial activity. *Journal of Ethnopharmacology*, *100*(1-2), 80–84. doi:10.1016/j.jep.2005.04.025 PMID:15964727

Rivera-Chavez, J., Gonzalez-Andrade, M., Gonzalez, M. C., Glenn, A. E., & Mata, R. (2013). Thielavins A, J and K: α-Glucosidase inhibitors from MEXU 27095, an endophytic fungus from *Hintonia latiflora*. *Phytochemistry*, *94*, 198–205. doi:10.1016/j.phytochem.2013.05.021 PMID:23809634

Russell, N. C., Hoelscher, D. M., & Lowenstein, N. (2007). Patients previously treated for lymphoma consume inadequate or excessive amounts of five key nutrients. *Journal of the Society for Integrative Oncology*, *5*(03), 118–124. doi:10.2310/7200.2007.009 PMID:17761131

Russo, E. B. (2001). Hemp for headache: An in-depth historical and scientific review of cannabis in migraine treatment. *Journal of Cannabis Therapeutics*, *1*(2), 21–92. doi:10.1300/J175v01n02_04

Russo, E. B. (2002). Cannabis treatments in obstetrics and gynecology: A historical review. *Journal of Cannabis Therapeutics*, *2*(3-4), 5–34. doi:10.1300/J175v02n03_02

Saleem, R., Ahmad, M., Hussain, S. A., Qazi, A. M., Ahmad, S. I., Qazi, M. H., & Hussein, S. N. (1999). Hypotensive, hypoglycemic and toxicological studies on the flavonol C-glycosides shamimin from *Bombax ceiba. Planta Medica*, *65*(4), 331–334. doi:10.1055/s-1999-14060 PMID:10364838

Sandhu, S. S., Abreu, I. N., Colombo, C. A., & Mazzafera, P. (2006). Pilocarpine content and molecular diversity in jaborandi. *Scientia Agricola*, *63*(5), 478–482. doi:10.1590/S0103-90162006000500010

Sandler, R. S., Halabi, S., Kaplan, E. B., Baron, J. A., Paskett, E., & Petrelli, N. J. (2001). Use of vitamins, minerals, and nutritional supplements by participants in a chemoprevention trial. *Cancer*, *91*(5), 1040–1045. doi:10.1002/1097-0142(20010301)91:5<1040::AID-CNCR1095>3.0.CO;2-N PMID:11251957

Scheindlin, S. (2010). Episodes in the story of physostigmine. *Molecular Interventions*, *10*(1), 5–10. doi:10.1124/mi.10.1.1 PMID:20124558

Schmidt, B. (2005). Methylxanthine therapy for apnea of prematurity: Evaluation of treatment benefits and risks at age 5 years in the international caffeine for apnea of prematurity (CAP) trial. *Biology of the Neonate*, *88*(3), 208–213. doi:10.1159/000087584 PMID:16210843

Schmidt, B., Roberts, R. S., Davis, P., Doyle, L. W., Barrington, K. J., Ohlsson, A., & Tin, W. et al. (2006). Caffeine therapy for apnea of prematurity. *The New England Journal of Medicine*, *354*(20), 2112–2121. doi:10.1056/NEJMoa054065 PMID:16707748

Schmidt, B., Roberts, R. S., Davis, P., Doyle, L. W., Barrington, K. J., Ohlsson, A., & Tin, W. et al. (2007). Long-term effects of caffeine therapy for apnea of prematurity. *The New England Journal of Medicine*, *357*(19), 1893–1902. doi:10.1056/NEJMoa073679 PMID:17989382

Scott, K. A., Shah, S., Dalgleish, A. G., & Liu, W. M. (2013). Enhancing the activity of cannabidiol and other cannabinoids in vitro through modifications to drug combinations and treatment schedules. *Anticancer Research*, *33*, 4373–4480. PMID:24123005

Seema, P. V., Sudha, B., Padayatti, P. S., Abraham, A., Raghu, K. G., & Paulose, C. S. (1996). Kinetic studies of purified malate dehydrogenase in liver of streptozotocin-diabetic rats and the effect of leaf extract of *Aegle marmelos* (L.) Correa ex Roxb. *Indian Journal of Experimental Biology*, *34*, 600–602. PMID:8792652

Selvamani, P., Latha, S., Elayaraja, K., Babu, P. S., Gupta, J. K., Pal, K., & Sen, D. J. (2008). Antidiabetic activity of the ethanol extract of *Capparis sepiaria* L leaves. *Indian Journal of Pharmaceutical Sciences*, *70*(3), 378–380. doi:10.4103/0250-474X.43008 PMID:20046752

Sevon, N., & Oksman-Caldentey, K. M. (2002). *Agrobacterium rhizogenes*-mediated transformation: Root cultures as a source of alkaloids. *Planta Medica*, *68*(10), 859–868. doi:10.1055/s-2002-34924 PMID:12391546

Sharma, A. K., Kumar, R., Mishra, A., & Gupta, R. (2010). Problems associated with clinical trials of Ayurvedic medicines. *Brazilian Journal of Pharmacognosy*, *20*, 276–281.

Sharma, G. L., & Bhutani, M. M. (1988). Plant based antiamoebic drugs; Part II. Amoebicidal activity of parthenin isolated from *Parthenium hysterophorus*. *Planta Medica*, *54*(02), 120–122. doi:10.1055/s-2006-962366 PMID:2900531

Sharma, R. (2009). Nutraceuticals and nutraceutical supplementation criteria in cancer: A literature survey. *Open Nutraceuticals Journal*, *2*(1), 92–106. doi:10.2174/1876396000902010092

Sharma, S. R., Dwivedi, S. K., & Swarup, D. (1997). Hypoglycemic, antihyperglycemic and hypolipidemic activities of *Caesalpinia bonducella* seeds in rats. *Journal of Ethnopharmacology*, *58*(1), 39–44. doi:10.1016/S0378-8741(97)00079-2 PMID:9324003

Sheela, C. G., & Augusti, K. T. (1992). Antidiabetic effects of S-allyl cysteine sulphoxide isolated from garlic *Allium sativum* Linn. *Indian Journal of Experimental Biology*, *30*, 523–526. PMID:1506036

Shiojima, K., Suzuki, H., Kodera, N., Ageta, H., Chang, H. C., & Chen, Y. P. (1996). Composite constituents: Thirty-nine triterpenoids including two novel compounds from *Ixeris chinensis*. *Chemical & Pharmaceutical Bulletin*, *44*(3), 509–514. doi:10.1248/cpb.44.509

Shukla, S., & Shukla, B. (1997). Aromatherapy in India: Yesterdays and Tomorrow. *Proceeding South Asian Countries Seminar on Medicinal Plants*.

Sicree, R., Shaw, J., & Zimmet, P. (2006). Diabetes and impaired glucose tolerance. In Diabetes Atlas. Gan D. International Diabetes Federation.

Singh, L. W. (2011). Traditional medicinal plants of Manipur as anti-diabetics. *Journal of Medicinal Plants Research*, *5*, 677–687.

Singh, S. N., Vats, P., Suri, S., Shyam, R., Kumria, M. M. L., Ranganathan, S., & Sridharan, K. (2001). Effect of an antidiabetic extract of *Catharanthus roseus* on enzymic activities in streptozotocin induced diabetic rats. *Journal of Ethnopharmacology*, *76*(3), 269–277. doi:10.1016/S0378-8741(01)00254-9 PMID:11448549

Sohn, H. Y., Son, K. H., Kwon, C. S., Kwon, G. S., & Kang, S. S. (2004). Antimicrobial and cytotoxic activity of 18 prenylated flavonoids isolated from medicinal plants: *Morus alba* L., *Morus mongolica* Schneider, *Broussnetia papyrifera* (L.) Vent,*Sophora flavescens* Ait and *Echinosophora koreensis* Nakai. *Phytomedicine*, *11*(7-8), 666–672. doi:10.1016/j.phymed.2003.09.005 PMID:15636183

Song, C. E. (Ed.). (2009). Cinchona alkaloids in synthesis and catalysis, ligands, immobilization and organocatalysis. Wiley-Vch Verlag GmbH & Co. KGaA. doi:doi:10.1002/9783527628179 doi:10.1002/9783527628179

Staniek, A., Woerdenbag, H. J., & Kayser, O. (2008). Endophytes: Exploiting biodiversity for the improvement of natural product-based drug discovery. *Journal of Plant Interactions*, *3*(2), 75–93. doi:10.1080/17429140801886293

Stevenson, R. (2004). Chemical harvest. *Chemistry & Industry*.

Stierle, A., Strobel, G., Stierle, D., Grothaus, P., & Bignami, G. (1995). The Search for a taxol-producing microorganism among the endophytic fungi of the pacific yew, *Taxus brevifolia*. *Journal of Natural Products*, *58*(9), 1315–1324. doi:10.1021/np50123a002 PMID:7494141

Stierle, A. A., & Stierle, D. B. (2000). Bioactive compounds from four endophytic Penicillium sp. of a Northwest Pacific yew tree. In A. R. Rahman (Ed.), *Studies in Natural Products Chemistry*. Elsevier Science B.V. doi:10.1016/S1572-5995(00)80058-7

Strobel, G., Daisy, B., Castillo, U., & Harper, J. (2004). Natural products from endophytic microorganisms. *Journal of Natural Products*, *67*(2), 257–268. doi:10.1021/np030397v PMID:14987067

Suba, V., Murugesan, T., Arunachalam, G., Mandal, S. C., & Saha, B. P. (2004). Anti-diabetic potential of *Barleria lupulina* extract in rats. *Phytomedicine*, *11*(2-3), 202–205. doi:10.1078/0944-7113-00316 PMID:15070173

Subramonium, A., Pushpangadan, P., Rajasekharan, S., Evans, D. A., Latha, P. G., & Valsaraj, R. (1996). Effects of *Artemisia pallens* Wall.on blood glucose levels in normal and alooxan-induced diabetic rats. *Journal of Ethnopharmacology*, *50*(1), 13–17. doi:10.1016/0378-8741(95)01329-6 PMID:8778502

Thakur, G. S., Sharma, R., Sanodiya, B. S., Pandey, M., Prasad, G. B. K. S., & Bisen, P. S. (2012). *Gymnema sylvestre*: An alternative therapeutic agent for management of diabetes. *Journal of Applied Pharmaceutical Science*, *2*, 1–6.

Theuns, H. G., Theuns, H. L., & Lousberg, R. J. J. (1986). Search for new natural sources of morphinans. *Economic Botany*, *40*(4), 485–497. doi:10.1007/BF02859662

Veronese, P., Li, X., Niu, X., Weller, S. C., Bressan, R. A., & Hasegawa, P. M. (2001). Bioengineering mint crop improvement. *Plant Cell, Tissue and Organ Culture*, *64*(2/3), 133–144. doi:10.1023/A:1010649207445

Vlietinck, A. J., De Bruyne, T., Apers, S., & Pieters, L. A. (1998). Plant-derived leading compounds for chemotherapy of human immunodeficiency virus (HIV) infection. *Planta Medica*, *64*(02), 97–109. doi:10.1055/s-2006-957384 PMID:9525100

Wan, J., Wilcock, A., & Coventry, M. J. (1998). The effect of essential oils of basil on the growth of Aeromonas hydrophila and Pseudomonas fluorescens. *Journal of Applied Microbiology*, *84*(2), 152–158. doi:10.1046/j.1365-2672.1998.00338.x PMID:9633630

Watkins, J. W., Schwarz, E. S., Arroyo-Plasencia, A. M., & Mullins, M. E. (2014). The use of physostigmine by toxicologists in anticholinergic toxicity. *Journal of Medical Toxicology; Official Journal of the American College of Medical Toxicology*, *11*(2), 179–184. doi:10.1007/s13181-014-0452-x PMID:25510306

Wheeler, G. S. (2005). Maintenance of a narrow host range by *Oxyops vitiosa*; a biological control agent of *Melaleuca quinquenervia*. *Biochemical Systematics and Ecology*, *33*(4), 365–383. doi:10.1016/j.bse.2004.10.010

Wild, S., Roglic, G., Green, A., Sicree, R., & King, H. (2004). Global prevalence of diabetes: Estimates for the year 2000 and projections for 2030. *Diabetes Care*, *27*(5), 1047–1053. doi:10.2337/diacare.27.5.1047 PMID:15111519

Windholz, M. (Ed.). (1983). The Merck Index (10th ed.). Rahway, NJ: Merck & Co.

World Health Organization. (1992). *Quality Control Methods for Medicinal Plant Materials*. Geneva: World Health Organization.

World Health Organization. (1996a). *Quality Assurance of Pharmaceuticals: A Compendium of Guidelines and Related Materials, Good Manufacturing Practices and Inspection*. Geneva: World Health Organization.

World Health Organization WHO. (1996b). *Guidelines for the Assessment of Herbal Medicines. WHO Technical Report Series*. Geneva: World Health Organization.

World Health Organization WHO. (2006). *Guidelines for the treatment of malaria*. World Health Organization.

Yoshikawa, M., Murakami, T., Kadoya, M., Matsuda, H., Muraoka, O., Yamahara, J., & Murakami, N. (1996). Medicinal foodstuff. III. Sugar beet. (1): Hypoglycemic oleanolic acid oligoglycosides, betavulgarosides I, II, III, and IV, from the root of *Beta vulgaris* L. (Chenopodiaceae). *Chemical & Pharmaceutical Bulletin, 44*(6), 1212–1217. doi:10.1248/cpb.44.1212 PMID:8814952

Zhang, B., Salituro, G., Szalkowski, D., Li, Z., Zhang, Y., Royo, I., & Moller, D. E. et al. (1999). Discovery of small molecule insulin mimetic with antidiabetic activity in mice. *Science, 284*(5416), 974–977. doi:10.1126/science.284.5416.974 PMID:10320380

Zhang, L., Xu, X., Yang, R., Chen, J., Wang, S., Yang, J., & Zhang, D. (2015). Paclitaxel attenuates renal interstitial fibroblast activation and interstitial fibrosis by inhibiting STAT3 signaling. *Drug Design. Development & Therapy, 9*, 2139–2148. doi:10.2147/DDDT.S81390 PMID:25931810

Zhang, P., Luo, S., Li, M., & Tan, S. (2015). Artesunate inhibits the growth and induces apoptosis of human gastric cancer cells by downregulating COX-2. *Onco Targets & Therapy, 8*, 845–854. doi:10.2147/OTT.S81041 PMID:25945055

Zhang, S., Wang, J., Xue, H., Deng, Q., Xing, F., & Ando, M. (2002). Three new guaianolides fromSiyekucai (*Ixeris chinensis*). *Journal of Natural Products, 65*(12), 1927–1929. doi:10.1021/np0202632 PMID:12502342

Chapter 9
Phytopharmaceutical Applications of Nutraceutical and Functional Foods

Dhan Prakash
Amity University, India

Charu Gupta
Amity University, India

ABSTRACT

Nutraceuticals are actually "Bioactive herbal formulations" that contains selective combinations of specific bioactive constituents of plants and/or their parts that possess health-promotive, disease preventing and medicinal properties. The important phytochemical constituents commonly found in plants are polyphenols, flavonoids, isoflavonoids, anthocyanidins, carotenoids, fibers, limonoids, glucosinolates, phytoestrogens, phytosterols and terpenoids. They play positive pharmacological activities in human health such as antioxidant activity, anti-microbial activity, anti-inflammatory, anti-allergic, anti-spasmodic, chemo-preventive, hepato-protective, neuro-protective, hypolipidemic, hypotensive, anti-aging, diabetes, osteoporosis, repair DNA damage, heart diseases, diuretic, Central Nervous System (CNS) stimulant, immuno-modulator, carminative, Thus the present chapter summarizes the phyto-pharmaceutical applications of nutraceuticals and functional foods and would lay emphasis on its importance for future generations for their well-being.

INTRODUCTION

Since the early 1990s, there has been a considerable shift in consumers' perspective toward nutraceuticals and functional foods. Currently, consumers are much more conscious and aware about health and many share the perception that the onset of many chronic diseases can be prevented with the proper intake of nutritious diet. Food supplements are not only being consumed for just meeting the recommended dietary allowance but also as a mechanism for performance enhancement and disease prevention (FICCI Newsletter; Sharma et al., 2014).

DOI: 10.4018/978-1-5225-0754-3.ch009

Consumers are now moving towards food products that are obtained from natural non-GMO (genetically modified organism) extracts. Nutraceuticals are those food derived substances in extracted form, which claim to provide medicinal and health benefits (Prakash & Kumar, 2011).

Globally, nutraceuticals are gaining prominence and becoming a part of the average consumer's daily diet. The key reasons for this have been the increased incidence of lifestyle diseases, increase in life expectancy and inadequate nutrition due to the current lifestyle. In fact, in developing nations, mortality due to nutrition related factors is nearly 40 percent, underscoring the need for nutraceutical products and to balance the nutritional intake of the individual (Prakash, Gupta, & Sharma, 2012).

Vision gain predicts the world market for functional foods and nutraceuticals will reach $241.25bn in 2015. Market growth has been supported by a significant increase in the world's ageing population as well as growing consciousness of health and wellness across the globe. Increasing usage of internet and social media has also driven the trend towards self-medication using functional foods and nutraceuticals. This has provided an important incentive for the global food industry, which is experiencing an increasing shift towards functional foods and nutraceuticals (Sharma & Prakash, 2013).

NUTRACEUTICALS: THEN AND NOW

Nutraceuticals are products that provide health and medicinal benefits, including the prevention and treatment of diseases in addition to the basic nutritional value found in foodstuff. Nutraceuticals are particularly of interest to the present generation because they have the potential to substantially reduce the expensive, high-tech, disease treatment approaches presently being employed in Western healthcare (Sharma & Prakash, 2013).

This category includes any food that we eat, having a particular health benefit that has been established through molecular and clinical research. In other words, a food can become a nutraceutical simply through the production of new scientific knowledge (Street, 2015).

Chemically the nutraceuticals may be classified as isoprenoid derivatives (terpenoids, carotenoids, saponins, tocotrienols, tocopherols, terpenes), phenolic compounds (couramines, tannins, lignins, anthocyanins, isoflavones, flavonones, flavanoids), carbohydrate derivatives (ascorbic acid, oligosaccharides, non-starch polysaccharides), fatty acid and structural lipids (n-3 PUFA, CLA, MUFA, sphingolipids, lecithins), amino acid derivatives (amino acids, allyl-S compounds, capsaicinoids, isothiocyanates, indoles, folate, choline), microbes (probiotics, prebiotics) and minerals (Ca, Zn, Cu, K, Se) (Prakash, Dhakarey, & Mishra, 2004; Sharma, 2009). They play a crucial role in maintaining optimal immune response, such that deficient or excessive intakes can have negative impact on health. Around the world, the governing bodies have accepted nutraceuticals as possible nutraceutical therapy in main stream of medical education and health (Sharma, 2009).

The major nutraceuticals mainly include vitamins and minerals and bioactive constituents from plant sources (phytochemicals). The vitamins A, B_6, B_{12}, D, E, folate have been reported as anti-cancer, immunoprotective and reducing cancer risk in individuals who used self-medication (Zhang et al., 2008).

Several preclinical and clinical trial studies have shown that the regular consumption of fruits, vegetables and whole grains, reduces the risk of chronic diseases associated with oxidative damage (Cieslik, Greda, & Adamus, 2006). Carotenoids, tocopherols, ascorbates, lipoic acids and polyphenols are strong natural antioxidants with free radical scavenging activity. Besides, there are several endogenous antioxidant enzymes like super oxide dismutase (SOD), catalase, glutathione peroxidase, glutathione reductase, minerals like Se, Mn, Cu, Zn, vitamins A, C and E, carotenoids, limonoids and polyphenols that exert synergistic actions in scavenging free radicals. Synthetic antioxidants such as butylated hydroxy anisole (BHA) and butylated hydroxy toluene (BHT) play a useful role in food and pharmaceutical industries (Kondratyuk & Pezzuto, 2004).

The interaction of nutraceuticals with food and drugs is another area, which should be taken into consideration. The effect of different processing methods on the biological availability and effectiveness of nutraceuticals remains to be determined. Similar to drugs, there should be stringent regulatory controls for nutraceuticals also.

Nutritional therapy and phyto-therapy have emerged as new concepts of health aid in recent years. Strong recommendations for consumption of nutraceuticals from plant origin have become progressively popular to improve health, and to prevent and treat diseases (Pandey, Meena, Rai, & Pandey-Rai, 2011).

Nature of Nutraceuticals

Nutraceuticals is a very broad term which includes a variety of substances/compounds ranging from essential plant nutrients, metals, and large polymers up to bacteria. Chemical nature of nutraceutical depends upon their structure and function. The chemical characteristics can be used for grouping nutraceuticals based upon their chemical nature. This approach allows nutraceuticals to be categorized under different molecular/elemental groups and sub groups. For example (1) Amino acid-based substances: amino acids, ally-S compounds, indole, folate and choline (2) Carbohydrates and derivatives: ascorbic acid, oligosaccharides, non-starch-polysaccharides (3) Fatty acids and structural lipids: lecithin, fatty acids, oil (4) Isoprenoid derivatives: carotenoids, saponins, tocopherols, simple terpenes (5) Phenolic substances: coumarins, tannins, lignin, anthocyanins, isoflavones, flavones, flavonols (6) Microbes: probiotics, prebiotics (7) Minerals: calcium, selenium, potassium, copper, zinc etc. (Pandey, Meena, Rai, & Pandey-Rai, 2011).

Nutraceuticals Development using Biotechnology

Biotechnological tools can also be used to develop and improve nutraceutical products and functional foods. Some of the benefits include increased enzyme or metabolite production from recombinant microorganisms, improvement of thermostability of these metabolites and enzymes and their ability to tolerate large pH ranges.

Genetic engineering has made it possible to isolate particular genes coding for enzymes or other metabolites of our interest, from organisms of unknown genetics. For example, it is widely believed that omega-3 fatty acids are beneficial against cardiovascular disease. Although there are sources of omega-3 fatty acids available in the market such as fish, flax seed and some vegetable oils.

Using biotechnology it may be possible to produce a vegetable oil that has ten or twenty times the amount of omega-3 fatty acids compared to present day oils. Such types of oil would be useful to include in the diet of patients prone to heart disease. Conventional plant-breeding methods can also improve nutraceutical quality and production by enhancing both agronomic and medicinal traits. In vitro propagation or tissue culture of plants holds tremendous potential for the production of high-quality plant-based medicines.

Besides these, nutritional genomics is a recent off-shoot of this genetic revolution in the area of nutraceutical development which includes nutrigenomics (the study of interaction of dietary components with the genome and the resulting proteomic and metabolomic changes) and nutrigenetics (understanding the gene-based differences in response to dietary components and developing nutraceuticals that are most compatible with health based on individual genetic makeup) (Ravi, 2007; Pandey, Meena, Rai, & Pandey-Rai, 2011).

FUNCTIONAL FOODS AS NATURAL HEALTH PRODUCTS

Functional foods bridge the gap between ordinary foods aimed to maintain adequate nutrition status and pharmaceutical agents, medicines aimed to diagnose, prevent, cure or treat an illness. In contrast to the efficacy area of medicines functional foods are developed for enhanced function of reduction of risk of disease (Arouma, 2001). Functional foods are similar in appearance to, or may be, a conventional food, consumed as part of a usual diet, which is demonstrated to have physiological benefits and/or to reduce the risk of chronic disease beyond basic nutritional functions.

They are developed through various means, such as fortification with vitamins and/or minerals, beyond mandatory requirements, to provide added health benefits (for example, fortified soy beverages and fruit juice with calcium); addition of bioactive ingredients (for example, margarine with phytosterols, muffins with beta-glucan, yogurts with probiotics, and drinks with herb blends); and enhancement with bioactive components through plant breeding, genetic modification, processing, or special livestock feeding techniques (for example, eggs, milk and meat with omega-3; canola oil high in carotenoids; and strawberries with enhanced levels of ellagic acid).

PHYTOPHARMACEUTICALS OF NUTRACEUTICAL IMPORTANCE

Polyphenols

In the recent years, there has been much awareness about functional foods and nutraceuticals fortified with natural polyphenols and their health benefits like their potent antioxidant activity, anti-carcinogenic, anti-inflammatory, anti-neurodegenerative, anti-diabetic, antiviral, skin photo-protective, antiallergic, anti-platelet, anti-aging, cytoprotective and DNA-protective properties. Polyphenolic compounds are plant nutraceuticals showing a huge structural diversity, including chlorogenic acids, hydrolyzable tannins, and flavonoids (flavonols, flavanones, flavan-3-ols, anthocyanidins, isoflavones, and flavones). Most of them occur as glycosylated derivatives in plants and foods, including fruits, vegetables, nuts, seeds, flowers and bark. A wide variety of dietary plants including grains, berries, legumes, tea, grapes, olive oil, cocoa, walnuts, peanuts, spices, fruits, vegetables etc. contain polyphenols (Tenore, Daglia, Ciampaglia, & Novellino, 2015). Polyphenols, with approximately 8000 structural variants, are characterized by the presence of aromatic rings bearing one or more hydroxyl moieties, which have proven pivotal roles in mediating their properties (Leiro et al., 2004). Although the knowledge of absorption, bioavailability and metabolism of polyphenols is not entirely known, it appears that some polyphenols are bioactive and are absorbed in their native or modified form by the microflora of the intestine. The active components of dietary phytochemicals (e.g. curcumin, resveratrol, capsaicin, catechins, vitamins and beta-carotene) are believed to suppress the inflammatory processes, moderate cell signaling pathways, proliferation, apoptosis, redox balance and most often appear to be protective against cancer, neurodegenerative disorders and cardiovascular diseases among others (Aggarwal and Shishodia, 2006; Rahman, Biswas, & Kirkham, 2006).

A wide variety of polyphenols have been reported to possess substantial skin photo-protective effects (Nichols & Katiyar, 2010). In order to become bioactive at human body, these polyphenols must undergo diverse intestinal transformations, due to the action of digestive enzymes, but also by the action of microbiota metabolism. After elimination of sugar tailoring (generating the corresponding aglycons) and diverse hydroxyl moieties, as well as further backbone reorganizations, the final absorbed compounds enter the portal vein circulation towards liver (where other enzymatic transformations take place) and from there to other organs, including behind the digestive tract or via blood towards urine excretion. During this transit along diverse tissues and organs, they are able to carry out strong antiviral, antibacterial, and anti-parasitic activities (Marin, Miguélez, Villar, & Lombó, 2015).

Flavonoids

Flavonoids are the most common group of polyphenolic compounds in the human diet. Major dietary sources of flavonoids include fruits, vegetables, cereals, dry legumes, tea, wine and chocolate (Spencer, Abd El Mohsen, Minihane, & Mathers, 2008). The main dietary groups of flavonoids are flavonols

Table 1. Phytopharmaceuticals of nutraceutical importance, their sources and health benefits

Phytochemicals	Source Plant	Health Benefits
α-linolenic acid (ALA)	Flax seeds	Cancer preventive, reduce risk of coronary heart disease
Allicin	Garlic, onion	Antibacterial, anticancer, antifungal, anti-inflammatory, chemopreventive, hepato-protective, hypolipidemic, hypotensive, and neuroprotective
Anthocyanins	Blackberry, cherry, orange, purple corn, raspberry, red grapes	Anti-allergic, anti-inflammatory, antioxidants, and pigments
Apigenin	Apple, artichoke, basil, celery, cherry, grapes, nuts, parsley	Anti-inflammatory, antioxidant, Antispasmodic, chemo-preventive, induce apoptosis, and inhibits breast and ovarian cancers
Caffeic acid	Artichoke, pear, basil, oregano	Anti-inflammatory, anti-fatigue and anti-stress **properties**
Carotene	Carrots, Leafy greens and red, orange and yellow vegetables, pumpkin	Anti-carcinogenic, enhances release of immunogenic cytokines IL-1 and TNF-alpha, provide cornea protection against UV light, stimulate DNA repair enzymes
Catechins	Tea	Antioxidant, CNS stimulant, and Diuretic
Curcumin	Turmeric	Anti-hypertensive, anti-inflammatory, antioxidant, and cancer preventive
Diosgenin	Fenugreek seeds	Hypolipidemic
Ellagic acid	Cranberry, grapes, pecans, pomegranates, raspberry, strawberry, walnuts	Anticancer, and antioxidant
Ferulic acid	Oats, rice, orange, pineapple, peanut	Protect against cancer, bone degeneration, menopausal symptoms (hot flushes)
Gallic acid	Tea, mango, strawberries, soy	Cytotoxic and anti-oxidative activities, Anti-leukemic, antioxidant, anticancer, anti-neoplastic, anti-inflammatory, anti-diabetic

continued on following page

Table 1. Continued

Phytochemicals	Source Plant	Health Benefits
Genistein	Alpha-alfa sprouts, red clover, chickpeas, peanuts	acts as a phytoestrogens, antioxidant, anti-cancer agent, heart health, and help people with metabolic syndrome
Lutein	Kale, spinach, red pepper, mango, papaya, kiwi, peaches, squash, honeydew melon, plum, avacado	Absorbs damaging blue light, protect against colon cancer
Lycopene	Apricots, papaya, pink guava, tomato, watermelon	Lowers risk of atherosclerosis and prostate cancer
Momorbicin	Karela (Bitter gourd)	Anti-diabetic
Myristicin	Nutmeg	Hypo-lipidemic
Piperine	Pepper	Aeromatic, analgesic, hepato-protective, and stomachic
Quercetin	Red onions, buckwheat, red grapes, green tea, apple skin	Strong antioxidant, reduces LDL oxidation, vasodilator and blood thinner
Resveratrol	Blueberry, peanuts, red grapes, and red wine	Antioxidant, prevents aging, cancer, diabetes and heart diseases
Rutin	Asparagus, buckwheat and citrus fruits	Strengthens capillary walls
Silymarin	Milk thistle (*Silybum marianum*)	Protects from UVB-induced carcinogenesis, and hepatoprotective
Stigmasterol	Soybean	Anticancer, hypolipidemic, prevention of osteoporosis
Sulforaphane, Glucosinolates	Broccoli sprouts, cabbage, cauliflower, collards, cruciferous vegetables, kale, radish, turnip	Antioxidant, prevent DNA damage, reduce risk of breast and prostate cancers
Ursolic acid	Apple, basil, cranberry, lavender, Oregano, rosemary	Anti-inflammatory, antimicrobial, and Antitumor
Withaferin, Withanolides	*Withania somnifera*	Anticancer, and immuno-modulator
Zingiberene	Ginger	Antibacterial, antifungal, carminative, and in treatment of dizziness

(Sharma, Prakash & Gupta, 2014)

(found in onions and broccoli); flavones (found in parsley and celery); isoflavones (found in soy and soy products); flavanones (found in citrus fruit and tomatoes); flavanols (abundant in green tea, red wine, chocolate); and anthocyanidins (in red wine and berry fruits).

Flavonoids are usually present and stored in plant tissues in the form of diverse derivatives, mostly as sugar O-conjugates at C2 (chalcones), at C3 (flavonols, anthocyanidins, and flavan-3-ols), or at C7 (flavanones, flavones, and isoflavones) positions. Most common bound sugars are glucose, galactose, rhamnose, xylose, rutinose, arabinopyranose, and arabinofuranose (Crozier, Jaganath, & Clifford, 2009). These modifications (and others as methylations and gallate tailoring) add extra structural stability to flavonoids during storage in vacuoles and chloroplasts (Marinova, Kleinschmidt, Weissenbock, & Klein, 2007). Once the plant, fruit, or seed is recollected, flavonoids usually have good stability in this conjugated state and keep high concentrations in food and beverages. All these modifications in chemical structure and sugar binding will determine their absorption and bioavailability (Lewandowska, Szewczyk, Hrabec, Janecka, & Gorlach, 2013; D'Archivio, Filesi, Vari, Scazzocchio, & Masella, 2010).

Among the biological activities of flavonoids are active against free radicals, free radical mediated cellular signaling, inflammation, allergies, platelet aggregation, microbes, ulcers, viruses, tumors and hepatotoxins. Proposed mechanisms by which they provide health benefits, in addition to being direct chemical protectants, involve modulatory effects on a variety of metabolic and signaling enzymes. Flavonoids have been shown to block the angiotensin converting enzyme (ACE) that raises blood pressure; they inhibit cyclooxygenase, which forms prostaglandins; and they block enzymes that produce estrogen. Certain flavonoids prevent platelet aggregation, reducing heart disease and thrombosis; and inhibit estrogen synthase, which binds estrogen to receptors in several tissues, thus decreasing the risk of estrogen related cancers. Bioactive properties such as free radical scavenging, inhibition of hydrolytic and oxidative enzymes, anti-inflammatory and anti viral action of flavonoids is also known (Hodek, Trebil, & Stiborova, 2002). Anti proliferative effects such as cancers, cardio vascular and inflammatory diseases of dietary flavonoids are recognized.

The major sources of flavonoids intake are tea (61%), onions (13%) and apples (10%), the other sources include cherry, tomato, broccoli, black grapes, and blueberries. There is inverse association between flavonoid intake and coronary heart disease mortality. Flavonoids in regularly consumed foods appeared to reduce the risk of death from coronary heart disease.

The capacity of flavonoids to act as antioxidants depends upon their molecular structure. The position of hydroxyl groups and other features in the chemical structure of flavonoids are important for their antioxidant and free radical scavenging activities. Quercetin, the most abundant dietary flavonol, is a potent antioxidant because it has all the right structural features for free radical scavenging activity (Kumar & Andy, 2012). Luteolin has anti-inflammatory, anti-mutagenic and antibacterial activities.

Apigenin is antibacterial, anti-inflammatory, diuretic, hypotensive, and also promotes smooth muscle relaxation.

Myricetin, a hexahydroxyflavone, exhibits antibacterial activity and has anti-gonadotropic activity, but apparently is not a mutagen.

The flavonol kaempferol, which is widely found in the diet, has anti-inflammatory and antibacterial activities and is directly mutagenic.

Quercetin, the most common flavonoid in higher plants, seems to contribute to the mutagenicity of kaempferol in the presence of microsomal metabolizing systems. Quercetin inhibits a number of enzymes, inhibits smooth muscle contraction and proliferation of rat lymphocytes. Although it is anti-inflammatory, antibacterial, antiviral and anti-hepatotoxic, it exhibits mutagenic activity and allergenic properties (Prakash & Gupta, 2009).

Catechins and gallic acids, major sources of catechins are grapes, berries, cocoa and green tea. Tea contains considerable amounts of gallic acid esters, such as epicatechin, epicatechingallate and epigallocatechingallate (EGCG). Numerous studies have suggested that these components provide protective benefits by their free radical scavenging ability and their inhibition of eicosanoid synthesis and platelet aggregation. The green tea provides protection against prostate cancer (Nichenametla, Taruscio, Barney, & Exon, 2006). In wines, catechins and procyanidins are involved in the astringency sensation. Catechin is one of the major phenolics in grapes and red wines, and it is considered to be responsible for part of the protective effect of red wine against atherosclerotic cardiovascular disease.

Isoflavonoids

Isoflavones are secondary vegetable substances, which can act as estrogens in the body and have protective functions. They exercise a balancing effect when the level of estrogens is low, such as during the menopause, and cause less menopause systems. Isoflavones can also reduce the effect of the estrogen on cells and skin layers when the hormone levels are high, and then essentially reduce the risk of estrogen linked cancers. Some isoflavones are termed as antioxidants, in particular soy isoflavones, when studied in populations eating soy protein, have indicated that there is a lower incidence of breast cancer and other common cancers because of its role in influencing sex hormone metabolism and biological activity through intracellular enzymes, protein synthesis, growth factor actions, malignant cell proliferations, differentiation and angiogenesis (Heber Berdanier, Dwyer, & Feldman, 2008).

Isoflavones are produced almost exclusively by the members of the Fabaceae (Leguminosae) family. Their main food sources are soy cheese, soy flour, soy bean, and tofu. Daidzein and genistein are among several known isoflavones. They should be integral part of everyone's diet as they help to reduce cholesterol, prevent atherosclerosis, protect or slow prostate and breast cancer growth, prevent the kind of cell mutation that causes DNA damage, inhibit blood supply to already existing tumors, ease menopause and lower the risk of osteoporosis (Trock, Hilakivi-Clarke, & Clarke, 2006). Soybeans flour is a rich source of isoflavones, which are a subclass of ubiquitous flavonoids. Isoflavones, which have potent antioxidant properties comparable to that of vitamin E, can reduce the long-term risk of cancer by preventing free radical damage to DNA. Genistein followed by daidzein is the most predominant antioxidant among soybean isoflavones (Udgata & Naik, 2007).

Isoflavones compounds have been found effective in the management of diabetes. It reduces low-density lipoprotein and triglycerides and hence minimizes the risk of coronary heart disease. Soy isoflavones was found useful for treatment of osteoporosis by inhibiting tyrosine kinase (Meghwal & Sahu, 2015).

Anthocyanins

Anthocyanins are the largest group of water-soluble pigments in the Plant Kingdom. They have been demonstrated to have potential health benefits and disease prevention properties and are known as potential antioxidants (Zafra-Stone et al., 2007). Consumption of anthocyanin-enriched foods is associated with a reduced risk of several diseases such as atherosclerosis (Xia et al., 2006) dyslipidemia (Qin et al., 2009), and diabetes (Ghosh & Konishi, 2007). Anthocyanins may appear red, purple, or blue depending on the pH. They are synthesized via the phenylpropanoid pathway; they are odorless and nearly flavorless, contributing to taste as a moderately astringent sensation. Anthocyanins occur in all tissues of higher plants, including leaves, stems, roots, flowers and fruits. Anthocyanins are derivatives of anthocyanidins, which include pendant sugars. Plants rich in anthocyanins are *Vaccinium* species, such as blueberry, cranberry, blackberry, cherry, red cabbage. The highest recorded amount is present in the seed coat of black soybean. Anthocyanins are considered secondary metabolites as a food additive. They are approved for use as a food additive in the European Union, Australia and New Zealand. The main anthocyanin compounds are pelargonidin, cyanidin and delphinidin. Cyanidin and its glycosides are natural dietary pigments which have been found with promising potential benefits to humans, especially in the prevention and treatment of diabetes mellitus (Akkarachiyasit, Charoenlertkul, Yibchok-Anun, & Adisakwattana, 2010).

Unlike other flavonoids that are absorbed and secreted, anthocyanins, the glycosylated versions of anthocyanidin aglycons (as cyanidin, pelargonidin, and malvidin), do not appear to undergo extensive metabolism of the parent glycosides to glucuronic, sulfo or methyl derivatives, and therefore their bioavailability is very low (Manach, Williamson, Morand, Scalbert, & Remesy, 2005). Procyanidins occur in monomeric as well as in oligomeric and polymeric forms and are the most abundant and bioactive dietary polyphenols, as they are responsible for most red, blue, and purple color in fruits (specially berries), flowers, and leaves, besides having an important antioxidant activity (Miladinovic et al., 2014; Burdulis et al., 2009).

All the anthocyanins and their metabolites tested significantly enhance growth of *Bifidobacterium sp., Lactobacillus sp.* and *Enterococcus sp.* Therefore anthocyanins and their metabolites could perform a positive modulation of intestinal bacterial populations (Hidalgo et al., 2012).

Phytoestrogens

Phytoestrogens are a diverse group of plant-derived compounds that structurally or functionally mimic mammalian estrogens and show potential benefits for human health hence, serve as potential alternatives to the synthetic selective estrogen receptor modulators and currently being used in hormone replacement therapy. Estrogens play many important physiological roles in men and women. In women, life is severely affected by a variety of estrogen-related conditions such as osteoporosis, cognitive and cardiovascular disease, increased risk of breast cancer and other symptoms that decrease the overall quality of life. Phytoestrogens are effective in maintaining bone mineral density, prevent bone loss, and help in the prevention and/ or treatment of such health related problems. They can be classified as flavonoids, isoflavonoids, coumestans, stilbenes, lignans and terpenoids. Terpenoids (ferutinine, tschimgine, and tschimganidine) found in the Umbelliferae family have estrogenic activities. The main dietary source of phytoestrogenic stilbenes is *trans*-resveratrol from red wine and peanuts. Plant-derived foods may be an adequate source for variety of phytoestrogens capable of producing a range of pharmacological effects and protection from various life threatening diseases (Prakash & Gupta, 2014a).

Animal experiments and pre-clinical models have provided strong evidence that phytoestrogens may have anti-diabetic function via both estrogen-dependent and estrogen-independent pathways. A number of epidemiological studies and clinical trials have thus been conducted in different populations linking two major types of phytoestrogens, isoflavones and lignans, to the prevention and management of diabetes. Although the current evidence is complex and inconsistent, habitual consumption of phytoestrogens, particularly their intact food sources, could be considered as a component of overall healthy dietary pattern for prevention and management of diabetes (Talaei & Pan, 2015).

Terpenoids

The terpenes, also known as isoprenoids, are the largest class of phytonutrients in green foods, and grains. These compounds are found in higher plants, mosses, liverworts, algae and lichens, as well as in insects, microbes or marine organisms. Terpenoids are derived from a common biosynthetic pathway based on mevalonate as parent, and are named terpenoids, terpenes or isoprenoids with the subgroup of steroids among them as a class (Bohlmann & Keeling, 2008). Their importance to plants relates to their necessity to fix carbon through photosynthetic reactions using photosensitizing pigments. Animals have evolved to utilize these compounds for hormonal and growth regulatory functions (vitamin A) and, as it is now being understood, the presence of these molecules in animal tissues also provides a measure of protection from certain diseases, especially those related to chronic damage and growth deregulation.

The diverse functional roles of some of the terpenoids are characterized as hormones (gibberellins), photosynthetic pigments (phytol, carotenoids), electron carriers (ubiquinone, plastoquinone), and mediators of polysaccharide assembly, as well as communication and defense mechanisms. Several biological actions have been reported for diterpenes including antibacterial, antifungal, anti-inflammatory, anti-leishmanial, cytotoxic and anti-tumour activities (Paduch, Kandefer-Szerszen, Trytek, & Fiedurek, 2007). Terpenes are also used as skin penetration enhancers, as well as natural insecticides and can be of use as protective substances in storing agriculture products. Terpenes have a unique antioxidant activity in their interaction with free radicals. The most studied terpene antioxidants are the tocotrienols and tocopherols. They are found naturally in whole grains and have effects on cancer cells. The tocotrienols are effective apoptotic inducers for human breast cancer cells. The impact of a diet of fruits, vegetables and grains on reduction of cancer risk may be explained by the actions of terpenes *in vivo* (Prakash & Kumar, 2011).

In cyanobacteria, they are synthesized from the methylerythritol-phosphate (MEP) pathway, using glyceraldehydes 3-phosphate and pyruvate produced by photosynthesis as substrates. The products of the MEP pathway are isopentenyl diphosphate and dimethylallyl diphosphate, which in turn form the basic building blocks for formation of all terpenoids. Many terpenoid compounds have useful properties and are of interest in the fields of pharmaceuticals and nutrition, and even potentially as future biofuels. The MEP pathway, its function and regulation, and the subsequent formation of terpenoids have not been fully elucidated in cyanobacteria, despite its relevance for biotechnological applications (Pattanaik & Lindberg, 2015).

Carotenoids

Carotenoids comprising carotenes and oxy-carotenoids as two main groups are fat-soluble pigments, widely distributed in nature. The distinctive pattern of alternating single and double bonds in the polyene backbone of carotenoids might be responsible to quench reactive oxygen species (ROS), while the nature of specific end groups on carotenoids may influence their polarity. Antioxidants help to control free radicals by quenching them by donating electrons to molecules before they damage other bio-molecules of the cell or by reducing their energy or stopping their formation by interrupting oxidizing chain reaction.

Carotenes along with xanthophylls, astaxanthin, lycopene and lutein seem to offer protection against lungs, colorectal, breast, uterine and prostate cancers. They help to prevent heart disease, supplementation along with vitamin C and E, reduce the risk of developing diabetes and to fight against Alzheimer's disease. They are generally regarded as safe (GRAS) but increased consumption of carotenoids may cause the skin to turn orange or yellow, known as "carotenodermia." This occurrence is completely benign and is unrelated to jaundice that can result from liver disease or other causes (Prakash & Gupta, 2014b).

Carotenoids are biosynthesized by bacteria, algae, fungi, and plants, but not by animals, which must obtain them from their food. These compounds are divided into two major classes based on their structural elements; carotenes, constituted by carbon and hydrogen (e.g. β-carotene, α-carotene and lycopene), and xanthophylls, constituted by carbon, hydrogen, and additionally oxygen (for example lutein, β-cryptoxanthin, zeaxanthin, astaxanthin and fucoxanthin). Carotenoids have good effect on human health, such as pro-vitamin A, antioxidant, anticancer, anti-obesity effect and anabolic effect on bone components. Currently, carotenoids are used commercially as feed additives, animal feed supplements, natural food colorants, nutrient supplement and, more recently, as nutraceuticals for cosmetic and pharmaceutical purposes. These compounds can be produced commercially by chemical synthesis, fermentation or isolation from the small number of abundant natural sources. Furthermore, commercial production of carotenoids from microorganisms competes mainly with synthetic manufacture by chemical synthesis (Jaswir, Noviendri, Hasrini, & Octavianti, 2011).

The nutraceutical industry synthetically manufactures five major carotenoids on an industrial scale (e.g. lycopene, β-carotene, canthaxanthin, zeaxanthin and astaxanthin) for use in a range of food products and cosmetics, such as vitamin supplements and health products and as feed additives for poultry, livestock, fish and crustaceans (Jackson, Braun, & Ernst, 2008). One of the most commercially valuable pigments, astaxanthin, is primarily synthesized by marine microorganisms, such as the green alga *Haematococcus pluvialis* and accumulates in fish such as salmon, thus, colouring their flesh red. Astaxanthin has been implicated as a potential therapeutic agent treating cardiovascular disease and prostatic cancer (Fassett & Coombes, 2011).

Lycopene

Lycopene, a carotenoid without provitamin-A activity, is present in many fruits and vegetables; however, tomatoes and processed tomato products constitute the major source of lycopene in North American diet. Among the carotenoids, lycopene is a major component found in the serum and other tissues. Dietary intakes of tomatoes and tomato products containing lycopene have been shown to be associated with decreased risk of chronic diseases such as cancer and cardiovascular diseases in several recent studies. Serum and tissue lycopene levels have also been inversely related with the chronic disease risk. Although the antioxidant properties of lycopene are thought to be primarily responsible for its beneficial properties, evidence is accumulating to suggest other mechanisms such as modulation of intercellular gap junction communication, hormonal and immune system and metabolic pathways may also be involved. Lycopene also has the ability to destroy free radicals that form when the body metabolizes oxygen (Rao & Shen, 2002; Gupta & Prakash, 2014).

Limonoids

Limonoids are heavily oxygenated, modified triterpenes dominant in Meliaceae and Rutaceae plant families. The term 'limonoid' is derived from limonin, which was first identified as the bitter constituent of *Citrus* seeds in 1841. This group of secondary metabolites exhibits a wide range of biological properties, including anticancer, antibacterial, antifungal, antimalarial and antiviral activities. Significant progress on the role of limonoids as promising candidates for cancer chemoprevention and/or therapy has been achieved in particular in recent years (Tundis, Loizzo, & Menichini, 2014). Citrus limonoids appear in large amounts in Citrus juices and tissues as water-soluble limonoid glucosides or in seeds as water-insoluble limonoid aglycones. For most Citrus species, limonin (1), followed by nomilin (2), is the most abundant aglycone, whereas the most representative glucoside is limonin glucoside (3).

Citrus limonoids were considered a major problem for the Citrus juice industry as they cause delayed bitterness of the juices at room temperature, thus lowering the quality and value of the commercial juice. Limonoids bitterness occurs gradually after juice processing. However, at present, these bitter compounds have gained significant importance because of their role in inhibition of several chronic diseases since it is possible to detect limonoids in human plasma after Citrus ingestion (Tian, Miller, Jayaprakasha, & Patil, 2007).

Potential cancer preventive constituents of sour orange (*C. aurantium*, Rutaceae) were isolated and identified as isolimonic acid and ichanexic acid. Both compounds exhibited differential inhibition at various concentrations (Kim et al., 2009). Besides anticancer activity, the other biological activities reported for limonoids are antioxidant, anti-inflammatory, neuroprotective, anti-plasmodial, antiviral and antimicrobial (Tundis, Loizzo, & Menichini, 2014).

Phytosterols

Phytosterols are a group of steroid alcohols and esters that occur naturally in plants as non-saponifiable fraction of plant oils. Phytosterols (including plant sterols and stanols) cannot be synthesized by humans, and all plant sterols and stanols in the human body therefore originate from the diet (Jong, Plat, & Mensink, 2003). Phytosterol and stanol (or phytosterols) consumption reduces intestinal cholesterol absorption, leading to decreased blood LDL-cholesterol levels and lowered cardiovascular disease risk. However, other biological roles for plant sterols and stanols have also been proposed. Considerable emerging evidence supports the inhibitory actions of phytosterols on lung, stomach, as well as ovarian and breast cancer. Phytosterols seem to act through multiple mechanisms of action, including inhibition of carcinogen production, cancer-cell growth, angiogenesis, invasion and metastasis, and through the promotion of apoptosis of cancerous cells. Plant sterols might also protect against certain types of cancer such as colon, breast and prostate (Awad & Fink, 2000).

Phytosterol consumption may also increase the activity of antioxidant enzymes and thereby reduce oxidative stress. In addition to altering cell-membrane structure and function, phytosterols probably promote apoptosis by lowering blood cholesterol levels. Moreover, consumption of phytosterols by healthy humans at the recommended level of 2 g per day does not cause any major health risks. In summary, mounting evidence supports a role for phytosterols in protecting against cancer development. Hence, phytosterols could be incorporated in diet not only to lower the cardiovascular disease risk, but also to potentially prevent cancer development (Woyengo, Ramprasath, & Jones, 2009).

The primary sources of phytosterols are vegetables, nuts, fruits and seeds. Seeds contain an average of 120 mg of plant sterols/100 g wet weight; vegetables contain 20 mg/100 g of wet weight and fruit about 15 mg/100 g wet weight. Sitosterol, campesterol and stigmasterol are most abundant in nature comprising 65%, 30%, and 3% of dietary phytosterol intake (John, Sorokin, & Thompson, 2007).

In animals, these exhibit anti-inflammatory, anti-neoplastic, anti-pyretic and immuno-modulating activity. Phytosterols were reported to block inflammatory enzymes, for example by modifying the prostaglandin pathways in a way that protected platelets. Phytosterols compete with cholesterol in the intestine for uptake, and aid in the elimination of cholesterol from the body. In the intestine, plant sterols are initially solubilized into a micelle form. These micelles interact with brush border cells and are transferred into enterocytes. Plant sterols are esterified within the enterocyte, assembled into chylomicrons and secreted into the lymphatics. They are excreted via the biliary system. The nonesterified phytosterols are transported back into the intestinal lumen by sterolin (1 and 2) pumps containing the ATP binding cassette (ABC) proteins encoded by the genes ABCG5 and ABCG8. These are expressed in the mucosal cells and the canalicular membrane, and they resecrete sterols, especially absorbed plant sterols, back into the intestinal lumen and from the liver into bile (von Bergmann, Sudhop, & Lutjohann, 2005). Saturated phytosterols appear to be more effective than unsaturated compounds in decreasing cholesterol concentrations in the body. Their actions reduce serum or plasma total cholesterol and low-density lipoprotein (LDL) cholesterol. Competition with cholesterol for absorption from the intestine is not unexpected as the structure of plant sterols is similar to that of cholesterol. In mammals, concentrations of plasma phytosterol are low because of their poor absorption from the intestine and their faster excretion from liver, and metabolism to bile acids, compared with cholesterol (Dillard & German, 2000). Available animal studies suggest that phytosterols reduce atherosclerosis in the Apo-E deficient mouse model. Human studies are mixed, and do not prove or disprove an increase in atherosclerotic risk that can be clearly related to serum phytosterol levels. It is reassuring that vegetarians who consume considerable plant sterols are at decreased risk of atherosclerosis cardiovascular diseases (ASCVD), but it is impossible to separate the effects of phytosterol excess from animal fat reduction in this population (John, Sorokin, & Thompson, 2007).

Glucosinolates

They are present in cruciferous vegetables, are activators of liver detoxification enzymes. These chemicals are responsible for the pungent aroma and bitter flavor of cruciferous vegetables. Consumption of cruciferous vegetables offers a phytochemical strategy for providing protection against carcinogenesis, mutagenesis and other forms of toxicity of electrophiles and reactive forms of oxygen. The sprouts of certain crucifers, including broccoli and cauliflower, contain higher amounts of glucoraphanin (the glucosinolate of sulforaphane) than do the corresponding mature plants. Crucifer sprouts may protect against the risk of cancer more effectively than the same quantity of mature vegetables of the same variety (Cartea & Velasco, 2008; Traka & Mithen, 2009). During food preparation, chewing, and digestion, the glucosinolates in cruciferous vegetables are broken down to form biologically active compounds such as indoles, nitriles, thiocyanates, and isothiocyanates (Hayes, Kelleher, & Eggleston, 2008). Indole-3-carbinol (an indole) and sulforaphane (an isothiocyanate) have been most frequently examined for their anticancer effects. Epidemiological studies indicate that consumption of brassica vegetables is associated with a reduced incidence of cancers at a number of sites including the lung, stomach, colon and rectum. Glucosinolates, the thioglucosides, present in brassica vegetables are thought to contribute to this phenomenon. Dietary glucosinolates have been reported to block formation of endogenous or exogenous carcinogens for preventing initiation of carcinogenesis (Vig, Rampal, Singh, & Arora, 2009). The mechanism of the protective effects is thought to involve the modulation of carcinogen metabolism by the induction of Phase 2 detoxification enzymes and inhibition of Phase 1 carcinogen-activating enzymes, thereby possibly influencing several processes related to chemical carcinogenesis, e.g. the metabolism, DNA binding and mutagenic activity of promutagens. A reducing effect on tumor formation has been shown in rats and mice, and studies carried out in humans using high but realistic human consumption amounts of indoles and brassica vegetables have shown putative positive effects on health. Indole-3-carbinol is a glucosinolate metabolite that inhibits organ-site carcinogenesis in rodent models. Its preventive effect on human mammary carcinogenesis may be due in part to its ability to regulate cell cycle progression, increase the formation of anti-proliferative estradiol metabolite and induce cellular apoptosis (Sharma, Prakash, & Gupta, 2014).

Fibers

Most plant foods in their native state contain indigestible residues that used to be classified as crude fibre, but are currently classified as dietary fibre (DF) and also known as non-starch polysaccharide (NSP). Dietary fibre is not a single entity but consists of a wide range of complex polysaccharides such as cellulose, gums, mucilages, hemicellulose and lignins with different chemical, physiochemical and physiological properties (Narasinga Rao, 2003). The Institute of Medicine defines DF as the non-digestible carbohydrates and lignin that are intrinsic and intact in plants (Food and Nutrition board, 2005).

Recently, the National Academy of Sciences (NAS) proposed a new definition for fiber (Food and Nutrition board, 2005). The new definition proposes that total fiber = dietary fiber + functional fiber. Fiber consists of non-digestible carbohydrates and lignin (a non-carbohydrate substance bound to fiber), which are intrinsic and intact in plants (e.g., gums, cellulose, oat bran, wheat bran), and functional fiber consists of isolated, non-digestible carbohydrates that have beneficial physiological effects in humans. Functional fibers may be extracted or modified from plants (e.g., resistant starch from green bananas and cooked, cooled potatoes) or may be derived from animal sources (e.g., chitin and chitosan found in crab and lobster shells). Functional fiber also must have a beneficial physiological effect in humans.

DF is usually divided into 2 major categories based on water solubility and viscosity. The physical properties of viscous and non-viscous DF in food determine their physiologic effects, which in turn are related to their known and potential health benefits. The roles of dietary fibers and nutraceuticals for primary prevention of cardiovascular disease from childhood have been well reported. Dietary fibers have important health benefits in childhood and research suggests that they may prevent obesity and lower blood cholesterol levels with a favourable impact on the risk of future cardiovascular disease incidence (Martino, Puddu, Pannarale, & Barilla, 2013).

Saponins

Triterpenoid and steroidal glycosides, referred to collectively as saponins, are bioactive compounds present naturally in many plants. They have considerable potential as pharmaceutical and/or nutraceutical agents in natural or synthetic form. Saponins are amphipathic glycosides found in many types of plants, and have been reported to produce a variety of beneficial biological effects when taken as dietary supplements. Currently, saponins are being studied for their hypo-cholesterolemic, anti-coagulant, anti-carcinogenic, hepatoprotective, hypoglycemic, immunomodulatory, neuroprotective, anti-inflammatory, anti-proliferative, hypolipemic and anti-oxidant activity (Rao & Gurfinkel, 2000).

Some saponins even have been used as flavour enhancer and sweeteners in foods and cigarettes. For example, the flavour enhancer, licorice root extract is rich in the saponin glycyrrhizin and saponins from the roots of *Glycyrrhiza glabra* and leaves of *Abrus precatorius* (Meena, Singh, Sharma, Kumari, & Rao, 2010) are 941-fold as sweet as sucrose and 60 times sweeter than cane sugar. Recent research has established saponins as the active components in many herbal medicines (Liu & Henkel, 2002) and highlighted their contributions to the health benefits of foods such as soybeans (Kerwin, 2004) and garlic (Matsuura, 2001). The commercial potential of saponins has resulted in the development of new processing strategies and re-evaluation of existing technologies (Muir, Paton, Ballantyne, & Aubin, 2002) for their extraction and concentration (Rickert, Meyer, Hu, & Murphy, 2004)

The main dietary sources of saponins are legumes (soybeans, chickpeas, mungbeans, peanuts, broad beans, kidney beans, lentils), they are also present in oats, allium species (leek, garlic), asparagus, tea, spinach, sugarbeet, and yam (Yücekutlu & Bildacı, 2008). Soap bark tree (*Quillaja saponaria*), fenugreek (*Trigonella foenum-graceum*), alfalfa (*Medicago sativa*), horse chestnut (*Aesculus hippocastanum*), licorice (*Glycyrrhiza glabra*), soapwort (*Saponaria officinalis*), Mojave yucca (*Yucca schidigera*), gypsophila genus (such as *Gypsophila paniculata*), sarsaparilla (*Smilax regelii*) and ginseng (*Panax ginseng*) are the main non-food sources of saponins used in health and industrial applications (Kharkwal et al., 2012).

Polysaccharides

Polysaccharides widely exist in plants, microorganisms, algae, and animals, are essential biomacromoleules in life activities and play important roles in cell-cell communication, cell adhesion, and molecular recognition in the immune system. Recently, some bioactive polysaccharides isolated from natural sources have attracted much attention in the field of biochemistry and pharmacology; especially plant polysaccharides have shown diverse biological activities such as wound healing, enhancement of the reticuloendothelial system, stimulation of the immune system, treatment of tumors and effects on the hematopoietic system. In folk medicine plants containing polysaccharides have been used as hypoglycemic (Lopez, 2007) and anti-inflammatory (Atherton, 2002). Traditionally, polysaccharides are used as thickening, emulsifying and stabilizing agents. But, nowadays, a huge market in healthy compounds has appeared with the production of oligo- or monosaccharide syrups, using physical methods or controlled enzymatic degradation of polysaccharides (*e.g.* starch). Some of them possess interesting biological properties e.g., oligodextrins (anti-ulcer agents, lowering serum cholesterol in low saturated fat diet), fructooligosaccharides (prebiotics, dietary fibre, stimulate mineral absorption, enhance defense mechanism) (Lopez, 2007; Sharma, Prakash, & Gupta, 2014).

Probiotics

The probiotics are the unconventional source of nutraceuticals and functional foods. The probiotics, prebiotics and synbiotics modifies the composition of the GI microbiota, restore the microbial balance and therefore have the potential to provide health benefits. The majority of probiotic microorganisms belong to the genera *Lactobacillus* and *Bifidobacterium* (Baffoni & Biavati, 2008). *Lactobacilli* and *Bifidobacteria* are Gram-positive lactic acid-producing bacteria that constitute a major part of the normal intestinal micro-flora in animals and humans. The number of *Bifidobacteria* in the colon of adults is 10^{10}–10^{11} CFU/g, but this number decreases with age. *Bifidobacteria* are non-motile, non-spore forming, Gram-positive rods with varying cell morphology. Most strains are strictly anaerobic.

Prebiotics and Lactic acid bacteria (LAB) (probiotics) have demonstrated beneficial effects with respect to the function of innate immunity, intestinal barrier function, and increased resistance to disease. The gut mucosa and microbiota are intimately linked in the maintenance of a functional interface between the host and the external environment (Henke & Bassler, 2004; Sansonetti, 2004). A combined supply of prebiotics and probiotics (synbiotics) has synergistic effects in enhancing immunity and facilitating intestinal barrier function.

The probiotic bacteria are used for the manufacture of a natural remedy, for controlling weight gain, preventing obesity, increasing satiety, prolonging satiation, reducing food intake, reducing fat deposition, improving energy metabolism, treating and enhancing insulin sensitivity and treating obesity. Animal studies have demonstrated the efficacy of some strains of lactic acid bacteria (LAB) to be able to lower serum cholesterol levels, presumably by breaking down bile in the gut, thus inhibiting its re-absorption (Sanders, 2000).

Lactobacillus (*Lb. sporogenes* and *Lb. acidophilus* NCFB 1748) and *Bifidobacterium* genus representatives have been reported to play a critical role in weight regulation as an anti-obesity effect in experimental models and humans. *Lactobacillus sporogenes* has the ability to lower cholesterol levels. It produces a significant reduction in low density lipoprotein (LDL) levels and a small but significant increase in high density lipoprotein (HDL) cholesterol (Mercenier, Pavan, & Pot, 2002).

Lactobacillus acidophilus ferments lactose into lactic acid, like many lactic acid bacteria. During digestion, *L. acidophilus* assists in the production of niacin, folic acid and pyridoxine. It also helps in bile de-conjugation, separating amino acids from bile acids, which can then be recycled by the body. *L. acidophilus* may provide additional health benefits, including improved gastrointestinal function, a boosted immune system, and a decrease in the frequency of vaginal yeast infections and relief from indigestion and diarrhea (Gupta & Prakash, 2014).

ROLE OF PHYTOPHARMACEUTICALS IN HEALTH AND DISEASES

Nutraceuticals (phytopharmaceuticals) have been claimed to have a physiological benefit or provide protection against several diseases and/or found to act as cardiovascular agents, anti-obese agents, anti-diabetics, anticancer agents, immune boosters, chronic inflammatory disorders and degenerative diseases. Nutraceuticals in the form of antioxidants, dietary fibers, omega-3 polyunsaturated fatty acids (n-3 PUFAs), vitamins, and minerals are recommended together with physical exercise for prevention and treatment of CVD (German & Walzem, 2000). Herbal stimulants, such as ephedrine, caffeine, mahuang-guarana, chitosan and green tea have proved effective in facilitating body weight loss (Schiller, Barranger, Schauss, & Nichols, 2001). Dietary fibers from psyllium have been used extensively both as pharmacological supplements, food ingredients, in processed food to aid weight reduction, for glucose control in diabetic patients and to reduce lipid levels in hyperlipidemia (Baljit, 2007).

Thus, nutraceuticals are currently receiving recognition as being beneficial in coronary heart disease, obesity, diabetes, cancer, osteoporosis and other chronic and degenerative diseases such as Parkinson's and Alzheimer's diseases. Evidences indicate that the mechanistic actions of natural compounds involve a wide array of biological processes, including activation of antioxidant defenses, signal transduction pathways, cell survival-associated gene expression, cell proliferation and differentiation and preservation of mitochondrial integrity. It appears that these properties play a crucial role in the protection against the pathologies of numerous age-related or chronic diseases (Mandel, Packer, Youdim, & Weinreb, 2005)

CONCLUSION

From foregoing it may be concluded that phytopharmaceuticals may play a key role in the development of nutraceuticals and functional foods, prevention or treatment of several diseases and maintenance of good general health in human. Dietary intake of phytochemicals promotes health benefits by protecting against chronic degenerative disorders, such as cancer, cardiovascular, and neurodegenerative diseases. These phytochemicals, either alone and/or in combination, have tremendous therapeutic potential in curing various ailments. Phytochemicals with nutraceutical properties present in food are of enormous significance due to their beneficial effects on human health since they offer protection against numerous diseases or disorders such as cancers, coronary heart disease, diabetes, high blood pressure, inflammation, microbial, viral and parasitic infections, psychotic diseases, spasmodic conditions, and ulcers. Thus phytopharmaceuticals can be regularly taken without any side effects. The future of nutraceuticals from both plant (phytonutrients) and animal origin holds exciting opportunities for the food industry to create novel food products containing bioactive food components. The government should persuade the food industry by investing more in the nutraceuticals and functional foods and gaining monetary rewards. However, the products should be designed and formulated as per the interest and tastes of the consumers.

ACKNOWLEDGMENT

Authors are grateful to Dr. Ashok K. Chauhan, Founder President, Amity Group of Institutions and Mr. Atul Chauhan, Chancellor, Amity University UP, Noida for the encouragement, research facilities and financial support.

REFERENCES

Aggarwal, B. B., & Shishodia, S. (2006). Molecular targets of dietary agents for prevention and therapy of cancer. *Biochemical Pharmacology*, *71*(10), 1397–1421. doi:10.1016/j.bcp.2006.02.009 PMID:16563357

Akkarachiyasit, S., Charoenlertkul, P., Yibchok-Anun, S., & Adisakwattana, S. (2010). Inhibitory activities of cyanidin and its glycosides and synergistic effect with acarbose against intestinal α-Glucosidase and pancreatic α-Amylase. *International Journal of Molecular Sciences*, *11*(9), 3387–3396. doi:10.3390/ijms11093387 PMID:20957102

Aruoma, O. (2001). In vitro and in vivo methods for the assessment of antioxidant activity. In *Proceedings of the EUROFOODCHEM 11th Meeting: Biologically-Active Phytochemicals in Food: Analysis, Metabolism, Bioavailability and Function*. The Royal Society of Chemistry.

Atherton, P. (2002). *Aloe vera*: Magic or medicine with antidiabetic potential. *Journal of Ethnopharmacology*, *81*, 81–100. PMID:12020931

Awad, A. B., & Fink, C. S. (2000). Phytosterols as anticancer dietary components: Evidence and mechanism of action. *The Journal of Nutrition*, *130*, 2127–2130. PMID:10958802

Baffoni, L., & Biavati, B. (2008). Ecologia microbica dell'apparato digerente. In B. Biavati & C. Sorlini (Eds.), *Microbiologia agroambientale* (pp. 147–162). Milan: Casa Editrice Ambrosiana.

Baljit, S. (2007). Psyllium as therapeutic and drug delivery agent. *International Journal of Pharmaceutics*, *334*(1-2), 1–14. doi:10.1016/j.ijpharm.2007.01.028 PMID:17329047

Bohlmann, J., & Keeling, C. I. (2008). Terpenoid biomaterials. *The Plant Journal*, *54*(4), 656–669. doi:10.1111/j.1365-313X.2008.03449.x PMID:18476870

Burdulis, D., Sarkinas, A., Jasutiene, I., Stackeviciene, E., Nikolajevas, L., & Janulis, V. (2009). Comparative study of anthocyanin composition, antimicrobial and antioxidant activity in bilberry (*Vaccinium myrtillus* L.) and blueberry (*Vaccinium corymbosum* L.) fruits. *Acta Poloniae Pharmaceutica-Drug Research*, *66*, 399–408. PMID:19702172

Cartea, M. E., & Velasco, P. (2008). Glucosinolates in Brassica foods: Bioavailability in food and significance for human health. *Phytochemistry Reviews*, *7*(2), 213–229. doi:10.1007/s11101-007-9072-2

Cieslik, E., Greda, A., & Adamus, W. (2006). Contents of polyphenols in fruits and vegetables. *Food Chemistry*, *94*(1), 135–142. doi:10.1016/j.foodchem.2004.11.015

Crozier, A., Jaganath, I. B., & Clifford, M. N. (2009). Dietary phenolics: Chemistry, bioavailability and effects on health. *Natural Product Reports*, *26*(8), 1001–1043. doi:10.1039/b802662a PMID:19636448

D'Archivio, M., Filesi, C., Vari, R., Scazzocchio, B., & Masella, R. (2010). Bioavailability of the polyphenols: Status and controversies. *International Journal of Molecular Sciences, 11*(4), 1321–1342. doi:10.3390/ijms11041321 PMID:20480022

Dillard, C. J., & German, J. B. (2000). Review Phytochemicals: Nutraceuticals and human health. *Journal of the Science of Food and Agriculture, 80*(12), 1744–1756. doi:10.1002/1097-0010(20000915)80:12<1744::AID-JSFA725>3.0.CO;2-W

Fassett, R. G., & Coombes, J. S. (2011). Astaxanthin: A potential therapeutic agent in cardiovascular disease. *Marine Drugs, 9*(12), 447–465. doi:10.3390/md9030447 PMID:21556169

Food and Nutrition Board, Institute of Medicine. (2005). *Dietary Reference Intakes for Energy, Carbohydrates, Fiber, Fat, Fatty Acids, Cholesterol, Protein, and Amino Acids*. Washington, DC: National Academies Press.

German, J. B., & Walzem, R. L. (2000). The health benefits of wine. *Annual Review of Nutrition, 20*(1), 561–593. doi:10.1146/annurev.nutr.20.1.561 PMID:10940346

Ghosh, D., & Konishi, T. (2007). Anthocyanins and anthocyanin-rich extracts: Role in diabetes and eye function. *Asia Pacific Journal of Clinical Nutrition, 16*, 200–208. PMID:17468073

Gupta, C., & Prakash, D. (2014). Phytonutrients as therapeutic agents. *Journal of Complementary and Integrative Medicine, 11*(3), 151–169. doi:10.1515/jcim-2013-0021 PMID:25051278

Hayes, J. D., Kelleher, M. O., & Eggleston, I. M. (2008). The cancer chemopreventive actions of phytochemicals derived from glucosinolates. *European Journal of Nutrition, 47*(S2), 73–88. doi:10.1007/s00394-008-2009-8 PMID:18458837

Heber, D., Berdanier, C. D., Dwyer, J. T., & Feldman, E. B. (2008). Plant Foods and Phytochemicals in human health. CRC Press.

Henke, J. M., & Bassler, B. L. (2004). Bacterial social engagements. *Trends in Cell Biology, 14*(11), 648–656. doi:10.1016/j.tcb.2004.09.012 PMID:15519854

Hidalgo, M., Oruna-Concha, M. J., Kolida, S., Walton, G. E., Kallithraka, S., Spencer, J. P., & de Pascual-Teresa, S. (2012). Metabolism of anthocyanins by human gut microflora and their influence on gut bacterial growth. *Journal of Agricultural and Food Chemistry, 60*(15), 3882–3890. doi:10.1021/jf3002153 PMID:22439618

Hodek, P., Trebil, P., & Stiborova, M. (2002). Flavonoids- potent and versatile biologically active compounds interacting with cytochromes. *Chemico-Biological Interactions, 139*(1), 1–21. doi:10.1016/S0009-2797(01)00285-X PMID:11803026

Jackson, H., Braun, C. L., & Ernst, H. (2008). The chemistry of novel xanthophyll carotenoids. *The American Journal of Cardiology, 101*(10), S50–S57. doi:10.1016/j.amjcard.2008.02.008 PMID:18474275

Jaswir, I., Noviendri, D., Hasrini, R. F., & Octavianti, F. (2011). Carotenoids: Sources, medicinal properties and their application in food and nutraceutical industry. *Journal of Medicinal Plants Research, 5*(33), 7119–7131.

John, S., Sorokin, A. V., & Thompson, P. D. (2007). Phytosterols and vascular disease. *Current Opinion in Lipidology, 18*(1), 35–40. doi:10.1097/MOL.0b013e328011e9e3 PMID:17218830

Jong, A., Plat, J., & Mensink, R. P. (2003). Metabolic effects of plant sterols and stanols. *The Journal of Nutritional Biochemistry, 14*(7), 362–369. doi:10.1016/S0955-2863(03)00002-0 PMID:12915216

Kerwin, S. M. (2004). Soy saponins and the anticancer effects of soybeans and soy-based foods. *Current Medicinal Chemistry, 4*, 263–272. PMID:15134504

Kharkwal, H., Panthari, P., Pant, M. K., Kharkwal, H., Kharkwal, A. C., & Joshi, D. D. (2012). Foaming Glycosides: A review. *IOSR Journal of Pharmacy, 2*(5), 23–28. doi:10.9790/3013-25202328

Kim, W., Fan, Y. Y., Smith, R., Patil, B., Jayaprakasha, G. K., McMurray, D. N., & Chapkin, R. S. (2009). Dietary curcumin and limonin suppress CD4+ T-cell proliferation and interleukin-2 production in mice. *The Journal of Nutrition, 139*(5), 1042–1048. doi:10.3945/jn.108.102772 PMID:19321585

Kondratyuk, T. P., & Pezzuto, J. M. (2004). Natural Product Polyphenols of Relevance to Human Health. *Pharmaceutical Biology, 42*(sup1), 46–63. doi:10.3109/13880200490893519

Kumar, S., & Andy, A. (2012). Health promoting bioactive chemicals from *Brassica. International Food Research Journal, 19*, 141–152.

Leiro, J., Alvarez, E., Arranz, J. A., Laguna, R., Uriarte, E., & Orallo, F. (2004). Effects of cis-resveratrol on inflammatory murine macrophages: Antioxidant activity and down regulation of inflammatory genes. *Journal of Leukocyte Biology, 75*(6), 1156–1165. doi:10.1189/jlb.1103561 PMID:14982945

Lewandowska, U., Szewczyk, K., Hrabec, E., Janecka, A., & Gorlach, S. (2013). Overview of metabolism and bioavailability enhancement of polyphenols. *Journal of Agricultural and Food Chemistry, 61*(50), 12183–12199. doi:10.1021/jf404439b PMID:24295170

Liu, J., & Henkel, T. (2002). Traditional Chineese medicine (TCM): Are polyphenols and saponins the key ingredients triggering biological activities? *Current Medicinal Chemistry, 9*(15), 1483–1485. doi:10.2174/0929867023369709 PMID:12173978

Lopez, J.L. (2007). Use of *Opuntia* Cactus as a Hypoglycemic. *Nutrition Bytes, 12*, Article 2.

Manach, C., Williamson, G., Morand, C., Scalbert, A., & Remesy, C. (2005). Bioavailability and bioefficacy of polyphenols in humans: Review of 97 bioavailability studies. *The American Journal of Clinical Nutrition, 81*(supplement 1), 230S–242S. PMID:15640486

Mandel, S., Packer, L., Youdim, M. B. H., & Weinreb, O. (2005). Proceedings from the Third Int. Conf. Mechanism of Action of Nutraceuticals. *The Journal of Nutritional Biochemistry, 16*, 513–520. doi:10.1016/j.jnutbio.2005.03.001 PMID:16115539

Marín, L., Miguélez, E. M., Villar, C. J., & Lombó, F. (2015). Bioavailability of Dietary Polyphenols and Gut Microbiota Metabolism: Antimicrobial Properties. BioMed Research International.

Marinova, K., Kleinschmidt, K., Weissenbock, G., & Klein, M. (2007). Flavonoid biosynthesis in barley primary leaves requires the presence of the vacuole and controls the activity of vacuolar flavonoid transport. *Plant Physiology, 144*(1), 432–444. doi:10.1104/pp.106.094748 PMID:17369433

Martino, F., Puddu, R. E., Pannarale, G., & Barilla, F. (2013). Dietary Fibers and Nutraceuticals for Primary Cardiovascular Prevention in Children and Adolescents: A Critical Review. *Food and Nutrition Sciences*, *4*(07), 39–47. doi:10.4236/fns.2013.47A006

Matsuura, H. (2001). Saponins in garlic as modifiers of the risk of cardiovascular disease. *The Journal of Nutrition*, *131*, 1000S–1005S. PMID:11238805

Meena, A. J., Singh, A., Sharma, K., Kumari, S., & Rao, M. M. (2010). Physicochemical and preliminary phytochemical studies on the Rhizomes of *Glycyrrhiza glabra* Linn. *International Journal of Pharmacy and Pharmaceutical Sciences*, *2*, 48–50.

Meghwal, M., & Sahu, C. K. (2015). Soy Isoflavonoids as Nutraceutical for Human Health: An Update. *Journal of Cell Science and Therapy*, *6*, 194. doi:10.4172/2157-7013.1000194

Mercenier, A., Pavan, S., & Pot, B. (2002). Probiotics as biotherapeutic agents: Present knowledge and future prospects. *Current Pharmaceutical Design*, *8*, 99–110. PMID:11812252

Miladinovic, B., Kostic, M., Savikin, K., Đorđević, B., Mihajilov-Krstev, T., Živanović, S., & Kitić, D. (2014). Chemical Profile and Antioxidative and Antimicrobial Activity of Juices and Extracts of 4 Black Currants Varieties (*Ribes nigrum* L.). *Journal of Food Science*, *79*(3), C301–C309. doi:10.1111/1750-3841.12364 PMID:24506271

Muir, A. D., Paton, D., Ballantyne, K., & Aubin., A. A. (2002). *US Patent, 6,355,249*. US Patent Office.

Narasinga Rao, B. S. (2003). Bioactive phytochemicals in Indian foods and their potential in health promotion and disease prevention. *Asia Pacific Journal of Clinical Nutrition*, *12*, 9–22. PMID:12737006

Nichenametla, S. N., Taruscio, T. G., Barney, D. L., & Exon, J. H. (2006). A review of the effects and mechanism of polyphenolics in cancer. *Critical Reviews in Food Science and Nutrition*, *46*(2), 161–183. doi:10.1080/10408390591000541 PMID:16431408

Nichols, J. A., & Katiyar, S. K. (2010). Skin photoprotection by natural polyphenols: Anti-inflammatory, anti-oxidant and DNA repair mechanisms. *Archives of Dermatological Research*, *302*(2), 71–83. doi:10.1007/s00403-009-1001-3 PMID:19898857

Paduch, R., Kandefer-Szerszen, M., Trytek, M., & Fiedurek, J. (2007). Terpenes: Substances useful in human healthcare. *Archivum Immunologiae et Therapiae Experimentalis*, *55*(5), 315–327. doi:10.1007/s00005-007-0039-1 PMID:18219762

Pandey, N., Meena, R. P., Rai, S. K., & Pandey-Rai, S. (2011). Medicinal plants derived nutraceuticals: A re-emerging health aid. *International Journal of Pharma and Bio Sciences*, *2*(4), 419–441.

Pattanaik, B., & Lindberg, P. (2015). Terpenoids and Their Biosynthesis in Cyanobacteria. *Life (Chicago, Ill.)*, *5*, 269–293. PMID:25615610

Prakash, D., Dhakarey, R., & Mishra, A. (2004). Carotenoids: The phytochemicals of nutraceutical importance. *Indian Journal of Agricultural Biochemistry*, *17*, 1–8.

Prakash, D., & Gupta, C. (2014a). Role of Phytoestrogens as Nutraceuticals in Human Health. In D. Prakash & G. Sharma (Eds.), *Phytochemicals of Nutraceutical Importance* (pp. 148–172). CABI International Publishers. doi:10.1079/9781780643632.0000

Prakash, D., & Gupta, C. (2014b). Carotenoids: Chemistry and Health Benefits. In D. Prakash & G. Sharma (Eds.), *Phytochemicals of Nutraceutical Importance* (pp. 181–195). CABI International Publishers. doi:10.1079/9781780643632.0000

Prakash, D., Gupta, C., & Sharma, G. (2012). Importance of Phytochemicals in Nutraceuticals. *Journal of Chinese Medicine Research and Development*, *1*(3), 70–78.

Prakash, D., & Gupta, K. R. (2009). The antioxidant phytochemicals of nutraceutical importance. *The Open Nutraceuticals Journal*, *2*(1), 20–35. doi:10.2174/1876396000902010020

Prakash, D., & Kumar, N. (2011). Cost Effective Natural Antioxidants. In R. R. Watson, J. K. Gerald, & V. R. Preedy (Eds.), *Nutrients, Dietary Supplements and Nutraceuticals* (pp. 163–188). Humana Press, Springer. doi:10.1007/978-1-60761-308-4_12

Qin, Y., Xia, M., Ma, J., Hao, Y., Liu, J., Mou, H., & Ling, W. et al. (2009). Anthocyanin supplementation improves serum LDL- and HDL-cholesterol concentrations associated with the inhibition of cholesteryl ester transfer protein in dyslipidemic subjects. *The American Journal of Clinical Nutrition*, *90*(3), 485–492. doi:10.3945/ajcn.2009.27814 PMID:19640950

Rahman, I., Biswas, S. K., & Kirkham, P. A. (2006). Regulation of inflammation and redox signaling by dietary polyphenols. *Biochemical Pharmacology*, *72*(11), 1439–1452. doi:10.1016/j.bcp.2006.07.004 PMID:16920072

Rao, A. V., & Gurfinkel, D. M. (2000). The bioactivity of saponins: Triterpenoid and steroidal glycosides. *Drug Metabolism and Drug Interactions*, *17*(1-4), 211–235. doi:10.1515/DMDI.2000.17.1-4.211 PMID:11201296

Rao, A. V., & Shen, H. (2002). Effect of low dose lycopene intake on lycopene bioavailability and oxidative stress. *Nutrition Research (New York, N.Y.)*, *22*(10), 1125–1131. doi:10.1016/S0271-5317(02)00430-X

Ravi Subbiah, M. T. (2007). Nutrigenetics and nutraceuticals: The next wave riding on personalized medicine. *Translational Research; the Journal of Laboratory and Clinical Medicine*, *149*(2), 55–61. doi:10.1016/j.trsl.2006.09.003 PMID:17240315

Rickert, D. A., Meyer, M. A., Hu, J., & Murphy, P. A. (2004). Effect of extraction pH and temperature on Isoflavone and saponin partitioning and profile during soy protein isolate production. *Journal of Food Science*, *69*(8), C623–C631. doi:10.1111/j.1365-2621.2004.tb09910.x

Sanders, M.E. (2000). Considerations for use of probiotic bacteria to modulate human health. *The Journal of Nutrition, 130*(Suppl 2), 384S–390S.

Sansonetti, P. J. (2004). War and peace at mucosal surfaces. *Nature Reviews. Immunology*, *4*(12), 953–964. doi:10.1038/nri1499 PMID:15573130

Schiller, R. N., Barranger, E., Schauss, A. G., & Nichols, E. (2001). Life style management of Obesity. *Journal of the American Medical Association, 4*, 34–41.

Sharma, G., & Prakash, D. (2013). Nutraceuticals: Defense against Diseases? *Scientific Reports*, *50*(09), 32–33.

Sharma, G., Prakash, D., & Gupta, C. (2014). Phytochemicals of Nutraceutical Importance: Do they Defend against diseases? In D. Prakash & G. Sharma (Eds.), *Phytochemicals of Nutraceutical Importance* (pp. 1–19). CABI International Publishers.

Sharma, R. (2009). Nutraceuticals and nutraceutical supplementation criteria in cancer: A literature survey. *The Open Nutraceuticals Journal*, *2*(1), 92–106. doi:10.2174/1876396000902010092

Spencer, J. P., Abd El Mohsen, M. M., Minihane, A. M., & Mathers, J. C. (2008). Biomarkers of the intake of dietary polyphenols: Strengths, limitations and application in nutrition research. *The British Journal of Nutrition*, *99*(01), 12–22. doi:10.1017/S0007114507798938 PMID:17666146

Street, A. (2015). Food as pharma: Marketing nutraceuticals to India's rural poor. *Critical Public Health*, *25*(3), 361–372. doi:10.1080/09581596.2014.966652 PMID:25866449

Talaei, M., & Pan, A. (2015). Role of phytoestrogens in prevention and management of type 2 diabetes. *World Journal of Diabetes*, *6*(2), 271–283. doi:10.4239/wjd.v6.i2.271 PMID:25789108

Tenore, G. C., Daglia, M., Ciampaglia, R., & Novellino, E. (2015). Exploring the nutraceutical potential of polyphenols from black, green and white tea infusions - an overview. *Current Pharmaceutical Biotechnology*, *16*(3), 265–271. doi:10.2174/138920101666150118133604 PMID:25601602

Tian, Q., Miller, E. G., Jayaprakasha, G. K., & Patil, B. S. (2007). An improved HPLC method for the analysis of citrus limonoids in culture media. *Journal of Chromatography B. Analytical Technolology & Biomedical Life Sciences*, *846*(1-2), 385–390. doi:10.1016/j.jchromb.2006.09.012

Traka, M., & Mithen, R. (2009). Glucosinolates, isothiocyanates and human health. *Phytochemistry Reviews*, *8*(1), 269–282. doi:10.1007/s11101-008-9103-7

Trock, B. J., Hilakivi-Clarke, L., & Clarke, R. (2006). Meta-analysis of soy intake and breast cancer risk. *Journal of the National Cancer Institute*, *98*(7), 459–471. doi:10.1093/jnci/djj102 PMID:16595782

Tundis, R., Loizzo, M. R., & Menichini, F. (2014). An Overview on Chemical Aspects and Potential Health Benefits of Limonoids and Their Derivatives. *Critical Reviews in Food Science and Nutrition*, *54*(2), 225–250. doi:10.1080/10408398.2011.581400 PMID:24188270

Udgata, J. R., & Naik, S. N. (2007). Soybean Isoflavones: Remedial nutraceuticals in Indian perspective. *Journal of Scientific and Industrial Research*, *66*, 11–18.

Vig, A. P., Rampal, G., Singh, T. S., & Arora, S. (2009). Bioprotective effects of glucosinolates- A review. *LWT Food Science and Technology*, *42*(10), 1561–1572. doi:10.1016/j.lwt.2009.05.023

Von Bergmann, K., Sudhop, T., & Lutjohann, D. (2005). Cholesterol and plant sterol absorption: Recent insights. *The American Journal of Cardiology*, *96*(1), 10D–14D. doi:10.1016/j.amjcard.2005.03.014 PMID:15992510

Woyengo, T. A., Ramprasath, V. R., & Jones, P. J. H. (2009). Anticancer effects of phytosterols. *European Journal of Clinical Nutrition*, *63*(7), 813–820. doi:10.1038/ejcn.2009.29 PMID:19491917

Xia, X., Ling, W., Ma, J., Xia, M., Hou, M., Wang, Q., & Tang, Z. et al. (2006). An anthocyanin-rich extract from black rice enhances atherosclerotic plaque stabilization in apolipoprotein E-deficient mice. *The Journal of Nutrition*, *136*, 2220–2225. PMID:16857844

Yücekutlu, A. N., & Bildacı, I. (2008). Determination of plant saponins and some of Gypsophila species: A review of the literature. *Hacettepe Journal of Biololgy & Chemistry*, *36*, 129–135.

Zafra-Stone, S., Yasmin, T., Bagchi, M., Chatterjee, A., Vinson, J. A., & Bagchi, D. (2007). Berry anthocyanins as novel antioxidants in human health and disease prevention. *Molecular Nutrition & Food Research*, *51*(6), 675–683. doi:10.1002/mnfr.200700002 PMID:17533652

Zhang, S. M., Cook, N. R., Albert, C. M., Gaziano, J. M., Buring, J. E., & Manson, J. E. (2008). Effect of combined folic acid, vitamin B6, and vitamin B12 on cancer risk in women: A randomized trial. *Journal of the American Medical Association*, *300*(17), 2012–2021. doi:10.1001/jama.2008.555 PMID:18984888

ADDITIONAL READING

Kowalski, J., Samojedny, A., Paul, M., Pietsz, G., & Wilczok, T. (2005). Effect of apigenin, kaempferol and resveratrol on the expression of interleukin-1 beta and tumor necrosis factor-alpha genes in J774.2 macrophages. *Pharmacological Reports*, *57*, 390–394. PMID:15985724

Section 6
Cosmeceuticals

Chapter 10
Cosmeceuticals:
Safety, Efficacy and Potential Benefits

Long Chiau Ming
University of Tasmania, Australia

Wei Chern Ang
University of Bath, UK

Quan Yang
University of Bath, UK

Premrutai Thitilertdecha
Mahidol University, Thailand

Tin Wui Wong
Universiti Teknologi MARA, Malaysia

Tahir Mehmood Khan
Monash University Malaysia, Malaysia

ABSTRACT

Cosmeceuticals are topical cosmetic-pharmaceutical hybrids used to maintain and improve appearance and beauty of the skin. The strong demand from the consumers to constantly look youthful and flawless has driven the research and development as well as sale volume of cosmeceuticals. Present studies show that many cosmetic products, which were assumed to be inert in the past, may modulate dermatological structure or function. The key players of cosmeceuticals are anti-aging therapy along with bleaching agent, sunscreen, and hair cosmeceuticals. This book chapter aims to explore the safety, toxicity and efficacy of these cosmeceuticals. Challenges and possible advancement potentials would be discussed. As patients are increasingly seeking advice from physicians and pharmacists regarding cosmeceuticals, the authors hope to provide health care professional and pharmaceutical scientists a resource that would aid to educate patients in using evidence-based cosmeceuticals to enhance their appearance and alleviate dermatological problems.

INTRODUCTION

The desire to be beautiful is an intrinsic nature of all human beings. Aesthetics is a branch of philosophy regarding appreciation of beauty (Gaut & Lopes, 2005): given a choice or even an opportunity, everyone wants to be aesthetically pleasing to oneself or in the eye of others. Physical attractiveness by itself, directly or indirectly influences self-confidence, success, power, happiness and satisfaction in life. Aesthetic needs had been included in Maslow's expanded hierarchy of needs, which is the need for oneself to be appreciative and to seek for beauty (Maslow & Frager, 1987).

DOI: 10.4018/978-1-5225-0754-3.ch010

In this respect, cosmetics are present in almost every society and civilization on earth across human history. Cosmetics spans across of human history, and is present in almost every society on earth. Cosmetics is derived from a Greek word, Kosmos which means "order" (Oumeish, 2001). In rough term, cosmetics is a field to restore order aesthetically. There are various means in cosmetics which include covering up, masking, camouflaging and concealing.

The Egyptians were among the first civilization to recognize the beneficial effects of cosmetics. The Ebers Papyrus, a medical papyrus of herbal knowledge written c. 1550 BC, have documented some cosmeceutical products. The Egyptian formulated a cosmeceutical consisted of honey and milk that claimed to alleviate skin conditions, while another formulation was made from equal portion of rush oil, frankincense, balantine oil, and wax claiming to "expel wrinkles from the face" (Ali & Finlayson, 2013; Oumeish, 2001). Back in Roman time, Galen was both a cosmetic scientist and a physician by profession. Cold emulsion consisted of olive oil and beeswax was invented by Galen for his patients to keep skin healthy.

In this book chapter the authors will carefully analyze the safety, toxicity and efficacy of the cosmeceuticals ingredients used. Challenges and possible advancement potentials of cosmeceuticals would be discussed.

BACKGROUND

Pharmaceuticals are drugs or drug(s)-containing products that prevent, mitigate, treat disease and /or affect the anatomy or physiological functions of the body. 'Cosmeceuticals' is a deliberate portmanteau of these two terms. 'Cosmeceuticals' are intended to connote drug-like benefits and perceptions from an otherwise cosmetic product (Oricha, 2010). Applied on the skin as usual cosmetic does, these cosmeceutical products are fortified with natural ingredients that could improve the skin's biological function just like pharmaceuticals. Essentially, cosmeceuticals bridge the gap between drugs and cosmetics.

Dr Albert M. Kligman coined the word "cosmeceuticals" in an address to Society of Cosmetic Chemists in 1984. (Kligman, 2005). Now, the term cosmeceutical was used to refer to skin products from simple moisturisers (as they themselves have effects on skin hydration) to prescription retinoids and almost everything in between. However, in most circumstances, the term cosmeceutical is solely reserved for enhanced moisturisers with active ingredients that provide substantial benefits to the skin.

Even till today, the cosmeceutical category is still considered not well defined thus ambiguous for pharmaceutical regulation and control. The term 'cosmeceuticals' is not recognized by US Food and Drug Administration (FDA) under the Federal Food, Drug and Cosmetic Act although being widely used in pharmaceutical and cosmetic markets (Draelos, 2009). Awareness of establishing quality control, industry standards and regulations in cosmetics or cosmeceuticals were recently initiated. To prove the significance of beneficial skin effect of a cosmeceuticals can be difficult if not impossible, compared to clinical trials of drugs of other route of administrations: there are simply no placebos to begin with as anything that is applied to the skin will have an effect in some ways on top of the baseline placebo effect (Sommerfeld, 2007)

REGULATION, REVIEW, SAFETY, AND EFFICACY OF COSMECEUTICALS INGREDIENTS

Issues of Regulatory Provisions on Cosmeceuticals

In United States (US), the Federal Food, Drug, and Cosmetic Act (FD&C Act) 2006, through sec. 201 (i), defines cosmetics as "*articles intended to be rubbed, poured, sprinkled, or sprayed on, introduced into, or otherwise applied to the human body for cleansing, beautifying, promoting attractiveness, or altering the appearance*" Among the products included in this definition are "skin moisturizers, perfumes, lipsticks, fingernail polishes, eye and facial makeup preparations, cleansing shampoos, permanent waves, hair colors, and deodorants, as well as any substance intended for use as a component of a cosmetic product" (FDA, 2015).

According to the same regulation, a drug is defined as something that can be used to diagnose, treat, mitigate and cure a disease. The definition of drug also covers non-food item that can change the body function (FDA, 2015). Due to the strong awareness on the use of natural and non-synthetic compound for personal beauty and youthfulness, the cosmetic industry is shifting towards introducing cosmeceutical products.

Thus the industry is actively researching particular active ingredients to make subtle claims of additives that purport to affect anatomical structure. For example, retinol, which has been proven to penetrate the epidermis had make the impression that consistent use will provide antioxidant benefit for the skin, resulting in retard of aging process (Decker & Graber, 2012). Such claims are often disseminated through mass media which the public or potential consumers are targeted bypassing scientific channels. The volume of new products churning out in the markets has exceeded the FDA's ability to investigate and/or regulate. Multiple new claims on certain products rarely change the FDA's requirements on such products.

In US, a product could be both a cosmetic and a drug provided fulfilling the requirements of both cosmetics and drugs (FDA, 2015). A shampoo is a cosmetic because its intended use is to "cleanse" the hair ("appearance"). If the shampoo is enhanced to be anti-dandruff containing antifungal for example ketoconazole, it is defined as a drug because of its intended use in dandruff "treatment". The anti-dandruff shampoo is considered both a cosmetic and a drug. Toothpastes that contain fluoride, deodorants that are anti-perspirants and moisturisers and makeup marketed with sun-protection claims must adhere to the intended use for both cosmetics and drugs. "Intended use" are achieved by: 1. Claims stated on the product labelling; 2. Consumer perception; 3. Active ingredients (FDA, 2015).

As for cosmeceuticals, FD&C Act does not recognize "cosmeceuticals" as a marketing categorization of product (FDA, 2015). Legally, a product could be classified as a drug, a cosmetic, or both, but not as "cosmeceutical".

Although the FDA does not have the authority to approve cosmetic products' ingredients, there are several regulations that prohibiting certain ingredients found in Title XXI of the Code of Federal Regulations (CFR), Parts 250.250 and 700.11-700.23 (US Government Publishing Office, 2015).The examples are bithionol (21 CFR 700.11), chlorofluorocarbon propellants (21 CFR 700.23), chloroform (21 CFR 700.18), halogenated salicylanilides (di-, tri-, metabromsalan and tetrachlorosalicylanilide) (21 CFR 700.15), hexachlorophene (21 CFR 250.250), mercury compounds (21 CFR 700.13), methylene chloride (21 CFR 700.19), prohibited cattle materials (21 CFR 700.27), vinyl chloride (21 CFR 700.14), and zirconium-containing complexes (21 CFR 700.16). Depending on the claims, the labeling of a product with the wording "sunscreen" or similar would render a product to be regulated as a drug or a drug/cosmetic, depending on the aims. Despite this, sunscreen ingredients could be used provided the labeling states the rationale sunscreen ingredient is used, with phrase such as, "contains a sunscreen to protect product color." If the equivalent explanation is absent, the product will be regulated as a drug.

Additionally, the CTFA (Cosmetic Toiletry and Fragrance Association, now the Personal Care Products Council) has established the Cosmetic Ingredient Review (CIR) expert panel, which has listed additional unsafe agents in cosmetic or cosmeceuticals. The following examples are as of December 2014: 4- methoxy-m- phenylenediamine, 4-methoxy-m-phenylenediamine hydrochloric acid, 4-methoxy-m-phenylenediamine sulfate, chloroacetamide, ethoxyethanol, ethoxyethanol acetate, formaldehyde, HC Blue No. 1, hydroquinone, methylene glycol, p-hydroxyanisole and pyrocatechol. The outputs of the CIR bear no legal weightage as the FDA will decide on the final verdict on regulations.

There is no mention of "cosmeceutical" term by both European Medicines Agency (EMA) and European Food Safety Authority (EFSA). Generally, cosmetics are evaluated by authorities in respective Member State. They are not evaluated nor licensed by the EMA itself (EMA, 2015). However, cosmetics must contain ingredient only in a European Commission database, CosIng (Cosmetic Ingredient database) which includes legal requirements from 3 resources: European Commission Regulation No 1223/2009; the latest revision of Inventory of Cosmetic Ingredients ; opinions by Scientific Committee for Consumer Safety (European Commission, 2015). At European Union level also, all products in the European Union must be registered in the Cosmetic Products Notification Portal (CPNP) before being marketed, not being animal-tested, have sufficient market surveillance by respective countries at the national level (European Commission, 2015).

The need of additional legislation to regulate the field of cosmeceuticals remains controversial. The Organization of Pharmaceutical and Food Safety Bureau (PFSB) of Japan had resolved this legal contradiction. It sensibly recognized a category of 'quasi-drugs' which cosmeceuticals could be categorized. In a nutshell, cosmeceuticals is considered a subclass of drug in US. In European Union and Japan, it is a subclass of cosmetics. There has yet to have legal definition anywhere in the world; expecting legislation harmonization regarding cosmeceutical US, European Union, Asia and other continents in the world would still be a long way (Table 1).

Table 1. The melanin production pathway

Process	Substance/ Compound (Mechanism Involved)
Premelanin Synthesis	Tretinoin (tyrosinase transcription)
During Melanin Synthesis	Ascorbic acid (product reduction and reactive oxygen species scavengers); ascorbic acid palmitate (product reduction and reactive oxygen species scavengers); HQ (tyrosinase inhibition); 4-hydroxyanisole (tyrosinase inhibition); arbutin (tyrosinase inhibition); aloesin (tyrosinase inhibition); azelaic acid (tyrosinase inhibition); kojic acid (tyrosinase inhibition);
Postmelanin Synthesis	Lecithins and neoglycoproteins (melanosome transfer inhibition); soymilk extracts (melanosome transfer inhibition); niacinamide (melanosome transfer inhibition); glycolic acid (skin turn over acceleration); retinoic acid (skin turn over acceleration); linoleic acid (tyrosinase degradation); α-linoleic acid (tyrosinase degradation);

SKIN WHITENING AND DEPIGMENTING COSMECEUTICALS

Hydroquinone

The most extensively and successfully used substance for hyperpigmentation treatment is the phenolic material, hydroquinone (HQ). HQ produces reversible depigmentation of the skin by suppression of melanocyte metabolic processes, in particular the inhibition of the enzymatic oxidation of tyrosine to DOPA (3,4dihydroxyphenylalanine). However, the user is advised to avoid sunlight because UV ray reverses this effect leading to repigmentation. It is offered over-the-counter in the United States in concentration of around 2%, and by prescription in strength of up to 4%. HQ cream, emulsion and gel formulations are indicated for the gradual treatment of ultraviolet-induced dyschromia (such as chloasma, melasma, freckles, senile lentigines) and skin discoloration caused by the use of oral contraceptives, hormone replacement therapy, skin trauma, or pregnancy. For melasma and post inflammatory hyperpigmentation, researches recommend that around 6-12 weeks of treatment period is essential (Rendon, Vazquez, & Micciantuono, 2013). Utilizing HQ in combo with various other naturally derived depigmenting substances, such as glycolic acid, vitamin C, or aloesin, could help minimize adverse effects and also boost efficiency. One of the most commonly utilized combinations is HQ with prescribed materials such as steroids andretinoids. However, it must be noted that up to 35% of HQ could be absorbed into blood circulation via topical applications (Bucks, McMaster, Guy, & Maibach, 1988) and adverse effects could derive from uncontrolled applications.

Alpha Hydroxyl Acids

There are numerous types and numerous sources of alpha hydroxyl acids (AHAs), such as glycolic acid, lactic acid, citric acid and malic acid. AHA has been used in topical preparations for hyperpigmentation and photo damaged skin. Mainly they contain keratolytic and humectant as well as melanin inhibition properties. Glycolic acid derivatives with similar properties and uses include ammonium glycolate and guanidine glycolate. In term of permeability through the skin, both lactic acid and glycolic acid are more advantageous because of theirs smaller molecular size.

Kornhauser et al reported that glycolic acid and lactic acids displayed ability to inhibit formation of melanin. The ability of reducing pigment is especially enhanced when both glycolic acid and lactic acids are combined together with hydroquinone (Kornhauser, Coelho, & Hearing, 2010). However, study had shown that AHAs at concentrations below 15% are not effective in inhibiting melanin synthesis; instead the pigmentation disappearance observed is mainly from skin exfoliation.

When utilized for post inflammatory hyper pigmentation, glycolic acid peels need to be initiated at much lower concentration. One research study that compared a 70% glycolic acid peel with a 1% tretinoin peel exposed comparable depigmentation results, however individuals experienced much more irritation with the glycolic acid peel. While this increased irritation did not induce post inflammatory hyper pigmentation in this research study, it absolutely has the possibility to induce this problem in darker skin types. Furthermore, a cream containing HQ 4% and glycolic acid 2% was effective when used alone or in combination with salicylic acid peels for treating photodamage on the neck and upper chest. For 12 weeks, 19 women applied the cream (Lustra®, which contains also vitamin C and vitamin E) to the neck and upper chest twice daily. Nine of the women also received salicylic acid peels at 3 week intervals. Both groups showed significant reductions in melanin and erythema and improvement in texture, dryness, tone, and clarity of skin ($p < 0.001$ to 0.5 for all categories). Neither treatment was obviously superior to the other (Gladstone et al., 2000).

In a recent study, glycolic acid, retinol, apple stem cell extract together with polyhydroxy acid gluconolactone, maltobionic acid, N-acetylglucosamine were combined as a 35% active ingredient of skin-care products including cleanser, day cream, night cream and eye cream. The twice-a-day regimen was tested in a randomized, double-blind, vehicle-controlled clinical trial using 69 volunteers. All clinician-graded aging symptoms, firmness and elasticity assessment, dermal density and total skin thickness showed significant improvements compared to vehicle control group. The authors contended that with a combination of 7 active substances at 35% concentration had synergistic actions that could alleviate skin aging (Farris, Edison, Brouda, Weinkauf, & Green, 2012).

Kojic Acid

Kojic acid (5-hydroxy-4-pyran-4-one-2-methyl), an all-natural compound generated by fungi or bacteria, such as *Aspergillus, Penicillium, or Acetobacter spp*, is existing in traditional Japanese fermented foods(Bentley, 2006). Kojic acid is reported to inhibit melanin production and is used in dermatology formulation for the treatment of hyperpigmentation disorders. However, the issue with kojic acid is that it is an exceptionally unpredictable component in aesthetic formulations. Thus kojic acid, most of the time is used along with HQ as well as glycolic acid for the treatment of skin pigmentation (Lim, 1999).

Addition of kojic acid to HQ and glycolic acid combination may improve efficacy in the treatment of melasma. Previous study conducted in China recruited 40 women received twice a day 2% HQ and 10% glycolic acid combination gel in one half of the face, and received 2% kojic acid, 2% hydroquinone, and 10% glycolic acid combination gel on the other half of the face in a double-blind randomized manner. After 12 weeks, patients with greater than 50% improvement in melasma were found in 60% of the side with kojic acid and 48% of the side without kojic acid. Both formula improved melasma, but the difference between the 2 was not statistically significant ($p=0.9$). Three patients developed redness and irritation and withdrew from the study. All patients experienced redness, stinging, and mild exfoliation on both sides of the face. The adverse effects were settled by the third week. Kojic acid did not worsen side effects and could be added to the treatment regimen if patients did not respond to the HQ and glycolic acid combination (Lim, 1999).

Azelaic Acid

Azelaic acid, a type of natural saturated dicarboxylic acid found serendipity from *Pityrosporum ovale* which is a type of fungus that can cause skin hypopigmentation, tinea versicolor. Azelaic acid is formulated as a cream or gel at concentration of between 15% to 20% which is indicated for pigmentation and acne. It could likewise hinder melanin manufacturing. A double-blind research study with 329 women showed that 20% azelaic acid lotion together with a broad-spectrum sun screen lotion produced 65% exceptional or good results versus melasma. Over the treatment duration of 24 weeks, the azelaic acid lotion had similar effects to 4% HQ lotion when it comes to general rating, decrease in sore dimension, and pigment intensity. Relatively large double-blind studies have reported that topical azelaic acid 20% cream is superior to topical HQ 2% cream and comparable in efficacy to HQ 4% cream in the treatment of melisma (Balina & Graupe, 1991; Fitton & Goa, 1991; Verallo-Rowell, Verallo, Graupe, Lopez-

Villafuerte, & Garcia-Lopez, 1989). The incidence of local adverse effects with 20% azelaic acid cream and 2% to 4% HQ were comparable (Fitton & Goa, 1991).

Other Depigmenting Cosmeceutical Ingredients

Paper mulberry essence is a popular skin-lightening substance in Europe and also South America that is acquired from the roots of the *Broussonetia papyrifera* tree. Paper mulberry generates little or no skin irritability, and is for that reason suitable for usage in people with darker skin types as well as in those which cannot put up with HQ. Soy-derived essences have been utilized in the therapy of varicolored hyperpigmentation and solar lentigines. Unpasteurized soymilk consists of Bowman-Birk and soy bean trypsin inhibitors, two serine protease inhibitors that disrupt the protease-activated receptor-2 pathway. These inhibitors efficiently lower melanin transfer as well as induce depigmentation. Soy additionally has actually an included advantage of shielding versus photo-damage with its powerful antioxidant activity. Alkyl esters of the organic item gentisic acid are also a type of tyrosinase inhibitors. The smaller esters (e.g. methyl as well as ethyl) were much more reliable. Sphingosylphosphorylcholine is becoming a powerful signaling-lipid conciliator. It significantly inhibits melanin synthesis in a concentration dependent fashion, and additionally, that it minimizes the activity of tyrosinase. Zinc alpha-2-glycoprotein prevents melanin manufacturing by B16 most cancers cells through posttranscriptional effects on tyrosinase protein. Cosmeceutical scientist had recently postulated that epidermal-derived zinc alpha-2-glycoprotein may influence normal regulation of melanin production *in vivo* considering that zinc alpha-2-glycoprotein is generally created by epidermal keratinocytes.

Safety and Related Adverse Drug Reactions

The most usual unfavorable effects linked with HQ are dermatitis and skin irritability, especially in higher concentrations of 4% or higher, or when combined with tretinoin. In a randomized, double-blind, comparative study of azelaic acid 20% and HQ 2% cream for the treatment of melasma in 155 patients, side effects from both preparations consisted of transient mild to moderate irritant reactions. Symptoms of burning, itching, and/or stinging occurred in 9 of 78 patients receiving hydroquinone (Verallo-Rowell et al., 1989). Transient erythema, mild burning, stinging, dryness and fissuring of paranasal and infra obital areas have been reported with HQ use (Fisher, 1983).

Ochronosis secondary to the application of hydroquinone-containing creams has been reported by several investigators. This paradoxical hyperpigmentation of the skin is usually associated with long-term use of HQ bleaching creams. The build-up of homogentisic acid in the dermis appears as hyperpigmentation. The hyperpigmentation usually fades following discontinuation of the cream; however, in severe cases, it may be irreversible. Patients with darker skin tone are at a higher risk for exogenous ochronosis. Ochronosis-like pigmentation described as pitch-black pigmentation and colloid millium formation was noted following the use of 2% hydroquinone-containing creams in 2 black American patients. These skin changes were accentuated in areas of sun exposure (Hoshaw, Zimmerman, & Menter, 1985). Furthermore, sarcoid-like ochronosis developed following treatment with HQ 4% cream for dark spots. A discrete, nonpruritic papular eruption was noted on both cheeks of the patient, which was successfully treated with tetracycline with resolution of the lesions in 3 months (Fisher, 1988). A contact dermatitis confirmed by HQ patch case of a 34-year old female who used a cream containing HQ and para-aminobenzoic acid (PABA) for treatment of chloasma been reported (Boyle & Kennedy, 1985; Romaguera & Grimalt, 1985).

Interestingly, fingernail staining due to hydroquinone-containing cream was reported in 2 older females. Both patients had applied HQ 2%-containing cream twice daily to the back of their hands for actinic lentigines. The staining was described as a brown discoloration (Mann & Harman, 1983).

Meanwhile, other active ingredients are less associated with adverse reactions. For example, azelaic acid is an optional prospect for skin lightening if an individual has acne and postinflammatory hyperpigmentation or has allergic reaction with hydroquinone. Topical retinoids might irritate the skin creating redness, dryness, swelling, shedding, as well as subjective sensations such as itching, painful, and also burning feeling. Ironically, kojic acid which is widely used in cosmeceutical products due to its low toxicity profile has actually been banned in Japan due to its possibility for triggering inflammation (García-Gavín, González-Vilas, Fernández-Redondo, & Toribio, 2010).

ANTIAGING COSMECEUTICALS

Photoaged skin has variable signs created by the dynamic of different cellular or non-cellular parts of the skin as well as by varying mechanisms. It is challenging to develop a cosmeceutical with multiple functions to comply with all the needs (American Academy of Dermatology, 2014). A few of the aforementioned cosmeceuticals, such as depigmenting, hydrating, and also antiwrinkle cosmeceuticals, have the capability to improve photoaging indicators (Bhattacharyya, Pathria, Mathison, Vargas, & Thomas, 2014). It is postulated that molecular mechanisms of photoaging are the same as chronological skin aging, which also occurs in all others organs (Bhattacharyya et al., 2014). Skin damage related to sun exposure may accelerate its intrinsic aging process; therefore, photoaging represents the superposition of the biological effects of sun irradiation over the intrinsic aging that occurs naturally over time.

One of the hugely popular product lines of cosmeceuticals are anti-aging or antiwrinkle which naturally are the main research and development areas of cosmetic and skincare companies. Packaged Facts (Rockville, MD), a renowned publisher in market studies on consumer products in the US, estimated that retail sales of cosmeceuticals in the US alone would worth USD 11.7 billion in 2016 (Packaged Facts, 2012). According to the Freedonia Group (Cleveland), an industry research company, the demand for cosmeceutical products in the US could potentially increase 5.8 percent annually through 2015 with a whooping total of US$6.5 billion. Anti-aging skin care products based on botanicals recorded the fastest market growth with antioxidants still pose as the products with the highest sale (The Freedonia Group, 2015).

The scientific basis of anti-aging cosmeceutical products mostly are developed based on sound biological grounds. For example, the last pathway to all the mechanism of aging involves interruption of the network of collagen as well as elastin (Sachs et al., 2013). In this respect, antiaging cosmeceuticals are aimed to repair and to maintain the anatomical maintenance and repair systems (Fisk, Agbai, Lev-Tov, & Sivamani, 2014). These give the basis of protein-based cosmeceutical such as cosmeceutical peptides. Cosmeceutical peptides may contain elements such as ascorbic acid (Vitamin C), neurotransmitter, signal peptides or carrier proteins. As much as 500 peptides have actually been characterized are thought to enhance growth factor (Lupo & Cole, 2007).

Wrinkle is among the crucial attributes of aging skin, besides photoaging and also chronological skin aging. The precise mechanism of wrinkle formation remained debatable. Generally, aged dermis has fragmented elastic fibers, lowered collagen, and also uneven types I and III collagens. Below a wrinkle, there is a lower amount of type IV collagen. Glycosaminoglycan's, specifically hyaluronic acid, exist in a low amount. The damage in collagen is associated with numerous kinds of collagen-degrading enzymes called matrix metalloproteinases (MMPs). The activation of metalloproteinases can cause the production of collagenase, gelatinase, as well as stromelysin. Elastins may also be degraded by MMP-2 (Choi, Park, Kim, Na, & Shin, 2014; Kim, Song, Lee, & Lee, 2014).

Retinoids

Retinoids are Vitamin A-derived substances that its topical treatment of aging skin and comedones has been proven effective. The underlying pharmacology action is by activation of retinoic acid receptors eliciting transcriptional activation of retinoic acid responsive genes products. It induces type I and type III procollagen gene expression in human skin which lead to an increased deposition of collagen fibrils in the dermis. It also retards collagen breakdown by inhibiting the metalloproteinases. Retinoids can reduce the inflammatory lesions comedones and microcomedo because it can regulate the desquamation of the follicular epithelium (Babamiri & Nassab, 2010; Higgins & Wesley, 2015).

Due to the well-published evidence of retinoids, various cosmeceutical companies started producing non-prescription products based on the natural-occurring or synthetic retinoids such as retinoic acid (tretinoin, the biological active form) retinol, retinaldehyde, as well as retinyl esters (the storage retinoids derivative). Naturally-occurring retinoids (retinol, retinaldehyde and retinoic acid) are all-trans-isomer. In term of nomenclature, all-trans retinol is known as retinol or Vitamin A; all-trans-retinaldehyde is described as retinal; and also all-trans-retinoic acid is known as retinoic acid or tretinoin. Artificial retinoids derivatives such as adapalene, bexarotene, tazarotene, as well as alitretinoin had been developed but it is utilized as prescription items and not as cosmeceutical.

Up until now, retinoic acid (tretinoin cream) has been marketed as lotion, cream, gel products in various strengths from 0.025% to 0.1% formulations. It is commonly believed that higher concentration of retinoic acid could lead to skin irritation. Retinoic acid was found improving surface roughness, fine lines as well as dyspigmentation. The stages of improvement can be observed over a course of 2-month treatment. Within the first week of therapy, user could notice tactile smoothening; implying the stratum corneum and spongiosis in the skin has become more compact. With the continuous use of up to 2 months, visibility of creases became less (Fisk et al., 2014). A trial of 30 patients had reported that an application of retinoic acid 0.05% cream over 6-months period on sun-damaged skin, an 80% boost in extracellular type I collagen was noted compared to just a 14% boost in vehicle-treated skin.

Retinol has been marketed as a cosmeceutical product at strengths higher than retinoic acid because retinol tends to cause less skin irritation. Furthermore, retinol needs *in vivo* enzymatic conversion to its active metabolite, retinoic acid (Oblong & Bisset). A comparative *in vivo* human skin study using retinol, tretinoin, and control vehicle, retinol 1.6% was discovered to considerably raise skin thickening equivalent to tretinoin 0.025% yet without causing tretinoin-associated erythema. However, the effect of retinol remained debatable. Certain studies have actually shown that retinol hinders UV induction of collagen-degrading enzymes. On the other hand, other studies showed that retinol at commercially available dosages have collagen-enhancing properties. The other disadvantages of using retinol are it undergoes degradation easily and it is comparatively more water soluble causing less penetration into the skin (Duell, Kang, & Voorhees, 1997; Kang et al., 1995). In order to counteract on these weaknesses, a novel retinol derivative with is more resistant towards degradation, retinyl N-formylaspartamate, was found to be effective in a clinical study (n=24) (Lee et al., 2006).

Similar to the comparison between retinol and retinoic acid, retinal has no reported incidence of local inflammation compared to retinoic acid. In a study, retinal 0.05% was compared with retinoic acid 0.05% and also with control vehicle: silicone duplicates of skin in the crow's feet area were executed at baseline, 18 weeks as well as 44 weeks using optical profilometry to examine wrinkles as well as roughness. At week 18, there was a statistically substantial reduction in creases as well as roughness in both the retinal and also retinoic acid arms; no enhancements were noted in the vehicle arm (Fort-Lacoste, Verscheure, Tisne-Versailles, & Navarro, 1999; Pechere, Pechere, Siegenthaler, Germanier, & Saurat, 1999).

Retinyl esters are the primary storage component of retinol in the epidermis. When retinol sources are reduced, retinyl esters will be hydrolyzed to retinol. In human body, retinyl esters mainly consist of retinyllinoleate (as the majority), retinyllaurate, retinylpalmitate and retinyloleate. Interestingly, even though retinyl esters are used as frequently as retinol, not much literature has reported on its uses and effects. Basically, it is unclear on its roles on anti-aging. The auto-regulatory nature of natural retinoids suggests that there is actually no need for expensive retinyl esters as retinol and retinoic acid will certainly be formed from retinoids substances.

Green Tea Extract

Green tea is produced by lightly steaming the fresh cut leaf of tea plant (*Camellia sinensis*). Compared to black tea or oolong tea which uses the same tea plant, green tea does not undergo oxidation process because it will inactivate the enzymes present in tea. These enzymes include polyphenols with potent antioxidant properties. Thus the antioxidant activity of green tea was six times greater than that of black tea. The major polyphenols in green tea are flavonoids (eg, catechin, epicatechin, epicatechingallate, epigallocatechin gallate, and proanthocyanidins). Green tea polyphenol hinders the activity of collagenase as well as enhances collagen biosynthesis of human fibroblasts as well as inhibit tyrosinase activity (Gao, Zhang, Wei, & Chen, 2008; Korkina, Pastore, Dellambra, & De Luca, 2013). Green tea polyphenol was reported to be able to safeguard UV-induced DNA damage in a variety of cell lines, consisting of skin fibroblasts and keratinocytes (Katiyar, Elmets, & Katiyar, 2007).

The green tea polyphenols that have been investigated for medicinal qualities due to antioxidant and other activities include epigallocatechin-3-gallate (EGCG) (the major constituent), epigallocatechin (EGC), epicatechin-3-gallate (ECG), epicatechin (EC), and catechin. EGCG was effective at preventing ultraviolet-induced skin damage which correlated with reduced lipid peroxidation, decreased collagenase mRNA expression and protein, and the inhibition of nuclear factor kappa-light-chain-enhancer of activated B cells and activator protein-1 (AP-1) binding. For example, topical application of EGCG inhibited dimer formation and reduced edema in a dose dependent manner when applied to the dorsal epidermis of mice prior to exposure to ultraviolet B. Then, by using a human keratinocyte cell line, EGCG inhibited ultraviolet B exposure and induced AP-1 activation and proto-oncogene transcription in a dose dependent manner. Meanwhile, in humans, pretreatment of skin with green tea extracts 30 minutes prior to ultraviolet B exposure resulted in a dose dependent protection against acute erythema formation. However, there has yet to be validated literature regarding the topical use of green tea or its derivatives on skin because the formulation of green tea polyphenols as viable ingredients as topical remain a challenge to comesceutical scientists due to its highly oxidative nature.

Ascorbic Acid and Magnesium-L-Ascorbyl-2-Phosphate (MAP)

Vitamin C, or L-ascorbic acid, exist as the main antioxidant in human skin and claimed to be the major free radical scavenger (Farris, 2005). Interestingly, study had shown that the increase of vitamin C in human skin is not proportionate to the oral intake of Vitamin C which is essential part of diet because human body does not form endogenous Vitamin C (Wang, Dhariwal, & Levine, 1992). Vitamin C plays an important role in protecting intracellular structures from oxidative stress and collagen biosynthesis. In fact, vitamin C is a cofactor for enzymes to hydroxylateproline and lysine in collagen which eventually stabilizes its triple helical structure. Further evidence also has shown that Vitamin C also affects directly collagen synthesis (Nusgens et al., 2001). It must be noted that Vitamin C disrupts pigment manufacturing at various oxidative steps in the melanin manufacturing pathway. It communicates with copper ions at the tyrosinase energetic site as well as lowers dopaquinone production.

Vitamin C has always been a much sought-after topically applied cosmeceutical because it is the only way to ensure its bioavailability in the target organ, which is skin itself. Without advance formulation development, Vitamin C is not available as cosmetic because it will oxidise upon air exposure. Esterified derivatives of L-ascorbic acid are the first attempt used in topical formulations to improve its stability. One of the successful examples of derivatives is magnesium ascorbyl phosphate and ascorbyl- 6-palmitate (Farris, 2005; Kobayashi, Takeana, Kanke, Itoh, & Ogata, 1998). The secure derivative referred to as MAP has been shown to have skin-lightening activity. Topically used vitamin C formulations may shield against ultraviolet-B radiation-induced phototoxicity as well as enhance hyperpigmentation disorders, such as melasma as well as post-inflammatory hyperpigmentation. Topical vitamin C is generally non-irritating, and also thus works in dark-skinned ethnic groups in which post-inflammatory hyperpigmentation is a worry. When made use of as a 10% cream, MAP revealed considerable lightening result in majority of clients with melasma and solar lentigines. MAP has been revealed to have a defensive effect versus skin harm caused by UV-B irradiation.

Other Antiaging Cosmeceutical

Dimethylaminoethanol (DMAE) is a precursor of neurotransmitter acetylcholine, with a structure analogue of choline (of B-complex vitamin). DMAE, when incorporated into a neuronal membrane as phosphatidyl-DMAE, may function as a free radical scavenger and act as a protectant for that neuronal membrane (Semsei & Zs-Nagy, 1985). In a randomized clinical trial, 3% DMAE face gel applied daily for 16 weeks has been proven to be well tolerated and effective in reduction of forehead lines and periorbital wrinkles. Follow-up study among DMAE gel users for up to 1 year had demonstrated a good safety profile. The improvement of skin firmness with possible augmentation of face muscle tone may be caused by DMAE's anti-inflammatory properties (Grossman, 2005). Other the other hand, paeoniflorin (In traditional Chinese medicine as Baishao), which is extracted from the roots of *Paeonia lactiflora* had been found to protect cells from DNA damage caused by UV-B in both human and hairless mouse keratinocytes culture. There is evidence exclusively from animal and *in vitro* studies that extracts of Paeonia from its root might possess antioxidative and free radical scavenging activities. A clinical trial of 8 weeks had revealed that 0.5% paeoniflorin-containing topical formulation lowered facial creases. These outcomes suggest that paeoniflorin contains potent antiaging and also antiwrinkle properties (J.-H. Choi et al., 2015; Q.-S. Wang, Gao, Cui, Gao, & Jiang, 2014).

SUNSCREENS COSMECEUTICALS

Both ultraviolet B (UVB) and ultraviolet A (UVA) radiation can cause sunburn, skin cancer, and premature skin aging. Ultraviolet radiation (UVR) exposure is one of the main factors accelerating skin aging, a condition called photoaging. Some immediate effects of excessive unprotected skin exposure to UVR are erythema, pigmentation or sun tanning which are caused by acute inflammatory skin modification. Physiologically, UVR exposure causes increased nitric oxide (NO) levels leading to nitrosative damage, inhibition of cell proliferation as well as cancer (Terra et al., 2015). For instance melanoma and non-melanoma skin cancers are both linked to sun exposure (Bauer, Diepgen, & Schmitt, 2011; Schmitt, Seidler, Diepgen, & Bauer, 2011). Therefore sunscreen plays an important role to prevent the damaging effect of UVR.

Generally, sunscreen agents can be categorized into organic and inorganic sunscreen based on their approach of protection. Organic sunscreen blocks ultraviolet radiation absorption while inorganic sun screen lotions serve as particle matter that reflect and scatter UVR. Some examples of the compounds used in cosmetics as UV-A filter are benzophenones, butyl methoxydibenzoyl, and meradimate. Similarly, UV-B filter examples are PABA derivatives, cinnamates, salicylates, octocrylene, as well as ensulizole. Furthermore, compounds such as calcitriol, caffeic acid, polyphenols compound and isoflavones also are slowly gaining ground as sunscreen compounds especially in cosmeceutical (Kullavanijaya & Lim, 2005). The inconvenience caused by organic sunscreen is the cream or lotion should be applied liberally over exposed areas 30 minutes prior to exposure for formulations containing benzophenones, salicylates, anthranilates, cinnamates, or dibenzoylmethanes. Similarly, sunscreen containing PABA or PABA esters need to be applied 2 hours prior to sun exposure.

PABA

PABA is a chemical sunscreen that is very effective in absorbing UVB from 200 to 320 nm and is most effective in a concentration of 5% in a 70% ethanol solution. For greatest efficacy, sunscreens containing PABA should be applied 2 hours prior to solar exposure to allow for penetration through the dermis and binding to proteins in the stratum corneum (FDA, 2011). Meanwhile, para-aminobenzoic acid esters (PABA esters) are chemical sunscreens that are derivatives of PABA and include such agents as padimate O (octyldimethyl PABA), padimate A (amyldimethyl PABA), and glyceryl PABA. PABA esters are very effective and as a group absorb UVB from 290 to 320 nm and are most effective in a concentration of 2.5 to 8% in 65% ethanol solution (FDA, 2011). The initial PABA dropped out of favor compound of sunscreen mainly as a result of staining and allergic contact reactions. There is a much greater existence of contact as well as photocontact allergy to PABA than to various other sunscreening representatives. The PABA derivatives additionally were stated to cause contact sensitization.

Benzophenones

Benzophenones such as oxybenzone, dioxybenzone, and sulisobenzone are chemical sunscreens that are fairly effective and as a group absorb UVB radiation from 250 to 400 nm. Due to the broader range of absorbing capability into the UVA range, benzophenones prevent photosensitivity reactions. As a single agent, the benzophenones possess a low degree of substantivity and are therefore generally combined with other sunscreening agents. When benzophenones are combined with other agents such as PABA,

PABA esters, and/or cinnamates, the combination has proven to be more effective than any single agent (FDA, 2011). Study had shown that 1% to 2% topically applied sunscreen can be absorbed through skin. For example, oxybenzone, contained in sunscreen, was recovered in urine after topical application of the sunscreen to the forearms of 9 volunteers over an duration of 10 hours (Hayden, Roberts, & Benson, 1997).

Anthranilates

Anthranilates, including such agents as methyl anthranilate, are chemical sunscreens that are weak UVB absorbers and absorb some UVA radiation. Methyl anthranilate in high concentration absorbs UV radiation from 290 to 320 nm. Anthranilates are generally combined with other UV absorbers to yield broad spectrum protection that is similar to benzophenones (FDA, 2011). Benzophenone derivates and anthranilates are effective at absorbing UVA radiation. Although the main protective wide range for benzophenone is in the UVA range, a second safety band is additionally kept in mind in the UVB range. The most frequently utilized benzophenone agents are oxybenzone and dioxybenzone. Although these substances are considerably less allergenic compared to PABA, they do nonetheless still carry a risk of photocontact and also call allergy. Anthranilates, such as menthylanthranilate, offer low-level, yet broad-spectrum coverage. They are frequently contributed to sun blocks to enhance security.

Cinnamate

Cinnamate sunscreens effectively absorb light throughout the UVB range but absorb little or no UVA light. Cinnamate sunscreens may therefore be used to prevent sunburn but are unlikely to prevent drug-related or other photosensitivity reactions associated with UVA light; combination with a benzophenone may give some added protection against such photosensitivity. Cinnamates may occasionally produce photosensitivity reactions (Lugović, Šitum, Ožanić-Bulić, & Sjerobabski-Masnec, 2007).

Inorganic sunscreen

The use of inorganic sunscreen has slowly increasing due to its proven safety profile because it is photostable and less frequent photoallergic reactions reported. Mainly its advantage is its excellent profiles against both UVA and UVB. Titanium dioxide, zinc oxide, ferric chloride, ichthyol, or red petrolatum are main examples of inorganic sunscreen. Its main mode of action is through scattering and reflecting all ultraviolet and visible radiation. Titanium dioxide provides overall UVA and UVB protection. Physical sunscreens reflect up to 99% of UV radiation throughout the entire spectrum (290 to 700 nm), thereby preventing or minimizing sunburns, photoaging, and tanning. Comparison in between zinc oxide and titanium dioxide showed that zinc oxide is superior for UVA defense in the 340-- 380nm range and also has the tendency to be much less pasty on the skin (Schalka et al., 2014).

Early formulations of bodily sunscreen representatives were not extensively accepted since the particulate concerns had to be included in high attentions, resulting in a non-transparent film on the skin in order to achieve adequate protection. These agents are visible, tend to melt in heat, and are difficult to remove. The current formulation of sunscreen utilises nanotechnology to give a translucent and smooth texture for the skin appearance yet provide sufficient sun protection. This is an improvement from previous formulation that contains high concentration of titanium dioxide or zinc oxide cream mixture which cause an opaque film on the skin as UV protectant barrier. Microfine zinc oxide (particle size less than 2 microns) also is transparent on the skin, is completely photostable, and protects throughout the ultraviolet spectrum (Antoniou, Kosmadaki, Stratigos, & Katsambas, 2008).

Safety and Related Adverse Drug Reactions

In a 7-month, randomized, placebo-controlled, double-blinded trial, 114 of 603 (18.9%) participants in a sunscreen trial complained of an adverse skin reaction (Foley, Nixon, Marks, Frowen, & Thompson, 1993). Fifteen were judged unrelated to the sunscreen product. Between 5 to 90 days of sunscreen use, the remaining 90 subjects reported affected with symptoms such as rash, pruritus, blistering, skin flakiness and dryness. Twenty-one percent of the reactions involved the face alone, and 27% involved the forearms and hands alone, and 52% had reactions at all sites. Symptoms resolved in the majority within 3 weeks after stopping the cream, in less than 48 hours in 11 subjects, and greater than 3 weeks in only 6 subjects. None of the 49 subjects patch tested were allergic to the active sunscreen ingredients (cinnamate and dibenzoylmethane derivatives).

HAIR LOSS AND HAIR CARE COSMECEUTICALS

According to The Freedonia Group (Cleveland), the demand for cosmeceutical hair care products was projected to increase by more than 3.8% per year through 2012 with an estimated market size of USD950 million in 2017 (The Freedonia Group, 2015). Female and also male pattern loss of hair could be heartbreaking both for patients and also for the doctors who treat them.

Grape Seed

The membrane (skin) of the grape seed (*Vitis Vinifera*) is a rich source of proanthocyanidins (also referred to as procyanidins), one of the most beneficial groups of plant flavonoids. The most active proanthocyanidins are those bound to other proanthocyanidins. Grape seed extract has been recognised for its collagen stabilization and cross-linking activity. An *in vitro* study had demonstrated that procyanidins inhibit the activities of some proteolytic enzymes (collagenase, elastase) involved in the degradation of the main structural components of the extravascular matrix, collagen, elastin and hyaluronic acid.

Topical application of a 1% procyanidin beta-2 tonic for hair growth among men with androgenetic alopecia were tested in a double-blind, placebo-controlled trial. 19 subjects received the active drug and 10 randomized to receive placebo which 78.9% of the treatment group showed an increase in mean hair diameter compared to 30% in the controlled group.

The evidence from this procyanidin study had elucidated the mechanisms involved in regulating hair growth. It had been shown that procyanidin beta-2 could reduce the expression of protein kinase C, a known inhibitor of hair growth and a higher amount of growth factors such as transforming growth factor beta, fibroblast growth factor-5, tumor necrosis factor alpha, interleukin-1 alpha, and interleukin-1 beta could retard hair growth.

Raspberry

Oil from raspberry (*Rubus idaeus*) seeds contains phytosterol 0.73% to 1.10%, with a saponification value of 187 to 192. The most abundant fatty acids from oil of raspberry seed, together comprising 96% of the total fatty acid, are linoleic, alpha- linolenic, and oleic acids. Anti-inflammatory activity of raspberry seed oil, notable for avoidance of gingivitis, rash, and eczema has led to it being patented for inclusion in cosmetics and pharmaceutical products. The hair growth enhancement property of raspberry extract is promoted by an increased levels of dermal insulin-like growth factor I and sensory neuron activation (Oomah, Ladet, Godfrey, Liang, & Girard, 2000). Cosmeceutical scientists *analyzed* raspberry ketone, a structurally similar fragrant substance consisted of in red raspberries. When used to the scalp, 0.01% raspberry ketone marketed hair growth in 50% of people with alopecia areata (n=10) after 5 months.

SOLUTIONS AND RECOMMENDATIONS

Theoretical Basis for Cosmetic Testing

Evidences had revealed that hypo-collagenesis is the main factor that influences cosmesceutical treatment outcome. Punch biopsies obtained pre-treatment and post-treatment were analyzed for the content of type I procollagen from five independent studies. The analysis revealed that volunteers with hypo-collagenesis responded 6.4 times more often than subjects with normo-collagenesis. Therefore, hypo-collagenesis is very likely the unique parameter predicting anti-aging cosmeceutical treatment outcome.

Revisiting the Role of Compounding Pharmacist

In recent years, in most countries around the world such as the USA, Canada and UK, as well as some of the Asian countries such as South Korea, Japan and Taiwan, the profession of pharmacy has shifted from product provision to patient centered care, where pharmacists directly contribute to clinical care and have a significant role in the promotion of the quality use of medicine (Anderson, 2002; Karen N. Eggleston, 2011; Shafie, Hassali, Azhar, & See, 2012). Traditionally, the physician determined the root cause of topical medical condition and then a compounding pharmacist prepare appropriate treatments. Now the compounding role of pharmacist had become very minimum except in certain European countries such as Germany. Majority of the products now are mass produced in factory in fixed concentration and combination of product. Now, compounding is mostly dominated by dermatologists who offer various ranges of individualised cosmeceuticals products to the clients who might not be able to gain maximum benefit from the commercialised product. The curriculum of pharmacy programme and training should shift certain emphasis to compounding technology such as topical formulations that can be prepared in community pharmacy and compatibility of excipient with the active ingredient when prepared as a capsule. This will facilitate the dispensing of individualised cosmeceutical regardless in the term of topical or capsule.

FUTURE RESEARCH DIRECTIONS

Dermatologists have a responsibility to help to achieve a healthy appearance of their patient's skin through proper skin care guidance. It is important for us to understand the science behind cosmeceuticals as they are increasingly being incorporated into the skin by daily use of skin care products. American Academy of Dermatology has anticipated the popularity of cosmeceuticals in the mainstream market. It initiated Work Group on Complementary and Alternative Medicine which comprises dermatologists and adviser to the regulatory and enforcement agency of cosmetics and cosmeceuticals. The group mainly provides guidance and validated data on the toxicity and efficacy data of commonly used complementary substances including cosmeceutical products. For cosmeceuticals, the mandatory stringent regulatory requirement and control are not essential thus dermatologists tend to be sceptical of the efficacy of cosmeceuticals. This report had shown that many cosmeceutical products had undergone the recommended double-blind vehicle-controlled studies to gain the necessary evidence of efficacy and toxicity.

A proven clinical data are driven by the fact that consumers are highly exposed to medical information via internet and demand for products that are plant and evidence based as well as environmental friendly. They will search for the user feedback and clinical report online before the purchase. Moreover, the consumers will scrutinize the product compositions and origin of the raw material to ensure the manufacturer utilize the natural and sustainable sources ingredients (Nohynek, Antignac, Re, & Toutain, 2010). It is the responsibility of the manufacturers to comply and even propose production and registration regulations for cosmeceutical products including packaging labeling and medicinal in regard to the active ingredients and concentration used. Eventually, the manufacturer that can offer innovative product that has validated safety, stability and efficacy profiles for different market demographic layers will be well accepted by the medical professionals and consumers. Identifying product niches, new actives and more effective delivery systems will no doubt give way to a plethora of cosmeceutical products with broader clinical applications.

CONCLUSION

Hyperpigmentation, hair loss, skin dryness and aging are common dermatologic disorders. Although various therapy alternatives are available, dealing with these disorders successfully within a short time frame remains to be a therapeutic challenge. The main active ingredient used cosmeceuticals is changing due to strong demand from consumers for a more potent and rapid acting compound. A current interest in organic ingredients has driven scientists to examine other agents, but while these items may induce less irritability, they have actually not demonstrated the success of pharmaceutical drugs such as HQ. Thus, multiple ingredients formulation providing synergistic effect is the current strategy of cosmeceuticals company. Furthermore, continuous scientific test and trial are needed to further substantiate the clinical claims of the products to ensure easy acceptance and popularity among the consumers.

REFERENCES

Ali, F. R., & Finlayson, A. E. (2013). Pharaonic trichology: The Ebers Papyrus. *JAMA Dermatology*, *149*(8), 920. doi:10.1001/jamadermatol.2013.4240 PMID:24026454

American Academy of Dermatology. (2014). *Cosmeceuticals*. Retrieved October 13, 2015, from http://www.aad.org/media-resources/stats-and-facts/cosmetic-treatments/cosmeceuticals

Anderson, S. (2002). The state of the world's pharmacy: A portrait of the pharmacy profession. *Journal of Interprofessional Care*, *16*(4), 391–404. doi:10.1080/1356182021000008337 PMID:12487847

Antoniou, C., Kosmadaki, M. G., Stratigos, A. J., & Katsambas, A. D. (2008). Sunscreens–what's important to know. *Journal of the European Academy of Dermatology and Venereology*, *22*(9), 1110–1119. doi:10.1111/j.1468-3083.2007.02580.x PMID:18482317

Babamiri, K., & Nassab, R. (2010). Cosmeceuticals: The evidence behind the retinoids. *Aesthetic Surgery Journal*, *30*(1), 74–77. doi:10.1177/1090820X09360704 PMID:20442078

Balina, L. M., & Graupe, K. (1991). The treatment of melasma. 20% azelaic acid versus 4% hydroquinone cream. *International Journal of Dermatology*, *30*(12), 893–895. doi:10.1111/j.1365-4362.1991.tb04362.x PMID:1816137

Bauer, A., Diepgen, T. L., & Schmitt, J. (2011). Is occupational solar ultraviolet irradiation a relevant risk factor for basal cell carcinoma? A systematic review and meta-analysis of the epidemiological literature. *The British Journal of Dermatology*, *165*(3), 612–625. PMID:21605109

Bentley, R. (2006). From miso, sake and shoyu to cosmetics: A century of science for kojic acid. *Natural Product Reports*, *23*(6), 1046–1062. doi:10.1039/b603758p PMID:17119644

Bhattacharyya, T. K., Pathria, M., Mathison, C., Vargas, M., & Thomas, J. R. (2014). Cosmeceutical effect on skin surface profiles and epidermis in UV-B-irradiated mice. *JAMA Facial Plastic Surgery*, *16*(4), 253–260. doi:10.1001/jamafacial.2013.2582 PMID:24874724

Boyle, J., & Kennedy, C. T. (1985). Leukoderma from hydroquinone. *Contact Dermatitis*, *13*(4), 287–288. doi:10.1111/j.1600-0536.1985.tb02578.x PMID:4085240

Bucks, D. A., McMaster, J. R., Guy, R. H., & Maibach, H. I. (1988). Percutaneous absorption of hydroquinone in humans: Effect of 1-dodecylazacycloheptan-2-one (azone) and the 2-ethylhexyl ester of 4-(dimethylamino) benzoic acid (escalol 507). *Journal of Toxicology and Environmental Health*, *24*(3), 279–289. doi:10.1080/15287398809531162 PMID:3260963

Choi, J.-H., Cho, C.-W., Kim, J.-H., Park, S. H., Chang, S., & Yu, Y.-B. (2015). Liquid crystal formulation and optimization of anti-microbial polyherbal ointment. *Journal of Nanoscience and Nanotechnology*, *15*(8), 5656–5659. doi:10.1166/jnn.2015.10461 PMID:26369133

Choi, Y. L., Park, E. J., Kim, E., Na, D. H., & Shin, Y. H. (2014). Dermal stability and in vitro skin permeation of collagen pentapeptides (KTTKS and palmitoyl-KTTKS). *Biomolecules & Therapeutics*, *22*(4), 321–327. doi:10.4062/biomolther.2014.053 PMID:25143811

Decker, A., & Graber, E. M. (2012). Over-the-counter acne treatments: A review. *The Journal of Clinical and Aesthetic Dermatology*, *5*(5), 32–40. PMID:22808307

Draelos, Z. D. (2009). Cosmeceuticals: Undefined, unclassified, and unregulated. *Clinics in Dermatology*, *27*(5), 431–434. doi:10.1016/j.clindermatol.2009.05.005 PMID:19695473

Duell, E. A., Kang, S., & Voorhees, J. J. (1997). Unoccluded retinol penetrates human skin in vivo more effectively than unoccluded retinyl palmitate or retinoic acid. *The Journal of Investigative Dermatology*, *109*(3), 301–305. doi:10.1111/1523-1747.ep12335788 PMID:9284094

European Commission. (2015). *Cosmetics*. Retrieved October 13, 2015, from http://ec.europa.eu/growth/sectors/cosmetics/index_en.htm

European Medicines Agency. (2015). *Frequently asked questions*. Retrieved October 11, 2015, from http://www.ema.europa.eu/ema/index.jsp?curl=pages/about_us/q_and_a/q_and_a_detail_000114.jsp

Farris, P. K. (2005). Topical vitamin C: A useful agent for treating photoaging and other dermatologic conditions. *Dermatologic Surgery*, *31*(7 Pt 2), 814–817. PMID:16029672

Farris, P. K., Edison, B. L., Brouda, I., Weinkauf, R. L., & Green, B. A. (2012). A high-potency, multimechanism skin care regimen provides significant antiaging effects: Results from a double-blind, vehicle-controlled clinical trial. *Journal of Drugs in Dermatology*, *11*(12), 1447–1454. PMID:23377515

FDA. (2015). Retrieved October 13, 2015, from http://www.fda.gov/RegulatoryInformation/Legislation/FederalFoodDrugandCosmeticActFDCAct/default.htm

Fisher, A. A. (1983). Current contact news. Hydroquinone uses and abnormal reactions. *Cutis*, *31*(3), 240–244, 250. PMID:6220868

Fisher, A. A. (1988). Tetracycline treatment for sarcoid-like ochronosis due to hydroquinone. *Cutis*, *42*(1), 19–20. PMID:3203531

Fisk, W. A., Agbai, O., Lev-Tov, H. A., & Sivamani, R. K. (2014). The use of botanically derived agents for hyperpigmentation: A systematic review. *Journal of the American Academy of Dermatology*, *70*(2), 352–365. doi:10.1016/j.jaad.2013.09.048 PMID:24280646

Fitton, A., & Goa, K. L. (1991). Azelaic acid. A review of its pharmacological properties and therapeutic efficacy in acne and hyperpigmentary skin disorders. *Drugs*, *41*(5), 780–798. doi:10.2165/00003495-199141050-00007 PMID:1712709

Foley, P., Nixon, R., Marks, R., Frowen, K., & Thompson, S. (1993). The frequency of reactions to sunscreens: Results of a longitudinal population-based study on the regular use of sunscreens in Australia. *The British Journal of Dermatology*, *128*(5), 512–518. doi:10.1111/j.1365-2133.1993.tb00227.x PMID:8504041

Food & Drug Administration. (2011). Labeling and effectiveness testing; sunscreen drug products for over-the-counter human use. Final rule. *Federal Register, 76*(117), 35620.

Fort-Lacoste, L., Verscheure, Y., Tisne-Versailles, J., & Navarro, R. (1999). Comedolytic effect of topical retinaldehyde in the rhino mouse model. *Dermatology (Basel, Switzerland)*, *199*(Suppl 1), 33–35. doi:10.1159/000051376 PMID:10473958

Gao, X. H., Zhang, L., Wei, H. C., & Chen, H. D. (2008). Efficacy and safety of innovative cosmeceuticals. *Clinics in Dermatology*, *26*(4), 367–374. doi:10.1016/j.clindermatol.2008.01.013 PMID:18691517

García-Gavín, J., González-Vilas, D., Fernández-Redondo, V., & Toribio, J. (2010). Pigmented contact dermatitis due to kojic acid. A paradoxical side effect of a skin lightener. *Contact Dermatitis*, *62*(1), 63–64. doi:10.1111/j.1600-0536.2009.01673.x PMID:20136888

Gaut, B. N., & Lopes, D. (Eds.). (2005). *The Routledge companion to aesthetics* (2nd ed.). London: Routledge.

Gladstone, H. B., Nguyen, S. L., Williams, R., Ottomeyer, T., Wortzman, M., Jeffers, M., & Moy, R. L. (2000). Efficacy of hydroquinone cream (USP 4%) used alone or in combination with salicylic acid peels in improving photodamage on the neck and upper chest. *Dermatologic Surgery*, *26*(4), 333–337. doi:10.1046/j.1524-4725.2000.99233.x PMID:10759820

Grossman, R. (2005). The role of dimethylaminoethanol in cosmetic dermatology. *American Journal of Clinical Dermatology*, *6*(1), 39–47. doi:10.2165/00128071-200506010-00005 PMID:15675889

Hayden, C. G., Roberts, M. S., & Benson, H. A. (1997). Systemic absorption of sunscreen after topical application. *Lancet*, *350*(9081), 863–864. doi:10.1016/S0140-6736(05)62032-6 PMID:9310609

Higgins, S., & Wesley, N. (2015). Topical retinoids and cosmeceuticals: Where is the scientific evidence to recommend products to patients? *Current Dermatology Reports*, *4*(2), 56–62. doi:10.1007/s13671-015-0102-9

Hoshaw, R. A., Zimmerman, K. G., & Menter, A. (1985). Ochronosislike pigmentation from hydroquinone bleaching creams in American blacks. *Archives of Dermatology*, *121*(1), 105–108. doi:10.1001/archderm.1985.01660010109032 PMID:3966811

Kang, S., Duell, E. A., Fisher, G. J., Datta, S. C., Wang, Z. Q., Reddy, A. P., & Voorhees, J. J. et al (1995). Application of retinol to human skin in vivo induces epidermal hyperplasia and cellular retinoid binding proteins characteristic of retinoic acid but without measurable retinoic acid levels or irritation. *The Journal of Investigative Dermatology*, *105*(4), 549–556. doi:10.1111/1523-1747.ep12323445 PMID:7561157

Karen, N., & Eggleston, W. H. S. (2011). Prescribing institutions: Explaining the evolution of physician dispensing. *Journal of Institutional Economics*, *8*(02), 247–270.

Katiyar, S., Elmets, C. A., & Katiyar, S. K. (2007). Green tea and skin cancer: Photoimmunology, angiogenesis and DNA repair. *The Journal of Nutritional Biochemistry*, *18*(5), 287–296. doi:10.1016/j.jnutbio.2006.08.004 PMID:17049833

Kim, M. S., Song, H. J., Lee, S. H., & Lee, C. K. (2014). Comparative study of various growth factors and cytokines on type I collagen and hyaluronan production in human dermal fibroblasts. *Journal of Cosmetic Dermatology*, *13*(1), 44–51. doi:10.1111/jocd.12073 PMID:24641605

Kligman, A. (2005). The future of cosmeceuticals: An interview with Albert Kligman, MD, PhD. Interview by Zoe Diana Draelos. *Dermatologic Surgery*, *31*(7 Pt 2), 890–891. PMID:16029684

Kobayashi, S., Takeana, M., Kanke, M., Itoh, S., & Ogata, E. (1998). Postadministration protective effect of magnesium-L-ascorbyl-phosphate on the development of UVB-induced cutaneous damage in mice. *Photochemistry and Photobiology*, *67*(6), 669–675. doi:10.1111/j.1751-1097.1998.tb09111.x PMID:9648533

Korkina, L. G., Pastore, S., Dellambra, E., & De Luca, C. (2013). New molecular and cellular targets for chemoprevention and treatment of skin tumors by plant polyphenols: A critical review. *Current Medicinal Chemistry*, *20*(7), 852–868. PMID:23210776

Kornhauser, A., Coelho, S. G., & Hearing, V. J. (2010). Applications of hydroxy acids: Classification, mechanisms, and photoactivity. *Journal of Clinical. Cosmetic and Investigational Dermatology*, *3*, 135–142. doi:10.2147/CCID.S9042

Kullavanijaya, P., & Lim, H. W. (2005). Photoprotection. *Journal of the American Academy of Dermatology*, *52*(6), 937–958. doi:10.1016/j.jaad.2004.07.063 PMID:15928611

Lee, M. S., Lee, K. H., Sin, H. S., Um, S. J., Kim, J. W., & Koh, B. K. (2006). A newly synthesized photostable retinol derivative (retinyl N-formyl aspartamate) for photodamaged skin: Profilometric evaluation of 24-week study. *Journal of the American Academy of Dermatology*, *55*(2), 220–224. doi:10.1016/j.jaad.2006.01.013 PMID:16844502

Lim, J. T. E., Frcpi, , & Fams, . (1999). Treatment of melasma using kojic acid in a gel containing hydroquinone and glycolic acid. *Dermatologic Surgery*, *25*(4), 282–284. doi:10.1046/j.1524-4725.1999.08236.x PMID:10417583

Lugović, L., Šitum, M., Ožanić-Bulić, S., & Sjerobabski-Masnec, I. (2007). Phototoxic and photoallergic skin reactions. *Collegium Antropologicum*, *31*(1), 63–67. PMID:17469754

Lupo, M. P., & Cole, A. L. (2007). Cosmeceutical peptides. *Dermatologic Therapy*, *20*(5), 343–349. doi:10.1111/j.1529-8019.2007.00148.x PMID:18045359

Mann, R., & Harman, R. (1983). Nail staining due to hydroquinone skin-lightening creams. *The British Journal of Dermatology*, *108*(3), 363–365. doi:10.1111/j.1365-2133.1983.tb03976.x PMID:6219692

Maslow, A. H., & Frager, R. (Eds.). (1987). *Motivation and Personality*. New York, London: Harper & Row.

Nohynek, G. J., Antignac, E., Re, T., & Toutain, H. (2010). Safety assessment of personal care products/cosmetics and their ingredients. *Toxicology and Applied Pharmacology*, *243*(2), 239–259. doi:10.1016/j.taap.2009.12.001 PMID:20005888

Nusgens, B. V., Humbert, P., Rougier, A., Colige, A. C., Haftek, M., Lambert, C. A., & Lapiere, C. M. et al. (2001). Topically applied vitamin C enhances the mRNA level of collagens I and III, their processing enzymes and tissue inhibitor of matrix metalloproteinase 1 in the human dermis. *The Journal of Investigative Dermatology*, *116*(6), 853–859. doi:10.1046/j.0022-202x.2001.01362.x PMID:11407971

Oblong, J. E., & Bisset, D. L. (2005). Retinoids. In Z. D. Draelos (Ed.), *Cosmeceuticals* (pp. 35–45). Philadelphia: Elsevier Saunders.

Oomah, B. D., Ladet, S., Godfrey, D. V., Liang, J., & Girard, B. (2000). Characteristics of raspberry (Rubus idaeus L.) seed oil. *Food Chemistry*, *69*(2), 187–193. doi:10.1016/S0308-8146(99)00260-5

Oricha, B. S. (2010). Cosmeceuticals: A review. *African Journal of Pharmacy and Pharmacology*, *4*(4), 127–129.

Oumeish, O. Y. (2001). The cultural and philosophical concepts of cosmetics in beauty and art through the medical history of mankind. *Clinics in Dermatology*, *19*(4), 375–386. doi:10.1016/S0738-081X(01)00194-8 PMID:11535377

Packaged Facts. (2012). *Cosmeceuticals in the U.S.* (6th ed.). Retrieved October 11, 2015, from http://www.marketresearch.com/Packaged-Facts-v768/Cosmeceuticals-Edition-6281775/

Pechere, M., Pechere, J. C., Siegenthaler, G., Germanier, L., & Saurat, J. H. (1999). Antibacterial activity of retinaldehyde against Propionibacterium acnes. *Dermatology (Basel, Switzerland)*, *199*(Suppl 1), 29–31. doi:10.1159/000051375 PMID:10473957

Rendon, M. I., Vazquez, Y., & Micciantuono, S. (2013). Cosmeceutical Skin Lighteners. In P. K. Farris (Ed.), *Cosmeceuticals and Cosmetic Practice* (pp. 218–225). New Orleans, LA: Wiley-Blackwell. doi:10.1002/9781118384824.ch22

Romaguera, C., & Grimalt, F. (1985). Leukoderma from hydroquinone. *Contact Dermatitis*, *12*(3), 183. doi:10.1111/j.1600-0536.1985.tb01101.x PMID:3995954

Sachs, D. L., Rittie, L., Chubb, H. A., Orringer, J., Fisher, G., & Voorhees, J. J. (2013). Hypo-collagenesis in photoaged skin predicts response to anti-aging cosmeceuticals. *Journal of Cosmetic Dermatology*, *12*(2), 108–115. doi:10.1111/jocd.12037 PMID:23725304

Schalka, S., Steiner, D., Ravelli, F. N., Steiner, T., Terena, A. C., Marçon, C. R., & Ponzio, H. et al. (2014). Brazilian consensus on photoprotection. *Anais Brasileiros de Dermatologia*, *89*(6), 1–74. doi:10.1590/abd1806-4841.20143971 PMID:25761256

Schmitt, J., Seidler, A., Diepgen, T. L., & Bauer, A. (2011). Occupational ultraviolet light exposure increases the risk for the development of cutaneous squamous cell carcinoma: A systematic review and meta-analysis. *The British Journal of Dermatology*, *164*(2), 291–307. doi:10.1111/j.1365-2133.2010.10118.x PMID:21054335

Semsei, I., & Zs-Nagy, I. (1985). Superoxide radical scavenging ability of centrophenoxine and its salt dependence in vitro. *Journal of Free Radicals in Biology & Medicine*, *1*(5-6), 403–408. doi:10.1016/0748-5514(85)90153-9 PMID:3018064

Shafie, A. A., Hassali, M. A., Azhar, S., & See, O. G. (2012). Separation of prescribing and dispensing in Malaysia: A summary of arguments. *Research in Social & Administrative Pharmacy*, *8*(3), 258–262. doi:10.1016/j.sapharm.2011.06.002 PMID:21824823

Sommerfeld, B. (2007). Randomised, placebo-controlled, double-blind, split-face study on the clinical efficacy of Tricutan on skin firmness. *Phytomedicine*, *14*(11), 711–715. doi:10.1016/j.phymed.2007.09.015 PMID:17923398

Terra, V. A., Souza-Neto, F. P., Frade, M. A., Ramalho, L. N., Andrade, T. A., Pasta, A. A., & Cecchini, A. L. et al. (2015). Genistein prevents ultraviolet B radiation-induced nitrosative skin injury and promotes cell proliferation. *Journal of Photochemistry and Photobiology. B, Biology*, *144*, 20–27. PMID:25668145

The Freedonia Group. (2015). *Cosmeceuticals to 2015 - demand and sales forecasts, market share, market size, market leaders*. Retrieved September 18 2015, from http://www.freedoniagroup.com/Cosmeceuticals.html

US Government Publishing Office. (2015). *Subpart B—Requirements for Specific Cosmetic Products*. Retrieved September 18 2015, from http://www.ecfr.gov/cgi-bin/text-idx?c=ecfr&sid=c108128827d21f2d274e894731665ef4&rgn=div6&view=text&node=21:7.0.1.2.10.2&idno=21

Verallo-Rowell, V. M., Verallo, V., Graupe, K., Lopez-Villafuerte, L., & Garcia-Lopez, M. (1989). Double-blind comparison of azelaic acid and hydroquinone in the treatment of melasma. *Acta Dermato-Venereologica, 143*, 58–61. PMID:2528260

Wang, Q.-S., Gao, T., Cui, Y.-L., Gao, L.-N., & Jiang, H.-L. (2014). Comparative studies of paeoniflorin and albiflorin from Paeonia lactiflora on anti-inflammatory activities. *Pharmaceutical Biology, 52*(9), 1189-1195.

Wang, Y. H., Dhariwal, K. R., & Levine, M. (1992). Ascorbic acid bioavailability in humans. Ascorbic acid in plasma, serum, and urine. *Annals of the New York Academy of Sciences, 669*(1), 383–386. doi:10.1111/j.1749-6632.1992.tb17130.x PMID:1444054

KEY TERMS AND DEFINITIONS

Alpha Hydroxyl Acids: An organic acid containing a hydroxyl group bonded to the carbon atom adjacent to the carboxylic acid group. Lactic acid, glycolic acid, malic acid and citric acid are commonly used alpha hydroxyl acids that exhibit exfoliative, keratolytic, humectant and whitening properties.

Cosmeceuticals: A term used to describe topical cosmetic-pharmaceutical hybrids intended to improve health and beauty of the skin. Cosmeceutical products are fortified with natural ingredients that could augment the skin's biological function just like pharmaceuticals.

Retinoids: Vitamin A-derived substances that are widely used as a topical treatment of aging skin and comedones. Naturally-occurring retinoids consist of all-trans-retinol, all-trans-retinaldehyde and all-trans-retinoic acid. All-trans retinol is likewise referred to as retinol or Vitamin A; all-trans-retinaldehyde is described as retinal; and also all-trans-retinoic acid is known as retinoic acid or tretinoin.

Chapter 11
Cosmeceuticals:
Camel and Other Milk – Natural Skin Maintenance

Reuven Yagil
Ben-Gurion University, Israel & Beauty Treat Organic Cosmetics Ltd., Israel

ABSTRACT

This chapter will deal with delivering of a substance in a natural product, milk, via the skin – cosmeceuticals, from a variety of sources, camels, equine, ruminant and breast milk. The large quantities of bacteria on the normal skin, both friendly and "bad" bacteria provide skin and body health. The activity of cosmeceuticals of camel milk is due to the specific milk components, whose efficacy is retained in skin preparations which have not been destroyed in their preparation. By using camel milk which is pathogen-free the preparations are probiotic by definition and rapidly penetrate the outer skin layers to be active in the deeper layers. Massage therapy has been shown to improve flexibility and range of motion and strengthen the immune system. A list of the organic substances used for making the cosmeceuticals is provided.

MILK COSMECEUTICALS: A NOVEL APPROACH FOR EXTERNAL DRUG DELIVERY

This chapter will deal with a novel approach to delivering natural active substances, milk, especially camel milk, on and via the skin, in the form of cosmeceuticals. The milk is not only a vehicle for added substances but naturally contains substances that are "skin-friendly and healthy". This work provides information how milk is active on and in the skin.

Transdermal drug delivery has made an important contribution to medical practice, but has yet to fully achieve its potential as an alternative to oral delivery and hypodermic injections. For thousands of years, people have placed substances on the skin for therapeutic effects and, in the modern era, a variety of topical formulations have been developed to treat local indications. The first transdermal system for systemic delivery—a three-day patch that delivers scopolamine to treat motion sickness—was approved for use in the United States in 1979. A decade later, nicotine patches became the first transdermal blockbuster to reduce smoking, raising the profile of transdermal delivery in medicine and for the public in

DOI: 10.4018/978-1-5225-0754-3.ch011

general. Today, there are 19 transdermal delivery systems for such drugs as estradiol, fentanyl, lidocaine and testosterone. It is common for women after menopause to have estrogen patches to help in preventing osteoporosis. However, the patches must not be placed on or close to the breasts in order to prevent breast cancer from occurring.

Perhaps the greatest challenge for transdermal delivery is that only a limited number of drugs are amenable to administration by this route.

Transdermal delivery offers compelling opportunities to improve vaccine administration. The most successful vaccine of all time—the smallpox vaccine, which eradicated the disease worldwide—was administered via the skin with the aid of a small needle device to breach the stratum corneum barrier.

Cosmeceuticals are the combination of cosmetics and pharmaceuticals with biologically active ingredients purporting to have medical or drug-like benefits (Yurystyn et al, 2014).

Cosmeceuticals contain active ingredients that are known to be beneficial to humans in some way. For example, vitamin C is a known antioxidant and when this is added to a lotion or cream the product is considered a cosmeceutical (see below).

Before presenting data about cosmeceuticals it is pertinent to provide data about our skin itself.

HUMAN SKIN

Skin is the largest body organ. It has three layers: the epidermis, the outermost layer of skin, which provides a waterproof barrier and creates our skin tone. The dermis, beneath the epidermis, contains tough connective tissue, hair follicles, and sweat glands. The deeper subcutaneous tissue (hypodermis) consists of fat and connective tissue.

There are around 1000 species of bacteria on human skin (De Noon, 2009) from 19 phyla. The total number of bacteria on an average human has been estimated at 1 trillion. Most are found in the superficial layers of the epidermis and the upper parts of hair follicles. The benefits of most bacteria can offer prevention of transient pathogenic organisms from colonizing the skin surface, either by competing for nutrients, secreting chemicals against them, or stimulating the skin's immune system (Kanodia et al, 2007.). Therefore, our "good bacteria" crowd out pathogenic bacteria, some even secreting a natural antibiotic to ward off these bad bacteria and secure more space for themselves. Note! When we wash our hands to remove pathogens, we are also removing bacteria that can help protect us against those same pathogens as well as other diseases.

Dehydrated skin is a condition where the skin has limited or a lack of moisture in the intracellular system of the skin. Skin dehydration can be problematic all year round. Your skin is more susceptible to dehydration in the winter due to aggressive environmental factors. It is very important to monitor the signs and symptoms regularly to treat it when needed. Age, location and amount of time spent outside are all factors that can impact the condition of your skin.

The skin can feel tight and you may feel a burning sensation. It will often get irritated and has a lesser ability to heal. The skin sometimes gets flaky and shows dry lines. The texture of the skin will be rough and will not look smooth anymore. A very common sign of dehydrated skin is extreme itching, which can even become painful.

Camel creams prevent further loss of moisture from the skin but drinking is the only way to reinstate body hydration.

When the outer skin layers are compromised, bacteria gain access and can cause infections.

FRAGRANCES OF COSMETICS

Although the first thing people do when checking a cosmetic is to smell it, the fragrance does not always mean it is a good product for the skin (Begoun, 2013).

Most fragrance ingredients impart scent through a volatile reaction, which almost always causes irritation and some amount of inflammation. Research has established that fragrances in skin-care products are among the most common cause of sensitizing and allergic reactions.

Some ingredients have a pleasant fragrance but cause no irritation and are good for skin. Other products may have no aroma because the fragrance is included to mask the odors of the real skin-care ingredients, which aren't necessarily pleasant.

Many beneficial skin-care ingredients (antioxidants, for example) have a natural fragrance, and some of them even smell pleasant. Distinguishing potent antioxidants (fighters of free radicals and skin aging) from those that are simply added to make you "shop with your nose" is not easy Like anything in skin care, the basic information is on the ingredient label, but because those ingredients read like a college chemistry course they are impossible for the layman to decipher.

Frequently used fragrance ingredients which should be avoided (some may come as a surprise) are:

- Linalool
- Citronellol
- Cinnamal
- Limonene
- Geraniol
- Eugenol
- Lavender oil (Lavandula angustifolia)
- Rose flower extract (Rosa damascene)
- Bergamot oil (Citrus bergamia)
- Ylang-ylang oil (Canaga odora)
- Lemon (Citrus limon)
- Lime (Citrus aurantifolia or Citrus medica)
- Orange (Citrus sinensis)
- Tangerine (Citrus tangerine)
- Peppermint (Mentha piperita)
- Spearmint (Mentha spicat)
- Menthol
- Cinnamon (Cinnamomum)

It is a fact that the first thing a buyer does when choosing a cosmetic is to smell it, mostly by opening a test sample when it is available. If it is not pleasant, it will not be purchased.

Skin reduces water loss and plays an important role in homeostasis and thermeostasis.

MILK

Cosmeceuticals deal with milk of a number of mammals. The most important is camel milk which now receives worldwide acceptance for both its nutritional and alternative medicine (CAM) properties (Yagil, 2013). The special CAM composition of camel milk explains its skin-friendly activity as a cosmeceutical. Equine (mares and donkey) milk, goat and breast milk will also be presented, as they also show good properties.

It is assumed that Cleopatra bathed in milk of camels (Piceno, 2011). The question is: was it to maintain her beauty by reducing wrinkles? Or was it to help control a skin ailment e.g. psoriasis brought about by stress? Camel milk would have been beneficial in both cases.

Camel Milk

Even though camel-milk cosmeceuticals have been shown to be very affective, obtaining the required regulations for marketing them has often proven to be virtually impossible. This is due to the complete lack of knowledge, by officials dealing with cosmetics, of both human skin and camel milk and the absence of a minimal idea of how cosmeceuticals work, creates a negative acceptance of camel milk and their cosmeceuticals. Hopefully, this publication will help rectify this lack of knowledge.

The relevant components that make the camel milk preparations skin-friendly and effective are presented in Yagil, 2000:

Fat

Low fat of 2% that is completely homogenized to very small particles and mainly omegas, poly-unsaturated-fatty acids (PUFAs). The small fat globules are attached to proteins and so are readily absorbed into the deeper skin layers without leaving a trace on the skin itself.

PUFAs help to reduce inflammation by giving rise to the potent signaling molecules, called eicosanoids and attenuates UV-induced photo-damage (any of a class of compounds (as the prostaglandins, leukotrienes, and thromboxanes) derived from polyunsaturated fatty acids (as arachidonic acid) and involved in cellular activity (Soberman & Christmas 2003,).

Findings also show that the production of antimicrobial peptides by adipocytes is an important element for protection against infections of the skin (Zhang et al, 2015).

PUFAs remove the typical signs of lupus on the skin, such as looking like a wolf (lupus), or a butterfly rash (personal observation).

When the skin is cut or scratched specialized immune-system cells, neutrophils and monocytes, destroy the pathogens (Mercola, 2009). However, this is not the body's only line of defense. The dermal fat cells or adipocytes – the ones just below the skin – may be the first responders against potential invaders.

Findings show that the production of antimicrobial peptides by adipocytes is an important element for protection against S. aureus infection of the skin (Zhang et al, 2015).

Therefore, the fat in camel milk is "friendly" on the skin and its absorption into the skin plays an important role in creating a healthy skin.

Lactose

There is no "lactose intolerance" when drinking camel milk. The lactase (enzyme) circulating in the human body easily breaks down camel-milk lactose in contrast to what happens with ruminant lactose. Lactose is a skin-conditioning agent – it acts as a humectant (Shah &Nickerson, 1978), retaining moisture in contrast to a drying agent, a desiccant. Humectants are hygroscopic substances. Lactose is, therefore, widely used in skincare products for its ability to hydrate skin.

Therefore, camel-milk-lactose in cosmeceuticals is healthy for the human skin.

Proteins

Camel milk does not contain the protein-allergens of ruminant milk (beta-casein and beta-lactoglobulin). Camel immunoglobulins are considered natural nanobodies (Gibbs, 2005), being 1/10 of the size of human ones and are far more active (Muyldermans, 2001), so easily pass into deeper skin layers as they pass through thick tissues (Hamers-Casterman et al, 1993). There are skin repair proteins and powerful bactericides, viricides and fungicides, which all make up the special defense system which will control infections of the skin and the inner layers. When the outer skin layers are compromised the camel-milk proteins help in repairing the damage and prevent infections.

Urea, formed from proteins, is widely used in skincare because of its hydrating properties. It is also a great and widely used preservative in cosmetics. It has been found to prevent sun radiation from aging the skin (Gloor et al, 2002).

Urea can be found in a large number of products, including the following:

- Facial moisturizers
- Facial cleansers
- Anti-aging creams
- Body lotions
- Eye creams
- Foundations
- Shampoos & conditioners, styling mousses and foams
- Acne treatments
- After-shave lotions
- Lip balm/treatments
- Mascara
- Sunless tanning products
- Antiperspirants/deodorants
- Cuticle treatments
- Nail polishes

However, urea has the tendency to cause allergic reactions which may be due to its release of formaldehyde. Those suffering from sensitive and infected skin are advised to steer clear of this ingredient. In fact, the American Academy of Dermatology has established diazolidinyl urea as a primary cause of contact dermatitis.

The proteins, attached to fat in camel milk prevent infections of the outer skin and deeper layers and unclog pores.

Lactoperoxidase, present in camel milk, is an enzyme that is very abundant in milk in general (lacto refers to milk). It has very strong, broad-spectrum antimicrobial activity and also helps to stabilize products.

Lactoferrin, found in camel milk, is something that has recently started to show up in beauty products. It is considered an antioxidant, which is why it is included in some hair care and skin care products (Combs, 2015).

Therefore, camel milk-proteins in cosmeceuticals are healthy for the various layers of the human skin and especially important if the epidermis is damaged.

VITAMINS

Camel milk contains many vitamins but is particularly noted for the high concentrations of vitamin C.

Vitamin C in camel milk has antioxidant and tissue repair protection activities that slow the rate of free-radical damage which causes skin dryness, and wrinkles (Escott-Stump, 2008).

Vitamin C is an essential water soluble vitamin that helps protect the immune system.

Over-exposure to ultraviolet radiation and environmental pollutants can accelerate skin aging by degrading collagen and triggering oxidative stress in the skin. Fortunately, the anti-aging benefits of a time-honored remedy used by ancient civilizations to heal the skin can help overcome these undesirable effects. Vitamin C is an essential component in the body's production of collagen and a potent antioxidant that can help rejuvenate aged and photo-damaged skin (Goldfaben, 2009). Collagen is found in the skin, joints and cartilage; by increasing the production of collagen, vitamin C strengthens the structural support and resiliency of skin thus helping to repair it. The vitamin C and protective proteins in camel milk, therefore, are efficient in treating sun-burn. The reaction is immediate (personal observation).

Vitamin C acts as a skincare treatment in the cosmeceutical industry. It reduces ageing, wrinkles, pigmentation, fine lines etc. and this will keeps the skin clear and healthy.

When the outer skin layer is disrupted vitamin C prevents infection and hastens repair.

In vitamin C deficiency the skin is dull and in the long term it can involve skin infections like dermatoses (Gopan, 2014).

Scurvy was associated with lack of fresh citrus fruit i.e. vitamin C on long boat trips, shown by formation of spots on the skin, spongy gums, and bleeding from the mucous membranes. Spots are most abundant on the thighs and legs, and a person with the ailment looks pale, feels depressed, and is partially immobilized. As scurvy advances, there can be open, suppurating wounds, loss of teeth, jaundice, fever, neuropathy and finally death from hemorrhage when blood vessels become extremely weak.

Therefore, the vitamin C, as well as other vitamins, in camel-milk cosmeceuticals are healthy for the human skin.

ELECTROLYTES

Although many active ingredients are used in cosmetic products for moisturizing and whitening the skin, they are often electrolytes, and the stabilities of oil in water (O/W) type emulsion formulae containing electrolytes are generally difficult to control (Maliepaard et al, 2013).

Camel milk contains high concentrations of calcium, magnesium and iron.

Magnesium slows down the aging process in the skin as it stabilizes DNA and RNA which are both negatively charged and are attracted to the positively charged magnesium. Magnesium is also needed for hair to grow properly because chronic stress can cause hair to fall out as a result of unstable blood sugar, chronic inflammation, insufficient nutrition or sleep deprivation.

- **Calcium:** Strengthens cell membranes & cleanses pores (mindful minerals, 2014).
- **Iron:** Helps production of melanin and promotes a healthy skin tone (mindful minerals, 2014).

SODIUM

Sodium is beneficial in maintaining PH balance, protecting the body against fluid loss. Sweat contains water but also urea, with little loss of sodium. Transport of water in the kidney is also accomplished by urea. Humans actively reabsorb urea from their kidneys.

In conclusion, all aspects of camel milk in the cosmeceuticals are beneficial for skin health and repairing damage.

The percentage of camel milk in the cosmeceuticals varies between 40% to 96%, depending on what health aspects are required and what substances are added to obtain the best effect. It should be noted that our cosmeceuticals are derived from pathogen-free milk, thus qualifying as probiotics rather than food additives. The importance, as explained before, is that good bacteria control the "bad" ones (Fahey, 2009).

Therefore, camel-milk cosmeceuticals are healthy for the human skin.

SKIN BEAUTY (COSMETIC) ACTIVITY

Cosmetics (also known as makeup or make-up) are care substances used to enhance the appearance or odor of the human body. They are generally mixtures of chemical compounds, some being derived from natural sources and many being synthetics.

In the U.S., the Food and Drug Administration (FDA), which regulates cosmetics, defines cosmetics as "intended to be applied to the human body for cleansing, beautifying, promoting attractiveness, or altering the appearance without affecting the body's structure or functions" (FDA, 2015). Camel milk cosmeceuticals provide health especially when the body's structure and function have been disrupted. There is no mention as to what is expected when the body structure and function ARE disrupted.

Castor oil was used by ancient Egypt as a protective balm .Skin creams made of beeswax, olive oil, and rosewater were all described by the Romans. Vaseline and lanolin were used in the nineteenth century. Nivea was used in 1911. However, note that the chemicals in cosmetics can trigger severe allergies, even with Nivea (Derbyshire 2015).

One of the most popular Traditional Chinese Medicines is the fungus Tremella fuciformis; used as a beauty product by women in China and Japan (Reshetnikov et al, 2000).

The fungus reportedly increases moisture retention in the skin and prevents senile degradation of micro-blood vessels in the skin, reducing wrinkles and smoothing fine lines.

Cosmetics include skin-care creams, lotions, powders, perfumes, lipsticks, nail polish, eye and facial makeup, towelettes, permanent waves, colored contact lenses, hair colors, hair sprays and gels, deodorants, hand sanitizers, baby products, bath oils, bubble baths, bath salts, butters and many other types of products.

Most cosmetics are distinguished by the area of the body intended for application.

Cosmetics can be liquid or cream emulsions; powders, both pressed and loose; dispersions; and anhydrous creams or sticks.

Skincare & Cosmetics: It has been said that glowing skin is the best make-up.

BLOOD FLOW TO SKIN

The thermoregulatory control of human skin blood flow is vital to the maintenance of normal body temperatures. The sympathetic neural control of skin blood flow includes the noradrenergic vasoconstrictor system and a sympathetic active vasodilator system (Charkoudian, 2003). Cutaneous sympathetic vasoconstrictor and vasodilator systems also participate in baroreflex control of blood pressure; this is particularly important during heat stress, when a large percentage of cardiac output is directed to the skin. Note that in maintaining body temperatures in extreme heat and activity a person can lose up to 4 liters sweat per hour, rapidly leading to heat-stroke. Of course, in cold circumstances there is a constriction of blood vessels to the skin, maintaining body heat. It is common knowledge that in very cold circumstances blood flow to the extremities is severely reduced and can lead to loss of extremities.

After menopause, changes in reproductive hormone levels substantially alter thermoregulatory control of skin blood flow, causing "hot flashes".

Skin Grafts

Healthy skin is taken from a site on the body called the donor site. Most people having a skin graft have a split thickness skin graft whereby the two top layers of skin are taken from the donor site (the epidermis) and the layer under the epidermis (the dermis.(

The donor site can be any area of the body. There are two types of skin grafts; the more common type is where a thin layer is removed from a healthy part of the body (the donor section) like peeling a potato, or a full thickness skin graft, which involves cutting skin away from the donor section. A full thickness skin graft is more risky, in terms of the body accepting the skin, yet it leaves only a scar line on the donor section

Hand Cream

Nothing shows your age like your hands, and nothing works as "our" hands.

Our (camel luxury) revolutionary non-greasy quick penetrating hand treatment with camel milk cosmeceuticals is the first ever product to combine Retinol, sunscreen and active materials (a complex lightening ingredient derived by fermentation of lactic acids with licorice extract). Vitamin A antioxidants in the formula simultaneously strengthen nails, whitens hyper-pigmentation caused by sun, change of hormones or age.

Your hands will look much healthier.

Camel milk is a natural source of Alpha-hydroxyl acids known to plump the skin and smooth fine lines. The preparations pass into the deeper layers of the skin, leaving the outer skin clean and healthy feeling. The fat, lactose, proteins, vitamins and electrolytes all are skin friendly, healthy and safe to use.

The stratum corneum contains a natural mixture of amino acids, lactates, urea and electrolytes, which also help retain water (Shah & Nickerson, 1978).

Skin Health Aspects of Camel Cosmeceuticals

It must be noted that it is accepted practice to state on a product that it has not been tested on animals to prevent the past exploitation of animals for making cosmetics. With camel milk cosmeceuticals the products are a natural secretion of the camels and cause the animals no harm.

Note: the "ceuticals" suggest a healing effect of the camel-milk cosmetics.

Skin disorders that have successfully been used as clinical vignettes with camel-milk cosmeceuticals are:

After successfully treating a child with seemingly incurable Atopic dermatitis by swabbing with camel milk; a cream containing 97% camel milk was introduced and was found to be as effective as the milk. No treated child ever had a recurrence of the dermatitis. However these products had to be stored frozen until used and kept refrigerated when in use (Yurystyn et al, 2014).

Later the cosmetic company, Beauty Treat, overcame the need for cooling and introduced many kinds of cosmeceuticals (personal observation).

CLINICAL VIGNETTES

The skin afflictions cured by camel milk are based on the special quality of camel milk and the knowledge of the diseases themselves. Short explanations about the diseases, the effects of camel-milk cosmeceuticals and its activity are presented below.

After finding that applying camel milk the skin cured Atopic dermatitis it was decided to produce a cream that would provide a suitable application for the many children suffering from this malady. A pharmacist working with camel milk succeeded in making a suitable product based on 96% camel milk. This was as close to milk as possible. The only problem was that it had to be refrigerated to maintain its activity. This was seen by many to be a drawback. However, as eye ointments and other medicinal creams are still kept refrigerated the creams were made and stored appropriately.

One woman with facial acne asked to try the creams. After a while she reported that she experienced skin peeling. After apologizing to her we learned that this, in fact, is desired as it is an ant-aging property much sought after. Thus the cosmetic side of the creams were born.

Contrary to popular belief, cosmetics are not just for the face. Most people don't think beyond nail polish when it comes to cosmetics for the body but actually the reality is that bodily flaws can lessen self-confidence While most people associate concealers with facial flaws, a new generation of solutions for the body has restored the confidence of many women who once found themselves hiding as much skin as possible under heavy clothing.

Spider veins, bruises, burns, stretch marks, scars and birth mark all require cosmetic treatment. Treating them can be considered as beautifying but also as medicinal hence the name of cosmeceuticals, covering both aspects.

Other cosmetic benefits are:

- **Sensitive Skin:** The camel milk products make the skin less sensitive and give a good feeling.

After shave balm calms the skin after shaving, the same as for sensitive skin.

Small amounts of the balm should be gently rubbed onto the face just before shaving and immediately afterwards.

Shampoo gives a soft feeling to the hair and skin feels healthy.

Clinical Benefits

Reports of a few results without mentioning places or names of people.

It must be stressed that in no case did we seek people who fitted our trials but we relied entirely on people who approached us with a skin problem requiring immediate attention. Our professional experience allowed us to decide on treatment regimens.

The preparation of the skin before application:

Taking into account that our skin is rich in bacteria, most of which are good, it is enough to use a clean dry cloth/towel to wipe the area. Do not use soap and water.

If cream is applied with a finger then clean the finger as well with a dry cloth. If another application is used the finger should still be cleaned because it is necessary to massage the cream into the skin.

Small circling movements are used for the massaging. The creams "disappear" into the skin.

REGIMENS FOR TREATMENTS

The preparation should be applied every hour for the first four hours, then twice after 2 hours then at least four times a day until cured.

Burns

The following incident was related to us: A man was on a long drive home in his truck. He stopped when he became aware that the radiator was overheating. He opened the bonnet and opened the cap on the radiator. As a result, the boiling water sprayed over his body, mainly on his chest. He went to the nearest doctor who advised him to go directly to a hospital as he had 3rd degree burns. As his truck was full of products which he had to deliver, he opted to drive another 200 km to his home, phoning to ask a doctor to meet him there. He remembered that he had been given some camel-milk creams which he had with him in his truck so he applied some to his chest. He claims the first application was extremely painful but every half hour he applied more of cream without any pain. When he arrived home the doctor examined him and was surprised to find a reddened skin but no sign of serious burns.

Another time a person riding a motor bike for tens of kilometers bought some creams for his family. After leaving us the chain on his motor bike came loose; while trying to fix it he burned himself badly on the palm of one hand. He was in terrible pain. He put some of the camel cream on the burn and went off to the nearest doctor. The doctor said he had a burn but not a bad one and there was no accompanying pain. No blister or other problem arose afterwards.

A number of women tell of touching a hot frying pan by mistake and getting burns. Application of the camel-milk creams alleviates the pain and the burn rapidly disappears without blistering.

Apply the creams every hour for a few hours. Tehn3 times a day for a few days.

- **Action:** The creams reduce the pain by repairing the damage and prevent infections.

Wounds

Open wound after open fracture: After falling off a ladder in his home, a man suffered an open wound fracture. The fracture was successfully treated with a plate but the open wound proved a problem. It was not repaired by stitching or clamps or even with skin-transplants. It was decided by a plastic surgeon to wait 6 months before attempting closure by long-term slow closing.

Camel-creams were applied directly to open wound, which elicited pain first time but the following applicants had no pain. After 3 days application it was observed that the wound was slowly closing. Each day the length and breadth of the wound was measured.

First there was a closing of the wound then a repair of the scarred skin until nothing was visible of the trauma.

After 6 weeks a visit to the plastic surgeon elicited the response that the wrong leg was shown as there were no signs of the wound.

Wounds after Child-Birth

Often during labor a women must undergo surgery to extend the opening for the new-born to exit. These wounds react very well to the camel-milk cosmeceuticals. Following a caesarean operation it often occurs that the wound opens and the hospital is not responsible for its treatment. Camel-milk cosmeceuticals give a rapid repair of the wounds.

Small wounds i.e. cuts during shaving/Balm prevents infection and has immediate healing of the wounds.

- **Cream Activity:** Pain relief, tissue repair, antibacterial.

It is proposed that an R&D trial be carried out with nanofiber technology to provide a covering for an open wound.

PSORIASIS

If the entire body is affected then drinking the milk is advised.

Localized Psoriasis

Localized on chest: When a man asked for help with localized psoriasis on his chest he was told that as it is a psychosomatic autoimmune disease it was assumed the creams would have no effect. After his desperate request to at least try, his chest was prepared used as written above. A day later there was a great decline in the feeling and reduction of the actual lesions. After 3 days it had cleared up.

After a young boy was successfully treated for localized psoriasis (joints of arms and legs).Before accompanying his parent on a sabbatical to another country where he did not know the language spoken, had no friends and was worried about his studies the parents took a number of creams, which they stored in their freezer.

After a time we received a letter from a woman telling us the following story. Her son developed psoriasis which was spreading all over his body, including his penis. The doctors could not find a way to control it. The mother tells that one day he returned from school to say that there was a new boy in the class who said that he once suffered from psoriasis. The mother contacted the parents who told them of the camel-milk creams. They agreed to give a container of creams to the mother. She writes that this was the only preparation that worked in halting the spread and repairing the existing psoriasis. She asked for more creams that were promptly sent to her.

Unfortunately the attending doctors would not accept the fact that the efficacy of the creams was responsible for the healing.

The activity of the camel-milk creams was due to immediate reduction of the itching, calming the person and then rehabilitating the immune attack on the skin by the antibodies in the creams.

The product should be massaged into the affected areas three times a day after dry cleaning of the area.

DANDRUFF

Camel-milk cosmeceuticals are absorbed into the underlying layers of the skin and repair damaged skin layers. Dandruff has a number of causes: not brushing the hair enough, a yeast WHAT, a fungus and in general a too rapid shedding of skin in the formation of flakes.

Dandruff can be a problem in persons who responsible for treating diseases or surgeons. Caps should be worn to prevent the flakes contaminating other people. Using the camel-shampoo, not necessarily with water and showering but rather 3 times a day rubbing the shampoo into the skin of the head leads to complete disappearance of the dandruff.

EYE INFECTIONS

It is known that a few drops of warm (not heated) camel milk into infected eyes brings relief. This has been shown to work with simple eye infections but also with more complicated ones.

In Africa this is done with breast milk.

HERPES

Oral

Oral herpes is a common infection of the mouth area. It is caused by the herpes simplex virus type 1 (HSV-1). Most people in the United States are infected with this virus by age 20.

After the first infection, the virus goes to sleep (becomes dormant) in the nerve tissues in the face. Sometimes, the virus later wakes up (reactivates), causing cold sores.

Camel-milk cosmeceuticals contain antiviral properties as part of the defense system.

Herpes virus type 2 (HSV-2) most often causes genital herpes. However, sometimes HSV-2 is spread to the mouth during oral sex, causing oral herpes.

Herpes viruses spread most easily from individuals with an active outbreak or sore. This virus may be spread through

- Intimate or personal contact with someone who is infected
- Touching an open herpes sore or something that has been in contact with the herpes virus, such as infected razors, towels, dishes, and other shared items.
- Parents may spread the virus to their children during regular daily activities.

Warning symptoms include:

- Itching of the lips or skin around mouth
- Burning near the lips or mouth area
- Tingling near the lips or mouth area.

With conventional treatment symptoms disappear after a few days. The signs may go away on their own without treatment in 1 to 2 weeks but can recur.

With camel-milk cosmeceuticals the symptoms disappear in a few hours and never return.

Genital Herpes

Genital herpes is a common and highly contagious infection usually spread through sex. This infection is usually caused by the herpes simplex virus-2 (HSV-2) or the herpes simplex virus-1 (HSV-1), the virus usually responsible for cold sores. Genital herpes treatment includes medicines to help sores heal faster and prevent outbreaks.

Genital herpes is common in the United States where about one out of every six people aged 14 to 49 years have genital herpes.

Most people who have herpes have no, or very mild symptoms. You may not notice mild symptoms or you may mistake them for another skin condition, such as a pimple or ingrown hair. Because of this, most people who have herpes do not know it.

Genital herpes sores usually appear as one or more blisters on or around the genitals

The blisters break and leave painful sores that may take weeks to heal. These symptoms are sometimes called "having an outbreak." The first time someone has an outbreak they may also have flu-like symptoms such as fever, body aches, or swollen glands.

To treat the area: Use a dry, clean towel to clean the area as well as the finger used to spread the cream. Gently rubbing camel creams onto the infected area gives rapid relief.

Repeat at least three times a day.

CONJUNCTIVITIS

Primarily caused by infection or allergy, conjunctivitis, better known as "pink eye," is the most common form of eye irritation. It is an inflammation of the white of the eye and eyelid lining, or, technically, inflammation of the conjunctiva, the transparent membrane that lines the inner eyelids and sheaths the globe of the eye. When the eye becomes irritated or infected, the tiny blood vessels dilate and turn red.

Symptoms:

- Redness in the eye
- A burning sensation
- Sensitivity to light
- Dryness
- Grittiness sensation
- Pain
- Itchy, scratchy feeling
- Watering of the eyes
- Sometimes a sticky discharge may cause the eyelashes and eyelids to stick together during sleep.

Bacterial (staph or strep), usually from hand-to-eye contact, and viral infections associated with a cold, sore throat, cold sore or measles, are causes for most conjunctivitis. Viral conjunctivitis tends to clear up of its own accord. Bacterial conjunctivitis produces a yellowish discharge that becomes crusty when you sleep. If the bacterial infection doesn't clear up after four days of using the compresses and other remedies listed below consult your doctor.

As with any infection, you will need to enhance your immune system to fight the infection.

Using camel-milk cosmeceuticals drops into the infected eyes at least 4 times a day will clear it up but should be continued for at least 5 days to prevent recurrence.

The abundant antibodies present in camel milk have shown to kill eye infections, ear infections, heal burns, eczema, and most intriguing of all, even to kill cancer cells,

Use warm (tepid) camel milk as an eyewash or as a compress.

VITILIGO

Vitiligo (vit-ih-LIE-go) is a disease that causes the loss of skin color in blotches. The extent and rate of color loss from vitiligo is unpredictable. It can affect the skin on any part of your body. It may also affect hair, the inside of the mouth and even the eyes.

Normally, the color of hair, skin and eyes is determined by melanin. Vitiligo occurs when the cells that produce melanin die or stop functioning. Melanin produced in middle part of hypophysis.

Research suggests vitiligo may arise from autoimmune conditions.

Camel cosmeceuticals contain substances which act positively on the hypophysis, are antiviral and antibacterial.

The creams should be applied three times a day and continued for two weeks after skin coloring returns to normal.

BODY MASSAGES: FEELING BEAUTY

As Cleopatra used camel milk baths it seems appropriate to consider whole body massages with camel-milk creams.

In all the massage techniques using camel-milk creams adds to the benefits and gives long-term relief.

Massage therapy has been shown to improve flexibility and range of motion, strengthen the immune system and relieve headaches and migraines in women. Research at The Touch Institute of the University of Miami School of Medicine found that massage therapy decreased the occurrence of headaches, sleep disturbances and distress symptoms while increasing serotonin levels in adults with migraine headaches.

VARIOUS TYPES OF MASSAGE

Swedish Massage

Swedish massage therapy is the modality that comes to mind when most people think about massage. As the best-known type of bodywork performed today, one of the primary goals of the Swedish massage technique is to relax the entire body.

But Swedish massage therapy goes beyond relaxation. Swedish massage is exceptionally beneficial for increasing the level of oxygen in the blood, decreasing muscle toxins, improving circulation and flexibility while easing tension.

Deep Tissue Massage

What Is Deep Tissue Massage Therapy?

Deep tissue massage therapy is similar to Swedish massage, but the deeper pressure is beneficial in releasing chronic muscle tension. The focus is on the deepest layers of muscle tissue, tendons and fascia (the protective layer surrounding muscles, bones and joints.)

A study in the Journal of Alternative and Complementary Medicine found that people's blood pressure fell after a single 45 to 60 minute deep tissue massage. Additionally, a 2010 meta-analysis in the Journal of Clinical Psychiatry found that massage modalities like deep tissue reduce stress hormone levels and heart rate while boosting mood and relaxation by triggering the release of oxytocin and serotonin.

Reflexology Massage

Benefits of Reflexology Massage

Reflexology Foot massage can be a deeply relaxing and therapeutic modality for those suffering from plantar fasciitis, ankle injuries or even everyday work and play.

Hot Stone Massage

Hot stone massage therapy melts away tension, eases muscle stiffness and increases circulation and metabolism. Each 1 ½ -hour hot stone massage therapy session promotes deeper muscle relaxation through the placement of smooth, water-heated stones at key points on the body. Our professional massage therapists also incorporate a customized massage, with the use of hot stones which offers enhanced benefits.

Geriatric Massage

Geriatric massage therapy is designed to address the specific needs of the elderly population. This type of massage for the elderly uses gentle and light application of massage techniques and can include passive stretching and a light oil or lotion to permit the muscles to be worked on without causing excessive friction to the skin. These techniques can help enhance blood circulation, combat depression, improve balance and flexibility, reduce the pain of arthritis, increase joint mobility, improve posture, and encourage overall well-being.

All massages should include camel-milk creams. They soften the skin, relieve pain and strengthen the skin.

Spa as Place for Massages

A good place for massages is together with a spa. It reduces and removes mouth wrinkles and laugh lines on the face.

Use a camel face cream by working it into the skin with your fingertips in upward motions. This helps to stimulate circulation, drain fluid from the lymphatic system and reduce the appearance of wrinkles. Camel milk contains natural anti-wrinkle components.

Generally, women are a lot more concerned about health than men. However men deal with all kinds of stress at work too, as well as added pressure from feeling responsible to provide more for their families. It's important for the men to care for their health so they don't age too quickly. A spa with good massage with camel creams gives clean and healthy skin.

ADDITIONS TO CAMEL MILK TO MAKE COSMECEUTICALS

Converting camel milk to cosmeceuticals requires additions of various substances. The choice of additive depends on what want to achieve. They are all organic and non-irritant.

Jojoba Oil: The jojoba plant grows in desert areas. The oil is in great demand for cosmeceuticals. Jojoba can be applied directly to the skin for acne, psoriasis, sunburn, and chapped skin. It is also used topically to encourage the regrowth of hair in people who are balding. Jojoba is used as an ingredient in shampoo; lipstick; makeup; cleansing products and in face, hand, and body lotions. Jojoba, when applied to the skin, is an emollient, which soothes skin and unclogs hair follicles.

Avocado Oil Avocado is a hidden treasure. Unlike the well-known tea tree oil, olive oil and lavender oil, avocado oil has yet to be discovered by many people for its great variety of health benefits. Among other things, avocado oil can be used as a beneficial skin care product, for special scalp treatments, medicinal purposes. Avocado oil is high in a substance called sterolin, which studies have shown to facilitate the softening of the skin and to reduce the incidence of age spot.;

Avocado oil is rich in antioxidants, making it useful for healing sun-damaged skin. Antioxidants like vitamins A, D and E in avocado cause the skin to be suppler, and are thus particularly good for dry or aged skin.

Avocado oil contains lecithin and potassium, which are all highly beneficial for the skin as well as the hair.

The other benefits of avocado oil are the fats but they are very similar to the fat found in camel milk.

Palm Oil is used for manufacturing cosmetics, soaps.

ANTIWRINKLE MOISTURIZING CREAMS

Besides camel milk the main ingredients are:

- **Ginseng Ext:** Different varieties of ginseng root have been used as treatments in Asia and North America for centuries. Ginseng is one of the most popular herbal medicines in the world.
- **Portulaca Oieracea Ext:** Portulaca oleracea (common purslane, also known as verdolaga, pigweed, little hogweed, red root, pursley, and moss rose) is an annual succulent in the family Portulacaceae, which may reach 40 cm in height.
- **Centella Asiatica Ext:** Centella asiatica, commonly known as centella and gotu kola, is a small, herbaceous, annual plant of the family Mackinlayaceae or subfamily Mackinlayoideae of family Apiaceae, and is native to wetlands in Asia.[2][3] It is used as a medicinal herb in Ayurvedic medicine, traditional African medicine, and traditional Chinese medicine. It is also known as the Asiatic pennywort or Indian pennywort in English.
- Simmondsia Chinensis Seed Oil.
- Persea Gratissima Oil organ.
- Olive Oil - Olea Europaea Oil organ.
- Palm Oil – Hydrogenated Palm Oil organ.
- Vitamin E – Tocopherol.

EYE-CREAM

- Cera Alba.
- Olive Oil - Olea Europaea Oil organic.
- Jojoba Oil - Simmondsia Chinensis Seed Oil organic.
- Avocado Oil - Persea Gratissima Oil organic.
- Almond Oil - Prunus Amygdalus Dulcis Oil organic.
- Wheat germ Oil - Triticum Vulgare Germ Oil organic.
- Carrot Seed Oil - Daucus Carota Sativa Seed Oil organic.
- Grape Seed Oil - Vitis Vinifera Seed Oil organic.
- Palm Oil – Hydrogenated Palm Oil organ organic.

- Shea Oil - Butyrospermum Parkii Oil organic.
- Vitamin E – Tocopherol.
- Fragrance.

SORES ABRASIONS

- Camel milk.
- Grape Seed Oil - Vitis Vinifera Seed Oil organic.
- Almond Oil - Prunus Amygdalus Dulcis Oil organic.
- Cera Alba.
- Olive Oil - Olea Europaea Oil organic.
- Palm Oil – Hydrogenated Palm Oil organic.
- Seaweed Spiralina.
- Tea Tree Oil - Melaleuca Alternifolia Leaf Oil organic.
- Lavender oil - Lavandula Angustifolia Oil organic.
- Vitamin E – Tocopherol.

GENITAL TRACT PROBLEMS

The vulva (Latin for womb or covering) consists of several layers that cover and protect the sexual organs and urinary opening. The fleshy outer lips of the vulva — the labia majora — are covered with pubic hair and contain fat that helps cushion the area. Inside the labia majora are the thinner, more pigmented and delicate flaps of skin called the labia minora.

Few physicians specialize in vulvar problems, and few medical schools provide much training in this field.

Crohn's disease, a chronic inflammatory intestinal disease, may cause abscesses or draining fistulas in the vulvar area, and vulvar skin problems are often one of its early symptoms. A mouth condition called lichen planus is another cause of vulva problems. (The term "lichen," as applied to skin disorders, refers fancifully to skin lesions that resemble lichen on rocks.) Long-term treatment with oral steroids, immune suppressants, or antibiotics also raises the risk for vulvar skin infection.

The vulva is the external part of a woman's genitals.

A woman may routinely pamper her face and work hard to keep it moisturized and irritation-free, but little is done for the more sensitive skin of her vulva, the external genital area surrounding her vagina?

Many women have been primed to think no further than "itch equals yeast infection." But with age and the decline in estrogen after menopause, we become more prone to a variety of conditions that irritate vulvar skin. These conditions aren't getting the medical attention they need — and women aren't getting the relief they deserve.

Some problems with the vulvar area include:

- Bacterial or fungal infections.
- Skin problems due to allergy.

- Vulvar cancer.
- Vulvodynia, or vulvar pain.

Symptoms may include redness, itching, pain, or cracks in the skin. Treatment depends on the cause.

Camel creams gently massaged into dry-cleaned skin removes itch and any other skin problem. It leaves vulva smooth and clean.

Vulval and vaginal problems in young girls often result in pruritus vulvae (itch affecting the female genital area). Causes and treatments differ slightly between prepubertal females and mature women.

The prepubertal vulva is thin, delicate, and has a neutral pH, meaning it is easily irritated.

Due to relatively high concentrations of vitamin C in camel=milk creams the pH is lowered, enhancing beneficial effects. Vitamin C is ascorbic acid. The sensitive skin and irritation are countered. Girls can apply the camel creams themselves at least twice-a-day.

Primary skin disease such as atopic dermatitis, seborrheic dermatitis, psoriasis, and lichen sclerosis may affect the vulva.

Infestations with pinworms, move from anus to vulva.

The vulva is subject to a range of skin problems, many of them inadvertently self-inflicted.

Many women have been primed to think no further than "itch equals yeast infection." But with age and the decline in estrogen after menopause, women become more prone to a variety of conditions that irritate vulvar skin. These conditions do not get the medical attention they need — and women aren't getting the relief they deserve.

BOYS' GENITAL PROBLEMS

Young boys can suffer from infections of the fore-skin. Jewish boys do not have this problem as the circumcision carried out at 8 days old removes the fore-skin.

It must be noted that the loss of the foreskin apparently reduces greatly the contraction of cervical cancer in women.

The foreskin should be gently cleaned in and out, best with a soft Q-tip. Apply the camel cream by hand by gently rubbing it into and around the fore-skin. Repeat every 2 hours for 5 times per day. The infection should clear up after the first day. Afterwards give the fore-skin a daily cleaning with warm soap and water.

1. There is a definite trend of camel-milk cosmeceuticals to enhance body beautifying activities.
2. There is a definite activity of camel-milk cosmeceuticals to cure many skin problems.
3. The activity of the camel-milk cosmeceuticals is rapid, curing many skin afflictions.

DANDRUFF

Simple dry skin is the most common cause of itchy, flaking dandruff. Oils and skin cells from the scalp can build up, causing dandruff (Benjamin, 2015). A yeast-like fungus (malassezia) lives on the scalps of most healthy adults without causing problems. But sometimes it grows out of control, feeding on the oils secreted by the hair follicles.

Massaging camel-milk shampoo rapidly into the scalp overcomes dandruff by rejuvenating the skin.

ACNE

Acne comes in different forms

- Mild acne, which refers to the whiteheads or blackheads that many people get at various times
- Moderate acne, which includes red inflamed pimples called papules and red pimples with white centers called pustules
- Severe acne, which causes nodules — painful, pus-filled cysts or lumps — to appear under the skin

The papules and pustules are removed by the skin repairing mechanisms and the bacteria are killed by the camel milk. The scars are repaired by the cell repairing properties in camel milk.

ACNE SCARS /SCARS IN GENERAL

Scars from acne may seem like double punishment — first having to deal with the pimples, now you have marks as a reminder (Goodman, 2006). Acne lesions or pimples occur when the hair follicles (or "pores") on the skin become plugged with oil and dead skin cells. A plugged follicle is the perfect place for bacteria to grow and create the red bumps and pus-filled red bumps known as pimples.

Lactoferrin, found in camel milk, is one of the most powerful natural antioxidants known. It can help destroy acne-causing bacteria and assist with cell growth promotion, and also has anti-inflammatory properties. As mentioned before, camel cosmeceuticals contain powerful antibacterial and antifungal factors, including lactoferrin, and can unplug blocked pores therefore they are effective against acne and the scar formation.

Burns are healed by the prevention of infections by the protective proteins; the skin healing activity creates an effective repair of the outer layer of the skin, preventing fluid loss. It has been reported that there is a rapid loss of pain (B Yagil personal observation, April, 2015).

Among the burns repaired by camel-cosmeceuticals are sun-burns.

Diaper rash is quickly overcome by applying camel milk cosmeceuticals whenever changing diapers.

Sore/cracked nipples during breast feeding- The mother can get relief when camel milk cosmeceuticals are gently massaged into the nipples before and after breast feeding. This does not cause changes in taste of the milk itself. Serious, open wounds are healed in a relatively short space of time. This is due to the anti-infectious components and the skin healing proteins.

Hemorrhoids are still considered a skin problem because a finger can reach the troubled spot. If not thrombosed, external hemorrhoids may cause few problems. However, when thrombosed, hemorrhoids may be very painful. A skin tag may remain after healing. If hemorrhoids are large and cause issues with hygiene, they may produce irritation of the surrounding skin, and thus itchiness around the anus.

After cleaning the area well with soap and water, gently massage camel milk cosmeceuticals into, and around, the painful area. After the first time, the swelling and pain diminish.

ATOPIC DERMATITIS

As mentioned before, the reason for making camel milk cosmeceuticals was based on finding that camel milk cures Atopic dermatitis in a short space of time.

The disease is not only rapidly overcome in children, even those with extreme itchy skins, but never returned in the past 10 years. In adults it is more difficult and time consuming. It is better to combine drinking camel milk with using some of the milk directly on the skin. The creams should be made with over 95% milk.

LOCALIZED PSORIASIS

The creams are very effective against localized psoriasis (general psoriasis requires drinking the camel milk). However, it should be noted that psoriasis is not only an autoimmune disease, which is controlled by drinking camel milk but is also a psychosomatic disease; recurring stress can create renewed flair-up of the psoriasis. Localized psoriasis affects certain body areas and the camel cosmeceuticals have been found to be very effective in curing the symptoms until further stress occurs. Recurring psoriasis can, therefore, be kept in check. The effectiveness is due to the antibodies in the creams being active "on site" and in the tissue repair substances.

TOES: TINEA PEDIS

Tinea pedis is a fungal infection of the feet, most frequently affecting the spaces between toes (inter-digital spaces).

It is transmitted by human to human contact in warm humid environments, for example through shared towels and on wet floors in swimming pools, changing rooms and gymnasia.

The antifungal properties in camel cosmeceuticals rapidly heal the fungus.

BREASTS

As breasts are considered "breast glands" surgery on them or to remove them is relatively simple. The same hormones that affect water metabolism also affect initiation and maintenance of lactation. This explains why the breasts of highly pregnant women suffering heat stress often secrete a liquid. It must be noted that breast milk contains large numbers of bacteria, required for a developing immune system and proper function of the infant's intestinal tract.

BACTRIAN (Camelus bactrianus) is the two-humped camel. The main difference between the milk of the one and two-humped camels is the high fat content of the latter animals. In the Bactrian camel the fat % can reach 12% as extra fat is required for the young living in cold climates. Use of creams has been found to have similar results as for the dromedary creams.

STEROIDS

Topical corticosteroids have been used for about 50 years, since the 1950s and their introduction was a milestone in dermatology (Tadicherla S, Ross K, Shenefelt PD, Fenske NA 2009). They are used to treat inflammatory skin conditions by suppressing the inflammatory reaction and relieving symptoms. However, they are not curative.

Note! Camel-milk cosmeceuticals not only combat infections but activate the defense response which also enhances the immune system activity, the opposite to steroid activity.

An Interesting finding was reported end June 2015 in which it was stated that a man being prepared for stem-cell treatment had pain in his legs (personal communication. Winter, Canada. June 2015). He massaged the camel-milk creams into his legs. This reduced the pain but also had an added benefit – it "led" to the stem-cell recovery taking a third of the time and getting double the amount of stem cells. This suggests that the immune activity mentioned in camel milk creams had a positive response in the body – an addition of a drug in a non-conventional way. This is also in agreement with the "New" idea of immune-treatment for treating cancer patients. The immune-activating activity in camel milk was previously described (Yagil, 2013).

SKIN ANTIBODIES

Two types of skin autoantibodies that detect different skin components are:

- Intercellular cement substance (Pemphigus antibodies)
- Basement membrane antibodies (Pemphigoid antibodies).

Facts about Pemphigus

The immune system manufactures antibodies, which attack viruses and harmful bacteria. With pemphigus, however, antibodies instead attack healthy cells in the skin or mucous. Camel milk has proven to be very effective in combatting pemphigus.

The Benefits of Raw Milk Cosmetics by Marcela De Vivo (2013)

Raw milk is natural and unmodified by any chemicals – unlike store-bought milk. Pasteurized (or "sterilized") milk does not have any beneficial activity on the skin because, as earlier explained, human skin contains many thousands of bacteria? Children in the past crawled on the floor and outside, putting their fingers in their mouths. This built up their immune systems. Nowadays practice of "sterility" has led to children suffering from many immune deficient problems.

The cells thought to be responsible for picking up the bacteria and transporting them to the breast are the dendritic cells. In non-breastfeeding people they are used to transport bacteria and bits of bacteria to the rest of the immune system to prepare a defense, and can sometimes carry entire live bacteria. Recent studies have shown that in mice bacteria from the gut translocate into lymph nodes and mammary glands during the late stages of pregnancy and the beginning of lactation. It has also been shown that if breastfeeding women are given a capsule of live (and safe!) bacteria to swallow, these bacteria can be isolated later from the breast milk (Wiley, 2013).

The aim of this chapter in a Handbook of Research on Novel Approaches for Drug Delivery is to provide relevant knowledge. Again I emphasize that the most important group who require this knowledge are the officials who decide on regulations for the marketing of cosmeceuticals. The FDA does not have to approve or review cosmetics, or what goes in them, before they are sold to the consumers (FDA, 2015). They must not be unsafe for their users. The camel milk cosmeceuticals are completely safe. Hopefully publications, like the present one, will educate the bureaucrats who show the 3-monkey syndrome of camel milk cosmeceuticals: "see nothing good; hear nothing good; say nothing good" As previously stated - they should realize the human skin is home to billions of bacteria" (De Noon, 2009). There is a growing body of research that suggests we should be thankful for that.

Dermatological research suggests that the bioactive ingredients used in cosmeceuticals have benefits beyond the traditional moisturizer. However, despite reports of benefits from some cosmeceutical products, there are no requirements to prove that these products live up to their claims.

If you are healthy, have a good immune system and the correct balance of skin microbiota – flora, the microorganisms that live on the skin – your chances of keeping pathogens under control are high. But if you are ill, have a weak immune system or the condition of your skin is compromised in any way, that is not the case. Of course when the skin is damaged then more demands are posed for safe and effective cosmeceuticals.

METHODS OF ADMINISTRATION OF CAMEL-MILK COSMECEUTICALS

- Creams – after gently washing the hands with camel-milk soaps- can be directly administered into open wounds.
- Spray canisters – after gentle cleaning of skin.
- Shampoo.

Damaged skin is an open door for infections. "Just look at burns victims," Power says. "They are very vulnerable to infections because their skin, their safety suit, is damaged."

The same thing happens if the skin is broken for some reason. Normally harmless bacteria penetrate to the inner layers, where they can cause chaos. That is when the application of a suitable cosmeceutical is imperative.

It must be noted that clinical trials constitute an excellent way to examine the efficacy of new drugs. However, camel milk has been used for ill people from the time that the prophet Mohammed advised ill people to drink it, thousands of years ago (Khan, 1974).

OTHER MAMMALIAN MILK USED AS COSMECEUTICALS

Breast Milk

It often is assumed that breast milk is sterile (no bacteria). However, in fact, breast milk contains a large amount of bacteria, which are essential for a child's development of his/her immune system and intestinal health. Scientists have discovered that breast milk contains more species of bacteria than originally expected — up to 1000 varieties (Gould, 2013).

The abundant antibodies present in breast milk have shown to kill eye and ear infections, heal burns and eczema, and most fascinating even kill cancer cells (Spatz, 2014).

Even though in Africa it is common to use breast milk itself for treating eye infections, new research has proven that breast milk, made into a lotion, is the latest alternative form of treatment for eczema, psoriasis, sunburns and itchy dry skin (Gauss, 2012). Although the idea of rubbing breast milk on your skin may seem rather unconventional, it is proving to be a safe and sometime superior treatment to other medicinal options. The antibodies found in breast milk will help aid in the onset of infection that can be secondary to persistent scratching.

There have been many discussions about creating banks of breast milk for infants whose mothers cannot, or prefer not to, breast feed. It will be imperative to establish that donors do not smoke, take any medications and have no diseases. This is important as it has been was found that breast-feeding women suffering from Mycobacterium avium paratuberculosis (MAP) infections – Crohn's Disease - excrete the bacteria in their milk (Yagil, 2013).

If this comes about it won't be long before breast milk will be used as cosmeceuticals. However, expressed breast milk must be rapidly frozen to prevent changes occurring.

Taking into account these data it is surprising that breast-milk banks pasteurize their milk Pasteurizing with the Holder Method (LTLT) involves heating the milk to 62.5°C/144.5°F and holding this for 30 minutes. Milk is gently heated in a shaking water bath using the Holder Method of pasteurization. Methods of pasteurization milk which eliminate bacteria while retaining the majority of the milk's beneficial components will be essential.

It is essential to stress the fact that bacteria are found in large numbers all over the human body wherever there is a channel to the outside world, for example in the gut, lungs, and surface of the skin. It is still believed by many persons, including doctors, that the inside of the human body is a bacteria-free environment unless an infection is raging. Again, it should be noted that as a product which is made within the human body like breast milk was rich in bacteria although it was traditionally thought to be sterile.

Recent studies have shown that in mice bacteria from the gut translocate into lymph nodes and mammary glands during the late stages of pregnancy and the beginning of lactation. It has also been shown that if breastfeeding women are given a capsule of live (and safe!) bacteria to swallow, these bacteria can be isolated later from the breast milk, as was the case, previously described, when mothers suffering from paratuberculosis secreted the bacteria in their milk.

Breast milk has been placed onto cuts, burns and small wounds to prevent infection and enhance skin healing. Breast milk has also applied to the skin to provide relief from insect bites, bee stings, chicken pox, poison ivy, poison oak and poison sumac. It has been used as a moisturizer to treat dry skin and eczema. It has also been used to relieve chapped lips, loosen cradle cap, and treat diaper rash: If rubbed into sore, cracked nipples, it is thought to relieve pain, prevent infection, and assist in healing.

Natural Ways to Maintain Beautiful, Youthful Body Skin (Rao, K 2013)

- Drink plenty of water.
- Eat foods with antioxidants
- Opt for natural skin products.
- Use non-toxic cleaning products
- Get enough vitamin C.

Although breast-milk cosmeceuticals may seem a good idea practically there are many drawbacks, the main being selection of suitable donors. This includes the age of the donors, their race, their origin and other factors, all of which could limit the use of their milk.

EQUINE MILK COSMECEUTICALS

Mare and Donkey Milk

Equus is a genus of mammals in the family Equidae, which includes horses, asses, and zebras.

Horse (Mare) Milk

Horse milk is becoming big business due to the upsurge in breeding horses (Burleson J.)

The first reason for the recent popularity of horse milk is not for cosmetics but for the medical aspects, especially for metabolic, gastrointestinal and liver problems, but also for recovering after surgery and severe illness, cholesterol problems, allergy to cows' milk, stress, skin problems, stiff joints or just to keep fit and well. Mare milk is certainly better than goat or cow milk but is similar to camel milk.

Mare milk supposedly strengthens the body, boosts the immune system and increases a person's energy and vitality. In the case of metabolic disorders, it stimulates internal cleansing, again, similar to the activity of camel milk.

As mare milk is high in vitamins that can be easily absorbed by the skin and stimulates skin saturation, the liquid has a very beneficial effect on human skin and hair (van der Burg et al, 2011). Horse milk contains chemicals that stimulate cell renewal and give the skin more resistance. Horse milk cosmetics, which contain a high percentage of horse milk, are therefore ideal for daily skin cleansing and hair care. People with dry, sensitive or problem skin types will, in particular, benefit from horse milk cosmetics. We do not animal test our products or ingredients.

Genghis Khan already knew about the effects of mare milk which he associated with the strength of his warriors, the health of his children and the beauty of his women.

Almost all cultures around the world keep a tight relationship between natural cosmetics, medicine and beauty (Jomana, 2015). Ancient cultures told us about the usage of mare milk for beauty purposes. In Central Europe, people cherished its healing effects. Already in ancient Rome, a bath with mare milk was luxury in times of considerable decadence. Nowadays we are able to afford this luxury again, as horse breeding is becoming very popular. Creams and lotions made from mare milk pamper our skin with the effects known for many centuries. Mare milk is a valuable treasure from nature. Its unique active ingredients support the human metabolism, the regeneration and regulation of the skin. The pH value of mare milk is similar to the one of the human skin and therefore ideal for the treatment of irritated and sensitive skin.

Mares' milk oil is considered an ingredient in Mongolian cosmetics because of its high content of polyunsaturated fatty acids which make it readily absorbed by human skin (Smaji, Soetaredja, & Ayeitra,, 2015).

The only drawback is that horses have only two teats and produce little milk, besides what the foal requires. Maintenance of horses is time consuming and requires good food and water.

Donkey (Ass) Milk

It is generally believed that asses' milk effaces wrinkles in the face, renders the skin more delicate, and preserves its whiteness: and it is a well-known fact, that some women are in the habit of washing their face with it seven times daily, strictly observing that number.

Donkey/asses' milk cosmetics have long been known (Yeomans, 2015).

Ass milk was in common use because it was readily available in farm animals.

CONCLUSION

Equine milk has cosmeceutical properties but the availability of the mare milk is problematical. Horses also require good food and much water. They also give relatively little milk through two teats and what is available usually just suffices for their offspring.

Cow Milk, Goat Milk

Cow milk is used for making cosmetics (McDougall, 2011).

A spa hotel in Germany is specializing in cow milk for a number of masks, creams and treatments claiming that these products have a regulating and regenerative effect on the skin.

Raw milk is natural and unmodified by any chemicals –unlike store-bought milk. Pasteurized (or "sterilized") milk is altered with added protein, and lactose. Conclusion: heating cow milk damages many beneficial properties for health, within and out of the body.

Goat milk protects the cell and influences cell regeneration positively. It contains high amounts of vitamins (A, B1, B2, C, D), minerals (Calcium, Sodium, Magnesium) and moisturizing factors such as Panthenol. Precious oils protect the skin from premature aging and soften the skin. The latest research on goat milk proves the importance of goat milk and its ingredients such as Coenzymes Q10 and more than 70 unsaturated fatty acids. Due to its low melting point of 37 Degrees Celsius goat butter can be absorbed easily also into the deeper layers of our skin. This has a positive impact on the absorption of highly effective natural essences (deJohn, 2012).

General Conclusions

The author has chosen suitable references but more data are available on the Internet.

When considering application of a healing substance to the skin, when it is whole and when the outer layer(s) is missing, it is advantageous to choose a natural, biological substance. The most obvious is milk.

The pros and cons of the various milks are presented above. It must be remembered that the specific milk is attuned to the young of that species and, therefore, has special qualities for those young.

In most cases the acquisition of the milk requires special housing, food, water sources and attention. Mothers' milk appears to be a good choice but there are so many medical and social demands that most milk is discarded. In addition there appears to be a reluctance to turn a breast-feeding woman into "a cow". Horse milk is a good solution but horses provide little milk (have only 2 teats), require good food, much water and much attention.

Camel milk is close to mothers' milk. Camel milk comes from animals adapted to marginal areas of the world. They require little food and food of poorer quality than of other animals. The price of camel milk is high so cosmeceuticals are economically attractive. There is a great upsurge in America to farm camels, even by those who no virtually nothing about managing them.

The components of camel milk are skin friendly, do not leave fatty stains and are readily absorbed through the skin. Camel milk cosmeceuticals also repair damaged skin and prevent the loss of liquids and prevent infections. Camel milk can be frozen and thawed, which other milks cannot, therefore can be stored until made into cosmeceuticals. This is a definite advantage.

Of all milks available as cosmeceuticals camel milk is readily available in marketable amounts, over 15 liters per camel per day (Yagil, 2013) all over the world.

It is not enough to make the products but there must be an understanding about the milk itself and what can be added to guarantee an efficient activity, be it for beautifying the skin or activity against a skin problem.

The medical world is finally confronting the evidence that we are surrounded, in and out, with bacteria. It is the "good" bacteria which initiate and maintain our immune system to function for our protection. Science should find how to nourish our "good" bacteria and not destroy them and then face the consequences of this folly. Camel milk immunoglobulins appear to be active on and in the skin.

It is convenient to accept the assumption that vigorous ant-bacterial activities in surgery wards in hospitals has allowed the upsurge of "bad bacteria" creating then problem of infections associated with sterile surgery.

For any help or suggestions the author is only an e-mail away.

My proclamation to the bureaucrats who deal with licensing camel-milk cosmeceuticals.

I have stated in this chapter that I, personally have been confronted by the complete incompetency of those making demands for licensing the products. An example was the demand that the milk must be pasteurized and that this must be confirmed by the "phosphatase test".

First of all the mere pasteurizing will destroy all bacteria, not only the pathogens, thus making it worthless based on the vast number of bacteria present on the skin, measured in trillions (De Noon, 2009). They should give more thought as how to prepare the skin for application. Pathogen-free milk should be the aim so that the cosmeceuticals will provide another pathogen-reducer because of the XX between the non-pathogen and pathogen-free (as explained in the article.

Secondly, and very important, the phosphatse test is not used in camels as even boiling the milk does not reduce phosphatase. This in contrast to goat milk which does not have phosphatase from the beginning so that any of its milk will show that it is pasteurized.

As far as possible the references are taken from the Internet as well as from the actual articles. The use of the Internet is a quick and easy way to keep a scientist up-to-date.

The strict demand that "medical" or "treatment" should not be used is nulled by the shown effects of the cosmeceuticals – as the name suggests.

Their incompetence comes from their strict following that "none are so blind as those that do not see". It is possible to find sensible restrictions to prevent con-men marketing bad products but that is not in the realm of the present officials.

REFERENCES

Begoun, P. (2003). *Don't Go to the Cosmetics Counter without Me*. Retrieved 13.6.2015, from www.paulas choice.com/expert-advice/sensitive-skin/fragrance-and-skin-care-smells-like-trouble

Benjamin, J. (2015). *Surprising Facts About Dandruff*. Retrieved 22.6.2015, from http://www.everydayhealth.com/news

Burg van der, L.J., Muller, I., & Sloet van Oldruitenborgh-Oosterbaan, M.M. (2011). Horse milking industry in The Netherlands and Flanders. *Tijdschrift voor Diergeneeskunde*, *136*, 257–261. PMID:21534278

Burleson, J. (n.d.). *Horse Milk*. Retrieved 10.6.2015, from http://www.burleson-arabians.com/horse_milk

Charkoudian, N. (2003). Skin blood flow in adult human thermoregulation: How it works, when it does not, and why. *Mayo Clinic Proceedings*, *78*(5), 603–612. doi:10.4065/78.5.603 PMID:12744548

Combs, T. (2015). *Animal Ingredients – What is Lactoferrin?* Retrieved 12.6.2015, from http://www.logicalharmony.net/animal-ingredients-what-is-lactoferrin

De John, A. (2012). *Benefits of goat milk acknowledged by beauty industry*. Retrieved 13.6.2105, from http://www.cosmeticsdesign.com/Market-Trends/Benefits-of-goat-s-milk-acknowledged-by-beauty-industry

De Noon, D. J. (2009). Human Skin Alive With Bacteria. *WebMD News Archive*. Retrieved 12.6.2015, from http://www.webmd.com/skin-problems-and-treatments/news/

De Vivo, M. (2013). The Benefits Of Raw Milk Cosmetics. *HelaD*. Retrieved 12.6.2015, from http://www.helladelicious.com/our-food/2013/03/the-benefits-of-raw-milk-cosmetics

Derbyshire, D. (n.d.). How your wrinkle cream could destroy. *Mail Online*. Retrieved 12.6.2015, from http://www.dailymail.co.uk/femail/article-2359596/How-wrinkle-cream-destroy-skin-Chemicals-cosmetics-trigger-severe-allergies.html#ixzz3Zj8FRcMf

Escott-Stump, S. (Ed.). (2008). *Nutrition and Diagnosis-Related Care* (6th ed.). Philadelphia: Wolters Kluwer Health Lippincott Williams & Wilkins.

Fahey, J. W., Haristoy, X., Dolan, P. M., Kensler, T. W., Scholtus, I., Stephenson, K. K., & Lozniewski, A. et al. (2002). Sulforaphane inhibits extracellular, intracellular, and antibiotic-resistant strains of Helicobacter pylori and prevents benzopyrene-induced stomach tumors. *Proceedings of the National Academy of Sciences of the United States of America*, *99*(11), 7610–7615. doi:10.1073/pnas.112203099 PMID:12032331

FDA-U.S. Food and Drug Administration Protecting and Promoting Your Health. (2015). Retrieved 1.6.2015, from http://www.fda.gov/cosmetics/guidanceregulation/default.htm

Gauss, D. (2012). *Breast Milk Lotion Recipe*. Retrieved 12.6.215, from http://www.justbreastfeeding.com/benefits-to-breastfeeding/breast-milk-lotion-recipe

Gibbs, W. (2005). Camel natural nanobodies. *Scientific American*, *293*(2), 78–83. doi:10.1038/scientificamerican0805-78 PMID:16053141

Gloor, M., Fluhr, J., Lehmann, L., Gehring, W., & Thieroff-Ekerdt, R. (2002). (20020. Do urea/ammonium lactate combinations achieve better skin protection and hydration than either component alone? *Skin Pharmacology and Applied Skin Physiology*, *15*(1), 35–43. doi:10.1159/000049387 PMID:11803256

Goldfaben, G. (2009). *Revitalize Aging Skin with Topical Vitamin C*. Life Extension Magazine.

Goodman, G. J. (2011). Treatment of acne scarring. *International Journal of Dermatology*, *50*(10), 1179–1194. doi:10.1111/j.1365-4632.2011.05029.x PMID:21950285

Gopan, A. (2014). *Sunheal*. Retrieved 15.6.2015, from http://goarticles.com/article/SUNHEAL-Best-for-Sun-Protection/9522049

Gould, S. E. (2013). The bacteria in breast milk. *Scientific American*, 7.

Hamers-Casterman, C., Atarouch, T., Muyldermans, S., Bendolman, N., & Hamers, R. (1993). Naturally occurring antibodies devoid of light chains. *Nature*, *363*(6428), 446–448. doi:10.1038/363446a0 PMID:8502296

Jomana. (2015). *Welcome to the World of Nature*. Retrieved 12.6.2015, fromhttp://www.s-jomana.com/eng

Kanodia, S., Fahey, L., Kast, W., & Martin-Kast, W. (2007). Mechanisms Used by Human Papillomaviruses to Escape the Host Immune Response. *Current Cancer Drug Targets*, *7*(1), 79–89. doi:10.2174/156800907780006869 PMID:17305480

Khan, M. M. (1974). Sahihal_Bukhari.The translation of the Meanings of the Koran. *Sahih Bukhari Book*, *7*, 582–590.

Maliepaard, M., Nofziger, C., Papaluca, M., Zineh, I., Uyama, Y., Prasad, K., & Paulmichl, M. et al. (2013). Pharmacogenetics in the evaluation of new drugs: A multiregional regulatory perspective. *Nature Reviews. Drug Discovery*, *12*(2), 103–115. doi:10.1038/nrd3931 PMID:23370249

McDougall, A. (2011). *Sustainable beauty the main theme at in-cosmetics*. Cosmetics design-Europe.com.

Mercola. (2009). *Top 12 Foods for Healthy Immune Response*. Retrieved 4.6.2015, from http://articles.mercola.com/sites/articles

Mindful Minerals. (n.d.). Retrieved 13.6.2015, from https://mindfulminerals.com

Muyldermans, S., Cambilla, C., & Wyns, L. (2001). Recognition of antigens by single-domain antibody, fractions: The superfluous luxury of paired domains. *Trends in Biochemical Sciences*, *26*(4), 230–235. doi:10.1016/S0968-0004(01)01790-X PMID:11295555

Piceno, J. (2011). *Smooth as silk skin. Cleopatra bathing in camel milk*. Retrieved 5.6.2015, from https://jenpiceno.wordpress.com/tag/cleopatras-beauty-secrets

Rao. (2013). *Maintaining good skin*. Retrieved 13.6.2015, from http://www.mindbodygreen.com/0-8355/15-natural-ways-to-maintain-beautiful-youthful-skin.html

Reshetnikov, S. V., Wasser, S. P., Duckman, I., & Tsukor, K. (2000). Medicinal value of the genus Tremella Pers. (Heterobasidiomycetes) (review). *International Journal of Medicinal Mushrooms*, *2*(3), 345–367. doi:10.1615/IntJMedMushr.v2.i3.10

Shah, N. O., & Nickerson, T. A. (1978). Functional properties of hydrolyzed lactose: Solubility, viscosity and humectant properties. *Journal of Food Science*, *43*(4), 1081–1084. doi:10.1111/j.1365-2621.1978.tb15238.x

Smaji, S., Soetaredja, F. E., & Ayeitra, A. (2015). Green chemistry for sustainability. In S. K. Sharma (Ed.), *SpringerBriefs in molecular science*. Springer SBM.

Soberman, R. J., & Christmas, P. (2003). The organization and consequences of eicosanoid signaling. *The Journal of Clinical Investigation*, *111*(8), 1107–1113. doi:10.1172/JCI200318338 PMID:12697726

Spatz, D. L. (2014). Changing Institutional Culture to Value Human Milk. *Advances in Neonatal Care*, *14*(4), 234–235. doi:10.1097/ANC.0000000000000128 PMID:25075920

Tadicherla, S., Ross, K., Shenefelt, P. D., & Fenske, N. A. (2009). Article. *Journal of Drugs in Dermatology*, *8*, 1093–1105. PMID:20027937

Wiley's Global Research. (2013). *Breast is best: Good bacteria arrive from mum's gut via breast milk*. Retrieved from www.sciencedaily.com

Yagil, R. (2000). Lactation in Camels. In T. K. Gahlot (Ed.), *Selected Topics on Camelids* (pp. 61–72). Bikaner, India: The Camel Publishers.

Yagil, R. (2013). Comparative Alternative Medicinal (CAM) Properties in Camel Milk for Treatment of Epidemic' Diseases. *Journal of Agricultural Science and Technology.*, *A3*, 575–580.

Yeomans, M. (2015). *Donkey milk cosmetics*. Retrieved 13.6.2015, from http://www.cosmeticsdesign-asia.com/Market-Trends/Donkey-milk-cosmetics-creme-de-la-creme-for-Asian-consumers

Yurystyn, E., Etzion, Z., van Creveld, C., & Yagil, R. (2014). Camel milk cosmeceuticals for comparative alternative medicine. *J Med. and Med. Res*, *2*, 8–12.

Zhang, L. J., Guerrero-Juarez, C. F., Hata, T., Bapat, S. P., Ramos, R., Plikus, M. V., & Gallo, R. L. (2015). Innate immunity. Dermal adipocytes protect against invasive Staphylococcus aureus skin infection. *Science*, *347*(6217), 67–71. doi:10.1126/science.1260972 PMID:25554785

Section 7

Red Blood Cells

Chapter 12
Resealed Erythrocytes as Drug Carriers and Its Therapeutic Applications

Prabhakar Singh
University of Allahabad, India

Sudhakar Singh
Kolkata Medical College, India

Rajesh Kumar Kesharwani
NIMS University, India

ABSTRACT

In this pharma innovative world, there are more than 30 drug delivery systems. Today's due to lacking the target specificity, the present scenario about drug delivery is emphasizing towards targeted drug delivery systems. Erythrocytes are the most common type of blood cells travel thousands of miles from wide to narrow pathways to deliver oxygen, drugs and nutrient during their lifetime. Red blood cells have strong and targeted potential carrier capabilities for varieties of drugs. Drug-loaded carrier erythrocytes or resealed erythrocytes are promising for various passive and active targeting. Resealed erythrocyte have advantage over several drug carrier models like biocompatibility, biodegradability without toxic products, inert intracellular environment, entrapping potential for a variety of chemicals, protection of the organism against toxic effects of the drug, able to circulate throughout the body, ideal zero-order drug-release kinetics, no undesired immune response against encapsulated drug etc. Resealed erythrocytes are rapidly taken up by macrophages of the Reticuloendothelial System (RES) of the liver, lung, and spleen of the body and hence drugs also. Resealed erythrocytes method of drugs delivery is secure and effective for drugs targeting specially for a longer period of time. This chapter will explain the different method of drug loading for resealed erythrocytes, their characterization, and applications in various therapies and associated health benefits.

DOI: 10.4018/978-1-5225-0754-3.ch012

INTRODUCTION

The emerging new drug delivery technologies are likely to have significant and lucrative impact on drug industries. Drugs delivery assembly suffers various limitation including the amount of molecule delivered and parallel adverse effects. To improve the targeting of drugs a number of attempts has been performed through engineering the properties of the drugs carrier system (Dinda, 2013). The present scenario about pharmaceutical research is aimed to develop drug delivery system with lower side effects and maximum therapeutic benefit. The major desirable properties of a drug carrier is being selective to a target tissue as well as to protect the drugs from premature bio-inactivation. New emerging drug targeting strategies through improving carrier towards tissue exhibit maximal therapeutic index with minimum adverse effects. In diverse drugs carrier, the cellular carriers fulfill maximum criteria desirable in clinical applications. Various carrier are being uses as drug targeting; however, cellular carriers like erythrocytes, platelets, leukocytes, fibroblasts, hepatocytes etc. evidenced themselves to have greater potential over other cellular carriers (Hamidi & Tajerzadeh, 2003, Rossi et al., 2005). Erythrocytes are most common type of blood cells travel thousands of miles from wide to narrow pathways to deliver oxygen, drugs and nutrient during their lifetime (Pandey & Rizvi, 2010). Erythrocytes have good potential carrier capabilities for varieties of drugs and could efficiently deliver various drugs to selected target cells (Gothoskar, 2004). Drug-loaded carrier erythrocytes or resealed erythrocytes are promising for precise drugs targeting.

Resealed erythrocytes as carrier for drugs provides secure and more effective drug targeting for longer period of time and have advantage over several drugs carrier models regarding the biocompatibility, biodegradability without toxic products, inert intracellular environment, entrapping potential for a variety of chemicals, protection of the organism against toxic effects of the drug, able to circulate throughout the body, ideal zero-order drug-release kinetics, no undesired immune response against encapsulated drug etc. (Gothoskar, 2004). Loading of drugs in erythrocytes are performed through process of collecting blood, isolating erythrocytes from blood, entrapping drug of interest in the erythrocytes then followed by resealing the resultant erythrocytes carriers (Green & Widder, 1987). Drug loading process in erythrocytes and sealing of them is based on the response of erythrocytes under osmotic condition (Jain & Jain, 1997). Drug loaded erythrocytes or resealed erythrocytes are biocompatible with large drug loading capacity, biodegradable, non-immunogenic which could circulate for long periods of time (months) through circulation of blood and can be easily targeted to macrophages. In clinical trial, use of resealed erythrocytes was extensively investigated *in vitro* and recently validated *in vivo* also.

BLOOD

Blood is mobile connective tissue composed of fluid called plasma and cells have been extensively uses in pathologies and research laboratory. Blood have several functions including transport of oxygen to cell for aerobic respiration, nutrients, drugs, and excretes toxic substances generated endogenously. Circulating nature of blood makes it universal and primary sample for assessing several organ functions test. Blood have two major components as cellular component (erythrocytes, white blood cells and platelets) and the solvent of cellular component called plasma. Cellular component are again fractionated major cell RBCs and WBCs and platelets (Guyton & Hall, 2006). Blood is a tissue of mesenchymal origin with liquid matrix. The matrix in which the cells are suspended is termed as plasma. This plasma holds the blood cells in form of a suspension. As whole plasma consists of 55% of blood volume and rest 45% is made up of formed elements (blood cells). The cellular component of blood are categories as red blood cells (RBCs) or erythrocytes, white blood cells (WBCs) and platelets.

Plasma

Plasma, the non-living fluid portion of blood is slightly alkaline (pH 7.40) containing an immense number of ions, inorganic molecules and organic molecules. Plasma transits to various parts of the body with several substances. It consists up to 5% of body weight, or roughly 3500 mL in a 70-kg man (Guyton & Hall, 2006). Generally, plasma clot in the absence of anticoagulant, and after clotting the remaining fluid is called serum. Serum has essentially the same composition as plasma except fibrinogen and clotting factors II, V, and VIII, and has a higher serotonin level. Plasma consists of 90-92% water, 0.9% mineral salt, sodium bicarbonate, nutrients (glucose, fatty acid, amino acids, nucleosides, etc.), 7 -8% plasma proteins, defence compound immunoglobulin, anticoagulant, vitamins, enzymes, dissolved gasses and excretory substances (Guyton & Hall, 2006).

The plasma protein consist albumin, globulin, and a fraction of fibrinogen. The globulin fraction is subdivided into α1, α2, β1, β2, and γ globulins and fibrinogen. Circulating antibodies in the γ globulin fraction of the plasma proteins are manufactured in the plasma cells. Most of the other plasma proteins are synthesized in the liver. Plasma protein provides 15% buffering capacity of blood due to presence of weak ionization of their substituent COOH and NH_2 groups. Albumin serves as a carrier for metals, ions, fatty acids, amino acids, bilirubin, enzymes, and drugs despite antioxidant potential (Guyton & Hall, 2006). Plasma protein used as marker of oxidative stress via measuring protein hydroperoxides, protein carbonyl (PCO), and advance oxidative protein products (AOPP) (Rizvi & Pandey, 2011, Singh & Rizvi, 2015).

Plasma lipid includes cholesterol, low density lipoprotein (LDL)-cholesterol, high density lipoprotein (HDL)-cholesterol, very low density lipoprotein (VLDL) cholesterol, triglycerides, phospholipids and free fatty acids. Phospholipids, LDL cholesterol and triglycerides are generally found to in higher amount and repeatedly used in diagnosis of fatty liver, atherosclerosis, or susceptibility for cardiac attack. Plasma proteins and lipids are good marker of oxidative stress implicated in several diseases (Mehdi & Rizvi, 2013, Singh & Rizvi, 2015). Carbohydrates content in plasma are mainly arise from the ingested food and dissociated glycan moiety form the cellular membrane. Plasma carbohydrates are presently uses to diagnose and evaluate various pathological conditions due to increasing the oxidative stress or with ageing (Mehdi et al., 2012).

Erythrocytes

Erythrocytes (Greek *erythros* for "red" and *kytos* for "hollow vessel", with -cyte translated as "cell" in modern usage) are unique circulating cells in the mammalian cells travels thousands of miles from wide to narrow pathways to deliver oxygen, drugs and nutrient during their life time. In normal men, the average number of RBCs per cubic millimeter is 5,200,000 (±300,000); in normal women, it is 4,700,000 (±300,000). Persons living at high altitudes have greater numbers of RBCs. RBCs have the ability to concentrate hemoglobin in the cell fluid up to about 34 grams in each 100 milliliters of cells. Millions of erythrocytes are produced every second, they developed in bone marrow and circulate for about 100-120 days in the human body however the mean erythrocyte lifespan of Wistar rats is 59.8 ±

Figure 1. Morphology of Erythrocytes: Side view & Top view

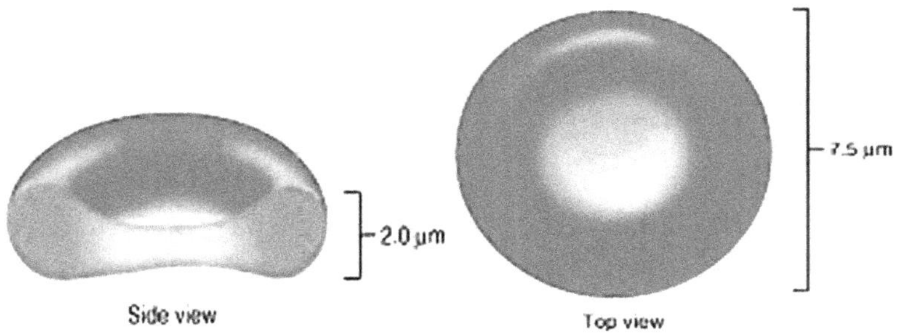

2.2 days and fixed during the modeling process, 60 days (Guyton & Hall, 1996). In most mammalian blood, mature RBCs are oval and flexible biconcave disks with lacking cell nucleus and most organelles to accommodate maximum space for hemoglobin. Normal erythrocytes are approximately 5.7 µm in diameter and a thick 2.5 µm at the thickest point and 1 µm or less in the center, discoid, and biconcave in cross (Figure 1) section (Guyton & J.E. Hall, 1996).

Erythrocyte Membrane

The erythrocyte membrane is composed of cholesterol and phospholipids, and secured an elastic network of skeletal proteins via trans-membrane proteins (Mohandas & Gallagher, 2008). Membrane is bilayer in nature and the composition of outer and inner layer is according to requirement. Glycolipids, phosphatidylcholine and sphingomyelin are located in the outer half of the bilayer; however, phosphatidylinositol, phosphatidylethanolamine and phosphatidylserine occur in the interior layer facing the cytoplasm (Mohandas & Gallagher, 2008). Due to membrane fluidity and flexibility erythrocytes can squeeze themself through much narrower than their diameter and can recover rapidly to their original shape. Phosphatidylcholine forms highly fluid lipid regions to induced fluidity, while sphingomyelin induces rigidity of membrane. Lipid domain controlling the fluidity is determined by the molar ratio of cholesterol to phospholipid, degree of unsaturation of phospholipid acyl chains and phosphatidylcholine sphingomyelin ratio (Mahmmoud, 2011).

An intact membrane skeleton is crucial for the mechanical and functional integrity of the RBCs because intact membrane skeleton determines RBCs viscoelastic properties to withstand the shear forces of the circulation and squeeze out through capillaries (Chassis et al., 1988). The membrane skeleton is constituted by a multi-protein network (ankyrin, anion exchanger (AE1 or band 3) and protein 4.1, 4.2 etc.) lying just beneath the plasma membrane (Lux & Palek, 1995). Band 3 and glycophorin A are most abundant glycated integral membrane protein whose concentration in the membrane varies according to the weather of living subject. Band 3 present as dimer, composed of two identical subunits in membrane and serves as a channel for the passive exchange of anions across the membrane like chloride shift. The tetrameric form of band 3 binds to ankyrin (Michaely & Bennett, 1995) and protein 4.2 (Rybicki et al., 1996) constituting the major attachment site of the RBCs membrane to the underlying cytoskeleton. A second site of attachment involves the glycophorin C complex with protein 4.1 and p55. Glycophorin A is 1TMS consisting carbohydrate cover 16 oligosaccharide chains and make up of 60 percent of the molecule's weight. Glycophorin have negative charge due to presence of sialic acid the sugar residue at the end of carbohydrate chain due to which RBCs repel each other and prevent the RBCs from clumping during circulation through the tiny capillaries (Mehdi et al., 2012).

Functions of Erythrocytes

In the 19th century, Hope Seyler identified hemoglobin and its crucial role in oxygen delivery to various parts of the body (Telen, 1993). In some lower animals, hemoglobin circulates as free protein in the plasma not enclosed in RBCs. The tetrameric hemoglobin molecule in turn is designed to unload oxygen cooperatively within the range of physiological tissue pO_2 (Sivilotti, 2004). Carbonic anhydrase, an important enzyme of erythrocytes catalyzes the reversible reaction between carbon dioxide (CO_2) and water to form carbonic acid (H_2CO_3) regulates the acid base balance in the blood. Despite these gaseous exchange, hormones, enzymes and nutrients transport function, blood actively remove toxic excretes of different cells, drugs of chemical inhaled, injected or ingested (Table 1) (Sivilotti, 2004).

When RBCs undergo shear stress during the circulation in constricted vessels, RBC release ATP which in turn relax and dilate the blood vessel to promote normal circulation of blood flow (Ristenpart et al., 2008). After deoxygenation of hemoglobin erythrocytes release S-nitrosothiols, which also acts as vasodilator for directing more blood in areas having less oxygen of the body (Diesen et al., 2008). Erythrocytes has also been found to synthesize nitric oxide is another vasodilator via using L-arginine as substrate (Kleinbongard et al., 2006). Shear stress on erythrocytes induced the nitric oxide synthase for nitric oxide synthesis and exportation of them is thought to involve in the regulation of vascular tonus (Ulke et al., 2009). Erythrocytes is also reported to produce hydrogen sulfide, a signaling gas which have similar effects like vasodilator through relaxing the vessel walls. It is believed that the cardio protective effects of garlic are due to erythrocytes converting its sulfur compounds into hydrogen sulfide (Benavides et al., 2007). For all these functions to run well, efficient and regulated transport of these molecules (O_2, CO_2 HCO^{3-}, Cl^-, S-nitrosothiols, nitric oxide) is very essential.

Table 1. Important biochemical reaction occurs in erythrocytes

Process	Chemical Reaction
Production of superoxide (by-product of various reactions)	$O_2 + e^- \rightarrow O_2^{\bullet-}$
NADPH-oxidase	$2\ O_2 + NADPH \rightarrow 2\ O_2^{\bullet-} + NADP + H^+$
Superoxide dismutase	$O_2^{\bullet-} + O_2^{\bullet-} + 2\ H^+ \rightarrow H_2O_2 + O_2$
Catalase	$H_2O_2 \rightarrow 2\ H_2O + O_2$
Myeloperoxidase	$H_2O_2 + X^- + H^+ \rightarrow HOX + H_2O$ ($X^- = Cl^-, Br^-, SCN^-$)
Glutathione peroxidase (Se-dependent)	$2\ GSH + R\text{-}O\text{-}OH \rightarrow GSSG + H_2O + ROH$
Fenton reaction	$Fe^{2+} + H_2O_2 \rightarrow Fe^{3+} + OH^{\bullet} + OH^-$
Iron-catalyzed Haber-Weiss reaction	$O_2^{\bullet-} + H_2O_2 \rightarrow O_2 + OH^{\bullet} + OH^-$
Glucose-6-phosphate dehydrogenase (G6PD)	$G6P + NADP \rightarrow 6$ Phosphogluconate $+ NADPH + H^+$
Glutathione reductase	$G\text{-}S\text{-}S\text{-}G + NADPH + H^+ \rightarrow 2\ GSH + NADP$

Life Span of Erythrocytes and Changes Associated with Erythrocyte Senescence

Worn-out erythrocytes are removed from circulation and destroyed in the spleen and liver, and the breakdown products are recycled. In human, erythrocytes are produced in red bone marrow under the regulation of a hemopoietic hormone erythropoietin by process called erythropoiesis (Torotra & Grabowski, 1993). RBCs are produced exclusively in the bone marrow until age of in younger age; however, most of cells continue to produce in marrow of vertebrae, sternum, ribs, and ilia. Blood cells are originated from pluripotential hematopoietic stem cells. Pluripotential cells differentiate in to committed stem cells which differentiate to form the other cells in the blood. Growth and differentiation of stem cells in to erythrocytes are controlled by multiple regulatory proteins as growth factor protein regulates the growth of stem cells and differentiation inducer induced the differentiation.

Erythropoiesis is process of production of erythrocytes from the committed stem cells through different process via different organs in about seven days. In healthy adult red bone marrow is the major site for the continuous synthesis of RBCs at a rate of 2 million per second. After the process of erythrocytes maturation steps, RBCs live in the blood for about 100-120 days (Guyton & Hall, 2006). Like animal aging erythrocytes passes through cellular aging as at the end of life erythrocytes become senescent and removed from the blood circulation. They become susceptible to selective recognition by macrophages and subsequent phagocytosis in the reticuloendothelial system (spleen, liver and bone marrow), thus removing old and defective cells and continually purging the blood. This process is termed eryptosis, or erythrocyte programmed cell death (Guyton & Hall, 2006).

Process of erythrocytes ageing induced changes in the membrane composition, fluidity and hence the activity of various enzymes and transport system (Rizvi et al., 2010). Progressive aging of erythrocytes increased the cellular density which could affect the properties of resealed erythrocytes. Aged cells shows a little decreases in the deformities index. Increases in the elastic modulus and surface viscosity in senescent erythrocytes has been observed as compare to young erythrocytes (Racca et al., 1999). There are studies which indicate a decrease in antigenic expression in the population of senescent erythrocytes of both blood group. One hypothesis that is related with erythrocytic senescence proposes that denatured/oxidized hemoglobin (hemichromes) arising late during an RBC's life span induces clustering of the integral membrane protein, band 3. In turn, band 3 clustering generates an epitope on the senescent cell surface leading to autologous IgG binding and consequent phagocytosis (Michael et al., 1999).

Oxidation of hemoglobin is caused by free radicals and ROS (reactive oxygen species) with progressive aging (Pandey & Rizvi, 2010). The progressive accumulation of oxidized hemoglobin covalently bound to the membrane skeleton not only disrupts membrane organization but also threatens eventual phospholipids oxidation via a calcium-promoted quasi-lipoxygenase activity. The emergence on the cell surface of a threshold concentration of oxidized phospholipids, principally phosphatidylserine, signals recognition by the CD36 macrophage receptor (Kiefer & Snyder, 2000).

Erythrocytes as Model Study

Erythrocytes have been extensively studied for their potential carrier capabilities for the delivery of nutrients, gasses, excretory products, toxic substances and drugs. Currently different types of mammalian erythrocytes have been used for research purpose, including erythrocytes of mice, cattle, pigs, dogs, sheep, goats, monkeys, chicken, rats and rabbits (Gothoskar, 2004). Erythrocytes are specialized cells perform critical functions in wide range of cellular environments. Due to absence of protein synthesizing machinery in erythrocytes they have additional impact on carrier capabilities for varieties of drugs.

RESEALED ERYTHROCYTES

Erythrocytes have water content 65% and rest of 35% are solid. Isotonic nature of plasma for erythrocytes protects them against osmosis. However, if medium is hypotonic erythrocyte get swelled and simultaneously lose their hemoglobin content. Erythrocytes without hemoglobin content are termed as ghost. There are three types of ghost has been recognized as (a) ghosts which reseal immediately after haemolysis, (b) resealed ghost after reversal of haemolysis by addition of alkali ions and, (c) erythrocytes ghost with leaky nature under different experimental conditions (Deloach et al., 1980, Ihler, 1983, Ihler & Tsang, 1987, Jain & Jain, 1997). During hypotonic shock and on resealing of erythrocytes hemoglobin is lost but cellular constituents are retained and erythrocytes called "resealed erythrocytes".

Encapsulation of adenosine triphosphate (ATP) in erythrocytes with was tried in 1953, by Gardos (Gardos, 1953). Ihler et al. and Zimmermann (1973) reported to use erythrocytes as drugs carrier; however, the term carrier erythrocytes was came in existence in 1979 which describe drug-loaded erythrocytes (Ihler, 1983, Zimmermann, 1973, Jain & Jain, 1997). It was found that several molecules leak rapidly from erythrocytes via membrane due to simple diffusion. However, principally drugs having nature of peptides, nucleic acids etc. may potential be entrapped in to erythrocytes. Erythrocytes have its own enzymatic activities which can be conveniently utilized to convert an inactive pro-drug into an active drug. These behavior of erythrocytes leads to design a number of pro-drugs with charged chemical groups making them non-diffusible or non-toxic. Red cells enzymes hydrolyze these chemical groups and converted pro-drug in to an active drug which can diffuse through erythrocytes membrane and released them in circulation or at specific sites. Hemoglobin free resealed erythrocytes with drugs serves as slow circulating depots to reticuloendothelial system (RES) (Zimmermann, 1983, Lewis & Alpar, 1984, Ropars et al., 1987, Jain & Jain, 1997).

Morphology of Resealed Erythrocytes

The survival and existence of resealed erythrocytes in biological system is affected by the membrane fluidity and biological behavior of resealed erythrocytes. The *in vitro* characterization of resealed erythrocytes is an important process to predict the biological properties of resealed erythrocytes in *in vivo*. Erythrocytes are flexible and they squeeze out themselves in narrow capillaries hence morphology of erythrocytes after loading of drugs and resealing decides their life span after their administration in body.

Morphological evaluation are usually performed through the microscope. Light microscopy has been reported to reveals no observable change in resealed cells; however, some spherocytes (spherical erythrocytes) has been detected (Talwar & Jain, 1992a, Jain et al., 1995, Jain et al., 1997). Increasing the resolution power, i.e. scanning electron microscopic (SEM) have shown that maximum drug loaded resealed erythrocytes are in their biconcave discoid shapes (Jrade et al., 1987), some form spherocytes with invagination in one point (stomatocytes) after the drug loading procedure (Garin et al., 1996). Smaller cells (microcyte) were also reported in some cases (Teisseire et al., 1987).

Deformities of erythrocytes has also been reported to modulate the life span of erythrocytes. Viscoelasticity of erythrocytes membrane, viscosity of the cell contents, and cellular surface-to-volume ratio are found to affects the rheological behavior of resealed erythrocytes in narrow capillaries and the RES (Jrade et al., 1987). Changes in the shape of resealed erythrocytes after drugs loading measured by the passage time of definite volume of resealed erythrocytes via a polycarbonate filter (pore size of 45 μm) or a capillary of 4 μm diameter (Jrade et al., 1987, Zanella et al., 1987). Turbidimetrically, chlorpromazine mediated shape changes is another approach to evaluate morphological changes (Hamidi et al., 2001).

PREPARATIVE METHODOLOGY

Source and Isolation of RBC

Erythrocytes isolated form mice, cattle, pigs, dogs, sheep, goats, monkeys, chicken, rats, and rabbits have been used for resealed erythrocytes or drugs encapsulated erythrocytes. Fresh erythrocytes isolated from whole blood has been found to have more encapsulation efficiency for the loading purposes of drugs. It has been also reported that young erythrocytes have higher capability then old erythrocytes. Fresh blood, collected from mammals chilled have to be store at 4 °C and less than of two days. The erythrocytes are harvested and washed with phosphate buffer saline by centrifugation. Mammalian erythrocytes have advantage over the other species erythrocytes due to lacking the nucleus and various cellular organelles such as their mitochondria, golgi apparatus and endoplasmic reticulum in their mature state. Erythrocytes consist nucleus during the early phases of erythropoiesis but the gradually disappear during development in order to provide more space for hemoglobin. Due to absence of nucleus and cellular organelles erythrocytes they do not contain DNA, cannot synthesize any RNA and also used to depend on ATP by the glycolysis (Ihler & Tsang, 1987). These properties of erythrocytes ensures that no virus can target erythrocytes for growth and propagation (Vienken et al., 1978).

Carrier erythrocytes are prepared collecting blood samples, separating erythrocytes from plasma, entrapping desire drug in the erythrocytes, and finally resealing the carriers (Green & Widder, 1987). Venous blood from different healthy volunteers or subjects can obtained in heparin by venipuncture. The blood was centrifuged at 800 × g for 10 min at 4°C. After the removal of plasma, buffy coat and upper 15% of the packed erythrocytes, the packed erythrocytes were washed twice with cold phosphate buffer saline at 4°C (0.9% NaCl, 10 mM Na_2HPO_4, pH 7.4). The washed erythrocytes are diluted with phosphate buffer saline and stored at 4°C until used (Singh et al., 2015, Singh & Rizvi, 2015).

Methodology of Drugs Loading

Various methods has been established to load drugs or other bioactive compounds in erythrocytes isolated from different mammals. Majorly includes physical method like electricalpulse method, osmosis-based systems, and chemical methods. Erythrocytes have capability to reverse the shape changes with or without accompanying volume change of erythrocytes and for reversible deformation under various stress.

Osmosis and Concept of Tonicity

Tonicity is a measure of the osmotic pressure of two solutions separated by a semi permeable membrane. Like osmotic pressure, tonicity is influenced only by solutes which cannot cross the semi permeable membrane. Higher the concentration of solute higher will be the tonocity of solution. Term is generally used when describing the response of cells immersed in an external solution. The process by which water moves across the semi permeable membrane from the region of higher solute concentration to the region of lower solute concentration is termed as osmosis. The process of osmosis is depended on erythrocytes response under the osmotic conditions. These methods exchanged the extra cellular solute having desired drugs with the cellular solute (hemoglobin) of erythrocytes before resealing. Hypo-osmotic methods are again classified in to hypotonic dilution methods, dialysis methods, Presswell method, and isotonic osmotic lyses.

Hypotonic Dilution

A hypotonic solution is that which contains a lesser concentration of impermeable solutes than the solution on the other side of the membrane. When a cell's cytoplasm is hypotonic than surrounding then water will be drawn out of the cytoplasm. If water molecules continue to diffuse into the cell, it will cause the cell to swell, and finally lysis will occur. Hypotonic dilution was the first method investigated for the encapsulation of chemicals into erythrocytes (Iher, 1973). In this methods, erythrocytes are exposed to hypotonic solution of 0.4% NaCl to escape of cellular contents in the exchange of hypotonic solution having desired drugs. This method was used to entrap β-glucosidase, β–galactosidase (Iher, 1973), asparginase (Updike & Wakamiya, 1983), and arginase (Adriaenssens et al., 1976), as well as bronchodilators salbutamol (Bhaskaran & Dhir, 1995). Hypotonic dilution methods is simplest and fastest (exchange of cellular content and hypotonic solution equilibrium is achieved with in one minute), but having lower capsulation efficacy (1 – 8%).

Dialysis

This methods are performed by erythrocyte dialyzer through which initially a desired haematocrit is achieved through suspending the washed erythrocytes with phosphate buffer (pH 7.4) having desired drug solution. This method provide good entrapment efficiency yet have disadvantages of time consuming and size distribution of loaded ghosts were not found to be homogeneous.

Press Well Dilution Method or Hypotonic Preswelling

This method was developed by Rechsteiner (1975) and again was modified by Jenner et al. (1981). Method is based on swelling the erythrocytes without the lyses due to suspending them in to slightly hypotonic solution (0.6% NaCl) and recovered the swollen erythrocytes by centrifugation at low speed. Then, a little volumes of drug solution are added to the point of erythrocytes lyses. Now cells placed in isotonic medium to make resealed erythrocytes. Press well dilution method are simple and fast with higher survival rate *in vivo* as long as native RBCs.

Isotonic Osmotic Lyses or Osmotic Pulse Method

Isotonic solutions contain equal concentrations of impermeable solutes on either side of the membrane. When cell cytoplasm is isotonic to surrounding no such change occur because there is no net movement of water across the cell membrane. Red blood cells are bound by a membrane which allows water to pass through while generally restricting the solutes. This process, causes cells to shrink due to loss of water (called exosmosis) when placed in hypertonic solutions. On the other hand, red cells absorb water (called endosmosis) when in a hypotonic medium. This results in swelling and ultimately hemolysis as the cell bursts. In isotonic osmotic lyses or osmotic pulse method erythrocytes are placed in high transerythrocytic membrane permeability solution which allow encapsulation of drugs through solution into erythrocytes via direct chemical potential gradient. Various chemical methods has adopted for isotonic hemolysis like ammonia chloride, urea solution, and polyethylene glycol (Davson & Danielli, 1970, Billah et al., 1977).

Electrical Breakdown/ Electro-Insertion/ Electroencapsulation

Zimmermann (1973) developed this method to encapsulate bioactive molecules. However, Kinosita & Tsong (1977a) suggested the use of transient electrolysis for required membrane permeability for drug loading. In this method optimum intensity of an electric field and optimal discharge time has been reported between 1–10 kW/cm and between 20–160 µs (Zimmermann et al., 1976, Kinosita & Tsong, 1977b, Zimmermann, 1983, Lewis & Alpar, 1984,, Tsong & Kinosita, 1985). Voltage (2kV/ cm for 20µ sec) mediated polarization induce electrical breakdown of erythrocytes membrane through formation of pore which helps in entrapment of drugs. Pore generation generally takes place at the lipid protein junction or lipoid regions in membrane and can be resealed by incubation in suitable solution at 37° C. In comparison with osmotic methods advantage of this method is the uniform distribution of loaded cells (Zimmermann, 1983). However, this process is very expensive.

Endocytosis

This method was reported by Schrier et al. (1975). In erythrocytes intracellular vesicles with desired drugs could be induce. This process can load virus (up to 1000 nm diameter), enzymes and small molecules. Intracellular vesicles derived from cytoplasm may release intracellular content in erythrocytes cytoplasm depending upon the nature of drugs. This method have been used to encapsulate primaquine and related 8-amino-quinolines, vinblastine, chlorpromazine and related phenothiazines, propranolol, tetracaine, hydrocortisone, and vitamin A (Tsong & Kinosita, 1977, DeLoach, 1983, Schrier, 1987)

Membrane Perturbation

This method is based on the ability of chemical to modulate membrane permeability of erythrocytes. Deuticke et al. (1973) has found that the erythrocytes membrane permeability increases when RBCs expose to polyene antibiotic such as amphotericin B. Antibiotics have ability to increase the permeability of erythrocytes membrane were exploited for loading of drugs in to erythrocytes e.g. Amphotericin-B interacts with the cholesterol in plasma membrane causing change in permeability for anti-leukemic drugs. Kitao et al., (1978) entrap the daunomycin (antineoplastic drug) in human and mouse erythrocytes. However, Lin et al. (1999) used halothane for the same purpose.

Lipid Fusion

Lipid vesicles are generally used to encapsulate the drugs and loaded to erythrocytes. Lipids vesicle tagged with specific phospholipids induced the drugs loading potential and functional properties of drugs loaded erythrocytes. This method was mainly used for entrapping inositol monophosphate which improve the oxygen carrying capacity of RBCs (Nicolau & Gersonde, 1997).

Red Cell Loader

Red cell loader was developed by the Magnani and co-workers, a novel method for loading of non-diffusible drugs into erythrocytes (Magnani et al., 1998). The loading process takes place in two sequential steps of hypotonic dilutions of washed RBCs and then an isotonic process for resealing the erythrocytes. This process of drugs entrapment have 30% of drug loading efficiency with 35–50% cell recovery despite normal survival of erythrocytes *in vivo*.

IN VITRO CHARACTERIZATION OF RESEALED ERYTHROCYTES

Characterization of resealed erythrocytes with drugs provide the significances of methods used to prepare the drug encapsulated erythrocytes. The following process could be used to evaluate and characterized the resealed erythrocytes-

Measuring Erythrocyte Sedimentation Rate (ESR)

Erythrocyte sedimentation rate determine the sedimentation rate of blood cells in a standard tube. It measure the suspension stability, size and number of the RBC in plasma or relative concentration of plasma protein (fibrinogen and α, β globulins). ESR is standardized as 0 to 15 mm/hr. for normal blood, higher rate indicates active but obscure disease processes (Teisseire et al., 1987).

Measuring Drug Content

Drugs contents was evaluated in erythrocytes. Initially erythrocytes were depolarized with acetonitrile and then centrifuge the whole content at 2500 rpm for 10 mins. Now supernatant was used to evaluate the drug content (Gothoskar, 2004).

In Vitro Release of Drug and Hemoglobin

In this process normal and resealed erythrocytes are incubated at room temperature in PBS in metabolic rotating wheel incubator path. Now sample was depolarized to evaluate the drugs content and hemoglobin. Hemoglobin can be measured by correlating the hemolysate solution with standard hemoglobin graph (Gothoskar, 2004).

Drug Release Pattern

Drug release pattern is the most important parameters to evaluate the properties of resealed erythrocytes. Hemoglobin is also reported to invariably release with drug form erythrocytes due to loss of cell membrane integrity, but drug releasing potential of erythrocytes is considerably higher than hemoglobin, reflects readily diffuses of drug. Size and polarity of the drug molecule are two factors that determine the drug release pattern (Eichler et al., 1987). It was found that cell lysis is not essential for the release of lipophilic drugs like phenytoin, dexamethasone (Eichler et al., 1987), methotrexate (Lewis & Alpar, 1984), primpquin (Talwar & Jain, 1992), and vitamin B-12 (Eichler et al., 1985). However, cell lysis is essential for non-diffusible or polar drugs like heparin, gentamicin and enalaprilat, and enzymes asparginase, peptides urogasterone and l-lysine-l-phenylalanine (Gothoskar, 2004). Cross-linking cell membrane with gluteraldehyde is reported to reduce the drugs release rate (Jenner et al., 1981, Talwar & Jain, 1992). Complex formation of drug with dextran and albumin also reduced the release rate (Ihler, 1983). Entrapment of biodegradable prodrug (cortisol-21- phosphate, o-acetyl propranolol, o-pivaloyl propranolol, and cytosine arabinoside monophosphate) has similar effects on drugs release pattern (Gothoskar, 2004).

Osmotic Fragility

The osmotic fragility test is a measure of the resistance of erythrocytes to hemolysis by osmotic stress. Osmotic stress is produced by exposing cell to NaCl solution of tonicity lower than that of plasma. The test consists of exposing red cells to decreasing strengths of hypotonic saline solutions and measuring the degree of hemolysis calorimetrically at room temperature (Pandey & Rizvi, 2014a). The osmotic fragility test ultimately tries to determine the concentration of solute inside the cell subjecting it to the hemolytic effects of solutions of different concentrations. Erythrocytes were added to tubes containing increasing concentrations of phosphate-buffered sodium chloride (0%, 0.1%, 0.2%, 0.3%, 0.5%, 0.7%, 0.8%, and 0.9%) solution at pH 7.4 in a final volume of 10 ml and incubated for 30 min at 37 °C. After centrifugation at 1500 x g for 10 min, absorbance of the supernatant was measured at 540 nm. Hemolysis in each tube was expressed as a percentage, using hemolysis in distilled water (0% NaCl) as 100% as shown below in Figure 2 (Pandey & Rizvi, 2014b).

Figure 2. Osmotic fragility

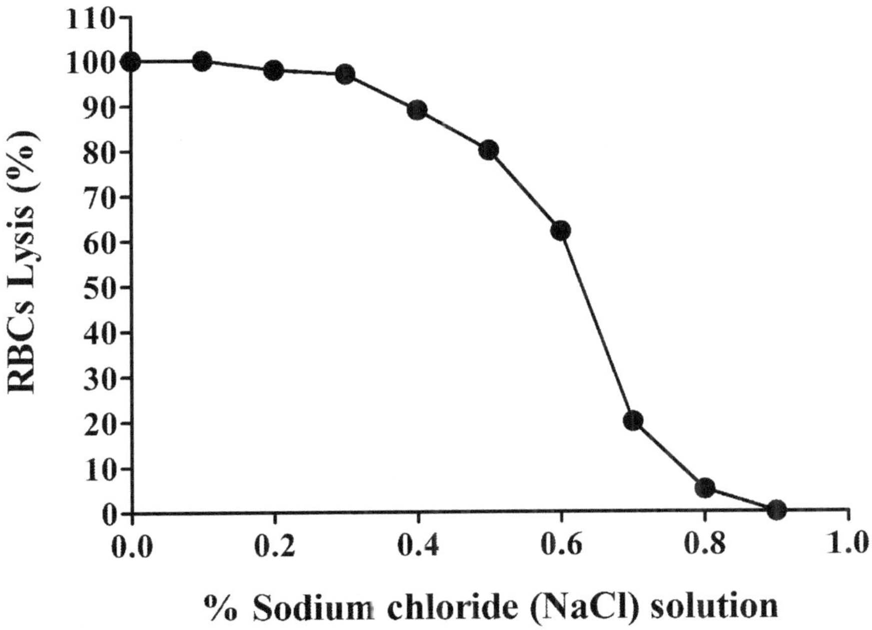

In osmotic fragility test % hemolysis values are calculated and finally plotted against concentration to give and sigmoidal curve. This sigmoidal shape of curve indicates that normal RBC varies in their resistance to hypotonic solution. The osmotic fragility of resealed erythrocytes is affected by concentration, type and process of drugs loading. Osmotic fragility indicate the changes in cell membrane integrity and their resistance towards osmotic pressure of the suspension medium.

Based on integrity and resistance of cell membrane another method, turbulence fragility measure the resistance of drugs loaded erythrocytes against hemolysis from turbulent flow within circulation by vigorously shaking (Hamidi et al., 2001) or by passing them through needles with smaller internal diameter (e.g., 30 gauge) (Talwar & Jain, 1992a, Talwar & Jain, 1992b, Jain et al., 1995, Jain et al., 1997). In above both method released hemoglobin and drug were determined and found that turbulent fragility is higher than osmotic fragility of resealed cells (Talwar & Jain, 1992a, Talwar & Jain, 1992b, Jain et al., 1995, Jain et al., 1997, Hamidi et al., 2001).

Morphological Evaluation

The plasma membrane of RBC is closely associated with a proteinaceous skeleton. This cytoskeleton and other features like excess membrane for given volume of cell make RBC (Mehdi et al., 2012). Erythrocyte membrane consists of approximately equal amounts of lipids proteins. Phospholipids and unesterified cholesterol constitute major portion of membrane lipids. Phosphatidylcholine are more abundant in the outer leaflet whereas phosphatidylethanolamine are more concentrated on the inner leaflet of the lipid bilayer. Cholesterol molecules are intercalated between the phospholipid molecules. The relative amounts of cholesterol & phospholipids are responsible for the fluid properties of the RBC membrane (Ballas & Krasnow, 1980). The distribution of lipids in both leaflet is asymmetrical. This asymmetry is maintained by action of flippase proteins (Daleke & Lyles, 2003). Morphological evaluation including changes in shape due to changes in membrane biochemical composition or altering the proteinaceous skeleton modulates the cellular compatibility to survive in various solution or pressure of narrow capillaries.

ADVANTAGE OF RESEALED ERYTHROCYTES (GOTHOSKAR, 2004)

- Able to circulate throughout the body
- The biocompatibility of resealed erythrocytes and no immunological responses.
- It degraded biologically and do not release any toxic substances.
- Generally in produced uniform and drugs carriers.
- Intracellular environment are inert hence protection of encapsulated dugs by endogenous chemicals
- Have capability to entrap wide variety of chemicals.
- It also protects the organism against side-effects of drugs
- It check the immune response by organism against the loaded drug
- Ideal for deal zero-order drug-release kinetics (Eichler et al., 1986)
- Ensures the dose sufficiency as a large amount of drugs can be loaded in the resealed erythrocytes.
- Resealed erythrocytes have larger life span comparatively other synthetic drugs carriers
- Easily monitoring and control of resealed erythrocytes during life span ranging from minutes to months (Summers, 1983).

APPLICATIONS OF RESEALED ERYTHROCYTES

Erythrocytes as carrier for drugs cover pharmacological as well as therapeutic targets. Resealed erythrocytes with drugs has been reported to have slow releasing tendency of drugs when intravenously injected (Gothoskar, 2004). Erythrocytes is used as circulating carriers to release drug for a long period of times as well as target specific for liver, spleen, and lymph nodes. Despite these the following are the major application of resealed erythrocytes as drugs carriers.

Slow Drug Release

Due to long life span or erythrocytes, resealed erythrocytes as drugs carrier could be used as circulating depots of various drugs including anti-tumor, anti-parasitic, antibiotics, cardiovascular drugs, vitamins and steroids (Jenner et al., 1981, Pitt et al., 1983, Eichler et al., 1985, Magnani et al., 1998). Slow drugs release propensity of resealed erythrocytes arise when drugs or selected methods for drugs loading do not changes the morphological and physiological properties of erythrocytes.

There are various mechanism which explain the drugs releasing properties-

- Passive diffusion
- Specialized carrier transporter at the membrane
- Macrophages of RES do phagocytosis of resealed erythrocytes with drugs and finally accumulated drugs into the macrophage interior fallowed by slow release pattern of drug (Talwar & Jain, 1992a, Jain & Jain, 1997).
- The subcutaneous injection resulted an accumulation of erythrocytes in lymph nodes followed by hemolysis to release the drug (Deloach et al., 1987).

Drug Targeting

Modification on the surface of erythrocytes has been used to target the organs of mononuclear phagocytic system or reticuloendothelial system (Alvarez et al., 1998). Site-specific and target-oriented drug delivery system exhibit maximal therapeutic index with minimum adverse effects.

Targeting RES Organs

Kupffer cells in liver and spleen has been found to rapidly clear the damaged erythrocytes from circulation. Modification in erythrocytes membrane induces the targeting specificity. In presence scenario, various approaches has been performed to modify the surface characteristics of erythrocytes membrane with the help of antibodies, gluteraldehyde, carbohydrates such as sialic acid, sulphydryl, chemical cross-linking (Alvarez et al., 1998). Sialic acids has been responsible to induced negative surface on erythrocytes reduce in erythrocytes membrane with aging (Mehdi et al., 2012).

Targeting the Liver

Enzyme Deficiency/Replacement Therapy

This methods is used to prevent the accumulation of glucocerebrosides in the liver and spleen by glucocerebrosidase-loaded erythrocytes (Deloach & Ihler, 1977). This methods used to overcome the allergic reactions, and toxic manifestations in exogenous enzyme therapy because resealed erythrocytes with enzymes can be treated as native cell.

Treatment of Hepatic Tumors

Antineoplastic drugs used in hepatic tumors like methotrexate (Zimmermann, 1983, Jaitely et al., 1996), bleomycin (Zimmermann, 1973), asparginase (Updike & Wakamiya, 1983, Jaitely et al., 1996), and Adriamycin have been found to delivered successfully by resealed erythrocytes (Benatti et al., 1987, Zocchi et al., 1988, Al-Achi & Boroujerdi, 1990, Jaitely et al., 1996).

Treatment of Parasitic Diseases

Parasitic infection involve the harboring of parasites in the RES organs which can be successfully treated by the drug loaded resealed erythrocytes due to selectively accumulation within RES organs. Results has been reported as favorable in animal models for anti-malarial (Summers, 1983), anti-leishmanial (Summers, 1983, Eichler et al., 1986, Berman, 1987), and anti-amoebic drugs (Talwar & Jain, 1992b, Jaitely et al., 1996).

Removal of RES Iron Overload

It was found that aged erythrocytes are destroyed in RES organs which in turn increased the accumulation of iron in these organs. Resealed erythrocytes with desferrioxamine induction has been found to reduce the excess iron accumulated in thalassemic patients (Berman, 1987, Jaitely et al., 1996,).

Removal of Toxic Agents

Resealed erythrocytes encapsulated with recombinant phosphodiestrase has been reported to reduce the organophosphorus intoxication (Pei et al., 1994). Cannon et al. (1994) also reported that carrier erythrocytes containing sodium thiosulfate and bovine rhodanase inhibited the cyanide intoxication.

Targeting Other Organs

Despite the RES targeting, resealed erythrocytes have been used to target other organs. Various method have been used for different organs like entrapment of paramagnetic particle with desired drugs, drugs with photosensitive material, attachment of antibody at erythrocytes membrane or use or ultrasound waves (Gothoskar, 2004).

Entrapment of paramagnetic particle in to erythrocytes could induced their localization under the influence of an external magnetic field to a particular location. Photosensitized erythrocytes are photo-triggered carrier use to deliver methotrexate in cancer treatment (Flynn et al., 1994). Targeted micro bubble destruction with ultrasound has also been used to deliver the colloidal particles and erythrocytes to tissue through rupturing of microvessel (Price et al., 1998).

Despite the above approaches following could also use for targeting different organs other than RES:

- Preparation of erythrocytes carrier having thermo responsive liposomes (localization could performed through an external thermal source)
- Intra-peritoneal injection for drug targeting to peritoneal macrophages
- Resealed cells pre-treated with lectin and loaded with antineoplastic drugs for improving target specificity to tumor cells.

Delivery of Antiviral Agents

Resealed erythrocytes have been used to deliver recombinant herpes simplex virus type 1 (HSV-1), deoxycytidine derivatives (Ihler, 1983), azidothymidine derivatives (Benatti et al., 1989), fludarabine phosphate (Fraternale et al., 1996), glycoprotein B (Chiarantini et al., 1995) and azathioprene, acyclovir (Magnani et al., 1998). Resealed erythrocytes has been used to deliver to anti-viral agents because most of them are either nucleotides or nucleoside analogs. Nucleosides have tendency to rapidly transported across the membrane; however, nucleotides have not, and hence exhibiting a prolonged release profiles.

Enzyme Therapy

Various biochemical derangement has been associated with the altered or deficient enzymes activity. Direct injection of enzymes into the body has been reported to induce the immunological response or deactivation due to other enzymes activity. Resealed erythrocytes overcome the above problem and act as a "circulating bioreactors" in which substrates enter, interact with enzymes, and generate products (Ihler et al., 1975, Adriaenssens et al., 1976, Zimmermann et al., 1976, Zimmermann, 1983, Alpar & Lewis, 1985, Fiorelli et al., 1987, Magnani et al., 1989, Jaitely et al., 1996) In addition, it can also accumulate enzymes in RES after hemolysis (Iher, 1973, Deloach & Ihler, 1977, Lewis & Alpar, 1984).

Following enzymes are being uses with resealed erythrocytes:

- β-glucoserebrosidase for the treatment of Gaucher's disease (Beutler et al., 1977)
- Aasparginase for the treatment of pediatric neoplasms.
- β -aminolevulinate dehydrogenase (ALA-D) against lead poisoning

Despite these, urease (Zimmermann et al., 1976), galactose-1-phosphate uridyl-transferase (Harris, 1977), uricase (Ihler et al., 1975), and acetaldehyde dehydrogenase (Tan, 1977) has also been reported to use in resealed erythrocytes.

Oxygen Delivery to Tissues

Hemoglobin is the red pigmented protein responsible for the oxygen transporting capacity of erythrocytes. Under normal condition the major fraction of oxygenated hemoglobin is recirculated with venous blood to the lungs. Use of this bound fraction has been reported in oxygen deficiency. 2,3-Diphosphoglycerate (2,3-DPG) a side glycolysis product through Rapoport-Luebering cycle has been reported to changes the binding affinity of hemoglobin for oxygen. Affinity of 2,3-DPG towards oxygen has been reported to much higher than that of hemoglobin (Guyton & Hall, 1996). Despite these 2,3-DPG, inositol hexophosphate (IHP) is also one of the modulator of binding affinity of hemoglobin for oxygen. IHP or 2,3-DPG loaded erythrocytes could beneficial under high altitude conditions, patient having reduced number of alveoli, reduction in oxygen carrying capacity, mutation or chemical modification associated with decrease in oxygen affinity for hemoglobin, oxygen-delivery capacity of stored blood and ischemia of myocardium, brain, or other tissues (Zimmermann, 1983, Villareal et al., 1987, Teisseire et al., 1987, Baron et al., 1987).

CURRENT NOVEL APPROACHES

Microinjection

Macromolecules such as DNA, RNA, and proteins are currently exploited in every field of therapeutics and research. Various models are present today; however, erythrocytes lacking of complex cellular components (e.g., nucleus) with relatively simple structure make them good candidates for the entrapment of macromolecules (Furusawa et al., 1974). In this microinjection methods, erythrocytes are used as microsyringes for injection of biomolecule or drugs to the host cells (Zimmermann, 1983). Above process takes place *in vitro* as culturing host eukaryotic cells coated with fusogenic agent (Sendai virus, or its glycoproteins or polyethylene glycol) are suspended with biomolecule or drugs loaded erythrocytes in an isotonic medium (Furusawa et al., 1974, Zimmermann, 1983, Schlegel & McEvoy, 1987). The microinjection process has been performed for micoroinject of DNA fragments (Lewis & Alpar, 1984), ferritin, latex particles, arginase (Kruse et al., 1981, Kruse et al., 1987), bovine and human serum albumin, and thymidine kinase (Wille & Willecke, 1976) to various cultured eukaryotic cells.

Erythrosomes

It is engineered vesicular systems which are chemically cross-linked to erythrocytes by modified reverse-phase evaporation technique. Erythrosomes has been hypothesized for macromolecular drugs encapsulation in erythrocytes (Cuppoletti et al., 1981, Jung, 1987, Vyas &. Dixit, 1999).

Nanoerythrosomes

Extrusion of erythrocyte ghosts has been associated with the production of small vesicles (diameter 100 nm) known as nanoerythrosomes. Specially used for daunorubicin which was found to with covalently conjugated with the help of gluteraldehyde spacer to nanoerythrosomes. Covalently conjugated daunorubicin to nanoerythrosomes has been reported to more active than free daunorubicin alone in *in vtiro* model as well as *in vivo* model (Moorjani et al., 1996, Lejeune et al., 1997).

IN VITRO STORAGE OF RESEALED ERYTHROCYTES

Resealed erythrocytes activity also depends to a greater extent on the medium and duration of their *in vitro* storage. Drug encapsulated erythrocytes and maintaining their life with drug content can be regulated by using appropriate *in vitro* storage methods. Hank's balanced salt solution (Lewis & Alpar, 1984, Lewis, 1984, Lewis & Desai, 1987, Jaitely et al., 1996, Hamidi et al., 2001,) and acid–citrate–dextrose media are has been reported to frequently uses as storage media for resealed erythrocytes (Zimmermann, 1983). Erythrocytes with drug remain viable regarding the physiological and carrier properties when stored in above media for at least 2 weeks at 4ºC (Lewis & Desai, 1987). Cells circulation life span was found to improve after addition of the purine nucleosides (Alpar & Irwin, 1987, Lewis & Desai, 1987) or calcium-chelating agents (Alpar & Irwin, 1987). Membrane stabilizing agents (dimethyl,3,3-di-thio-bispropionamide, dimethyl sulfoxide, toluene-2-4- diisocyanate, gluteraldehyde) exposure to drug loaded cells followed by sintered glass filtration and lyophilization has been reported to significantly increase the resealed erythrocytes stability upon storage (Jain & Jain, 1997, Talwar & Jain, 1992a, Talwar & Jain, 1992b, Bhaskaran & Dhir, 1995). Lyophilized powder has been found to stable without any detectable changes for at least one month. The major drawback of this method is the lower circulation life span of resealed erythrocytes. Despite this method encapsulation of a prodrug (Talwar & Jain, 1992a), high glycerol freezing technique (Zanella et al., 1987, Fiorelli et al., 1987), and reversible immobilization in alginate or gelatin gels (Zimmermann, 1983, Lewis & Alpar, 1984, Lewis, 1984) are other progressive methods use to perform for increasing storage stability of resealed erythrocytes.

CONCLUSION

Resealed erythrocytes are promising for precise and safe drugs delivery. In presence scenario methodologies applied for drugs encapsulation and preparation of resealed erythrocytes need some optimization for making it usual drugs carriers. The concept of resealed erythrocytes can be also extended to increase the bioavailable of various molecule including biopharmaceuticals. Above chapter prompt us to conclude that resealed erythrocytes is an effective carriers to deliver the various drugs and bioactive molecule, and much remains to be explored regarding the potential of resealed erythrocytes.

CONFLICT OF INTEREST

None

ACKNOWLEDGMENT

Prabhakar Singh acknowledges the support of Council of Scientific and Industrial Research (CSIR), New Delhi, India for providing Senior Research Fellowship. Rajesh Kumar Kesharwani acknowledges the Indian Council of Medical Research (ICMR), New Delhi, India for providing financial support as Senior Research Fellowship (SRF).

REFERENCES

Adriaenssens, K., Karcher, D., Lowenthal, A., & Terheggen, H. G. (1976). Use of enzyme-loaded erythrocytes in in-vitro correction of arginase-deficient erythrocytes in familial hyperargininemia. *Clinical Chemistry*, *22*(3), 323–326. PMID:1253407

Al-Achi, A., & Boroujerdi, M. (1990). Pharmacokinetics and Tissue Uptake of Doxorubicin Associated with Erythrocyte-Membrane: Erythrocyte Ghosts versus Erythrocyte-Vesicles. *Drug Development and Industrial Pharmacy*, *16*(15), 2199–2219. doi:10.3109/03639049009043795

Alpar, H. O., & Irwin, W. J. (1987). Some Unique Applications of Erythrocytes as Carrier Systems. [series]. *Advances in the Biosciences*, *67*, 1–9.

Alpar, H. O., & Lewis, D. A. (1985). Therapeutic Efficacy of Asparaginase Encapsulated in Intact Erythrocytes. *Biochemical Pharmacology*, *34*(2), 257–261. doi:10.1016/0006-2952(85)90133-9 PMID:3966927

Alvarez, F. J., Jordán, J. A., Calleja, P., Lotero, L. A., Olmos, G., Díez, J. C., & Tejedor, M. C. (1998). Cross-Linking Treatment of Loaded Erythrocytes Increases delivery of Encapsulated Substance to Macrophages. *Biotechnology and Applied Biochemistry*, *27*(pt 2), 139–143. PMID:9569609

Ballas, S. K., & Krasnow, S. H. (1990). Structure of erythrocyte membrane and its transport functions. *Annals of Clinical and Laboratory Science*, *10*(3), 209–219. PMID:6249177

Baron, J. F., Vicaut, E., Stucker, O., Villereal, M. C., Ropars, C., Teisserie, B., & Duvelleroy, M. (1987). Isolated Heart as a Model to Study the Effects of the Decrease in Oxygen Hemoglobin Affinity.[series]. *Advances in the Biosciences*, *67*, 73–78.

Benatti, U. (1987). Comparative Tissue Distribution and Metabolism of Free Versus Erythrocyte-Encapsulated Adriamycin in the Mouse. *Advanced Biosciences, 67*, 129-136.

Benatti, U., Zocchi, E., Tonetti, M., Guida, L., Polvani, C., & De Flora, A. (1987). Enhanced antitumor activity of adriamycin by encapsulation in mouse erythrocytes targeted to liver and lungs. *Pharmacological Research*, *2*, 27–33. PMID:2631085

Benavides, G. A., Squadrito, G. L., Mills, R. W., Patel, H. D., Isbell, T. S., Patel, R. P., & Kraus, D. W. et al. (2007). Hydrogen sulfide mediates the vasoactivity of garlic. *Proceedings of the National Academy of Sciences of the United States of America*, *104*(46), 17977–17982. doi:10.1073/pnas.0705710104 PMID:17951430

Berman, J. D. (1987). Antileishmanial Activity of Red Cell Encapsulated Drugs.[series]. *Advances in the Biosciences*, *67*, 145–152.

Beutler, E., Dale, G. L., Guinto, D. E., & Kuhl, W. (1977). Enzyme Replacement Therapy in Gaucher's Disease. Preliminary Clinical Trial of a New Enzyme Preparation. *Proceedings of the National Academy of Sciences of the United States of America*, *74*(10), 4620–4623. doi:10.1073/pnas.74.10.4620 PMID:200923

Bhaskaran, S., & Dhir, S. S. (1995). Resealed Erythrocytes as Carriers of Salbutamol Sulphate. *Indian Journal of Pharmaceutical Sciences*, *57*, 240–242.

Billah, M. M., Finean, J. B., Coleman, R., & Michell, R. H. (1977). Permeability characteristics of erythrocyte ghosts prepared under isoionic conditions by a glycol-induced osmotic lysis. *Biochimica et Biophysica Acta*, *465*(3), 515–526. doi:10.1016/0005-2736(77)90269-3 PMID:13834

Cannon, E. P., Leung, P., Hawkins, A., Petrikovics, I., DeLoach, J., & Way, J. L. (1994). Antagonism of Cyanide Intoxication with Murine Carrier Erythrocytes Containing Bovine Rhodanese and Sodium Thiosulfate. *Journal of Toxicology and Environmental Health*, *41*(3), 267–274. doi:10.1080/15287399409531842 PMID:8126749

Chassaigne, R. M., & Nicoulau, C. (1987). *Advances in the BioSciences*. Oxford, UK: Pergamon Press.

Chassis, J. A., Agre, P., & Mohandas, N. (1988). Decreased membrane mechanical stability and *in vivo* loss of surface area reflect spectrin deficiencies in hereditary spherocytosis. *The Journal of Clinical Investigation*, *2*(2), 617–623. doi:10.1172/JCI113640 PMID:3403720

Chiarantini, L., Rossi, L., Fraternale, A., & Magnani, M. (1995). Modulated red blood cell survival by membrane protein clustering. *Molecular and Cellular Biochemistry*, *144*(1), 53–59. doi:10.1007/BF00926740 PMID:7791745

Cuppoletti, J., Mayhew, E., Zobel, C. R., & Jung, C. Y. (1981). Erythrosomes: Large Proteoliposomes Derived from Cross-Linked Human Erythrocyte Cytoskeletons and Exogenous Lipid. *Proceedings of the National Academy of Sciences of the United States of America*, *78*(5), 2786–2790. doi:10.1073/pnas.78.5.2786 PMID:6789323

Daleke, D. L., Hess, D. T., & Stamler, J. S. (2008). Hypoxic vasodilation by red blood cells: Evidence for an s-nitrosothiol-based signal. *Circulation Research*, *103*(5), 545–553. doi:10.1161/CIRCRESAHA.108.176867 PMID:18658051

Daleke, D. L., & Lyles, J. V. (2000). Identification and purification of aminophospholipid flippases. *Biochimica et Biophysica Acta*, *1486*(1), 108–127. doi:10.1016/S1388-1981(00)00052-4 PMID:10856717

Davson, H., & Danielli, J. F. (1970). *Dannen Conn*. Hanfer Publishing Co.

Deloach, J. R. (1983). Encapsulation of Exogenous Agents in Erythrocytes and the Circulating Survival of Carrier Erythrocytes. *Journal of Applied Biochemistry*, *5*(3), 149–157. PMID:6438049

Deloach, J. R. (1987). Subcutaneous Administration of [35-S] r-IL-2 in Mice Carrier Erythrocytes: Alteration of IL-2 Pharmacokinetics. *Advances in the Biosciences*, *67*, 183–190.

Deloach, J. R., & Doleskey, R. (1987). Preparation and Properties of Microcytic Carrier Erythrocytes from Sheep and Goats. *Advances in the Biosciences*, *67*, 199–212.

Deloach, J. R., Harris, R. L., & Ihler, G. M. (1980). An Erythrocyte Encapsulator Dialyzer Used in Preparing Large Quantities of Erythrocyte Ghosts and Encapsulation of a Pesticide in Erythrocyte Ghosts. *Analytical Biochemistry*, *102*(1), 220–227. doi:10.1016/0003-2697(80)90342-5 PMID:6766688

Deloach, J. R., & Ihler, G. M. (1977). A Dialysis Procedure for Loading of Erythrocytes with Enzymes and Lipids. *Biochimica et Biophysica Acta*, *496*(1), 136–145. doi:10.1016/0304-4165(77)90121-0 PMID:836891

Dinda, S. C., & Pattnaik, G. (2013). Nanobiotechnology-based drug delivery in brain targeting. *Current Pharmaceutical Biotechnology*, *14*(15), 1264–1274. doi:10.2174/1389201015666140608143719 PMID:24910011

Eichler, H. C., Gasic, S., Daum, B., Bacher, S., & Sreger, G. (1987). In Vitro Drug Release From Human Carrier Erythrocytes. *Advances in the Biosciences*, *67*, 11–15.

Eichler, H. G., Gasicm, S., Bauer, K., Korn, A., & Bacher, S. (1986). *In Vivo* Clearance of Antibody-Sensitized Human Drug Carrier Erythrocytes. *Clinical Pharmacology and Therapeutics*, *40*(3), 300–303. doi:10.1038/clpt.1986.180 PMID:3091309

Eichler, H. G., Raffesberg, W., Gasic, S., Korn, A., & Bauer, K. (1985). Release of Vitamin B 12 from Carrier Erythrocytes *In Vitro. Research in Experimental Medicine. Zeitschrift fur die Gesamte Experimentelle Medizin Einschliesslich Experimenteller Chirurgie*, *185*(4), 341–344. doi:10.1007/BF01851959 PMID:4048655

Fiorelli, G., Fargion, S., Piperno, A., Cappellini, M. D., Rossi, F., Sabionedda, L., & Zanella, A. (1987). Transfusion of Thalasemic Patients with Desferrioxamine Loaded Standard Red Blood Cell Units. *Advanced Biosciences67*, 47-54.

Flynn, G., McHale, L., & McHale, A. P. (1994). Methotrexate-Loaded, Photosensitized Erythrocytes: A Photo-Activatable Carrier/Delivery System for Use in Cancer Therapy. *Cancer Letters*, *82*(2), 225–229. doi:10.1016/0304-3835(94)90016-7 PMID:8050095

Fraternale, A., Rossi, L., & Magnani, M. (1996). Encapsulation, Metabolism, and Release of 2-Fluoro-Ara-AMP from Human Erythrocytes. *Biochimica et Biophysica Acta*, *1291*(2), 149–154. doi:10.1016/0304-4165(96)00059-1 PMID:8898876

Furusawa, M., Nishimura, T., Yamaizumi, M., & Okada, Y. (1974). Injection of foreign substances into single cells by cell fusion. *Nature*, *249*(456), 449–450. doi:10.1038/249449a0 PMID:4365359

Gardos, G. (1956). Akkumulation de Kalium Onen Durch Menschiche Blutkorperchen. *Acta Physiologica Academiae Scientiarum Hungaricae*, *6*, 191–196.

Garín, M. I., López, R. M., Sanz, S., Pinilla, M., & Luque, J. (1996). Erythrocytes as carriers for recombinant human erythropoietin. *Pharmaceutical Research*, *13*(6), 869–874. doi:10.1023/A:1016049027661 PMID:8792424

Gothoskar, A. V. (2004). Resealed Erythrocytes: A Review. *Pharmaceutical Technology*, 140-158.

Green, R., & Widder, K. J. (1987). *Methods in Enzymology*. San Diego, CA: Academic Press.

Guyton, A. C., & Hall, J. E. (1996). *Red Blood Cells, Anemia and Polycytemia. In Textbook of Medical Physiology* (pp. 425–433). Philadelphia, PA: W.B. Saunders.

Guyton, A. C., & Hall, J. E. (1996). *Transport of Oxygen and Carbon Dioxide in the Blood and Body Fluids. In Textbook of Medical Physiology* (pp. 513–523). Philadelphia, PA: W.B. Saunders.

Guyton, A. C., & Hall, J. E. (2006). *Textbook of Medical Physiology* (11th ed.). Elsevier Inc.

Hamidi, M., & Tajerzadeh, H. (2003). Carrier erythrocytes: An overview. *Drug Delivery*, *10*(1), 9–20. doi:10.1080/713840329 PMID:12554359

Hamidi, M., Tajerzadeh, H., Dehpour, A. R., Rouini, M. R., & Ejtemaee-Mehr, S. (2001). *In vitro* characterization of human intact erythrocytes loaded by enalaprilat. *Drug Delivery*, *8*(4), 223–230. doi:10.1080/107175401317245903 PMID:11757780

Harris, R. C. (1977). Enzyme Replacement in Red Cells. *The New England Journal of Medicine*, *296*(16), 942–943. doi:10.1056/NEJM197704212961618 PMID:846521

Iher, G. M., Glew, R. M., & Schnure, F. W. (1973). Enzyme Loading of Erythrocytes. *Proceedings of the National Academy of Sciences of the United States of America*, *70*(9), 2663–2666. doi:10.1073/pnas.70.9.2663 PMID:4354859

Ihler, G., Lantzy, A., Purpura, J., & Glew, R. H. (1975). Enzymatic Degradation of Uricase-Loaded Human Erythrocytes. *The Journal of Clinical Investigation*, *56*(3), 595–602. doi:10.1172/JCI108129 PMID:1159075

Ihler, G. M. (1983). Erythrocyte Carriers. *Pharmacology & Therapeutics*, *20*(2), 151–169. doi:10.1016/0163-7258(83)90037-2 PMID:6351110

Ihler, G. M., & Tsang, H. C. W. (1987). Hypotonic Hemolysis Methods For Entrapment of Agents in Resealed Erythrocytes.[series]. *Methods in Enzymology*, *149*, 221–229. doi:10.1016/0076-6879(87)49059-9 PMID:3121983

Jain, S., & Jain, N. K. (1997). Engineered Erythrocytes as a Drug Delivery System. *Indian Journal of Pharmaceutical Sciences*, *59*, 275–281.

Jain, S., Jain, S. K., & Dixit, V. K. (1995). Erythrocytes Based Delivery of Isoniazid: Preparation and *In Vitro* Characterization. *Indian Drugs*, *32*, 471–476.

Jain, S., Jain, S. K., & Dixit, V. K. (1997). Magnetically Guided Rat Erythrocytes Bearing Isoniazid: Preparation, Characterization, and Evaluation. *Drug Development and Industrial Pharmacy*, *23*(10), 999–1006. doi:10.3109/03639049709149153

Jaitely, V., Kanaujia, P., Venkatesan, N., Jain, S., & Vyas, S. P. (1996). Resealed Erythrocytes: Drug Carrier Potentials and Biomedical Applications. *Indian Drugs*, *33*, 589–594.

Jenner, D. J., Lewis, D. A., Pitt, E., & Offord, R. A. (1981). The Effect of the Intravenous Administration of Corticosteroids Encapsulated in Intact Erythrocytes on Adjuvant Arthritis in the Rat. *British Journal of Pharmacology*, *73*, 212P–213P.

Jrade, M., Villereal, M. C., Boynard, M., & Ropars, C. (1987). Rheological Approach to Human Red Blood Cell Carriers Desferrioxamine Encapsulation. *Advances in the Biosciences*, *67*, 29–36.

Jung, C. Y. (1987). *Methods in Enzymology*. New York, NY: Academic Press.

Kiefer, C. R., & Snyder, L. M. (2000). Oxidation and erythrocyte senescence. *Current Opinion in Hematology*, *7*(2), 113–116. doi:10.1097/00062752-200003000-00007 PMID:10698298

Kim, D. M., & Zolinev, C. (1973). The Influence of Amphotericin-B on the Permeability of Mammalian Erythrocytes to Nonelectrolytes, anions and Cations. *Biochimica et Biophysica Acta*, *318*(3), 345–359. doi:10.1016/0005-2736(73)90199-5

Kinosita, K., & Tsong, T. Y. (1977a). Hemolysis of Human Erythrocytes by a Transient Electric Field. *Proceedings of the National Academy of Sciences of the United States of America*, *74*(5), 1923–1927. doi:10.1073/pnas.74.5.1923 PMID:266714

Kinosita, K., & Tsong, T. Y. (1977b). Formation and Resealing of Pores of Controlled Sizes in Human Erythrocyte Membrane. *Nature*, *268*(5619), 438–441. doi:10.1038/268438a0 PMID:895849

Kitao, T., Hattori, K., & Takeshita, M. (1978). Agglutination of Leukemic Cells and Daunomycin Entrapped Erythrocytes with Lectin *In Vitro* and *In Vivo*. *Experimentia*, *341*(1), 94–95. doi:10.1007/BF01921924 PMID:620752

Kleinbongard, P., Schulz, R., Rassaf, T., Lauer, T., Dejam, A., Jax, T., & Kelm, M. et al. (2006). Red blood cells express a functional endothelial nitric oxide synthase. *Blood*, *107*(7), 2943–2951. doi:10.1182/blood-2005-10-3992 PMID:16368881

Kruse, C. A., James, G. T., Cederbaum, S. D., et al., (1987). Arginase-Loaded Erythrocyte Carriers: Their Fusion to Host Cells with Viral Fusogenic Proteins and Subcellular Localization of Arginase. *Advanced Biosciences, 67*, 113-122

Kruse, C. A., Spector, E. B., Cederbaum, S. D., Wisnieski, B. J., & Popják, G. (1981). Microinjection of Arginase into Enzyme-Deficient Cells with the Isolated Glycoprotein of Sendai Virus as Fusogen. *Biochimica et Biophysica Acta*, *645*(2), 339–345. doi:10.1016/0005-2736(81)90205-4 PMID:6268159

Lejeune, A., Poyet, P., Gaudreault, R. C., & Gicquaud, C. (1997). Nanoerythrosomes, A New Derivative of Erythrocyte Ghost: III. Is Phagocytosis Involved in the Mechanism of Action? *Anticancer Research*, *17*, 5A. PMID:9413209

Lewis, D. A. (1984). Red Blood Cells for Drug Delivery. *Pharmaceutics Journal*, *233*, 384–385.

Lewis, D. A., & Alpar, H. O. (1984). Therapeutic Possibilities of Drugs Encapsulated in Erythrocytes. *International Journal of Pharmaceutics*, *22*(2-3), 137–146. doi:10.1016/0378-5173(84)90017-6

Lewis, D. A., & Desai, J. (1987). The Use of Animal Models in the Encapsulation of Drugs in Erythrocytes.[series]. *Advances in the Biosciences*, *67*, 213–222.

Lin, W., Mota de Freitas, D., Zhang, Q., & Olsen, K. W. (1999). Nuclear magnetic resonance and oxygen affinity study of cesium binding in human erythrocytes. *Archives of Biochemistry and Biophysics*, *369*(1), 78–88. doi:10.1006/abbi.1999.1285 PMID:10462442

Lux, S. E., & Palek, J. (1995). Disorders of the red cell membrane. In *Blood: Principles and Practice of Hematology*. Academic Press.

Magnani, M., Laguerre, M., Rossi, L., Bianchi, M., Ninfali, P., Mangani, F., & Ropars, C. (1989). Acetaldehyde dehydrogenase-loaded erythrocytes as bioreactors for the removal of blood acetaldehyde. *Alcoholism, Clinical and Experimental Research*, *13*(6), 849–859. doi:10.1111/j.1530-0277.1989.tb00436.x PMID:2690672

Magnani, M., Rossi, L., D'ascenzo, M., Panzani, I., Bigi, L., & Zanella, A. (1998). Erythrocyte engineering for drug delivery and targeting. *Biotechnology and Applied Biochemistry*, *28*(Pt 1), 1–6. PMID:9693082

Mahmmoud, Y. A. (2011). Curcumin is a lipid dependent inhibitor of the Na, K-ATPase that likely interacts at the protein-lipid interface. *Biochimica et Biophysica Acta*, *1808*(1), 466–473. doi:10.1016/j.bbamem.2010.09.021 PMID:20888791

Mehdi, M. M., & Rizvi, S. I. (2013). Plasma protein hydroperoxides during aging in humans: Correlation with paraoxonase 1 (PON1) arylesterase activity and plasma total thiols. *Archives of Medical Research*, *44*(2), 136–141. doi:10.1016/j.arcmed.2013.01.003 PMID:23376056

Mehdi, M. M., Singh, P., & Rizvi, S. I. (2012). Erythrocyte sialic acid content during aging in humans: Correlation with markers of oxidative stress. *Disease Markers*, *32*(3), 179–186. doi:10.1155/2012/293429 PMID:22377734

Michaely, P., & Bennett, V. (1995). The ANK repeats of erythrocyte ankyrin form two distinct but cooperative binding sites for the erythrocyte anion exchanger. *The Journal of Biological Chemistry*, *270*(37), 22050–22057. doi:10.1074/jbc.270.37.22050 PMID:7665627

Mohandas, N., & Gallagher, P. G. (2008). Red cell membrane: Past, present, and future. *Blood*, *112*(10), 3939–3948. doi:10.1182/blood-2008-07-161166 PMID:18988878

Moorjani, M., Lejeune, A., Gicquaud, C., Lacroix, J., Poyet, P., & Gaudreault, R. C. (1996). Nanoerythrosomes, a new derivative of erythrocyte ghost II: Identification of the mechanism of action. *Anticancer Research*, *16*(5A), 2831–2836. PMID:8917393

Nicolau, C., & Gersonde, K. (1979). Incorporation of Inositol Hexaphosphate into Intact Red Blood Cells, I: Fusion of Effector-Containing Lipid Vesicles with Erythrocytes. *Naturwissenschaften*, *66*(11), 563–566. doi:10.1007/BF00368810 PMID:514370

Pandey, K. B., & Rizvi, S. I. (2010). Markers of oxidative stress in erythrocytes and plasma during aging in humans. *Oxidative Medicine and Cellular Longevity*, *3*(1), 2–12. doi:10.4161/oxim.3.1.10476 PMID:20716923

Pandey, K. B., & Rizvi, S. I. (2014a). Resveratrol *in vitro* ameliorates tert-butyl hydroperoxide-induced alterations in erythrocyte membranes from young and older humans. *Applied Physiology, Nutrition, and Metabolism*, *31*, 1–5. PMID:24914573

Pandey, K. B., & Rizvi, S. I. (2014b). Role of resveratrol in regulation of membrane transporters and integrity of human erythrocytes. *Biochemical and Biophysical Research Communications*, *453*(3), 521–526. doi:10.1016/j.bbrc.2014.09.117 PMID:25285638

Pei, L., Omburo, G., McGuinn, W. D., Petrikovics, I., Dave, K., Raushel, F. M., & Way, J. L. et al. (1994). Encapsulation of phosphotriesterase within murine erythrocytes. *Toxicology and Applied Pharmacology, 124*(2), 296–301. doi:10.1006/taap.1994.1035 PMID:8122276

Pitt, E., Lewis, D. A., & Offord, R. (1983). The Use of Corticosteroids Encapsulated in Erythrocytes in the Treatment of Adjuvant Induced Arthritis in the Rat. *Biochemical Pharmacology, 132*(22), 3355–3358. doi:10.1016/0006-2952(83)90362-3 PMID:6651860

Price, R. J., Skyba, D. M., Kaul, S., & Skalak, T. C. (1998). Delivery of Colloidal Particles and Red Blood Cells to Tissue through Microvessel Ruptures Created by Targeted Microbubble Destruction with Ultrasound. *Circulation, 98*(13), 1264–1267. doi:10.1161/01.CIR.98.13.1264 PMID:9751673

Racca, A., Biondi, C., Cotorruelo, C., Galizzi, S., Rasia, R. J., Stoltz, J. F., & Valverde, J. (1999). Senescent erythrocytes: Modification of rheologic properties, antigenic expression and interaction with monocytes. *Medicina, 59*(1), 33–37. PMID:10349116

Rechsteiner, M. C. (1975). Uptake of Protein by Red Cells. *Experimental Cell Research, 43*(2), 487–492. doi:10.1016/0014-4827(75)90478-4 PMID:1098917

Rettig, M. P., Low, P. S., Gimm, J. A., Mohandas, N., Wang, J., & Christian, J. A. (1999). Evaluation of biochemical changes during in vivo erythrocyte senescence in the dog. *Blood, 93*(1), 376–384. PMID:9864184

Rizvi, S. I., & Pandey, K. B. (2011). Activation of the erythrocyte plasma membrane redox system by resveratrol: A possible mechanism for antioxidant properties. *Pharmacological Reports, 62*(4), 726–732. doi:10.1016/S1734-1140(10)70330-3 PMID:20885013

Rossi, L., Serafini, S., Pierigé, F., Antonelli, A., Cerasi, A., Fraternale, A., & Magnani, M. et al. (2005). Erythrocyte-based drug delivery. *Expert Opinion on Drug Delivery, 2*(2), 311–322. doi:10.1517/17425247.2.2.311 PMID:16296756

Rybicki, A. C., Schwartz, R. S., Hustedt, E. J., & Cobb, C. E. (1996). Increased rotational mobility and extractability of band 3 from protein 4.2-deficient erythrocyte membranes: Evidence of a role for protein 4.2 in strengthening the band 3-cytoskeleton linkage. *Blood, 88*, 2745–2753. PMID:8839871

Schlegel, R. A., & McEvoy L. (1987). Red Cell-Mediated Microinjection. *Methods in Enzymology, 149*, 293-301.

Schriei, S. L., Bensch, K. G., Johnson, M., & Junga, I. (1975). Energized endocytosis in human erythrocyte ghosts. *The Journal of Clinical Investigation, 56*(1), 8–22. doi:10.1172/JCI108083 PMID:124748

Schrier, S. L. (1987). Shape Changes and Deformability in Human Erythrocyte Membranes. *The Journal of Laboratory and Clinical Medicine, 110*(6), 791–797. PMID:3500247

Singh, P., Kesharwani, R. K., Misra, K., & Rizvi, S. I. (2015). (in press). The modulation effects of curcumin on erythrocyte Na^+/K^+-ATPase activity. *Journal of Advanced Research*. doi:10.1016/j.jare.2014.12.007

Singh, P., & Rizvi, S. I. (2015). Role of curcumin in modulating plasma PON1 arylesterase activity and susceptibility to LDL oxidation in oxidatively challenged wistar rats. *Letters in Drug Design & Discovery, 12*(4), 319–323. doi:10.2174/1570180811666141016000539

Sivilotti, M. L. (2004). Oxidant stress and haemolysis of the human erythrocyte. *Toxicological Reviews*, *23*(3), 169–188. doi:10.2165/00139709-200423030-00004 PMID:15862084

Summers, M. P. (1983). Recent Advances in Drug Delivery. *The Pharmaceutical Journal*, *230*, 643–645.

Talwar, N., & Jain, N. K. (1992). Erythrocytes as Carriers of Metronidazole: *In-Vitro* Characterization. *Drug Development and Industrial Pharmacy*, *18*(16), 1799–1812. doi:10.3109/03639049209040903

Talwar, N., & Jain, N. K. (1992). Erythrocytes as Carriers of Primaquin Preparation: Characterization and Evaluation. *Journal of Controlled Release*, *20*(2), 133–142. doi:10.1016/0168-3659(92)90159-O

Tan, C. (1972). L-Asparaginase in Leukemia. *Hospital Practice*, *7*, 99–103.

Teisseire, B. (1987). In Vivo Consequences of Rightward Shift of the Hemoglobin Dissociation Curve. Advanced Biosciences, 67, 89-94.

Telen, M. J. (1993). The mature erythrocyte. In Wintrobe's Clinical Hematology (9th Ed.). Lea & Febiger.

Torotra, G. J., & Grabowski, S. R. (1993). *The Cardiovascular System: The Blood. Principles of Anatomy and Physiology* (7th ed.). New York: Harper Collins College Publishers.

Tsong, T. Y., & Kinosita, K. Jr. (1985). Use of Voltage Pulses for the Pore, Opening and Drug Loading, and the Subsequent Resealing of Red, Blood Cells. *Bibliotheca Haematologica*, *51*, 108–114. PMID:4004753

Ulker, P., Sati, L., Celik-Ozenci, C., Meiselman, H. J., & Baskurt, O. K. (2009). Mechanical stimulation of nitric oxide synthesizing mechanisms in erythrocytes. *Biorheology*, *46*(2), 121–132. PMID:19458415

Updike, S. J., & Wakamiya, R. T. (1983). Infusion of Red Blood Cell-Loaded Asparaginase in Monkey. *The Journal of Laboratory and Clinical Medicine*, *101*, 679–691. PMID:6187874

Vienken, J., Jeltsch, E., & Zimmermann, U. (1978). Penetration and Entrapment of Large Particles in Erythrocytes by Electrical Breakdown Techniques. *Cytobiologie*, *17*, 182–186. PMID:689250

Villareal, M. C. (1987). Modification of Cardiac Parameters in Piglets After Infusion of IHP-Loaded Red Blood Cells.[series]. *Advances in the Biosciences*, *67*, 81–88.

Vyas, S. P., & Dixit, V. K. (1999). Pharmaceutical Biotechnology 1. CBS Publishers & Distributors.

Vyas, S. P., & Khar, R. K. (2002). *Resealed Erythrocytes in Targeted and Controlled Drug Delivery: Novel Carrier Systems*. CBS Publishers and Distributors.

Wan, J., Ristenpart, W. D., & Stone, H. A. (2008). Dynamics of shear-induced ATP release from red blood cells. *Proceedings of the National Academy of Sciences of the United States of America*, *105*(43), 16432–16437. doi:10.1073/pnas.0805779105 PMID:18922780

Wille, W., & Willecke, K. (1976). Retention of Purified Proteins in Resealed Human Erythrocyte Ghosts and Transfer by Fusion into Cultured Murine Cells. *FEBS Letters*, *65*(1), 59–62. doi:10.1016/0014-5793(76)80621-7 PMID:1278411

Zanella, A. (1987). Desferrioxamine Loading of Red Cells for Transfusion. *Advanced Biosciences*, *67*, 17–27.

Zimmermann, U. (1973). *Jahresbericht der Kernforschungsanlage Julich GmbH*. Julich: Nuclear Research Center.

Zimmermann, U. (1983). Cellular Drug-Carrier Systems and Their Possible Targeting. In *Targeted Drugs* (pp. 153–200). New York, NY: John Wiley & Sons.

Zimmermann, U., Pilwat, G., & Riemann, F. (1975). Preparation of Erythrocyte Ghosts by Dielectric Breakdown of the Cell Membrane. *Biochimica et Biophysica Acta*, *375*(2), 209–219. doi:10.1016/0005-2736(75)90189-3 PMID:1168495

Zimmermann, U., Riemann, F., & Pilwat, G. (1976). Enzyme Loading of Electrically Homogenous Human Red Blood Cell Ghosts Prepared by Dielectric Breakdown. *Biochimica et Biophysica Acta*, *436*(2), 460–474. doi:10.1016/0005-2736(76)90208-X PMID:1276224

Zocchi, E., Tonetti, M., Polvani, C., Guida, L., Benatti, U., & De Flora, A. (1988). *In-Vivo* Liver and Lung Targeting of Adriamycin Encapsulated in Glutaraldehyde-Treated Murine Erythrocytes. *Biotechnology and Applied Biochemistry*, *10*, 555–562. PMID:3148305

Section 8
Herbals

Chapter 13
New Herbal Approaches for the Treatment of Diabetic Kidney Diseases and Its Therapeutic Implications

Durgavati Yadav
Institute of Medical Sciences, India

Shivani Srivastava
Institute of Medical Sciences, India

Vivek Pandey
Institute of Medical Science, India

Yamini Bhusan Tripathi
Institute of Medical Science, India

ABSTRACT

Diabetic Kidney Diseases (DKD) is a very serious complication of diabetes. There is recent steep rise in the prevalence of metabolic syndrome and DKD worldwide. Factors responsible for intraglomerular hypertension include activation of various vasoactive systems, polyol pathway, oxidative stress, inflammation and protein kinase C. Sodium-Dependent Glucose Co-Transporter (SGLT-2) inhibitors, DPP-IV (Dipeptidyl peptidase-4) inhibitors are being develop to manage the hyperglycemia and oxidative stress induced inflammatory cascade. Herbal drugs have gained increasing popularity; are complex mixtures of polyphenols and phytochemicals from any raw or processed part of a plant, including leaves. Herbal drugs in this modern era are preferred due to its lesser side effects. Various preparations are presently used for ameliorating the effect of DKD. Since, medicinal plants have been reported to affect various metabolic receptors, enzymes and signaling cascade. Above book chapter explains the involvement of different phytochemicals in biological pathway associated with the kidney damage.

INTRODUCTION

Diabetes is a metabolic syndrome which now becomes a growing epidemic in most of the developed and developing countries. Diabetes is of two types; Type 1 diabetes i.e. if individual's body is not able to make enough insulin. It usually starts when the person is a child or young, but it can happen to anyone. It is treated by taking daily insulin shots or using an insulin pump and by following a restricted diet plan

DOI: 10.4018/978-1-5225-0754-3.ch013

with care. About 5-10% of cases of the diabetes are Type 1. Type 2 diabetes; body makes some insulin but cannot use it properly. It is partially preventable and is typically brought on by poor diet and lack of exercise. Heredity may be one of the reasons; but it usually starts when the person is above the age of 40, but it can happen earlier also. It is treated with exercise, weight loss and meal planning. People with Type 2 diabetes generally requires insulin, but oral medications are given (called hypoglycemics) are prescribed if diet and exercise alone do not control the disease. Type 2 is the most common type of diabetes.

Diabetic kidney diseases (DKDs) are one of the serious and common complications of diabetes and part of the chronic kidney diseases (Tripathi & Yadav, 2013). Presently modern medicine is using diabetic kidney diseases (DKD) instead of diabetic nephropathy for which cure has not been yet found. Much research has been conducted in both basic sciences and clinical therapeutics, enhancing our understanding of the pathophysiology of diabetic nephropathy and expanded horizon of the potential therapies available. A better understanding of the pathogenesis of DKDs is therefore necessary to develop more effective therapies.

EPIDEMIOLOGY

The recent steep rise in the prevalence of metabolic syndrome and of Type 2 diabetes worldwide is extremely pronounced in Asian nations and is particularly dramatically increasing in India. This gave India the dubious distinction of the "diabetes capital of the world". In urban Indians, the overt nephropathy and microalbuminuria was found to be 2.2 and 26.9%, respectively (Ritz & Zeng, 2011). Diabetic kidney diseases are the most common causes of chronic kidney failure and end-stage kidney diseases in the United States (Mehdi & Toto, 2009).

Factors responsible for intraglomerular hypertension include activation of various vasoactive systems, such as endothelial systems and the RAAS. Polyol pathway, oxidative stress, inflammation and PKC pathways which are involved in making it a syndrome; with serious complications. These changes results to high secretion of fibrotic cytokines such as transforming growth factor β resulting to furtherance of haemodynamic changes (Sharma & Sharma,2013). The earliest clinical evidence of nephropathy is an increase in microalbuminuria (defined as >30 mg/day) into the macroalbuminuria range (>300 mg/day) (Toth-Manikowski &Atta, 2015). Renal function is compromised even prior to the onset of initial damage to the kidney. There occurs several oxidation and reduction changes that appears early and continue as chronic damage progresses, highlighting the complexities of the disease. Besides the classical anti-diabetic drugs such as sulfonyl urea, begonides, α- glucosidase inhibitors, PPAR-γ agonists (Peroxisome proliferator activated receptor), Sodium dependent glucose co-transport (SGLT-2) inhibitors, aldose reductase inhibitors, DPP-IV (Dipeptidyl peptidase-4) inhibitors etc are being developed to manage hyper-glycemia (Pathak and Bridgeman, 2010).

Increasing evidence from both experimental and clinical studies suggests that there is a close relationship between hyperglycemia and oxidative stress induced inflammatory cascade. People with diabetes are at higher risk of vascular, peripheral and cardiovascular diseases. Evidence of kidney damages are albuminuria, proteinuria, haematuria, decrease in creatinine clearance and structural abnormalities found on the kidney imaging tests. AGEs cause thickening of extracellular matrix, decrease in function of glomerulus. An estimated GFR < 45 mL/min/ 1.73 m^2 is associated with higher risks of renal, cardiovascular and other clinical manifestations irrespective of the age. Herbal drugs in this modern era are preferred due to its lesser side effects. But new herbal multitargeted molecular therapeutics is required. Various herbal and medicinal plant preparations are presently used for ameliorating the effect of chronic renal damage. There are lists of pharmacological tools and their mechanistic action which are implied in the effective treatment of DKD. Ancient Ayurvedic systems, Chinese herbal medicines, folklore treatments around the various corners of the world are being investigated in newer dimensions for better prospects. Examples include Chiahuang-Yishen formula for chronic kidney diseases including diabetic nephropathy.

RISK FACTORS IN DKDs

Not all the diabetics develop kidney disease but those who develop it, their progression is very variable with time factor. The major lifestyle risk factors include high blood pressure, glycemia and dyslipidemia while less extreme risk factors are age, race and genetic makeup. Creatinine is widely used biomarker for kidney function; it is inaccurate at detecting mild renal impairment and levels differ with muscle mass and protein intake. DKDs are likely to develop in patients with a family history (Macisaac, Ekinci, & Jerums, 2014). Few racial groups are at higher risk such as Afro-Americans, Mexicans (Young, Maynard, Boyko, 1991).A meta-analysis of diabetic studies identified 24 genetic variants in 16 genes which are linked to DKD. These include a variety of genes; ACE, ALR2, APOC1, APOE, EPO, CARS, CPVL/CHN2, FRMD3, UNC13B and GREM1. In another study of subgroup of Type 2 of diabetic Asians, ELMOI, CCR5 and CNDP1are also important finding relevantto the study (Mooyart et al., 2011).Other meta-analyses implicated polymorphic genes of ADIPOQ, PAI-1, TGF-β, PPAR-γ etc in the growth of DKD. The inherent polymorphism varies with different groups of wide ethnicity (Sun et al., 2014).

STAGES IN DIABETIC KIDNEY DISEASES

Approximately 25% to 40% of patients with Diabetes Mellitus (DM) ultimately develop DKD, which progresses through five stages.

Stage 1 – Hyperfiltration (Glomerular Hypertrophy): (Very early diabetes). Increased demand of filtration on kidneys is indicated by an above normal Glomerular Filtration Rate (GFR).

Stage 2 – Hyperfiltration (Mesangial Expansion / Basement Membrane Thickening): GFR remains in elevated level or returned to the normal but glomerular damage has progressed to significant microalbuminuria. Patients excrete more than 30 mg of albumin in the urine over a 24 hrs period. Excessive micro or macroalbuminuria will finally leads to End-Stage Renal Disease (ESRD). All diabetics should be screened for microalbuminuria on a routine or yearly basis.

Stage 3 – Microalbuminuria (Mesangial Sclerosis, Dipstickpositive Diabetes): Glomerular damage has progressed to clinical albuminuria. Urine is "dipstick positive," containing more than 300 mg of albumin in a 24-hour period. Hypertension i.e. high blood pressure typically develops during stage 3.

Stage 4 – Overt-Proteinuria Hypertension (Progressive Sclerosis): Late-stage diabetes Glomerular deterioration showed a continuous rise with increasing amounts of protein albumin and kidneys' filtering process begun to decline steadily; Blood Urea Nitrogen (BUN) and Creatinine (Cr) has begun to increase. The Glomerular Filtration Rate (GFR) decreases about 10% annually. Almost all the patients developed hypertension at stage 4.

Stage 5 – ESRD (Fibrosis/Sclerosis): GFR has fallen to approximately 10 milliliters per minute (<10 mL/min) and renal replacement therapy (i.e., hemodialysis, peritoneal dialysis, kidney transplantation) is required.

PATHOLOGY AND PATHOPHYSIOLOGY OF DIABETIC KIDNEY DISEASES

DKDs are characterized by various structural and functional changes in the human physiology. In glomeruli, there is mesangial expansion, thickening of the basement membrane and characteristically nodular glomerulosclerosis (Kimmelstiel-Wilson nodules). In early stages of DKD, tubular hypertrophy is present but eventually interstitial fibrosis with tubular atrophy develops, along with hyalinosis. In advanced cases, there is an infiltration of macrophages and T-lymphocytes in the interstitial spaces. Ultrastructurally, there is podocyte loss and reduced endothelial cell fenestration (Weil et al., 2012). Pathogenesis in DKD patients with several linked physiological connections are given in Figure 1.

HEMODYNAMIC PATHWAY

It includes an imbalance in an afferent and an efferent arteriolar resistance resulting in the increased glomerular hydrostatic pressure and excess hyperfiltration. Activation of renin-angiotensin system (RAS) increases angiotensin II levels, leading to an efferent arteriolar vasoconstriction. It causes production of proinflammatory and profibrotic molecules through multiple cellular mechanisms. High angiotensin converting enzyme (ACE) levels are associated with greater albuminuria and kidney damage in diabetic mice and humans (Wong et al.,2007). Increased levels of endothelin-1 and urotensin II also contribute to vasoconstriction of the vessels. Various dysregulation of nitric oxide and nitric oxide synthase has been described in DKD. Nitric oxide mediates endothelium-dependent vasodilatation. Nitric oxide in cells is formed from L-arginine by endothelial nitric oxide synthase. In an experiment it was shown that diabetic endothelial nitric oxide synthase knockout mice develop more severe glomerular lesions and proteinuria compared to wild-type mice (Kosugi et al., 2010).

ACEIs (Angiotensin converting Enzyme Inhibitors) and ARBs (Angiotensin II receptor blocker) have a long track record in reducing the rate of the creatinine, albuminuria and progression to DKD, ESRD and death (Bakris, S3-10, 2008). ET-1 (a powerful vasoconstrictor) has various physiologic functions in the kidney that mimic RAS including vasoconstriction and hence playing a role in hypertension, endothelial dysfunction, inflammation and fibrosis (Toth- Manikowski & Atta, 2005). Increased ET-1 expression activates a signaling cascade which leads to mesangial hypertrophy and proliferation as well as extracellular matrix (ECM) thickening. It is also thought to activate receptors that directly increase glomerular permeability, hence leading to the worsening albuminuria and progression of DKD.

METABOLIC PATHWAY

Oxidative stress and generation of reactive oxygen species (ROS) damages DNA and protein or function as signaling amplifiers to activate cellular stress pathways such as PKC, MAPK etc (Trachootham, Lu, Ogaswara, Rivera-Del Valle & Huang, 2008). Polyol pathway activation, aldose reductase converting excess glucose to sorbitol and its subsequent conversion to fructose by enzyme sorbitol dehydrogenase contributes to oxidative stress by increasing the NADH/NAD^+ ratio (Figure 2). A recently described novel mechanism of insult to cells also involves endogenous fructose production with activation of enzyme fructokinase in the proximal tubules of the organ kidney. The formation of advanced glycation end-products (AGE) by nonenzymatic binding of glucose to proteins, lipids and nucleic acids leads to alteration of protein structure and function, oxidative stress; and expression of proinflammatory cytokines and growth factors (Singh, Bali, Singh & Jaggi, 2014).

THE POLYOL PATHWAY

The polyol pathway is upregulated as a result of increased continous and persistent hyperglycemic condition. The reduction of glucose to sorbitol results in decreased intracellular NADPH levels, an important cofactor involved in regenerating the antioxidant ie reduced glutathione (GSH). A decreased level of GSH contributes to increased intracellular oxidative stress which in turn causes increased cell stress and apoptosis (Circu & Aw, 2012) and then oxidation of sorbitol to fructose sugar produces increased intracellular NADH: NAD^+ ratio which further inhibits the process of glycolysis. The increased NADH:NAD^+ ratio also increases the formation of methylglyoxal and second messenger ie diacylglycerol, precursors of the AGEs and PKC pathways (Brownlee M, 2001). Finally, the end products of the polyol pathway, fructose has been emerged as a potentially nephrotoxic. In an experimentally developed diabetic murine

Figure 2. Glycolysis pathway as affected by hyperglycemic condition leading to accumulation of ECM and generation of free radicles

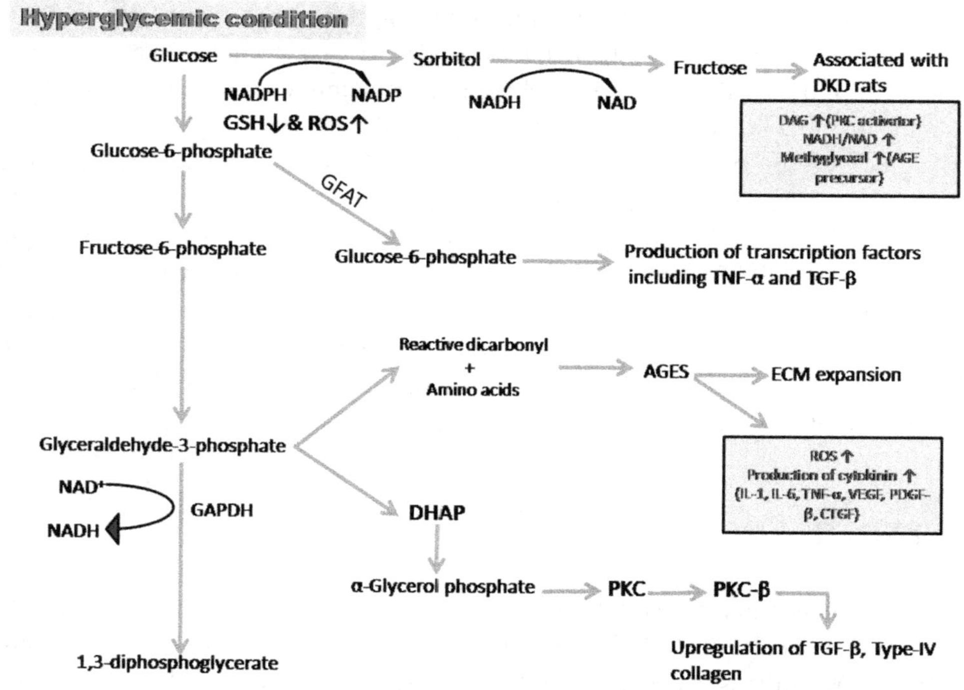

model, the endogenously produced fructose through polyol pathway led to increase in proteinuria, decline in GFR and increased glomerular capsule & proximal tubular injury when compared to mice with lower levels of endogenous fructose. Making the matter more worse, these mice expressed more superoxide levels and the inflammatory cytokines like NF-κB (2013, Forbes &Cooper).

HEXOSAMINE PATHWAY

The hexosamine pathway originates from the third step of the glycolysis, fructose-6-phosphate, is converted to glucosamine-6-phosphate by the enzyme glutamine: fructose-6-phosphate amidotransferase (GFAT) Figure 2. Glucosamine-6-phosphate is then used as a substrate to increase transcription of inflammatory cytokines tumor necrosis factor-(TNF-α) and transforming growth factor-β1 (TGF-β1) (Liu, Kelm, Straunch, 2009). Increased TGF-β1 levels are responsible for promoting renal cell hypertrophy and increase in the components of the mesangial matrix. These are the two most important pathological hallmarks of the DKD (Chen et al., 2001) whereas TNF-α is an important inflammatory cytokine (Liu, Kelm, Straunch, 2009).

ADVANCED GLYCATION END PRODUCTS (AGEs)

AGEs products are the outcome of irreversible glycation of proteins that occurs in the presence of intracellular hyperglycemic condition (Lim, 2014; Brownlee, 2001; Sheetz, 2002). Increase in the uptake of glucose to the proximal tubular cells via sodium glucose co-transporter 2 (SGLT2) stimulates free radical generation and RAGE expression; thereby aggravating the AGE induced apoptosis in this cell type. AGEs work through three mechanisms to induce final damages and are primarily responsible for the production of AGE precursors. In the first step, there is intracellular protein modification in the kidney cells; oxidation of glucose to form glyoxal and then breakdown of Amadori products; finally aberrant glycolysis which shunts glyceraldehydes-3-phospahate to make methylglyoxal (Verspohl, 2012). In the second step, its abnormal behaviour with other matrix components and with the receptors of the matrix proteins for e.g. integrins on cell surface. In the final third step, binding of AGE receptors generates ROS and NF-kB activated gene expression. When AGEs are formed, they damage renal cells by modifying or impairing the function of both intracellular and extracellular proteins (Sheetz & King, 2002). AGEs modifies both matrix proteins; laminin and Type IV collagen and increases the permeability of the glomerular basement membrane (Forbes, Cooper, Oldfield & Thomas, 2003) leading to increased excretion of protein in the urine. They also cause rise in the expression of fibronectin and collagen Types I and IV which leads to the increased density and expansion of the extracellular matrix in the kidney (Huang, 2001; Sakurai, 2003). AGEs bind themselves to various proinflammatory receptors which activate the downstream production of cytokines (IL-18, IL-1, IL-6, TNF-α, TGF-β1, VEGF, platelet-derived growth factor- β (PDGF-β), connective tissue growth factor (CTGF), generation of excess ROS (Alicic, 2014; Tan,2008). VEGF is required for endothelial cell survival, podocytes integrity and overall health of the mesangial cells whereas CTGF is a profibrotic agent; both have been implicated in DKD (Tufro & Veron, 2012; Mason, 2009).

THE PKC PATHWAY

Protein kinase has 12 isoforms. Nine PKCs are activated by DAG which is formed by excess production of glyceraldehydes-3-phosphate. High cellular glycemic index drives the conversion of glyceraldehyde-3-phosphate into dihydroxyacetone phosphate (DHAP) and finally diacylglycerol (DAG) which is a co-factor for activation of PKC (Noh & King, 2007). PKC pathway stems from the fourth step in glycolysis as shown in Figure 3.

In the presence of hyperglycemic state, DAG is chronically upregulated and gives its contribution to sustained activation of PKC (Craven, Davidson & DeRubertis, 1990). Protein kinase C contributes to DKD; it increases the prostaglandin E_2activity levels and nitric oxide (Bank & Aynedjian, 1993). This change further leads to vasodilation of the afferent arteriole and augmentation of angiotensin II's actions on the efferent arteriole (Ruan & Arendshorst, 1996; Nagahama, 2000). These complex actions combining together contribute to glomerular hyperfiltration (Noh &King, 2007). In the final stages of DKD, there is a progressive deficiency in level of nitric oxide which has been associated with severerity of proteinuria, decreasing renal function and high blood pressure. PKC mediates excess production of VEGF which is again linked to intra-renal blood flow abnormality and capillary permeability and is thought to play a role in the development of microalbuminuria (Menne et al., 2004). The activation of PKC increases CTGF and TGF-β levels in the tissue as well as the production of fibronectins and type IV collagen and opens gate to GBM thickening and ECM build up (Noh &King, 2007).

GROWTH FACTORS AND CYTOKINES

Activation of TGF-β and its relating cytokines like CTGF induces ECM formation and fibrosis. In most of the kidney biopsies, glomerular expression of TGF-β1 and CTGF were higher in diabetics as compared to controls and correlated with albuminuria and proteinuria. PDGF expression is also downregulated in

Figure 3. Different pathways activated when there is hyperglycemic condition

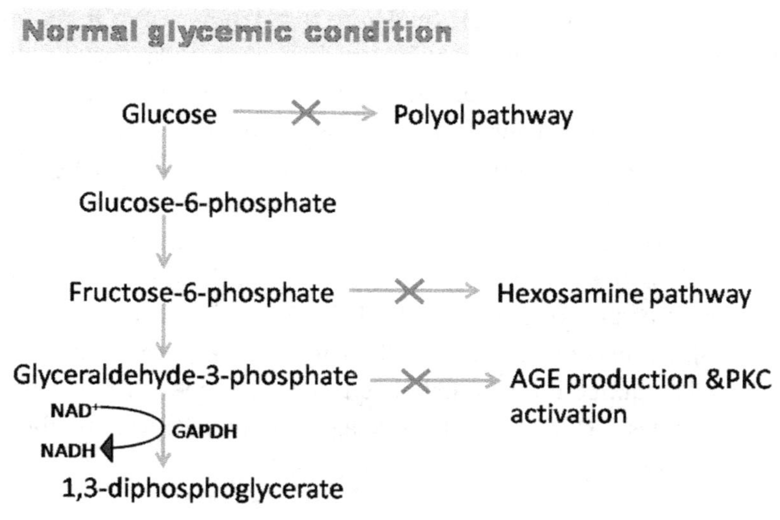

DKD, which influences chemotaxis, vascular tonicity and aggregation of the platelets. VEGF is very crucial in the angiogenesis process but it also mediate vasodilatation and leukocyte trafficking in DKD.

CELL SIGNALING AND TRANSCRIPTION FACTORS

Increased renal gene transcription of PKC-β showed a strong relationship with glycemic control (Langham et al., 2008). There are various different groups of transcription factors which get involved during the changes and lead to the organ damage as shown in Figure 4.

PKC activation has wide ranging effects, including the action of angiotensin II, dysregulation of nitric oxide, endothelial dysfunction and activation of MAPK and NF-κB (Noh & King, 2007). MAPKs are cell signaling intracellular kinases involved in various cellular responses. They form a chain of cascade in number of nuclear transcription factors, including NF-κB, which finally regulates gene expression of other cytokines, chemokines and adhesion molecules in the cell. The p38-α isoform activation in p38 MAPK pathway is strongly associated with renal inflammation and DKD (Sakai, 2005; Adhikary, 2004). It may be mentioned to be an important role for toll-like receptors (TLR 2, TLR 4) and B7-1 costimulatory signaling in modulating inflammation and injuries (Fiorina, 2014; Mudaliar, 2013). Transcription factors bind to the promoter regions of genes and modulate transcription of mRNA. The factor NF-κB had been widely acknowledged in case of DKD. Activation of NF-κB factor in the renal biopsies correlates with severity of proteinuria and glycemic control index (Schmid et al., 2006).

ROLE OF INFLAMMATION

There is recruitment and activation of innate immune cells with extensive elaboration of proinflammatory cytokines in DKD (Lim & Tesch, 2012). Macrophages and T-lymphocytes of the immune system are active in early diabetic glomeruli while their interstitial infiltration generally develops in later stages. However, the absence of lymphocytes did not prevent fibrosis and declining renal function in experimental DKD (Lim et al., 2010). Strategies involving compromise on the part of renal leukocyte recruitment, its proliferation and activation have demonstrated that macrophages mediate in DKD (Chow, 2007; Lim, 2009). Recently attention is being focused on the subset of regulatory T-cells (T_{reg}) type, which may play

Figure 4. Involvement of transcription factors in the metabolic pathways

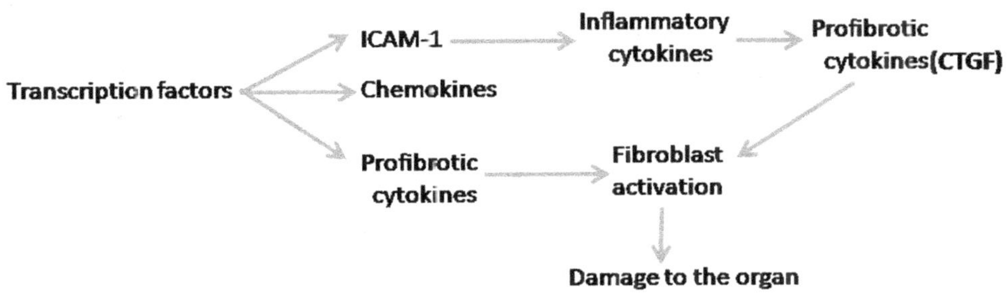

a protective role in DKD. T_{reg} cell numbers are increased in experimentally induced diabetic mice (Lim, 2010; Xu, 2009). They have also demonstrated an anti-inflammatory function, which further reduces the metabolic abnormalities and insulin resistance in a mouse model of Type 2 diabetes (Ilan et al., 2010). In case of humans, renal macrophage accumulation was associated with the severity of glomerulosclerosis.

The main proinflammatory cytokines which are implicated in DKD are ICAM-1, IL-1, IL-6, IL-18, TNF-α, MCP-1 etc. These cytokines are increased in diabetic patients and showed correlation with albuminuria and glomerular pathology (Lim & Tesch, 2010). The inflammatory pathways are a consequence of a chronically activated innate immune system and a low-grade inflammatory state with diabetes (Eller, 2011; Xu, 2009). NF-κB is an important transcription factor which regulates the expression of multiple genes related to apoptosis, inflammation, immunity, chemo-attractant protein-1and localizes to glomerular, interstitial and tubular epithelial cells in human kidney. Hyperglycemic conditions manifold increases the expression of expression of NF-κB (Holman, 2008; Perkovic, 2013). The NF-κB activation in DKD correlates with proteinuria and interstitial cell infiltration (Ilan, 2010; Perkovic, 2013). Proteinuria again known to further stimulate NF-κB and contributes to persistent proteinuria in a cyclic fashion. The Janus kinase/signal transducers and activators of transcription (JAK/STAT) signaling pathway (Duckworth et al., 2009) are activated by reactive oxygen species induced by hyperglycemic states and is associated with hypertrophy of mesangial cells. It was demonstrated that JAK-2 mRNA levels are inversely correlated with estimated glomerular filtration rate (eGFR) in patients with diabetic kidney diseases (Gerstein et al., 2008). Some inflammatory cytokines such as TNF-α and interleukins (eg IL-1, IL-6 and IL-18) are expressed in higher and in greater proportions in kidneys of diabetics as compared to non-diabetic controls. In an experimental induced diabetic rat models, rise in the expression of TNF-α and IL-6 was also associated with increased kidney weight and urine albumin excretion (Ismail-Beigi et al., 2010). SerumIL-18 and TNF-α levels are positively correlated with the degree of proteinuria in the diabetic patients (Ohga, 2007; Zhang, 2008. At cellular level, these cytokines increases the permeability of vascular endothelial cells, causes glomerular hypertrophy, GBM thickening, induces apoptosis of endothelial cells and directly leads to the toxicity in renal cells (Kodera, 2014; Mori, 2014; Fujita, 2014; Cherney 2014).

ALTERNATIVE PATHWAYS OF DKD

Autophagy is a highly conserved protective mechanism which allows cells to maintain homeostasis during cell starvation or oxidative stress (Tarnov et al., 2004). It involves the intracellular degradation of cytotoxic proteins and organelles by lysosomes whenever a cell is experiencing stress (de Galan et al., 2009). There was decreased autophagic activity which has been clearly explained in both metabolic disorders such as obesity and diabetes (Hayat, M.A., 2014). Renal podocytes are known to have a high basal level of autophagy (Brenner et al., 2001). In vi*tro stud*ies of podocytes exposed to high glucose conditions demonstrated defective autophagy which resulted in podocyte injury. Another evolutionary conserved mechanism is linked to the sodium-glucose transporter-2 (SGLT-2) in the proximal tubule. It is a very low-affinity and high-capacity transporter and is responsible for >90% of glucose reabsorption in the proximal tubules (Barnett, 2004; Lv, 2012). Experimentally knockout animalwithSGLT-2 gene loses approximately 60% of their filtered glucose into the urine. In hyperglycemia, there is upregulation of SLGT-2 expression which is believed to be the evolutionary benefit as it allows for glucose reabsorption and hence energy conservation for both the body and brain.

HISTOPATHOLOGICAL CHANGES IN CHRONIC KIDNEY DISEASES

Clinical manifestations of the diabetic kidney diseases are strongly related to the structural changes, especially with the degree of mesangial expansion in both Type 1 and Type 2 diabetes; and several important structural and functional changes are involved. Kidney is a part of the urinary system which is responsible for the excretion of the body's waste products and maintaining the proper balance of water and electrolytes. The functional unit of kidney is nephron, comprising of renal corpuscles and renal tubules. The Bowman's capsule and glomerulus filters the blood components selectively. The filteration in glomerulus is collectively performed by endothelial cells, intact glomerular basement membrane (GBM) and visceral epithelium that is podocytes. These three components working together prevent the passage of negatively charged molecules larger than albumin (about 3.6 nm) through this barrier. Albumin acts as an osmotic balancer of the blood.

GBM plays a very crucial role in both structural support and functional operation of the glomerulus. GBM is mainly comprises of integrins proteins such as laminin and collagen type-IV. The width of the GBM is double the thickness of the human basement membranes and is found in the range of 300-350 nm. At initial stages, glomerular volume goes high upto 70% and filtration surface area is increased by 80% as compared with the glomeruli of non-diabetic patients. One of the early physiological changes in diabetic patients are the occurrence of glomerular hyperfiltration accompanied by hypertrophied glomerulus. The first detectable and measurable change is GBM thickening, which can be detected as early as 1.5 to 2.5 years after the onset of the diabetes. Thickening in the tubular basement membrane (TBM) is closely parallels that of GBM thickening.

Mesangial expansion, predominant due to an increase in mesangial matrix, an advent rise in the matrix component of the mesangium can be detected as early as 8-9 years after diabetes onset. These structural and functional changes do not develop at the same rate in all the patients. Whenever, there is renal insufficiency, there would be marked mesangial expansion and GBM thickening. Mesangial expansion and diabetic glomerulosclerosis can be associated with nodular lesions consisting of marked areas of formed large, round, fibrillar mesangial zones i.e. nodule and compression of the associated glomerular capillaries (Kimmelstiel-Wilson nodules) (Figure 1). Both GBM and TBM thickenings are consequences of ECM accumulation with increased deposition of the type-IV and type-VI collagen, laminins and fibronectins (Berkholtz et al.,2006) due to their excess production, declined degradation or both.

The glomerular filtration barrier is composed of fenestrated endothelium, GBM, podocytes and slit diaphragms. Disintegration and insult to anyone or more elements of this filtration complex leads to proteinuria (Bianchi et al., 2006). Podocyte detachment from GBM, apoptosis, necrosis or loss of adhesive power plays a central role in the pathogenesis of albuminuria. In most of the renal glomerular disorders, proteinuria is finally associated with foot processes effacement. Numerous Glomerular disorders, collapsing glomerulopathy, lupus nephritis, chronic renal impairment and DKD have injured podocytes. A chronic hyperglycemic condition is necessary for DKD lesions and renal functional disturbances to develop.

It is essential to evaluate renal tissue using appropriate standards for renal biopsy for diagnosis. Staining is done by H & E (hematoxylin andeosin), Periodic acid- Schiff's (PAS), Periodic acid methenamine silver and Mason trichome for light microscopy. Kidney biopsy sections should contain at least 10 glomeruli per slide excluding incomplete glomeruli along the edge. In immunofluorescence technique different antibodies are used for eg IgA, IgM, IgG, CDs (Cluster of differentiation), C3, C1q and light chains to rule out non diabetic kidney diseases (Wesseling & Crowe, 2013). Electron microscopy must be accompanied for an accurate diagnosis of DKD. A patient should carry a clinical diagnosis of DKD with supportive information. DKD can lead to any nephritic disease.

DKD classification on criteria of glomerular damage:

CLASS I: THICKENING OF THE GLOMERULAR BASEMENT MEMBRANE OR PREDIABETIC LESIONS

The mechanisms involved in the development of diabetic lesions or thickening of basement membrane are not properly understood; but many of them are implicated by hyperglycemia. The microangiopathy leads to thickening of the GBM but also the expansion of the mesangial matrix and thickening of the tubular basement membrane. GBM thickening is a first prominent change change in Type 1 and Type 2; and increases with time duration of the disease.GBM thickening results fromaccumulations of proteins (types IV and VI collagen, laminins etc), their decreased degradation or both.

CLASS II: MESANGIAL EXPANSION, MILD (iia) OR SEVERE (iib)

Mesangial expansion is defined as an increase in extracellular material in the mesangium such that the width of the interspaces exceeds two mesangial cell nuclei in at least two lobules of the glomerulus. Generally the difference between mild and severe form of mesangial expansion is based the expanded mesangial area is smaller or larger than the mean area of capillary lumen. Expansion of cellular and matrix components in the mesangium is a hallmark of Type 1 and Type2 diabetes. Mesangium expansion restricts and distorts glomerular capillaries and diminishes the capillary filtration surface.

CLASS III: NODULAR SCLEROSIS (KIMMMELSTEIL-WILSON LESIONS)

Kimmelstiel-Wilson lesions appear in both Type 1 and Type 2 diabetes as lobular, round to oval mesangial lesions with hyaline acellular core which is rounded peripherally by sparse, crescent-shaped mesangial nuclei. While developing nodular sclerotic lesions in initial stages of DKD; two important processes take place: lytic changes in the mesangial area called mesangiolysis and detachment of the endothelial cells from GBM. Kimmelstiel-Wilson lesions are found in combination with mesangial expansion. The occurrence of Kimmelstiel-Wilson lesions is widely considered transition from an early or moderately advanced stage to a progressively higher advanced stage of the disease.

CLASS IV: ADVANCED DIABETIC GLOMERULOSCLEROSIS

Class IV implies advanced DKD and designates more than 50% of global glomerulosclerosis in which there is clinical or pathologic evidence that the sclerosis is attributable to DKD. Glomerulosclerosis is the end point of multifactorial mechanisms that lead to excessive accumulation of ECM in the mesangial space, which through various stages of mesangial expansion leads to the development of Kimmelstiel-Wilson lesions finally resulting in glomerulosclerosis. The presence of mononuclear cells in the interstitium is a widely recognized finding in DKD. Mesangiolysis is defined as disintegration of mesangium with the resultant balooned appearance of a glomerular tuft while the dilated lumens of simple tufts are filled with many red blood cells. Mesangiolysis was mostly observed in end stages regardless of acute or chronic disease.

THE FILTRATION BARRIER: A MULTICOMPONENT APPARATUS

Each capillary of a GBM is lined by fenestrated endothelium and covered by visceral epithelial cells or podocytes. The podocyte slit diaphragm is the final barrier in the GFB to filtration of macromolecules. It possesses interdigitating foot processes (primary, secondary and tertiary) which are separated by filtration slits/pores and is a specialized intercellular junction spanning the filtration slit. Filtration of blood components occurs via the endothelial fenestrae, across the basement membrane and through the filtration slits into collecting duct to form final urine. The glomerular filtration barrier (GFB) acting as a molecular sieve; is permeable to water, small solutes in plasma and maintains charge selectivity for proteins and larger molecules (Jarad & Miner, 2009). Importantly, when microalbuminuria like protein excretions are detectable then glomerular filtration rate (GFR) has passed through the state of hyperfiltration. Alterations in the components of filtration barrier play a part in the development of DKD and other pathological conditions. Chronic hyperglycaemic condition induces the morphological alteration in podocyte expression pattern, podocyte-integrin expression, altered and decreased MMP-2 & MMP-3 expression; finally rise in expression of tissue inhibitor of metalloproteinase (TIMP). Other factors contributing to renal matrix accumulation include VEGF, PDGF which are highly expressed in mesangial and visceral epithelial cells.

ENDOCRINOLOGICAL SIGNIFICANCE

DKD have characteristics that distinguish it from other forms of the chronic kidney diseases. Patients are generally anemic in DKD than in non-diabetic CKD. Erythropoiesis and proteinuria inhibitors, with losses of iron-carrying proteins, have been variably implied in the cause of CKD. Progressive fibrosis of the kidney precludes the increase of endogenous erythropoietin production in response to increasing levels of hypoxia sensed by the organ. DKD patients become highly vulnerable to the anemia when inflammation with proteinuria or both are diagnosed clinically. This is an important risk multiplier for diabetics with high prevalence rates of heart failure.

Endocrinologists have supported the confounding of glycemic control in the presence of renal impairment. When gluconeogenesis and glycogenolysis cell processes are impaired, with onset of insulin resistance; diabetic individuals are more susceptible to hypoglycemia. Hyperglycemia from insulin resistance promoting volume depletion strongly activates the sympathetic nervous system and brings about diabetic ketoacidosis. Continuous activation of renin-angiotensin-aldosterone system (RAAS) from ongoing sympathetic nervous system stimulation further aggravates proteinuria and renal fibrosis (Remuzzi et al., 2005).

Another endocrinological aspect which is more apparent in DKD is adynamic bone disease (ABD). This form of mineral and bone disorder is characterized by a marked decrement in bone turnover in the absence of osteoid accumulation. ABD occurs more frequently; this low-volume bone disorder is associated with lower parathyroid hormone levels, increase in fracture risk and calcified cardiovascularity. The pathophysiology of ABD in diabetics remains very mysterious. Improper absorption of calcium and phosphorus in bone makes them to migrate to vascular sites causing coronary and peripheral arterial diseases. Expansion in mesangiun caused by increased matrix secretion and cell enlargement is the initial change seen in light microscopy, while electron microscopy showed a thickened basement membrane and podocyte effacement Figure 5.

TREATMENT MODALITIES IN MODERN MEDICINE

There are different classes of compounds which are presently in use for the treatment of diabetic kidney disease. Orally given hypoglycemic drugs presently prepared in pharmaceutical world shown in Table 1 and novel agents used in treatment of diabetes related complications in Table 2.

Figure 5. (A) Light microscopy with hematoxylin & Eosin staining revealing extensive mesangial expansion without any marked increase in cellularity. A Kimmelstiel-Wilson (KW) lesion is shown here and refers to the nodular glomerulosclerosis that can be seen in late disease but is not as common as diffuse diabetic glomerulosclerosis. (B) KW lesions are spherical and eosinophilic with a central hypocellular or acellular area. Mesangial expansion and KW lesions are both due to increased extracellular matrix production. (C) Electron microscopy shows a thickened basement membrane and (D) podocyte foot process effacement. (Source: Lim A K H, 2014)

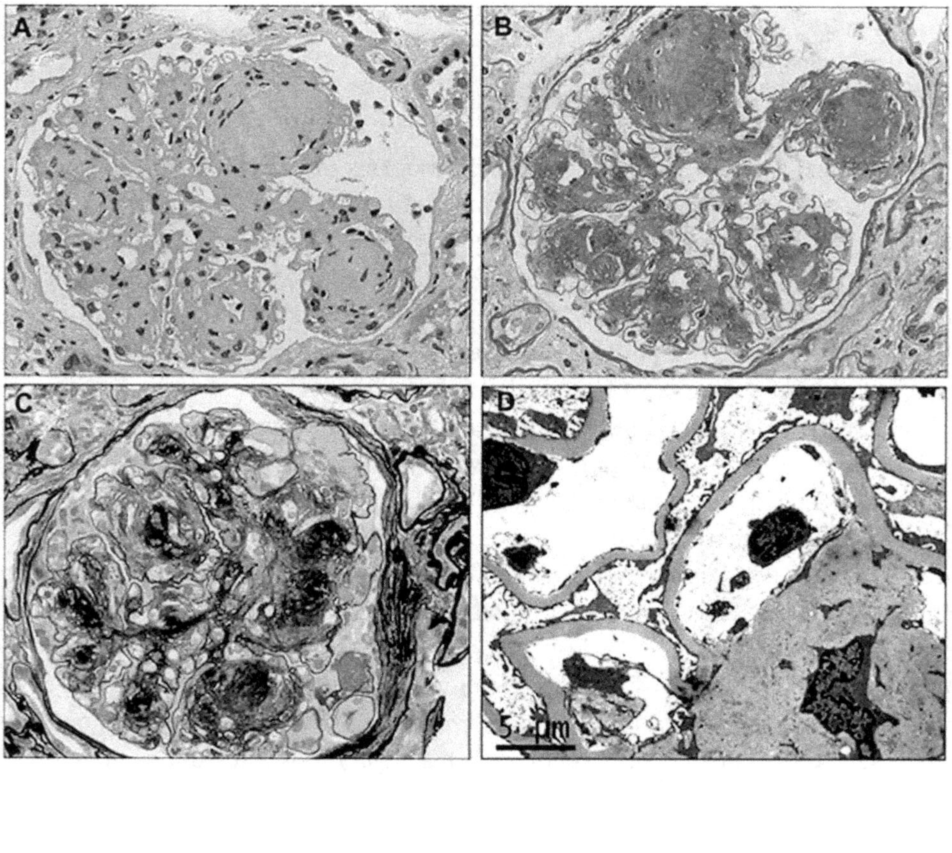

Table 1. Orally given hypoglycemic drugs

Class of compounds	First generation	Second generation	Adverse Effects
1. Sulphonyl ureas	Tolbutamide, Chlopropamide	Gilbenclamide, Glipizide, Gliclazide, Glimeperide	Hypoglycemia, non specific side effects (nausea, vomiting, diarrhea, headache, weight gain.
2. Biguanides	Phenformin, Metformin		Lactic acidosis, Abdominal pain, anorexia, mild diarrhea, Vit B_{12} deficiency
3. Meglitinide analogues	Repaglinide, Nateglinide		Dizziness, joint pain, flu like symptoms, nausea.
4. Thiazolidindiones	Rosiglitazone, Pioglitazone		Nausea, dizziness.
5.α-Glucosidase inhibitors	Acarbose, Miglitol		Produce flatulence, loose stools

Table 2. Summary of novel agents in diabetes related diseases

Category	Mechanism of action	Drugs
1. AGE inhibitors	Blocks AGE formation, enhances breakdown, or breaks crosslinks.	Aminoguanidine Pyridoxamine Alegebrium
2. Aldose reductase	Reduces sorbitol formation by the polyol pathway.	EpalrestatPonalrestat Tolrestat
3. Antifibrosis	Reduces TGF-β signaling and TNF-α levels but the exact mechanism needs to be discovered.	Pirfenidone
4. Antioxidative stress	Activation of nuclear transcription factor Nrf2.	Bardoxolone
5. Direct renin inhibitors	Blocks the conversion of angiotensinogen to angiotensin.	Aliskiren
6. Endothelin inhibitors	Predominantly blocks Predominantly blocks endothelin receptor on vascular endothelium.	Atrasentan, Avosentan
7. Glycosaminoglycans	Reduces heparan sulphate degradation in GBM and has anti-inflammatory actions.	Sulodexide
8. Vasopeptidase inhibitors	Blocks ACE and neutral endopeptidase while Palosuran blocks urotensin II receptor.	Palosuran Omapatrilat Ilepatril
9. PKC inhibitors	Blocks PKC-β intracellular signaling.	Ruboxistaurin
10. Phosphodiesterase inhibitors	Increases cellular cAMP with broad effects. Cilostazol blocks PDE3, pentoxifylline is nonspecific and also blocks the adenosine receptor.	Cilostazol Pentoxifylline

DRUGS MECHANISM OF ACTION

- **Sulphonylurea:** Sulphonylurea is an antidiabetic drug with stimulating effect on pancreas β-cells to secrete insulin. They induce channel closure by binding to the SUR subunit of ATP-sensitive potassium (K_{ATP}) ion channel.
- **Biguanides:** Biguanides has the ability to inhibit Gluconeogenesis; inhibitory effect which in turn is correlated well with its ability to inhibit pyruvate oxidation.
- **Meglitinide Analogues:** Meglitinide analogues belong to a new family of insulin secretagogues that acts synergistically with long-acting insulin (NPH insulin at bedtime), metformin and thiazolidinediones (pioglitazone and rosiglitazone). It acts by inhibiting the action of ATP-sensitive potassium ion channels of the β-cell membrane via binding to a receptor which is distinct from that of the sulphonylureas (SUR1/KIR 6.2).

- **Thiazolidindiones:** It improves insulin sensitivity through the mechanism involving activation of γ isoform of the peroxisome proliferator-activated receptor (PPAR-γ), a nuclear receptor.
- **α-Glucosidase Inhibitors:** Acarbose, Miglitol, Voglibose are some of the examples of α- glucosidase inhibitor which helps in delaying the absorption of carbohydrates from the small bowel which leads to the lower effect on postprandial blood glucose and insulin levels.

MARKERS OF THE CHRONIC DIABETIC RENAL FAILURE

There is dire need of biomarkers for the early detection of chronic kidney diseases, since it has multifactorial complexicities. In present scenario, proteinuria is the most important and widely used marker for the clinical detection of chronic kidney diseases. Low-grade albuminuria is a lesser predictor of disease progression than macroalbuminuria (Perkins et al., 2007). Therefore, there is keen interest in scientific world for finding biomarkers to detect DKD earlier and identify risk of progression while urine micro RNA profiling studies are fairly preliminary (Argyropoulos, 2013; Di-Stefano, 2013). The most promising biomarker currently is serum TNF-α receptor level which predicts the progression of CKD and ESRD, both in Type 1 and Type 2 diabetics. Markers are listed in Table 3.

Markers with their short description are given in the following sections.

HS-CRP (HIGH SENSITIVITY CRP) AND CRP (C - REACTIVE PROTEIN)

Both tests measure the same protein in the blood. CRP is a protein that increases in the blood with inflammation. CRP structure is annular ring shaped, pentameric protein found in the plasma; rises during inflammation. It is synthesized by the liver in response to factors released by macrophages and adipocytes; a member of the pentraxin family of proteins. Its physiological role is to bind to lysophosphatidylcholine expressed on the surface of dead or dying cells in order to activate complement system via the C1Q complex. Hs-CRP test is for healthy people to determine the risk of cardiovascular diseases. It measures the CRP in the range from 0.5 to 10 mg/L. Hs-CRP is a useful test for determining risk of CVD, heart attacks, strokes and that hs-CRP can play a role in the evaluation process before a person develops these health problems. High levels of hs-CRP in healthy individuals is found to be a predictive of an increased risk of future heart attack, stroke, sudden cardiac death or peripheral arterial diseases even when cholesterol levels is in normal range.

IL-18 (INTERLEUKIN-18)

Interleukin-18 (also known as interferon-gamma inducing factor) is a protein which is encoded by the *IL18* gene in humans and is an important proinflammatory cytokine. It belongs to cytokine of IL-1 superfamily which is produced by macrophages, dendritic cells, monocytes, neutrophils and epithelial cells of the organs. It works by binding to the interleukin-18 receptor and together with IL-12 induces cell-mediated immunity following an infection with microbial products like lipopolysaccharide (LPS). After stimulation with IL-18, natural killer (NK) cells and certain T cells release an important cytokine called interferon-γ (IFN-γ) or type II interferon that plays an important role in activating the macrophages

Table 3. Biomarkers for determining chronic kidney damage

Pathophysiology	Markers	Importance
1. Inflammation	Hs-CRP & CRP	Cardiac risk markers, they help to determine a person's risk of developing cardiovascular diseases.
	IL-18	Proinflammatory cytokine predictor of nephropathy and cardiovascular diseases in diabetes Type 2.
	TIMP-β 1	Glycoprotein which inhibits metalloproteinases (MMPs).
	PTX3	Deficiency increases the risk of DKD.
2. Fibrosis	TGF-β1	(TGF-β) is a key regulator of extracellular matrix protein synthesis and is secreted as latent complexes.
3. Oxidative stress	TBARS,MDA	Free radical generation, Cell membrane damage indicator.
	Protein carbonyl	Cell protein damage indicator.
	AGEs	Leads to thickening of extracellular matrix.
	Urinary 8-hydroxydeoxy guanosine 4 hydroxy nonenal	Oxidative stress derived DNA damage marker.
	Antioxidant enzymes (SOD, CAT, GPx)	Free radical generation.
	ADMA	Interferes with L-arginine in the production of NO which is involved in normal endothelial function. Indicator of progression of Type 1 diabetic nephropathy and microalbuminuria.
	Protein reduced thiols	Outcomes of free radical generation.
4. Kidney function	β-Trace protein	Potent inhibitor of platelet aggregation and involved in smooth muscle contraction, indicator of GFR.
	Cystatin C	It is an important extracellular inhibitor of cysteine proteinases.
5. Glomerular injury	Podocin	It is a component of slit diaphragms of podocytes which function as filtration barrier of the kidney glomerulus.
	Nephrin	It is a component of slit diaphragms of podocytes forming filtration barrier.
	Podocalyxin	It is the major constituent of the glycocalyx of podocytes, negatively charged and keeps adjacent foot processes separated, by keeping urinary filtration barrier open.
6. Tubulo-interstitial injury	NGAL	Early marker released in high amount to combat insult caused by kidney injury (Innate immunity).
	KIM-1	It is a membrane protein with extracellular immunoglobulin and mucin domains which maintains the integrity of epithelial cells.
	NAG	Predicts both micro and macro – albuminuria in Type 1 diabetic.
	L-FABT	Correlated with degree of urinary protein excretion.

or other cells. IL-12 has been shown to inhibit IL-4 dependent IgE and IgG1 production and enhances IgG2a production in B cells. IL-18 binding protein (IL18BP) can specifically interact with this cytokine and thus negatively regulate its biological activity. It also induces severe inflammatory reactions, suggesting its role in inflammatory disorders. The action of IL-18 on basophils and mast cells causes complex physiological reactions including allergic reactions. IL-18 activity is inhibited by IL-18BP protein found in serum.

TIMP-β 1(TISSUE INHIBITOR OF METALLOPROTEINASES-β 1)

Tissue inhibitor of metalloproteinases 1 (TIMP-1) is a matrix metalloproteinase (MMP)-independent regulator of growth and apoptosis in various cell types. They are widely distributed in the animal kingdom and the human genome contains four paralogous genes encoding different forms like TIMPs-1 to TIMP-4. RNA interference of TIMP-1 has revealed that endogenous TIMP-1 suppresses the proliferation, metabolic activity and osteogenic differentiating capacity of human mesenchymal stem cells (hMSCs). TIMPs are independent of metalloproteinases; these include effects on the cell growth & differentiation, cell movement, angiogenesis, apoptosis, synaptic plasticity etc. ECM composition variations are crucial for repair, morphogenesis, tissue remodeling, embryonic development etc. ECM catabolism activities are performed by proteases like matrix metalloproteinases (MMPs), which includes collagenases, gelatinases, matrilysins, stromelysins, membrane-type MMPs and ADAMTS (a disintegrin and metalloproteinase with thrombospondin domains) metalloproteinases. TIMPs are endogenous inhibitors of these metalloproteinases and are consequently important regulators of ECM formation, remodeling of the tissue and other cellular responses.

PTX3 (PENTRAXIN-3)

Pentraxin-related protein PTX3 also known as TNF-inducible gene 14 protein (TSG-14) is a protein; in humans is encoded by the *PTX3* gene. It is a member of the pentraxin superfamily. It is rapidly produced and released by different cell types, particularly involved are mononuclear phagocytes, dendritic cells (DCs), fibroblasts and endothelial cells in response to primary inflammatory signals [e.g., toll-like receptor (TLR) engagement, TNF-α, IL-1β].PTX3 binds with high affinity to the complement component C1q, the extracellular matrix component, TNF-α induced protein 6 (TNFAIP6; also called TNF-stimulated gene 6, TSG-6) and few selected microorganisms, including *Aspergillus fumigates* and *Pseudomonas* species. PTX3 activates the classical pathway of complement activation and accelerates the pathogen recognition by macrophages and dendritic cells. Its synthesis is stimulated by endothelial cells, macrophages, myeloid cells, dendritic cells by cytokines and endotoxins such as bacterial products, interleukin-1 etc.

TGF-β1 (TRANSFORMING GROWTH FACTOR-β1)

TGF-β1 is a polypeptide member of the transforming growth factor beta superfamily of cytokines. It is a secreted protein which performs many cellular processes like controlling of cell growth, cell proliferation, cell differentiation and cell death.TGF-β1 is encoded by *TGFB1* gene in humans. It acts synergistically with TGFA in inducing transformation and also acts as a negative autocrine growth factor. Dysregulation of TGF-β activation and defective signaling results in apoptosis. Many cells synthesize TGF-β and all of them have specific receptors that are TGF-β1, TGF-β2 and TGF-β3; all function through the same receptor signaling pathways. TGF-β1 with a molecular mass of 25 KDa has a potential role in wound healing. It plays an important role in controlling the immune system and shows different activities on different types of cell or cells at different stages of the development. TGF-β1 is secreted by many immune or leucocyte cells. Increased expression of transforming growth factor-β1 (TGF-β1) in glomerular mesangial cells augments extracellular matrix accumulation and hypertrophy during the progression of DKD.

TBARS (THIOBARBITURIC REACTIVE SUBSTANCES) AND MDA (MALONDIALDEHYDE)

Thiobarbituric acid reactive substances are formed as a byproduct of lipid peroxidation assayed by TBARS assay method. Reactive oxygen species have extremely short half-lives, so they are difficult to measure directly. Instead, the formed end products of damage produced by oxidative stress are measured e.g TBARS. Since the TBAR assay measures the end-point oxidative damage, it is very useful to determine the overall impact of oxidative stress-inducing while MDA is a low-molecular-weight end product formed via the decomposition of certain primary and secondary lipid peroxidation. However, only certain lipid peroxidation products generate MDA and it is neither the sole end product of fatty acid peroxide formation and decomposition, nor a complete substance generated exclusively through lipid peroxidation. Use of MDA analysis in studies of lipid peroxidation require caution, discretion and (especially in biological systems) correlative data from other indices of fatty peroxide formation and decomposition.

PROTEIN CARBONYL

Oxidative stress is an imbalance towards the pro-oxidant side of the pro-oxidant/antioxidant homeostasis found in several human diseases. These diseases include in which high levels of protein carbonyl (CO) groups have been observed including rheumatoid arthritis, diabetes, chronic renal failure, sepsis and respiratory distress syndrome. The usage of protein CO groups as biomarkers of oxidative stress has advantages in comparison to the measurement of other oxidation products because of the relative early formation and the relative stability of carbonylated proteins. Detection of protein assays containing CO groups involves derivatisation of the carbonyl group with 2, 4-dinitrophenylhydrazine (DNPH), which leads to the formation of stable product named dinitrophenyl (DNP) hydrazone. Their detection can be determined through various means such as spectrophotometric assay, enzyme- linked immunosorbent assay (ELISA) and one-dimensional or two-dimensional electrophoresis followed by Western blot. ROS leading to protein oxidation include radical species such as superoxide ($O_2^{\cdot-}$), hydroxyl ($OH^{\cdot}$), peroxyl ($RO_2^{\cdot}$), alkoxyl ($RO^{\cdot}$), hydro-peroxyl ($HO_2^{\cdot}$) and non-radical species such as hydrogen peroxide (H_2O_2), hypo-chlorous acid (HOCl), ozone (O_3), singlet oxygen ($^1O_2$) and peroxynitrite ($ONOO^-$). Carbonyl (CO) groups (aldehydes and ketones) are produced on protein side chains (especially Arg, Lys, Pro and Thr) on oxidation. These moieties are chemically stable which is useful for both their detection and storage. Protein carbonyl assays give the advantage of using no special or expensive equipment; they can be performed in any normally equipped biochemistry laboratory.

AGEs (ADVANCED GLYCATION END PRODUCTS)

AGEs are the risk factor in the development of many degenerative diseases (for eg diabetes, atherosclerosis, chronic renal failure, Alzheimer's disease etc). AGEs are formed both outside and inside of the body. Specifically, it start from the glycation reaction; addition of a carbohydrate to a protein without the involvement of an enzyme. Glycation, makes cell stiffer, unfit for the cellular function and premature aging. The mechanism by which AGEs induce damage is through a process called cross-linking that causes intracellular damage and apoptosis. They can form photosensitizers in crystalline lens, causes cataract development in later stages. Proteins inside the cells are usually glycated through their lysine residues. Histones found in the nucleus are richest in lysine and therefore form the glycated protein N (6)-Carboxymethyllysine (CML). AGEs receptors are found on many cells which include endothelial cells, smooth muscles cells of the immune system from tissue such as lung, liver and kidney. Receptor, when binding to AGEs, contributes to age- and diabetes-related chronic inflammatory diseases such as myocardial infarction, nephropathy, retinopathy, atherosclerosis, asthama, periodontitis, neuropathy etc.

URINARY 8-HYDROXY GUANOSINE 4 HYDROXY NONENAL

It is widely agreed that, increased generation of ROS cause toxic effects by oxidative damage of macromolecules, such as proteins, lipids and DNA. Reaction of ROS with purine and pyrimidine bases of DNA will generate several products; 8-OHdG is one of the major product of nucleotide oxidation ie oxidized derivative of deoxyguanosine. Concentrations of 8-oxo-dG within a cell are a measurement of oxidative stress.

ANTIOXIDANT ENZYMES (SUPEROXIDE DISMUTASE, CATALASE AND GLUTATHIONE PEROXIDASE)

Reactive oxygen species (ROS) are well recognized for playing a dual role as both deleterious and beneficial species. Cells generate ROS normally by regulated enzymes, such as nitric oxide synthase etc. Beneficial effects of ROS usually occur at moderate or low concentrations involving physiological cellular responses, in defense against pathological agents, in the function of cellular signaling pathways and in an induction of a mitogenic response. In contrast, overproduction of ROS [arising either from mitochondrial electron transport chain or excessive stimulation of NAD(P)H] results in oxidative stress to the cell or tissue. When antioxidant capacity exceeds the normal production inside cells, it gives rise to oxidative stress which causes damage to essential macromolecules resulting in abnormal gene expression, disturbance in receptor activity, apoptosis, immunity deviations, mutagenesis and protein or lipofuscin deposition. Antioxidant enzymes catalyze the decomposition of reactive oxygen species. Three unique antioxidant enzymes, SOD, glutathione peroxidase (GPx) and CAT help in combating oxidative stress. SOD is a group of metalloenzymes whose function is to protect cells from the toxic effects of endogenously generated superoxide radicals. GPx is a selenocysteine-dependent enzyme that protects against oxidative injury and they are the most important hydrogen peroxide (H_2O_2)-removing enzymes in all mammalian cells. CAT is an essential enzyme in the decomposition of intracellular H_2O_2. It promotes the breakdown of H_2O_2 into water and oxygen without producing free radicals. CAT is located in peroxisomes; found essentially in all aerobic cells. Catalase is an unusual enzyme although hydrogen peroxide is its only substrate still it follows ping-pong mechanism.

ADMA (ASSYMETRIC DIMETHYLARGININE)

ADMA is a naturally occurring chemical found in the plasma. It is a metabolic byproduct of continuous post translational protein modification processes in the cytoplasm of all human cells. It is closely related to the structure of L-arginine; a conditional essential amino acid. ADMA interferes with L-arginine in the production of nitric oxide, a key component involved in normal endothelial cell function, produced by dendritic cells as a defensive mechanism, endothelial homeostasis and cardiovascular health. This reaction is catalyzed by an enzyme called S-adenosylmethionine protein N-methyltransferases (protein methylases I & II) and methyl groups are transferred to create ADMA; which is derived from the methyl group donor S-adenosylmethionine. S-adenosylmethionine is an important intermediate in the metabolism of homocysteine. After synthesis it migrates into the extracellular space then to the plasma and can be measured by using high-performance liquid chromatography. ADMA concentrations are substantially elevated by native or oxidized LDL cholesterol. The elimination of ADMA occurs through urine excretion and metabolism by the enzyme dimethylarginine dimethylaminohydrolase (DDAH). Polyphenol antioxidants also play role in down-regulating homocysteine. ADMA's role has been linked with elevated levels of homocysteine. Whilst approaches at modifying the latter one with oral supplements of folic acid were strongly suggested. Endothelial layer or endothelium plays very crucial role in maintaining the structure and vascular tone. NO is major vasoactive substances, its low level is associated with impaired endothelial function. ADMA levels are increased in people with chronic renal and heart failure, atherosclerosis, hypertension, hypercholesteromia and diabetes mellitus. It is associated with three-fold increased risk of future mortality in patients undergoing hemodialysis.

PROTEIN REDUCED THIOLS

Oxidation and reduction of cysteine residues is emerging as an important post-translational control of protein function. The cysteine side chain is considered the most potent nucleophile of all amino-acid side chains under physiological conditions. This reactivity is due to the presence of a thiol functional group. Thiol is a sulfur analogue of alcohol, the smaller difference in electronegativity between the sulfur atom and the hydrogen atom makes the S-H bond less polarized than the O-H bond, leading to a diminished propensity to form hydrogen bonds. They are more acidic in comparison to alcohols, and this property can be explained by the weakness of the sulphur hydrogen bond. This gives information about the antioxidant status of the cellular processes.

β-TRACE PROTEIN (BTP)

BTP also known as prostaglandin D_2 synthase is a low-molecular weight glycoprotein (MW 25.2 kDa) was initially isolated from cerebrospinal fluid and served as a marker of cerebrospinal fluid leakage. The half-life of BTP is approximately 1.2 hr and it is easily filtered through the glomerular basement membrane with minimal non-renal elimination owing to its low MW and absence of protein binding. BTP serum levels increases progressively with the reduction in GFR. Low-molecular weight proteins in serum are better markers for detecting reduced GFR than the conventional measurement of serum creatinine. Recently, it has been identified as potential marker for renal function. β-Trace protein is synthesized mainly in the central nervous system by glial cells and the choroid plexus and forms one of the principal constituents of the cerebrospinal fluid. It catalyzes the reaction from prostaglandin H_2 to prostaglandin D_2, which plays a central role in nociception, temperature and sleep regulation pattern.

CYSTATIN C (CYSTATIN 3)

Cystatin C (γ-trace, post γ-globulin or neuroendocrine basic polypeptide)is a protein encoded by CST3 gene; mainly used as a biomarker for kidney function. In humans, all cells with a nucleus produce Cystatin C as a chain of 120 amino acids. It is a potent inhibitor of lysosomal enzymes and probably one of the most important extracellular inhibitors of cysteine proteases. Glomerular filtration rate (GFR), a marker of kidney health, is best measured by injecting compounds such as inulin, radioisotopes such as ^{51}chromium-EDTA, ^{125}I-iothalamate, ^{99m}Tc-DTPA or radiocontrast agents such as isohexol, but these techniques are mostly complicated, costly, time -consuming and have potential side-effects. Cystatin C has a low molecular weight with 13.3 KDa and is removed from the bloodstream by glomerular filtration in the kidneys. If kidney function and glomerular filtration rate decline, its blood level rises. Cystatin C levels are less dependent on age, sex, race and muscle mass as compared to creatinine. It has been suggested that Cystatin C might predict the risk of developing chronic kidney disease, thereby signaling a state of 'preclinical' kidney dysfunction.

PODOCIN

Podocin is a protein component of the filtration slits of podocytes. Glomerular endothelial cells, the glomerular basement membrane and the filtration slits function as the filtration barrier of the kidney glomerulus. Podocin is a new member of the stomatin family which consists of hairpin-like integral membrane proteins with intracellular $NH_{(2)}$ and COOH- terminus. Glomerular podocytes express podocin but its subcellular distribution and interaction with other proteins are unknown. Podocin localizes to the podocyte foot process membrane at the insertion site of the slit diaphragm and accumulates in an oligomeric form lipid rafts. It mediates the recruitment of nephrin into specialized microdomains of the plasma membrane and important for the function of the glomerular filter. It has been shown that nephrin and podocin are associated with detergent-resistant membranes at the filtration slit that represent special types of lipid rafts. Several studies have shown that deletion of the raft-associated protein tyrosine kinase results in a severe proteinuria in mice. Lipid rafts consist of dynamic assemblies of cholesterol and sphingolipids in the exoplasmic face of the lipid bilayer of the plasma membrane.

NEPHRIN

Nephrin is an Ig-like transmembrane protein necessary for the proper functioning of the renal filtration barrier which consists of fenestrated endothelial cells, glomerular basement membrane and podocytes of the epithelial cells. It is a structural component of the slit diaphragm and essential for maintaining glomerular permeability. A defect in the nephrin gene, NPHS1is associated with congenital nephrotic syndrome of the Finnish type and causes massive amounts of protein to be leaked into the urine. This protein is also required for cardiovascular development. One of the important protein ie CD2-associated protein (CD2AP) is necessary for normal glomerular permeability; a putative nephrin adapter molecule. Podocytes form a tight web like structure on top of GBM with their interdigitating foot processes joined by a slit diaphragm and disruption of nephrin/podocin is a final common pathway leading to foot processes effacement in the proteinuric diseases.

PODOCALYXIN

Podocalyxin, a sialoglycoprotein, is the major constituent of the glycocalyx of podocytes in the glomerulus (Bowman's capsule). It is a member of the CD_{34} family of transmembrane sialomucins. It coats the secondary foot processes of the podocytes. It is negatively charged and functions to keep adjacent foot processes separated; keeping the urinary filtration barrier open. It has a role in the opening of vascular lumens and regulation of vascular permeability. Podocalyxin is upregulated in a number of cancers and is frequently associated with poor prognosis. Sialylated, O-glycosylated glycoforms of podocalyxin expressed by colon carcinoma cells possess L-selectin and E-selectin binding activity and may be pivotal to the metastatic spread of colon carcinoma cells. At the cellular level podocalyxin has shown to regulate the size and topology of apical cell domains and act as a potent inducer of microvillus formation.

NGAL (NEUTROPHIL GELATINASE ASSOCIATED LIPOCALIN)/ LIPOCALIN-2 (LCN2)/ ONCOGENE 24p3

It is a protein that in humans is encoded by the *LCN2* gene (Kjeldsen et al., 1993). NGAL is involved in innate immunity by sequestrating iron that in turn limits bacterial growth. It is expressed in neutrophils and in low levels in the kidney, prostate and epithelia of the respiratory and alimentary tracts. NGAL is used as a biomarker of kidney injury. The binding of NGAL to bacterial siderophores is very important in the innate immune response to bacterial infection. Upon encountering invading bacteria the toll-like receptors on immune cells stimulate the synthesis and secretion of NGAL. Secreted NGAL then limits bacterial growth by sequestering iron-containing siderophores (Flo et al., 2004, Schmidt et al., 2007).

NGAL also functions as a growth factor. In the case of acute kidney injury (AKI), NGAL is secreted in high levels into the blood and urine within 2 hours of injury. NGAL is protease resistant and small; hence the protein is easily excreted and detected in the urine. NGAL can also be used as an early diagnosis for procedures such as chronic kidney disease, contrast induced nephropathy and kidney transplants (Goldstein, 2011). Serum creatinine is a marker of kidney function, whereas NGAL is a marker of kidney injury. Individuals positive for NGAL tend to have higher incidence of going renal replacement therapy. Renal expression of NGAL increases in the kidneys after injury for a variety of reasons. It is possible to measure NGAL in serum or urine in the range of 25 to 5,000 ng/mL by current laboratory tests. Low levels for NGAL have been considered to be 20 ng/mL, medium levels 200 ng/mL and high levels 1200 ng/mL (Lippy et al., 2012).

KIM-1(KIDNEY INJURY MOLECULE-1)

Kidney Injury Molecule-1 (KIM-1) is a type 1 transmembrane protein, with an immunoglobulin and mucin domain, whose expression is markedly up-regulated in the proximal tubule in the post-ischemic rat kidney. KIM-1 is not detectable in the normal human and rodent kidney but is increased in expression more than any other protein in the injured kidney and is localized predominantly to the apical membrane of the surviving proximal epithelial cells (Ichimura et al. 2008).

NAG (N-ACETYL β-GLUCOSAMINIDASE)

The urinary excretion of enzymes, in particular N-acetyl-β-D-glucosaminidase (NAGase), is considered a relatively simple, cheap, fast and non-invasive method in the detection of renal tubular function under various conditions. NAGase is an enzyme in lysosome which is contained abundantly in the renal tubular epithelia and is related to the degradation of mucopolysaccharides and glycoproteins. The determination of urinary NAGase provides a very sensitive and reliable indicator of renal damage, such as injury or dysfunction due to diabetes mellitus, nephrotic syndrome, inflammation, vesicoureteral reflux, urinary tract infection, hypercalciuria, urolithiasis, nephrocalcinosis, perinatal asphyxia, hypoxia, hypertension, heavy metals poisoning, and treatment with aminoglycosides, valproate or other nephrotoxic drugs.

L-FABT (LIVER TYPE FATTY ACIDS BINDING PROTEIN)

Liver-type fatty acid binding protein (L-FABP) is found in the cytoplasm of human proximal tubular cells. L-FABP binds fatty acids and transports them to mitochondria or peroxisomes where the fatty acids are β-oxidized, and participates in intracellular fatty acid homeostasis (Veerkamp et al., 1993). Moreover, L-FABP has a high affinity for and capacity to bind long-chain fatty acid oxidation products and thus is an effective endogenous antioxidant (Wang et al., 2005). FABP1 encodes the fatty acid-binding protein found in liver. Fatty acid binding proteins are a family of small, highly conserved, cytoplasmic proteins that bind long-chain fatty acids and other hydrophobic ligands. It is thought that FABPs roles include fatty acid uptake, transport, and metabolism.

We need better biomarkers that can identify the early diagnosis of diabetic nephropathy progression. Transcriptome analysis of human diabetic kidney diseases reveals the importance of biomarkers for the screening of the disease (Woroniecka et al., 2011).

HERBAL APPROACHES TO DIABETIC KIDNEY DISEASES

Herbal medicine is also known as botanical medicine, herbology, herblore, phytotherapy, medical herbalism. Sometimes it is extended to include certain animal parts, minerals, shells, fungal and bee products.

All plants produce different chemical compounds in their normal cellular metabolic activity. One is primary metabolites required for cellular function and other is secondary metabolites for special function that is not required for basic function. They are produced in very small quantities. Coloured pigments harvest light, minimizing radiation loss and attract pollinators. Many common weeds such as dandelion, chiraita, chickweed have important medicinal properties. Secondary metabolite gives specific property to the plant characteristics. They may act as poison to repel predators or pheromones to attract pollinators. Phytoalexins secretion helps in fighting fungal and bacterial attacks to plants. Allelochemicals inhibit the growth of rival plants by competing for soil, water and light. The synthetic biochemical pathways of plants are up and/ down-regulated in response to the long term weather conditions, herbivores, pollinators etc. Chemical profile of the plant varies according to the changing conditions overtime.

Plants synthesize variety of phytochemicals, some are commercially very important like rubber. But most of the compounds are derivatives of following biochemical motifs.

- **Alkaloids:** They contains one or more nitrogen heterocyclic ring as an integral part of their structure. They produce striking physiological properties. Some alkaloids stimulate the central nervous system while others cause paralysis; some act as pain relievers, others as local anesthetics. Most alkaloids are toxic. Examples are nicotine, quinine, strychnine (*Nux vomica*). Strychnine present in single fruit of *Nux vomica* is enough to kill twenty humans. But in lower doses, it is used as medicine.
- **Polyphenols:** These are organic compounds containing multiple phenolic structural units. The number and characteristics of these phenolic groups give unique biological and therapeutic properties to the plant. Examples are ellagic acid, tannic acid. Tannins are bitter polyphenolic compound.
- **Flavonoids:** They comprise of large group of secondary metabolites with two phenyl rings and heterocyclic rings. Two important examples are quercetin and kaemferol. They are important pigments for plant colouration and attract pollinators. They function as radical scavengers and posses metal-chelating properties.
- **Terpenes:** These are unsaturated compound joined together by isoprene units. Terpenes containing oxygen or other functional groups are called as terpenoids; they can be linear (eg β-carotene) or cyclic (eg menthol). They are responsible for imparting particular aroma to the plant species. They find use in perfumes, essential oils and medicines. They are building blocks for phytol tail of chlorophyll, cytokinins, steroids etc. Common spices which contain terpenes are clove, ginger, cinnamon.
- **Saponins:** They are the group of organic compounds that form persistent froth when shaken with water even in dilute solution. They cause hemolysis of the red blood cells: they are used as surfactant and emulsifying agent; their small part is absorbed when taken orally but they enhance the absorption of other drugs. They improve liver function, physical and mental performance, immune function and metabolism; also has adaptogenic effect. Glycosides: They are plant molecules in which sugar is bound to the anomeric functional group via glycosidic bond. Glycosides can be linked by O- (O-glycoside), N- (N-glycosamine), S-(thioglycoside), C- glycosides. Disaccharides are glycosides. Many plants store chemicals in the form of inactive glycosides. Example is sinigrin, salicin, oleandrin.

These secondary metabolites further usually refined to produce drugs.

Phytochemical screening of various extracts used in the treatment revealed the presence of tannins, flavonoids and phenolic compounds in most of the herbals applied in the research (see Table 4).

Table 4. Herbals applied for the treatment of diabetic kidney diseases

Recent Herbal Developments	Mechanism of action	References
1. Coenzyme Q10	Stabilizes the imbalance of antioxidant enzymes.	Maheshwari, Balaraman, Sen &Seth, 2014.
2. *Averrhoe carambola*	Decreases AGEs in the extracellular matrix.	Zheng et al., 2013.
3. Shemyan Kangfu (Chinese patents)	Decreases proteinuria.	Wang et al., 2013, trials
4. Yiqi Huaju Qingli	Reduces microalbuminuria	Wang et al., 2013
5. Mouten cortex	Reduces oxidative stress.	Zhang et al., 2014.
6. Chaihuan -Yishen	Decreases proteinuria.	
7. *Dioscorea bulbifera*	Controls blood pressure	Singh et al., 2013.
8. Huang Qi Elixir	Reduces proteinuria.	Xiang Tu et al., 2013.
9. Cortex Mori, dry root of *Morus alba* Linn.	Lowers blood sugar.	Yu Liu, Fang & Zhang, 2014.
10. *Pueraria tuberosa*	Balances antioxidant enzymes in the kidney.	Tripathi & Nagwani, 2010
11. *Cinnamomum cassia*	Balances antioxidant enzymes in the kidney.	Yan et al., 2015.
12. Zhen-wu-tang	Suppresses hyperactivity of renin-angiotensin system by modulating nephrin and podocin expressions.	Cai et al., 2010.
13. Loganin	Lead to reduced levels of AGE in kidney by downregulating its protein receptors.	Liu et al., 2015
14. Xiexin decoction combinations	Inflammation inhibition by NF-kB	Wu et al., 2014
15. *Ginkgo biloba*	Reduces glomerulosclerosis	Tang et al., 2014
16. *Cassia tora* (seeds)	Inhibition of AGEs accumulation	Kim et al., 2014
17. *Murraya paniculata*	Decreased expression of TGF-β1 and CTGF protein	Zou et al., 2014

ROUTES OF HERBAL DRUG ADMINISTRATION

Herbs can be administered in various forms, these include the following:

- **Decoctions:** It is a long-term boiled extract of roots, rhizomes, stems or bark.
- **Extracts:** These include liquid extracts, dry extracts and nebusilates. Liquid extracts are low percentage ethanolic liquids than tinctures. They are usually made by vacuum distilling tinctures. Dry extracts are plant material extracts which are evaporated into a dry mass. They can be further refined to a capsule or tablet. Nebulisates are dry extracts prepared by freeze drying.
- **Herbal Wines and Elixirs:** These are alcoholic extract of herbs; usually with an ethanolic percentage of 12-38%. Herbal wine is a maceration of herbs in wine while an elixir is a maceration of herbs in spirits (e.g., vodka, grappa, etc).

- **Inhalation:** As in aromatherapy it is used as a mood changing treatment to fight sinus infection or cough or to cleanse the skin on a deeper level (steam not direct inhalation).
- **Macerates:** These are cold infusion of plants with high mucilage-content such as sage, thyme, etc. Plants parts are chopped and added to cold water. They are left to stand for 7-12 hrs (depending on herb used). For most of the macerates 10 hrs is used.
- **Syrups:** Extracts of these herbs are made with honey or syrups. Sixty five parts of sugar are mixed with thirty five parts of water and herb. Whole is then boiled and macerated for three weeks
- **Tinctures:** They are obtained by combining 100% pure ethanol (or a mixture of 100% ethanol with water) with the herb. Alcoholic extracts of herbs such as *Echinacea* extract. A completed tincture has 25% of ethanol percentage (sometimes up to 90%). Sometimes tincture is applied to preparations using other solvents than ethanol. Nux vomica (strychnine).
- **Tisanes:** These are hot water extracts of herb, such as chamomile.
- **Vinegars:** These are prepared as the same way as tinctures by using a solution of acetic acid as solvent.
- **Whole Herb Consumption:** Either dried form (herbal powder) or fresh juice (fresh leaves and other plant parts).

Chemical compounds found in the plants mediate their effects on human body by binding to the receptor molecules present in the body; herbal medicines do not differ greatly from conventional drugs in terms of their mechanism of action. All plants produce various chemical compounds as part of their normal metabolic activities. These are divided into primary metabolites such as sugar and fats, found in all plants and secondary metabolites, compounds not essential for basic function; found in a smaller range of plants for specific purposes e.g. defense mechanisms (see Table 5).

Still inspite of modern research studies there is a wide search for new biomarkers to better diagnose patients with CKD according to the risk of the progression stages and mortality which is an underway process. Management of hypertension, glycosuria, lipid intake, consumption of dietary proteins is required for better outcomes in future with herbal assimilation of modern Ayurveda.

Last but not least nutritional management is of utmost importance for the prevention of DKDs and an important part of alternative medicine and therapy. It includes following points-

1. Maintenance of normal blood glucose level by food intake and exercise.
2. Achieving optimal blood pressure and serum lipids to reduce risk of cardiovascular diseases.
3. Management of body weight.
4. Maintaining biochemical parameters and fluid status.
5. Prevention of malnutrition to control gastroparesis.

CONCLUSION

Totally, herbal dependent approches can't cure the disease but definitely it will alter the lifestyle phenomenon by increasing the longevity. There is need for multitargeted approaches and their wise selec-

Table 5. Classification of bioactive compounds in different plants for DKDs

Categories	Example	Plant source	Mechanism of action	Reference
Lignans (polyphenolic compounds)	Vanillic acid	*Cladophora socialis*	↓ protein tyrosinase phosphatase-1β activity	Feng et al., 2007
	Cinnamaldehyde	*Cinnamonum zeylanicum*	↓oxidative stress, ↑insulin sensitivity	Mishra et al., 2010
Flavonoids or flavonols	Catechins	*Camellia, Zeylanicum*	↓ oxidative stress	Ramshini and Ayoubi, 2014
	Myrcetin	*Psidium guajava*	↓ oxidative stress, inflammation and glycative stress	Lin &Yin, 2012
	Apigain 6-Cβ-L fucopyranoside	*Averrhoe carambola*	↑insulin secretion	Cazarolli et al., 2009
	Quercetin	*Vaccinium vitis-idaea, Allium cepa*	↑AMPK pathway	Eid et al., 2010
	Steptogenin 4-o-β- D glucoside	*Morus alba*	↓ hyperglycemia	Zhang et al., 2009
	Cinchona	*Eriobotrya japonica*	↑insulin secretion	Qa'dan et al., 2009
Tannins	Proanthocyanidins	Grapes and berries	↓ AGEs, CTGF	Li et al., 2009
	Geranium	*Nephelium lappaceum*	↓hyperglycemia	Palanasamy et al., 2011
Terpenes	Auraptene	Citrus fruits	↓ MMP-1	Kuroyamy et al., 2008
	Karavitoside XI	*Momordica charantia*	↑AMPK pathway	Tan et al., 2008
	Triterpenoid	*Psidium guajava*	↑ insulin sensitivity	Kuang et al., 2012
Saponins	Ginsenoside	*Pomax jinseng*	↓ oxidative stress, ↓ AGEs	Kang et al., 2010
Others	Polysachharides	*Pueraria tuberosa*	↓malondialdehyde, ↑lipoprotein, ↓oxidative stress	Nagwani & Tripathi, 2010
	Curcumin	*Curcuma longa*	↓oxidative stress, ↓AGEs, ↓ NF-kB	Sharma et al., 2006

tion in different aspects of the disease. The nutrition management is fundamental for the prevention of diabetic kidney disease to ESRD. Thus, medicinal plants have been reported to affect metabolic enzymes involved in diabetegenesis correcting the imbalanced glucose metabolic disturbances, improving the glucose uptake, inhibiting gluconeogenic enzymes and modulating glycolytic and lipolytic pathways.

REFERENCES

Adhikary, L., Chow, F., Nikolic-Paterson, D. J., Stambe, C., Dowling, J., Atkins, R. C., & Tesch, G. H. (2004). Abnormal p38 mitogen-activated protein kinase signalling in human and experimental diabetic nephropathy. *Diabetologia*, *47*(7), 1210–1222. doi:10.1007/s00125-004-1437-0 PMID:15232685

Alicic, R. Z., & Tuttle, K. R. (2014). Novel therapies for diabetic kidney disease. *Advances in Chronic Kidney Disease*, *21*(2), 121–133. doi:10.1053/j.ackd.2014.01.007 PMID:24602462

Bakris, G.L. (2008). Slowing Nephropathy Progression: Focus on Proteinuria Reduction. *Clinical Journal of the American Society of Nephrology, 3*, S3-S10.

Bank, N., & Aynedjian, H. S. (1993). Role of EDRF (nitric oxide) in diabetic renal hyperfiltration. *Kidney International*, *43*(6), 1306–1312. doi:10.1038/ki.1993.183 PMID:8315943

Barnett, A. H., Bain, S. C., Bouter, P., Karlberg, B., Madsbad, S., Jervell, J., & Mustonen, J. (2004). Angiotensin-receptor blockade versus converting-enzyme inhibition in type 2 diabetes and nephropathy. *TheNew England Journal of Medicine*, *351*(19), 1952–1961. doi:10.1056/NEJMoa042274 PMID:15516696

Berkholtz, C. B., Lai, B. E., Woodruff, T. K., & Shea, L. D. (2006). Distribution of extracellular matrix proteins type I collagen, type IV collagen, fibronectin, and laminin in mouse folliculogenesis. *Histochemistry and Cell Biology*, *126*(5), 583–592. doi:10.1007/s00418-006-0194-1 PMID:16758163

Bianchi, S., Bigazzi, R., & Campese, V. M. (2006). Long-term effects of spironolactone on proteinuria and kidney function in patients with chronic kidney disease. *Kidney International*, *70*(12), 2116–2123. doi:10.1038/sj.ki.5001854 PMID:17035949

Brenner, B. M., Cooper, M. E., de Zeeuw, D., Keane, W. F., Mitch, W. E., Parving, H. H., & Shahinfar, S. et al. (2001). Effects of losartan on renal and cardiovascular outcomes in patients with type 2 diabetes and nephropathy. *The New England Journal of Medicine*, *345*(12), 861–869. doi:10.1056/NEJMoa011161 PMID:11565518

Brownlee, M. (2001). Biochemistry and molecular cell biology of diabetic complications. *Nature*, *414*(6865), 813–820. doi:10.1038/414813a PMID:11742414

Cai, Y., Chen, J., Jiang, J., Cao, W., & He, L. (2010). Zhen-wu-tang, a blended traditional Chinese herbal medicine, ameliorates proteinuria and renal damage of streptozotocin-induced diabetic nephropathy in rats. *Journal of Ethnopharmacology*, *131*(1), 88–94. doi:10.1016/j.jep.2010.06.004 PMID:20547220

Cazarolli, L. H., Folador, P., Moresco, H. H., Brighente, I. M. C., Pizzolatti, M. G., & Silva, F. R. M. B. (2009). Stimulatory effect of apigenin-6-C-beta-L-fucopyranoside on insulin secretion and glycogen synthesis. *European Journal of Medicinal Chemistry*, *44*(11), 4668–4673. doi:10.1016/j.ejmech.2009.07.001 PMID:19625113

Chen, S., Hong, S. W., Cruz, I. M. C., Isono, M., Casaretto, A., & Ziyadeh, F. N. (2001). Proteins, growth factors, and progression of kidney disease the key role of the transforming growth factor-b system in the pathogenesis of diabetic nephropathy. *Renal Failure*, *23*, 471–481. doi:10.1081/JDI-100104730 PMID:11499562

Cherney, D. Z. I., Perkins, B. A., Soleymanlou, N., Maione, M., Lai, V., Lee, A., & von Eynatten, M. et al. (2014). Renal hemodynamic effect of sodium-glucose co-transporter 2 inhibition in patients with type 1 diabetes mellitus. *Circulation*, *129*(5), 587–597. doi:10.1161/CIRCULATIONAHA.113.005081 PMID:24334175

Chow, F. Y., Nikolic-Paterson, D. J., Ma, F. Y., Ozols, E., Rollins, B. J., & Tesch, G. H. (2007). Monocyte chemo-attractant protein-1-induced tissue inflammation is critical for the development of renal injury but not type 2 diabetes in obese db/db mice. *Diabetologia*, *50*(2), 471–480. doi:10.1007/s00125-006-0497-8 PMID:17160673

Circu, M. L., & Aw, T. Y. (2012). Glutathione and modulation of cell apoptosis,*Biochimica et Biophysica Acta (BBA) -. Molecular Cell Research, 1823*, 1767–1777.

Craven, P. A., Davidson, C. M., & De-Rubertis, F. R. (1990). Increase in diacylglycerol mass in isolated glomeruli by glucose from de novo synthesis of glycerolipids. *Diabetes, 39*(6), 667–674. doi:10.2337/diab.39.6.667 PMID:2347431

de Galan, B. E., Zoungas, S., Chalmers, J., Dufouil, C., Pillai, A., & Cooper, M. (2009). …Woodward, M. Cognitive function and risks of cardiovascular disease and hypoglycaemia in patients with type 2 diabetes: the Action in Diabetes and Vascular Disease: Preterax and Diamicron Modified Release Controlled Evaluation (ADVANCE) trial. *Diabetologia, 52*(11), 2328–2336. doi:10.1007/s00125-009-1484-7 PMID:19688336

Duckworth, W., Abraira, C., Moritz, T., Reda, D., Emanuele, N., Reaven, P. D., & Huang, G. D. et al. (2009). Glucose control and vascular complications in veterans with type 2 diabetes. *The New England Journal of Medicine, 360*(2), 129–139. doi:10.1056/NEJMoa0808431 PMID:19092145

Eid, H. M., Martineau, L. C., Saleem, A., Muhammad, A., Vallerand, D., Benhaddou-Andaloussi, A., & Haddad, P. S. et al. (2010). Stimulation of AMP-activated protein kinase and enhancement of basal glucose uptake in muscle cells by quercetin and quercetin glycosides, active principles of the antidiabetic medicinal plant Vaccinium vitis-idaea. *Molecular Nutrition & Food Research, 54*(7), 991–1003. doi:10.1002/mnfr.200900218 PMID:20087853

Eller, K., Kirsch, A., Wolf, A. M., Sopper, S., Tagwerker, A., Stanzl, U., & Eller, P. et al. (2011). Potential role of regulatory T cells in reversing obesity-linked insulin resistance and diabetic nephropathy. *Diabetes, 60*(11), 2954–2962. doi:10.2337/db11-0358 PMID:21911743

Feng, Y., Carroll, A. R., Addepalli, R., Fechner, G., Avery, V. M., & Quinn, R. J. (2007). Vanillic acid derivatives from the green algae *Cladophora socialis* as potent protein tyrosine phosphatase 1B inhibitors. *Journal of Natural Products, 70*(11), 1790–1792. doi:10.1021/np070225o PMID:17949055

Fiorina, P., Vergani, A., Bassi, R., Niewczas, M., Altintas, M. M., Pezzolesi, M. G., & Sayegh, M. H. et al. (2014). Role of Podocyte B7-1 in Diabetic Nephropathy. *Journal of the American Society of Nephrology, 25*(7), 1415–1429. doi:10.1681/ASN.2013050518 PMID:24676639

Flo, T. H., Smith, K. D., Sato, S., Rodriguez, D. J., Holmes, M. A., Strong, R. K., & Aderem, A. et al. (2004). Lipocalin-2 Mediates an Innate Immune Response to Bacterial Infection by Sequestrating Iron. *Nature, 432*(7019), 917–921. doi:10.1038/nature03104 PMID:15531878

Forbes, J. M., & Cooper, M. E. (2013). Mechanisms of diabetic complications. *Physiological Reviews, 93*(1), 137–188. doi:10.1152/physrev.00045.2011 PMID:23303908

Forbes, J. M., Cooper, M. E., Oldfield, M. D., & Thomas, M. C. (2003). Role of advanced glycation end products in diabetic nephropathy. *Journal of the American Society of Nephrology, 14*(90003), S254–S258. doi:10.1097/01.ASN.0000077413.41276.17 PMID:12874442

Fujita, H., Taniai, H., Murayama, H., Ohshiro, H., Hayashi, H., Sato, S., & Yamada, Y. et al. (2013). DPP-4 inhibition with alogliptin on top of angiotensin II type 1 receptor blockade ameliorates albuminuria via up-regulation of SDF-1α in type 2 diabetic patients with incipient nephropathy. *Endocrine Journal*, *61*(2), 159–166. doi:10.1507/endocrj.EJ13-0305 PMID:24225429

Fukami, K., Yamagishi, S. I., Ueda, S., & Okuda, S. (2008). Role of AGEs in diabetic nephropathy. *Current Pharmaceutical Design*, *14*(10), 946–952. doi:10.2174/138161208784139710 PMID:18473844

Gerstein, H. C., Miller, M. E., Byington, R. P., Goff, D. C., Bigger, J. T., Buse, J. B., & Friedewald, W. T. et al. (2008). Effects of intensive glucose lowering in type 2 diabetes. *The New England Journal of Medicine*, *358*(24), 2545–2559. doi:10.1056/NEJMoa0802743 PMID:18539917

Goldstein, S. L. (2011). Acute kidney injury biomarkers: Renal angina and the need for a renal troponin I. *BMC Medicine*, *9*(1), 135. doi:10.1186/1741-7015-9-135 PMID:22189039

Hayat, M. A. (2013). Introduction to Autophagy: Cancer, Other Pathologies, Inflammation, Immunity, Infection, and Aging: Vol. 1-4. *Autophagy: Cancer, Other Pathologies, Inflammation, Immunity, Infection, and Aging*. Elsevier Inc.

Holman, R. R., Paul, S. K., Bethel, M. A., Matthews, D. R., & Neil, H. A. (2013). 10-year follow-up of intensive glucose control in type 2 diabetes. *The New England Journal of Medicine*, *359*(15), 1577–1589. doi:10.1056/NEJMoa0806470 PMID:18784090

Huang, J. S., Guh, J. Y., Chen, J. C., Hung, W. C., Lai, Y. H., & Chuang, L. Y. (2001). Role of receptor for advanced glycation end-product (RAGE) and the JAK/STAT-signaling pathway in AGE-induced collagen production in NRK-49F cells. *Journal of Cellular Biochemistry*, *81*(1), 102–113. doi:10.1002/1097-4644(20010401)81:1<102::AID-JCB1027>3.0.CO;2-Y PMID:11180401

Ilan, Y., Maron, R., Tukpah, A.-M., Maioli, T. U., Murugaiyan, G., Yang, K., & Weiner, H. L. (2010). Induction of regulatory T cells decreases adipose inflammation and alleviates insulin resistance in ob/ob mice. *Proceedings of the National Academy of Sciences of the United States of America*, *107*(21), 9765–9770. doi:10.1073/pnas.0908771107 PMID:20445103

Ismail-Beigi, F., Craven, T., Banerji, M. A., Basile, J., Calles, J., Cohen, R. M., & Hamilton, B. et al. (2010). Effect of intensive treatment of hyperglycaemia on microvascular outcomes in type 2 diabetes: An analysis of the ACCORD randomised trial. *Lancet*, *376*(9739), 419–430. doi:10.1016/S0140-6736(10)60576-4 PMID:20594588

Jarad, G., & Miner, J. H. (2009). Update on the glomerular filtration barrier. *Current Opinion in Nephrology and Hypertension*, *18*(3), 226–232. doi:10.1097/MNH.0b013e3283296044 PMID:19374010

Kang, K. S., Yamabe, N., Kim, H. Y., Park, J. H., & Yokozawa, T. (2010). Effects of heat-processed ginseng and its active component ginsenoside 20(S)-Rg3 on the progression of renal damage and dysfunction in type 2 diabetic Otsuka Long- Evans Tokushima Fatty rats. *Biological & Pharmaceutical Bulletin*, *33*(6), 1077–1081. doi:10.1248/bpb.33.1077 PMID:20522983

Kim, Y. S., Sohn, E., Lee, Y. M., Kim, C.-S., & Kim, J. S. (2014). Extract of *Cassiae semen* attenuates diabetic nephropathy via inhibition of advanced glycation end products accumulation in streptozotocin-induced diabetic rats. *Phytomedicine*, *21*(5), 734–739. doi:10.1016/j.phymed.2013.11.002 PMID:24374123

Kjeldsen, L., Johnsen, A. H., Sengeløv, H., & Borregaard, N. (1993). Isolation and primary structure of NGAL, a novel protein associated with human neutrophil gelatinase. *The Journal of Biological Chemistry*, *268*(14), 10425–10432. PMID:7683678

Kodera, R., Shikata, K., Takatsuka, T., Oda, K., Miyamoto, S., Kajitani, N., & Makino, H. et al. (2014). Dipeptidyl peptidase-4 inhibitor ameliorates early renal injury through its anti-inflammatory action in a rat model of type 1 diabetes. *Biochemical and Biophysical Research Communications*, *443*(3), 828–833. doi:10.1016/j.bbrc.2013.12.049 PMID:24342619

Kosugi, T., Heinig, M., Nakayama, T., Matsuo, S., & Nakagawa, T. (2010). eNOS Knockout Mice with Advanced Diabetic Nephropathy Have Less Benefit from Renin-Angiotensin Blockade than from Aldosterone Receptor Antagonists. *American Journal of Pathology*, *176*(2), 619–629. doi:10.2353/ajpath.2010.090578 PMID:20042665

Kuang, Q. T., Zhao, J. J., Ye, C. L., Wang, J. R., Ye, K. H., Zhang, X. Q., & Ye, W. C. et al. (2012). Nephro-protective effects of total triterpenoids from *Psidium guajava* leaves on type 2 diabetic rats. *Journal of Chinese Medicinal Materials*, *35*, 94–97. PMID:22734419

Kuroyanagi, K., Kang, M. S., Goto, T., Hirai, S., Ohyama, K., Kusudo, T., & Kawada, T. et al. (2008). *Citrus auraptene* acts as an agonist for PPARs and enhances adiponectin production and MCP-1 reduction in 3T3-L1 adipocytes. *Biochemical and Biophysical Research Communications*, *366*(1), 219–225. doi:10.1016/j.bbrc.2007.11.119 PMID:18060855

Langham, R. G., Kelly, D. J., Gow, R. M., Zhang, Y., Cox, A. J., Qi, W., & Gilbert, R. E. et al. (2008). Increased renal gene transcription of protein kinase C-beta in human diabetic nephropathy: Relationship to long-term glycaemic control. *Diabetologia*, *51*(4), 668–674. doi:10.1007/s00125-008-0927-x PMID:18278479

Li, X., Xiao, Y., Gao, H., Li, B., Xu, L., Cheng, M., & Ma, Y. et al. (2009). Grape seed proanthocyanidins ameliorate diabetic nephropathy via modulation of levels of AGE, RAGE and CTGF. *Nephron. Experimental Nephrology*, *111*(2), e31–e41. doi:10.1159/000191103 PMID:19142024

Lim, A. K., Ma, F. Y., Nikolic-Paterson, D. J., Kitching, A. R., Thomas, M. C., & Tesch, G. H. (2010). Lymphocytes promote albuminuria, but not renal dysfunction or histological damage in a mouse model of diabetic renal injury. *Diabetologia*, *53*(8), 1772–1782. doi:10.1007/s00125-010-1757-1 PMID:20422398

Lim, A. K., Ma, F. Y., Nikolic-Paterson, D. J., Thomas, M. C., Hurst, L. A., & Tesch, G. H. (2009). Antibody blockade of c-fms suppresses the progression of inflammation and injury in early diabetic nephropathy in obese db/db mice. *Diabetologia*, *52*(8), 1669–1679. doi:10.1007/s00125-009-1399-3 PMID:19466391

Lim, A. K., & Tesch, G. H. (2012). Inflammation in diabetic nephropathy. *Mediators of Inflammation*. PMID:22969168

Lim, A. K. H. (2014). Diabetic nephropathy- complications and treatment. *International Journal of Nephrology and Renovascular Disease*, *7*, 361–381. doi:10.2147/IJNRD.S40172 PMID:25342915

Lin, C. Y., & Yin, M. C. (2012). Renal Protective Effects of Extracts from Guava Fruit (Psidium guajava L.) in Diabetic Mice. *Plant Foods for Human Nutrition (Dordrecht, Netherlands)*, *67*(3), 303–308. doi:10.1007/s11130-012-0294-0 PMID:22581156

Lippi, G., Aloe, R., Storelli, A., Cervellin, G., & Trenti, T. (2012). Evaluation of NGAL Test™, a fully-automated neutrophil gelatinase-associated lipocalin (NGAL) immunoassay on Beckman Coulter AU 5822. *Clinical Chemistry and Laboratory Medicine*, *50*(9), 1581–1584. doi:10.1515/cclm.2011.839 PMID:22962213

Liu, H. Y., Fang, M., & Zhang, Y. Q. (2014). *In Vivo Hypoglycaemic Effect and Inhibitory Mechanism of the Branch Bark Extract of the Mulberry on STZ-Induced Diabetic Mice*. The Scientific World Journal.

Liu, K., Xu, H., Lv, G., Liu, B., Lee, M. K. K., Lu, C., & Wu, Y. et al. (2015). Loganin attenuates diabetic nephropathy in C57BL/6J mice with diabetes induced by streptozotocin and fed with diets containing high level of advanced glycation end products. *Life Sciences*, *123*, 78–85. doi:10.1016/j.lfs.2014.12.028 PMID:25623853

Liu, X., Kelm, R. J., & Strauch, A. R. (2009). Transforming Growth Factor β1-mediated Activation of the Smooth Muscle α-Actin Gene in Human Pulmonary Myofibroblasts Is Inhibited by Tumor Necrosis Factor-α via Mitogen-activated Protein Kinase 1-dependent Induction of the Egr-1 Transcriptional Repressor. *Molecular Biology of the Cell*, *20*, 2174–2185. doi:10.1091/mbc.E08-10-0994 PMID:19261809

Lv, J., Perkovic, V., Foote, C. V., Craig, M. E., Craig, J. C., & Strippoli, G. F. (2012). Antihypertensive agents for preventing diabetic kidney disease. *Cochrane Database of Systematic Reviews*, *12*, CD004136. PMID:23235603

Macisaac, R. J., Ekinci, E. I., & Jerums, G. (2014). Markers of and risk factors for the development and progression of diabetic kidney disease. *American Journal of Kidney Diseases*, *63*(2), S39–S62. doi:10.1053/j.ajkd.2013.10.048 PMID:24461729

Maheshwari, R. A., Balaraman, R., Sen, A. K., & Seth, A. K. (2014). Effect of coenzyme Q10 alone and its combination with metformin on streptozotocin-nicotinamide-induced diabetic nephropathy in rats. *Indian Journal of Pharmacology*, *46*(6), 627–632. doi:10.4103/0253-7613.144924 PMID:25538335

Manikowski, S. T., & Atta, M. G. (2013). Diabetic Kidney Disease: Pathophysiology and Therapeutic Targets. Journal of Diabetes Research.

Manikowski, S.T., & Atta, M.G. (2015) Diabetic Kidney Disease: Pathophysiology and Therapeutic Targets. *Journal of Diabetes Research.*

Mason, R. M. (2009). Connective tissue growth factor (CCN2), a pathogenic factor in diabetic nephropathy. What does it do? How does it do it? *Journal of Cell Communication and Signaling*, *3*(2), 95–104. doi:10.1007/s12079-009-0038-6 PMID:19214781

Mehdi, U., & Toto, R. D. (2009). Anemia, Diabetes, and Chronic Kidney Disease. *Diabetes Care*, *32*(7), 1320–1326. doi:10.2337/dc08-0779 PMID:19564475

Menne, J., Park, J. K., Boehne, M., Elger, M., Lindschau, C., Kirsch, T., & Haller, H. et al. (2004). Diminished loss of proteoglycans and lack of albuminuria in protein kinase C-??-deficient diabetic mice. *Diabetes*, *53*(8), 2101–2109. doi:10.2337/diabetes.53.8.2101 PMID:15277392

Mishra, A., Bhatti, R., Singh, A., & Singh Ishar, M. P. (2010). Ameliorative effect of the cinnamon oil from *Cinnamomum zeylanicum* upon early stage diabetic nephropathy. *Planta Medica*, *76*(5), 412–417. doi:10.1055/s-0029-1186237 PMID:19876811

Mooyaart, A. L., Valk, E. J. J., & Van, E. S. (2011). Genetic associations in diabetic nephropathy: A meta-analysis. *Diabetologia*, *54*(3), 544–553. doi:10.1007/s00125-010-1996-1 PMID:21127830

Mori, H., Okada, Y., Arao, T., & Tanaka, Y. (2014). Sitagliptin improves albuminuria in patients with type 2 diabetes mellitus. *Journal of Diabetes and Investigation*, *5*(3), 313–319. doi:10.1111/jdi.12142 PMID:24843780

Mudaliar, H., Pollock, C., Komala, M. G., Chadban, S., Wu, H., & Panchapakesan, U. (2013). The role of Toll-like receptor proteins (TLR) 2 and 4 in mediatinginflammation in proximal tubules. *American Journal ofPhysiology. Renal Physiology*, *305*(2), F143–F154. doi:10.1152/ajprenal.00398.2012 PMID:23576640

Nagahama, T., Hayashi, K., Ozawa, Y., Takenaka, T., & Saruta, T. (2000). Role of protein kinase C in angiotensin II-induced constriction of renal microvessels. *Kidney International*, *57*(1), 215–223. doi:10.1046/j.1523-1755.2000.00822.x PMID:10620202

Nagwani, S., & Tripathi, Y. B. (2010). Amelioration of cisplatin induced nephrotoxicity by PTY: A herbal preparation. *Food and Chemical Toxicology*, *48*(8-9), 2253–2258. doi:10.1016/j.fct.2010.05.057 PMID:20510324

Noh, H., & King, G. L. (2007). The role of protein kinase C activation in diabetic nephropathy. *Kidney International*, *106*, S49–S53. doi:10.1038/sj.ki.5002386 PMID:17653211

Noh, H., & King, G. L. (2007). The role of protein kinase C activation in diabetic nephropathy. *Kidney International. Supplement*, *106*, S49–S53. doi:10.1038/sj.ki.5002386 PMID:17653211

Ohga, S., Shikata, K., Yozai, K., Okada, S., Ogawa, D., Usui, H., & Makino, H. et al. (2007). Thiazolidinedione ameliorates renal injury in experimental diabetic rats through anti-inflammatory effects mediated by inhibition of NF-kB activation. *American Journal of Physiology. Renal Physiology*, *292*(4), F1141–F1150. doi:10.1152/ajprenal.00288.2005 PMID:17190910

Palanisamy, U. D., Ling, L. T., Manaharan, T., & Appleton, D. (2011). Rapid isolation of geraniin from *Nephelium lappaceum* rind waste and its hyperglycemic activity. *Food Chemistry*, *127*(1), 21–27. doi:10.1016/j.foodchem.2010.12.070

Pathak, R., & Bridgeman, M. B. (2010). Dipeptidyl Peptidase-4 (DPP-4) Inhibitors in the Management of Diabetes. *Pharmacy and Therapeutics*, *35*, 509–513. PMID:20975810

Perkin, B.A., Ficociello, L.H., Ostrander, B.E., Silva, K.H., Weinberg, J., Warram, J. H.& Krolewski, A.S. (2007). Microalbuminuria and the risk for early progressive renal function decline in type 1 diabetes. *Journal ofthe American Society of Nephrology*, *18*, 1353-1361.

Perkovic, V., Heerspink, H. L., Chalmers, J., Woodward, M., Jun, M., Li, Q., & Zoungas, S. et al. (2013). Intensive glucose control improves kidney outcomes in patients with type 2 diabetes. *Kidney International, 83*(3), 517–523. doi:10.1038/ki.2012.401 PMID:23302714

Qa'dan, F., Verspohl, E. J., Nahrstedt, A., Petereit, F., & Matalka, K. Z. (2009). Cinchonain Ib isolated from *Eriobotrya japonica* induces insulin secretion in vitro and in vivo. *Journal of Ethnopharmacology, 124*(2), 224-227.

Ramshini, H., & Ayoubi, F. (2014). Inhibitory Effect of *Cinnamomum Zeylanicum* and *Camellia sinensis* Extracts on the Hen Egg-White Lysozyme Fibrillation. *Journal of Kerman University of Medical Sciences, 21*(4), 3–9.

Ranasinghe, P., Pigera, S., Premakumara, G., Galappaththy, P., Constantine, G. R., & Katulanda, P. (2013). Medicinal properties of "true" cinnamon (Cinnamomum zeylanicum): A systematic review. *BMC Complementary and Alternative Medicine, 13*(1), 275. doi:10.1186/1472-6882-13-275 PMID:24148965

Remuzzi, G., Perico, N., Macia, M., & Ruggenenti, P. (2005). The role of renin-angiotensin-aldosterone system in the progression of chronic kidney disease. *Kidney International. Supplement, 99*, S57–S65. doi:10.1111/j.1523-1755.2005.09911.x PMID:16336578

Ritz, E., & Zeng, X. (2011). Diabetic nephropathy – Epidemiology in Asia and the current state of treatment. *Indian Journal of Nephrology, 21*(2), 75–84. doi:10.4103/0971-4065.82122 PMID:21769168

Ruan, X., & Arendshorst, W. J. (1996). Role of protein kinase C in angiotensin II-induced renal vasoconstriction in genetically hypertensive rats. *The American Journal of Physiology, 270*, F945–F952. PMID:8764313

Sakai, N., Wada, T., Furuichi, K., Iwata, Y., Yoshimoto, K., Kitagawa, K., & Yokoyama, H. et al. (2005). Involvement of extracellular signal-regulated kinase and p38 in human diabetic nephropathy. *American Journal of Kidney Diseases, 45*(1), 54–65. doi:10.1053/j.ajkd.2004.08.039 PMID:15696444

Schmid, H., Boucherot, A., Yasuda, Y., Henger, A., Brunner, B., Eichinger, F., & Kretzler, M. et al. (2006). Modular activation of nuclear factor-kappa B transcriptional programs in humandiabetic nephropathy. *Diabetes, 55*(11), 2993–3003. doi:10.2337/db06-0477 PMID:17065335

Schmidt-Ott, K. M., Mori, K., Li, J. Y., Kalandadze, A., Cohen, D. J., Devarajan, P., & Barasch, J. (2007). Dual action of neutrophil gelatinase-associated lipocalin. *Journal of the American Society of Nephrology, 18*(2), 407–413. doi:10.1681/ASN.2006080882 PMID:17229907

Sharma, P.L., & Sharma V. (2013). Role of Different Molecular Pathways in the Development of Diabetes Induced Nephropathy. *Journal of Diabetes & Metabolism, S9.*

Sharma, S., Kulkarni, S. K., & Chopra, K. (2006). Curcumin, the active principle of turmeric (Curcuma longa), ameliorates diabetic nephropathy in rats. *Clinical and Experimental Pharmacology & Physiology, 33*(10), 940–945. doi:10.1111/j.1440-1681.2006.04468.x PMID:17002671

Sheetz, M. J., & King, G. L. (2002). Molecular understanding of hyperglycemia's adverse effects for diabetic complications. *Journal of the American Medical Association, 288*(20), 2579–2588. doi:10.1001/jama.288.20.2579 PMID:12444865

Singh, R. G., Rajak, M., & Ghosh, B. (2013). Comparative evaluation of fosinopril and herbal drug Dioscorea bulbifera in patients of diabetic nephropathy. *Saudi Journal of Kidney Diseases and Transplantation*, *24*(4), 737–742. doi:10.4103/1319-2442.113866 PMID:23816723

Singh, V. P., Bali, A., Singh, N., & Jaggi, A. S. (2014). Advanced Glycation End Products and Diabetic Complications. *TheKorean Journal of Physiology and Pharmacology*, *18*(1), 1–14. doi:10.4196/kjpp.2014.18.1.1 PMID:24634591

Smith, S. R., Svetkey, L. P., & Dennis, V. W. (1991). Racial differences in the incidence and progression of renal diseases. *Kidney International*, *40*(5), 815–822. doi:10.1038/ki.1991.281 PMID:1762285

Tan, A. L. Y., Forbes, J. M., & Cooper, M. E. (2007). AGE, RAGE, and ROS in Diabetic Nephropathy. *Seminars in Nephrology*, *27*(2), 130–143. doi:10.1016/j.semnephrol.2007.01.006 PMID:17418682

Tan, M. J., Ye, J. M., Turner, N., Hohnen-Behrens, C., Ke, C. Q., Tang, C. P., & Ye, Y. et al. (2008). Antidiabetic Activities of Triterpenoids Isolated from Bitter Melon Associated with Activation of the AMPK Pathway. *Chemistry & Biology*, *15*(3), 263–273. doi:10.1016/j.chembiol.2008.01.013 PMID:18355726

Tan, Y., Wang, B., Keum, J.-S., & Jaffa, A. A. (2005). Mechanisms through which bradykinin promotes glomerular injury in diabetes. *American Journal of Physiology. Renal Physiology*, *288*(3), F483–F492. doi:10.1152/ajprenal.00165.2004 PMID:15692059

Tang, D., Yu, Y., Zheng, X., Wu, J., Li, Y., Wu, X., & Yin, X. et al. (2014). Comparative investigation of in vitro biotransformation of 14 components in Ginkgo biloba extract in normal, diabetes and diabetic nephropathy rat intestinal bacteria matrix. *Journal of Pharmaceutical and Biomedical Analysis*, *100*, 1–10. doi:10.1016/j.jpba.2014.07.022 PMID:25117949

Tarnow, L., Rossing, P., Carstensen, B., & Parving, H. H. (2004). Improved survival in patients obtaining remission of nephrotic range albuminuria in diabetic nephropathy. *Kidney International*, *66*(3), 1180–1186. doi:10.1111/j.1523-1755.2004.00870.x PMID:15327415

Trachootham, D., Lu, W., Ogasawara, M. A., Valle, N. R. D., & Huang, P. (2008). Redox Regulation of Cell Survival. *Antioxidants & Redox Signalling*, *10*(8), 1343–1374. doi:10.1089/ars.2007.1957 PMID:18522489

Tripathi, Y. B., Nagwani, S., Mishra, P., Jha, A., & Rai, S. P. (2012). Protective effect of Pueraria tuberosa DC. Embedded biscuit on cisplatin-induced nephrotoxicity in mice. *Journal of Natural Medicines*, *66*(1), 109–118. doi:10.1007/s11418-011-0559-1 PMID:21717089

Tripathi, Y. B., & Yadav, D. (2013). Diabetic Nephropathy: Causes and Managements Recent Patents on Endocrine. *Metabolic & Immune Drug Discovery*, *7*, 57–64.

Tu, X., Liu, F., Jordan, J. B., Ye, X. F., Fu, P., Wang, F., & Zhong, S. (2013). *'Huang Qi Elixir'* for proteinuria in patients with diabetic nephropathy: A study protocol for a randomized controlled pilot trial. *Trials*, *14*(1), 223. doi:10.1186/1745-6215-14-223 PMID:23866835

Tufro, A., & Veron, D. (2012). VEGF and Podocytes in Diabetic Nephropathy. *Seminars in Nephrology*, *32*(4), 385–393. doi:10.1016/j.semnephrol.2012.06.010 PMID:22958493

Turnbull, F. M., Abraira, C., Anderson, R. J., Byington, R. P., Chalmers, J. P., Duckworth, W. C., & Woodward, M. et al. (2009). Intensive glucose control and macrovascular outcomes in type 2 diabetes. *Diabetologia*, *52*(11), 2288–2298. doi:10.1007/s00125-009-1470-0 PMID:19655124

Veerkamp, J. H., van Kuppevelt, T. H., Maatman, R. G., & Prinsen, C. F. (1993). Structural and functional aspects of cytosolic fatty acid-binding proteins. *Prostaglandins, Leukotrienes, and Essential Fatty Acids*, *49*(6), 887–906. doi:10.1016/0952-3278(93)90174-U PMID:8140117

Verspohl, E. J. (2012). Novel pharmacological approaches to the treatment of type 2 diabetes. *Pharmacological Reviews*, *64*(2), 188–237. doi:10.1124/pr.110.003319 PMID:22407617

Wang, G., Gong, Y., Anderson, J., Sun, D., Minuk, G., Roberts, M. S., & Burczynski, F. J. (2005). Antioxidative function of L-FABP in L-FABP stably transfected Chang liver cells. *Hepatology (Baltimore, Md.)*, *42*(4), 871–879. doi:10.1002/hep.20857 PMID:16175609

Wang, H., Mu, W., Zhai, J., Xing, D. S., Wang, J., Deng, Y., … Shang, H. (2013). *The key role of Shenyan Kangfu tablets, a Chinese patent medicine for diabetic nephropathy: study protocol for a randomized, double-blind and placebo-controlled clinical trial*. Academic Press.

Wang, T. Z., Chen, Y., He, Y. M., Fu, X. D., Wang, Y., Xu, Y. Q., & Wang, W. J. et al. (2013). Effects of Chinese herbal medicine Yiqi Huaju Qingli Formula in metabolic syndrome patients with microalbuminuria: A randomized placebo-controlled trial. *Journal of Internal Medicine*, *11*, 175–183. PMID:23743161

Wesseling, C., & Crowe, J. (2013). The Epidemic of Chronic Kidney Disease of Unknown Etiology in Mesoamerica: A Call for Interdisciplinary Research and Action. *American Journal of Public Health*, 1-4. Retrieved from http://www.ncbi.nlm.nih.gov/pubmed/24028232

Wolf, G., Chen, S., & Ziyadeh, F. N. (2005). From the periphery of the glomerular capillary wall toward the center of disease: Podocyte injury comes of age in diabetic nephropathy. *Diabetes*, *54*(6), 1626–1634. doi:10.2337/diabetes.54.6.1626 PMID:15919782

Wong, D. W., Oudit, G. Y., Reich, H., Kassiri, J., Zhou, J., Liu, Q. C., & Scholey, J. W. et al. (2007). Loss of Angiotensin-Converting Enzyme-2 (*Ace2*) Accelerates Diabetic Kidney Injury. *American Journal of Pathology*, *171*(2), 438–451. doi:10.2353/ajpath.2007.060977 PMID:17600118

Woroniecka, K. I., Park, A. S., Mohtat, D., Thomas, D. B., Pullman, J. M., & Susztak, K. (2011). Transcriptome analysis of human diabetic kidney disease. *Diabetes*, *60*(9), 2354–2369. doi:10.2337/db10-1181 PMID:21752957

Wu, J.-S., Liu, Y., Shi, R., Lu, X., Ma, Y.-M., & Cheng, N.-N. (2014). Effects of combinations of Xiexin decoction constituents on diabetic nephropathy in rats. *Journal of Ethnopharmacology*, *157*, 126–133. PMID:25278183

Xu, J., Su, H. L., Wang, J. H., & Zhang, C. H. (2009). Role of CD4+CD25+Foxp3+ regulatory T cells in type 2 diabetic nephropathy. *Journal of the Southern Medical University*, *29*, 137–139. PMID:19218134

Yan, Y. M., Fang, P., Yang, M. T., Li, N., Lu, Q., & Cheng, Y. X. (2015). Anti-diabetic nephropathy compounds from *Cinnamomum cassia*. *Journal of Ethnopharmacology*, *13*(165), 141–147. doi:10.1016/j.jep.2015.01.049 PMID:25725434

Young, B. A., Maynard, C., & Boyko, E. J. (2003). Racial differences in diabetic nephropathy, cardiovascular disease, and mortality in a national population of veterans. *Diabetes Care*, *26*(8), 2392–2399. doi:10.2337/diacare.26.8.2392 PMID:12882868

Zhang, H., Saha, J., Byun, J., Schin, M., Lorenz, M., Kennedy, R. T., & Brosius, F. C. et al. (2008). … Brosius, F.C. Rosiglitazone reduces renal and plasma markers of oxidative injury and reverses urinary metabolite abnormalities in the amelioration of diabetic nephropathy. *American Journal of Physiology. Renal Physiology*, *295*(4), F1071–F1081. doi:10.1152/ajprenal.90208.2008 PMID:18667486

Zhang, M., Chen, M., Zhang, H. Q., Sun, S., Xia, B., & Wu, F. H. (2009). In vivo hypoglycemic effects of phenolics from the root bark of *Morus alba*. *Fitoterapia*, *80*(8), 475–477. doi:10.1016/j.fitote.2009.06.009 PMID:19545615

Zhang, M., Feng, L., Gu, J., Ma, L., Qin, D., Wu, C., & Jia, X. (2014). The attenuation of Moutan Cortex on oxidative stress for renal injury in AGEs-induced mesangial cell dysfunction and streptozotocin-induced diabetic nephropathy rats. *Oxidative Medicine and Cellular Longevity*. PMID:24876912

Zheng, N., Lin, X., Wen, Q., Kintoko, , Zhang, S., Huang, J., & Huang, R. et al. (2013). Effect of 2-dodecyl-6-methoxycyclohexa-2,5-diene-1,4-dione, isolated from Averrhoa carambola L. (Oxalidaceae) roots, on advanced glycation end-product-mediated renal injury in type 2 diabetic KK Ay mice. *Toxicology Letters*, *10*(1), 77–84. doi:10.1016/j.toxlet.2013.03.001 PMID:23500658

Zou, J., Yu, X., Qu, S., Li, X., Jin, Y., & Sui, D. (2014). Protective effect of total flavonoids extracted from the leaves of *Murraya paniculata* (L.) Jack on diabetic nephropathy in rats. *Food and Chemical Toxicology*, *64*, 231–237. doi:10.1016/j.fct.2013.11.043 PMID:24309143

KEY TERMS AND DEFINITIONS

Diabetic Kidney Diseases (DKDs): It is also known as Diabetic nephropathy. It is a disease that causes the damage of millions of tiny blood vessel clusters leading to the damage of delicate renal filtering system. It develops in severity of the cases of diabetic patients of Type 1 or Type 2.

Glomerular Filtration Rate (GFR): It is described as the rate of volume of the fluid filtered to remove excess wastes and fluids from the kidney glomerular capillaries into the Bowman's capsule per unit time.

Hyperglycemia: It means high (*hyper*) glucose (*gly*) or high blood sugar in the blood stream. It occurs due to the inability of the body to remove glucose from the blood so that cells can use it for energy, this adverse condition arises due to abnormal synthesis or utilization of insulin, often leads to the diabetes.

Metabolic Syndrome: Also known as syndrome X, insulin resistance or dysmetabolic syndrome. It is a cluster of biochemical and chemical metabolic risk factors that come together in a single individual, leading to disorder of energy utilization and storage. Occurrence of any three out of five abnormalities viz., abdominal (central) obesity, hypertension, elevated fasting plasma glucose, high serum triglycerides and low level of high density lipoprotein (HDL) results in cardiovascular disease and diabetes as the main part of metabolic syndrome.

Oxidative Stress: Oxidative stress is the phenomenon of imbalance between production of free radicals, also known as reactive intermediates e.g. O_2^-(superoxide radical), OH^-(hydroxyl radical), H_2O_2

(hydrogen peroxide) and the ability of the biological systems to counteract or detoxify their harmful effect on components of the cells which includes proteins, lipids, and DNA by neutralization through antioxidants.

Proteinuria: Proteinuria indicates the appearance of abnormal quantities of serum proteins in urine. It includes microalbuminuria and macroalbuminuria. It is a sign of chronic kidney diseases (CKDs) and EDRD.

Podocytes: It is an epithelial cell of the visceral layer of Bowman capsule that wrap around the capillaries of the glomerulus through long processes as foot projections called *pedicel* and leave slits between them.

APPENDIX: ABBREVIATIONS

AMPK = AMP- activated protein kinase
NAD^+ = Oxidised Nicotinamide Adenine Dinucleotide.
NADH = Reduced Nicotinamide Adenine Dinucleotide.
NADP = Nicotinamide Adenine Dinucleotide Phosphate.
NADPH = Reduced Nicotinamide Adenine Dinucleotide Phosphate.
GSH = Reduced Glutathione.
ROS = Reactive Oxygen Species.
AGE = Advanced Glycation End product.
PKC = Protein Kinase C.
DAG = Diacylglycerol.
DKD = Diabetic Kidney Diseases.
GAPDH = Glyceraldehyde 3-Phosphate Dehydrogenase.
IL = Interleukin.
VEGF = Vascular Endothelial Growth Factor.
PDGF = Platelet Derived Growth Factor.
CTGF = Connective Tissue Growth Factor.
DHAP = Dihydroxy Acetone Phosphate.
ECM = Extracellular Matrix.
TNF-α = Tissue Necrosis Factor- α.
GFAT = Glutamine Fructose-6-Phosphate Amidotransferase.
↑ = Increase.
↓ = Decrease.
OS = Oxidative Stress.
ICAM-1/ CD 54 = Intercellular Adhesion Molecule-1
CTGF/ CCN2 = Connective Tissue Growth Factor.
VEGF = Vascular Endothelial Growth Factor.
PDGF = Platelet Derived Growth Factor.
GFR = Glomerular Filtration Rate

Compilation of References

Aarøe, J., Torbjørn, L., & Vanessa, D. (2010). Gene expression profiling of peripheral blood cells for early detection of breast cancer. *Breast Cancer Research*, *12*, R7. PMID:20078854

Abdel-Hassan, I. A., Abdel-Barry, J. A., & Mohammeda, S. T. (2000). The hypoglycemic and antihyperglycemic effect of *Citrullus colocynthis* fruit aqueous extract in normal and alloxan induced diabetic rats. *Journal of Ethnopharmacology*, *71*(1-2), 1–2. doi:10.1016/S0378-8741(99)00215-9 PMID:10904143

Abu-Shakra, M., & Shoenfeld, Y. (2001). Azathioprine therapy for patients with systemic lupus erythematosus. *Lupus*, *10*(3), 152–153. doi:10.1191/096120301676669495 PMID:11315344

Acuna-Castroviejo, D., Escames, G., Tapias, V., & Rivas, I. (2006). Melatonin, mitochondria and neuroprotection. In *Montilla, Pedro; Túnez, Isaac. Melatonin: Present and Future* (pp. 1–33). New York: Nova Science Publishers.

Adelman, G., Rane, S. G., & Villa, K. F. (2013). The cost burden of multiple sclerosis in the United States: A systematic review of the literature. *Journal of Medical Economics*, *16*(5), 639–647. doi:10.3111/13696998.2013.778268 PMID:23425293

Adhikary, L., Chow, F., Nikolic-Paterson, D. J., Stambe, C., Dowling, J., Atkins, R. C., & Tesch, G. H. (2004). Abnormal p38 mitogen-activated protein kinase signalling in human and experimental diabetic nephropathy. *Diabetologia*, *47*(7), 1210–1222. doi:10.1007/s00125-004-1437-0 PMID:15232685

Adriaenssens, K., Karcher, D., Lowenthal, A., & Terheggen, H. G. (1976). Use of enzyme-loaded erythrocytes in in-vitro correction of arginase-deficient erythrocytes in familial hyperargininemia. *Clinical Chemistry*, *22*(3), 323–326. PMID:1253407

Affuso, F., Mercurio, V., & Ruvolo, A. (2012). Anutraceutical combination improves insulin sensitivity in patients with metabolic syndrome. *World J Cardiol*, *4*(3), 77–83. doi:10.4330/wjc.v4.i3.77 PMID:22451856

Aggarwal, B. B., & Shishodia, S. (2006). Molecular targets of dietary agents for prevention and therapy of cancer. *Biochemical Pharmacology*, *71*(10), 1397–1421. doi:10.1016/j.bcp.2006.02.009 PMID:16563357

Ahmad, A., Ali, S. M., Ahmad, M. U., Sheikh, S., & Ahmad, I. (2010). Orally administered endoxifen is a new therapeutic agent for breast cancer. *Breast Cancer Research and Treatment*, *122*(2), 579–584. doi:10.1007/s10549-009-0704-7 PMID:20052538

Ai, J., Huang, H., Lv, X., Tang, Z., Chen, M., Chen, T., & Zhou, Q. et al. (2011). FLNA and PGK1 are two potential markers for progression in hepatocellular carcinoma. *Cellular Physiology and Biochemistry*, *27*, 207–216. PMID:21471709

Ajibola, A., Chamunorwa, J. P., & Erlwanger, K. H. (2012). Nutraceutical values of natural honey and its contribution to human health and wealth. *Nutrition and Metabolism*, *9*(61), 1–12. PMID:22716101

Ajith, T. A., & Janardhanan, K. K. (2007). Indian medicinal mushrooms as a source of antioxidant and antitumor agents. *Journal of Clinical Biochemistry and Nutrition*, *40*(3), 157–162. doi:10.3164/jcbn.40.157 PMID:18398492

Akkarachiyasit, S., Charoenlertkul, P., Yibchok-Anun, S., & Adisakwattana, S. (2010). Inhibitory activities of cyanidin and its glycosides and synergistic effect with acarbose against intestinal α-Glucosidase and pancreatic α-Amylase. *International Journal of Molecular Sciences*, *11*(9), 3387–3396. doi:10.3390/ijms11093387 PMID:20957102

Al-Achi, A., & Boroujerdi, M. (1990). Pharmacokinetics and Tissue Uptake of Doxorubicin Associated with Erythrocyte-Membrane: Erythrocyte Ghosts versus Erythrocyte-Vesicles. *Drug Development and Industrial Pharmacy*, *16*(15), 2199–2219. doi:10.3109/03639049009043795

Alicic, R. Z., & Tuttle, K. R. (2014). Novel therapies for diabetic kidney disease. *Advances in Chronic Kidney Disease*, *21*(2), 121–133. doi:10.1053/j.ackd.2014.01.007 PMID:24602462

Ali, F. R., & Finlayson, A. E. (2013). Pharaonic trichology: The Ebers Papyrus. *JAMA Dermatology*, *149*(8), 920. doi:10.1001/jamadermatol.2013.4240 PMID:24026454

Allison, A. C. (2005). Mechanisms of action of mycophenolate mofetil. *Lupus*, *14*(Suppl 1), s2–s8. doi:10.1177/096120330501400102 PMID:15803924

Almaraz, N., Campos, M. G., Avila, J. A., Naranjo, N., Herrera, J., & Gonzalez, L. S. (2007). Antioxidant activity of polyphenolic extract of monofloral honeybee collected pollen from mesquite (Prosopisjuliflora, Leguminosae). *Journal of Food Composition and Analysis*, *20*(2), 119–124. doi:10.1016/j.jfca.2006.08.001

Alpan, O., Bachelder, E., Isil, E., Arnheiter, H., & Matzinger, P. (2004). 'Educated' dendritic cells act as messengers from memory to naive T helper cells. *Nature Immunology*, *5*(6), 615–622. doi:10.1038/ni1077 PMID:15156140

Alpar, H. O., & Irwin, W. J. (1987). Some Unique Applications of Erythrocytes as Carrier Systems.[series]. *Advances in the Biosciences*, *67*, 1–9.

Alpar, H. O., & Lewis, D. A. (1985). Therapeutic Efficacy of Asparaginase Encapsulated in Intact Erythrocytes. *Biochemical Pharmacology*, *34*(2), 257–261. doi:10.1016/0006-2952(85)90133-9 PMID:3966927

Altman, R. B. (1998). Bioinformatics in support of molecular medicine. In *Proceedings of American Medical Informatics Association Symposium (AMIA'98)* (pp. 53-61).

Altun, A., & Ugur-Altun, B. (2007). Melatonin: Therapeutic and clinical utilization. *International Journal of Clinical Practice*, *61*(5), 835–845. doi:10.1111/j.1742-1241.2006.01191.x PMID:17298593

Alvarez, F. J., Jordán, J. A., Calleja, P., Lotero, L. A., Olmos, G., Díez, J. C., & Tejedor, M. C. (1998). Cross-Linking Treatment of Loaded Erythrocytes Increases delivery of Encapsulated Substance to Macrophages. *Biotechnology and Applied Biochemistry*, *27*(pt 2), 139–143. PMID:9569609

Alzheimer's Association. (2013a). *Alzheimer's disease facts and figures*. Author.

Alzheimer's Association. (2013b). *The role of plaques and tangles*. Author.

Amado, R. G., Wolf, M., Peeters, M., Van Cutsem, E., Siena, S., Freeman, D. J., & Chang, D. D. et al. (2008). Wild-type KRAS is required for panitumumab efficacy in patients with metastatic colorectal cancer. *Journal of Clinical Oncology*, *26*(10), 1626–1634. doi:10.1200/JCO.2007.14.7116 PMID:18316791

Amalraj, T., & Ignachimuthu, S. (1998). Hypoglycemic activity of *Cajanus cajan* (seeds) in mice. *Indian Journal of Experimental Biology*, *36*, 1032–1033. PMID:10356965

Ambrosini, A., Di Lorenzo, C., Coppola, G., & Pierelli, F. (2013). Use of *Vitex agnus-castus* in migrainous women with premenstrual syndrome: An open-label clinical observation. *Acta Neurologica Belgica*, *113*(1), 25–29. doi:10.1007/s13760-012-0111-4 PMID:22791378

Ameer, O., Salman, I., Quek, K., & Asmawi, M. (2015). Loranthus ferrugineus: A Mistletoe from Traditional Uses to Laboratory Bench. *Journal of Pharmacopuncture*, *18*(1), 7–18. doi:10.3831/KPI.2015.18.001 PMID:25830054

American Academy of Dermatology. (2014). *Cosmeceuticals*. Retrieved October 13, 2015, from http://www.aad.org/media-resources/stats-and-facts/cosmetic-treatments/cosmeceuticals

Amissah-Arthur, M. B., & Gordon, C. (2010). Contemporary treatment of systemic lupus erythematosus: An update for clinicians. *Ther Adv Chronic Dis*, *1*(4), 163–175. doi:10.1177/2040622310380100 PMID:23251736

Amuka, O. (2013). An overview in support of continued research into phytomedicine: past, present and future. In A. Garib-Famkim & J. N. Eloff (Eds.), *Chemistry for Sustainable development in Africa* (pp. 3–15). Heidelberg, Germany: Springer- Verlag. doi:10.1007/978-3-642-29642-0_1

Anantha-Narayana, D. B. (2013). Approaches to pre-formulation R and D for PP emanating from herb based traditional Ayurvedic processes. *Journal of Ayurveda and Integrative Medicine*, *4*(1), 4–8. doi:10.4103/0975-9476.109542 PMID:23741154

Anderson, S. (2002). The state of the world's pharmacy: A portrait of the pharmacy profession. *Journal of Interprofessional Care*, *16*(4), 391–404. doi:10.1080/1356182021000008337 PMID:12487847

Andrews, K. W., Schweitzer, A., Zhao, C., Holden, J., Roseland, J., Brandt, M., & Yetley, E. (2006). Caffeine, theobromine and theophylline content of commonly purchased weight loss and sport performance enhancing dietary supplements. *Experimental Biology*, 1–5.

Andri, R., & Jacques, F. (2011). Personalized hepatitis C therapy: Opportunities and pitfalls. *Expert Review of Molecular Diagnostics*, *11*(2), 127–129. PMID:21405961

Andy, L. T. Y., Quing-Yu, H. E., & Jen, F. U. C. (2003). Proteomic technology and its biomedical application. *Acta Biochimica et Biophysica Sinica*, *35*, 965–975. PMID:14614532

Anjum, F., Bukhari, S. A., Shahid, M., Bokhari, T. H., & Talpur, M. M. A. (2014). Exploration of Nutraceutical Potential of Herbal Oil Formulated from Parasitic Plant. *African Journal of Traditional, Complementary, and Alternative Medicines*, *11*(1), 78–86. PMID:24653557

Annenkov, A., & Chernajovsky, Y. (2000). Engineering mouse T lymphocytes specific to type II collagen by transduction with a chimeric receptor consisting of a single chain Fv and TCR zeta. *Gene Therapy*, *7*, 714–722. PMID:10800096

Antonio, G., Tesser, C., & Moretti-Pires, R. (2014). Phytotherapy in primary health care. *Revista de Saude Publica*, *48*(3), 541–553. PMID:25119949

Antoniou, C., Kosmadaki, M. G., Stratigos, A. J., & Katsambas, A. D. (2008). Sunscreens–what's important to know. *Journal of the European Academy of Dermatology and Venereology*, *22*(9), 1110–1119. doi:10.1111/j.1468-3083.2007.02580.x PMID:18482317

Anton, N., Benoit, J. P., & Saulnier, P. (2008). Design and production of nanoparticles formulated from nano-emulsion templates-a review. *Journal of Controlled Release*, *128*(3), 185–199. doi:10.1016/j.jconrel.2008.02.007 PMID:18374443

Anwar, F., Przybylski, R., Rudzinska, M., Gruczynska, E., & Bain, J. (2008). Fatty acid, tocopherol and sterol compositions of Canadian prairie fruit seed lipids. *Journal of the American Oil Chemists' Society*, *85*(10), 953–959. doi:10.1007/s11746-008-1276-0

Apweiler, R., Aslanidis, C., Deufel, T., Gerstner, A., Hansen, J., Hochstrasser, D., & Maser, E. et al. (2009). Approaching clinical proteomics: Current state and future fields of application in cellular proteomics. *Cytometry. Part A*, *75*, 816–832. PMID:19739086

Arai, I., Amagaya, S., Komatsu, Y., Okada, M., Hayashi, T., Kasai, M., & Momose, Y. et al. (1999). Improving effects of the extracts from *Eugenia uniflora* on hyperglycemia and hypertriglyceridemia in mice. *Journal of Ethnopharmacology*, *68*(1-3), 307–314. doi:10.1016/S0378-8741(99)00066-5 PMID:10624893

Arai, S. (1996). Studies on functional foods in Japan–State of the art. *Bioscience, Biotechnology, and Biochemistry*, *60*(1), 9–15. doi:10.1271/bbb.60.9 PMID:8824819

Archer, D. L., & Glinsmann, W. H. (1985). Intestinal infection and malnutrition initiate Acquired Immune Deficiency Syndrome (AIDS). *Nutrition Research (New York, N.Y.)*, *5*(1), 9–19. doi:10.1016/S0271-5317(85)80014-2

Arnao, M. B., & Hernández-Ruiz, J. (2006). The physiological function of melatonin in plants. *Plant Signaling & Behavior*, *1*(3), 89–95. doi:10.4161/psb.1.3.2640 PMID:19521488

Arteaga, C. L., Sliwkowski, M. X., Osborne, C. K., Perez, E. A., Puglisi, F., & Gianni, L. (2012). Treatment of HER2-positive breast cancer: Current status and future perspectives.[Review]. *Nature Reviews Clinical Oncology*, *9*(1), 16–32. doi:10.1038/nrclinonc.2011.177 PMID:22124364

Aruoma, O. (2001). In vitro and in vivo methods for the assessment of antioxidant activity. In *Proceedings of the EUROFOODCHEM 11th Meeting: Biologically-Active Phytochemicals in Food: Analysis, Metabolism, Bioavailability and Function*. The Royal Society of Chemistry.

Asquith, D. L., Miller, A. M., McInnes, I. B., & Liew, F. Y. (2009). Animal models of rheumatoid arthritis. *European Journal of Immunology*, *39*(8), 2040–2044. doi:10.1002/eji.200939578 PMID:19672892

Atherton, P. (2002). *Aloe vera*: Magic or medicine with antidiabetic potential. *Journal of Ethnopharmacology*, *81*, 81–100. PMID:12020931

Atkinson, M. A., Eisenbarth, G. S., & Michels, A. W. (2014). Type 1 diabetes. *Lancet*, *383*(9911), 69–82. doi:10.1016/S0140-6736(13)60591-7 PMID:23890997

Augusti, K. T. (1973). Studies on the effects of a hypoglycemic principle from *Allium cepa* Linn. *The Indian Journal of Medical Research*, *61*, 1066–1071. PMID:4757998

Augustine, A. C., & D'Souza, L. (1997). Regeneration of an anticarcinogenic herb, *Curculigo orchioides* (Gaertn.). *In Vitro Cellular & Developmental Biology. Plant*, *33*(2), 111–113. doi:10.1007/s11627-997-0006-x

Awad, A. B., & Fink, C. S. (2000). Phytosterols as anticancer dietary components: Evidence and mechanism of action. *The Journal of Nutrition*, *130*, 2127–2130. PMID:10958802

Aybak, M., & Sermet, A. (1995). Effect of oral pyridoxine hydrochloride supplementation on arterial blood pressure in patients with essential hypertension. *Arzneimittel-Forschung*, *45*, 1271–1273. PMID:8595083

Babaee, N., Moslemi, D., Khalilpour, M., Vejdani, F., Monghadamnia, Y., Bijani, A., & Moghadamnia, A. et al. (2013). Antioxidant capacity of *calendula officinalis* flowers extract and prevention of radiation induced oropharyngeal mucositis in patients with head and neck cancers: A randomized controlled clinical study. *DARU Journal of Pharmaceutical Sciences.*, *21*(1), 18–24. PMID:23497687

Babamiri, K., & Nassab, R. (2010). Cosmeceuticals: The evidence behind the retinoids. *Aesthetic Surgery Journal*, *30*(1), 74–77. doi:10.1177/1090820X09360704 PMID:20442078

Baban, C. K., Cronin, M., O'Hanlon, D., O'Sullivan, G. C., & Tangney, M. (2010). Bacteria as vectors for gene therapy of cancer. *Bioengineered Bugs*, *1*(6), 385–394. PMID:21468205

Babaoglu, M. O., Bayar, B., Aynacioglu, A. S., Kerb, R., Abali, H., Celik, I., & Bozkurt, A. (2005). Association of the ABCB1 3435C>T polymorphism with antiemetic efficacy of 5-hydroxytryptamine type 3 antagonists. *Clinical Pharmacology and Therapeutics*, *78*(6), 619–626. doi:10.1016/j.clpt.2005.08.015 PMID:16338277

Babayan, V. K. (1987). Medium chain triglycerides and structural lipids. *Lipids*, *22*(6), 417–420. doi:10.1007/BF02537271 PMID:3112486

Bachelder, E. M., Beaudette, T. T., Broaders, K. E., Paramonov, S. E., Dashe, J., & Frechet, J. M. (2008). Acid-degradable polyurethane particles for protein-based vaccines: Biological evaluation and in vitro analysis of particle degradation products. *Molecular Pharmaceutics*, *5*(5), 876–884. doi:10.1021/mp800068x PMID:18710254

Bacon, C. W., & White, J. F. (2000). *Microbial Endophytes*. New York: Marcel Deker Inc.

Baek, J. Y., Lee, J. M., & Lee, S. C. (2008). Extraction of nutraceutical compounds from licorice roots with subcritical water. *Separation and Purification Technology*, *63*(3), 661–664. doi:10.1016/j.seppur.2008.07.005

Baffoni, L., & Biavati, B. (2008). Ecologia microbica dell'apparato digerente. In B. Biavati & C. Sorlini (Eds.), *Microbiologia agroambientale* (pp. 147–162). Milan: Casa Editrice Ambrosiana.

Bahl, N. (1983). Medicinal value of edible fungi. In *Proceeding of the International Conference on Science and Cultivation Technology of Edible Fungi*. Indian Mushroom Science.

Baichwal, R. S. (1999). Developments in nutraceuticals. *Pharmacy Times*, *1*, 19–20.

Bajaj, Y. P. S. (1998). Biotechnology for the improvement of medicinal plants. *Acta Horticulturae*, *457*(457), 37–45. doi:10.17660/ActaHortic.1998.457.4

Bakkali, F., Averbeck, S., Averbeck, D., & Idaomar, M. (2008). Biological effects of essential oils-A review. *Food and Chemical Toxicology*, *46*(2), 446–475. doi:10.1016/j.fct.2007.09.106 PMID:17996351

Bakris, G.L. (2008). Slowing Nephropathy Progression: Focus on Proteinuria Reduction. *Clinical Journal of the American Society of Nephrology, 3*, S3-S10.

Balachandran, V. P., Cavnar, M. J., Zeng, S., Bamboat, Z. M., Ocuin, L. M., Obaid, H., & DeMatteo, R. P. et al. (2011). Imatinib potentiates antitumor T cell responses in gastrointestinal stromal tumor through the inhibition of Ido. *Nature Medicine*, *17*(9), 1094–1100. doi:10.1038/nm.2438 PMID:21873989

Balina, L. M., & Graupe, K. (1991). The treatment of melasma. 20% azelaic acid versus 4% hydroquinone cream. *International Journal of Dermatology*, *30*(12), 893–895. doi:10.1111/j.1365-4362.1991.tb04362.x PMID:1816137

Baljit, S. (2007). Psyllium as therapeutic and drug delivery agent. *International Journal of Pharmaceutics*, *334*(1-2), 1–14. doi:10.1016/j.ijpharm.2007.01.028 PMID:17329047

Ballas, S. K., & Krasnow, S. H. (1990). Structure of erythrocyte membrane and its transport functions. *Annals of Clinical and Laboratory Science*, *10*(3), 209–219. PMID:6249177

Bandaranayake, W. M. (2006). Quality Control, Screening, Toxicity, and Regulation of Herbal Drugs. In Modern Phytomedicine: Turning Medicinal Plants into Drugs (pp. 25-57). Weinheim, Germany: Wiley-VCH Verlag GmbH & Co. KGaA.

Bank, N., & Aynedjian, H. S. (1993). Role of EDRF (nitric oxide) in diabetic renal hyperfiltration. *Kidney International*, *43*(6), 1306–1312. doi:10.1038/ki.1993.183 PMID:8315943

Baragob, A. A., AlMalki, W. H., Shahid, I., Bakhdhar, F. A., Bafhaid, H. S., & Eldeen, O. I. (2014). The hypoglycemic effect of the aqueous extract of the fruits of *Balanites aegypticea* in Alloxan-induced diabetic rats. *Pharmacognosy Research*, *6*(1), 1–5. doi:10.4103/0974-8490.122909 PMID:24497735

Baranyi, L., Slepushkin, V., & Dropulic, B. (2013). Ex vivo gene therapy: utilization of genetic vectors for the generation of genetically modified cell products for therapy. In *Gene Therapy of Cancer* (3rd ed.; pp. 3–18). San Diego, CA: Elsevier.

Bardhan, P. K., Khan, W. A., Salam, A., Saha, D., Golman, D., Harris, M. S., & Chaturvedi, P. (2009). *Safety and efficacy of a novel anti-secretory anti-diarrheal agent Crofelemer (NP-303), in treatment of adult infectious diarrhea and cholera, with or without the use of antibiotics. 13th International Conference on Emerging Infectious Diseases in the Pacific Rim*, Kolkata, India.

Barnes, P. J., & Pauwels, R. A. (1994). Theophylline in the management of asthma: Time for reappraisal? *The European Respiratory Journal*, *7*(3), 579–591. doi:10.1183/09031936.94.07030579 PMID:8013614

Barnett, A. H., Bain, S. C., Bouter, P., Karlberg, B., Madsbad, S., Jervell, J., & Mustonen, J. (2004). Angiotensin-receptor blockade versus converting-enzyme inhibition in type 2 diabetes and nephropathy. *TheNew England Journal of Medicine*, *351*(19), 1952–1961. doi:10.1056/NEJMoa042274 PMID:15516696

Baron, J. F., Vicaut, E., Stucker, O., Villereal, M. C., Ropars, C., Teisserie, B., & Duvelleroy, M. (1987). Isolated Heart as a Model to Study the Effects of the Decrease in Oxygen Hemoglobin Affinity.[series]. *Advances in the Biosciences*, *67*, 73–78.

Bar-Or, A., Pachner, A., Menguy-Vacheron, F., Kaplan, J., & Wiendl, H. (2014). Teriflunomide and its mechanism of action in multiple sclerosis. *Drugs*, *74*(6), 659–674. doi:10.1007/s40265-014-0212-x PMID:24740824

Barreca, M. L., De Luca, L., Iraci, N., Rao, A., Ferro, S., Maga, G., & Chimirri, A. (2007). Structure-based pharmacophore identification of new chemical scaffolds as non-nucleoside reverse transcriptase inhibitors. *Journal of Chemical Information and Modeling*, *47*(2), 557–562. doi:10.1021/ci600320q PMID:17274611

Basch, E., Prestrud, A. A., Hesketh, P. J., Kris, M. G., Feyer, P. C., & Somerfield, M. R. et al. American Society of Clinical, O. (2011). Antiemetics: American Society of Clinical Oncology clinical practice guideline update. *Journal of Clinical Oncology*, *29*(31), 4189–4198. PMID:21947834

Baselga, J., Cortes, J., Kim, S. B., Im, S. A., Hegg, R., Im, Y. H., & Group, C. S. et al. (2012). Pertuzumab plus trastuzumab plus docetaxel for metastatic breast cancer. *The New England Journal of Medicine*, *366*(2), 109–119. doi:10.1056/NEJMoa1113216 PMID:22149875

Bastianetto, S., & Quirion, R. (2002). Natural extracts as possible protective agents of brain aging. *Neurobiological Aging*, *23*(5), 891–897. doi:10.1016/S0197-4580(02)00024-6 PMID:12392793

Bauer, R., & Tittel, G. (1996). Quality assessment of herbal preparations as a precondition of pharmacological and clinical studies. *Phytomedicine, 2*, 193-198.

Bauer, A., Diepgen, T. L., & Schmitt, J. (2011). Is occupational solar ultraviolet irradiation a relevant risk factor for basal cell carcinoma? A systematic review and meta-analysis of the epidemiological literature. *The British Journal of Dermatology*, *165*(3), 612–625. PMID:21605109

Bauer, R. (1998). Quality criteria and standardization of PP: Can acceptable drug standards be achived. *Drug Information Journal*, *32*, 101–110.

Bax, M., Huizinga, T. W., & Toes, R. E. (2014). The pathogenic potential of autoreactive antibodies in rheumatoid arthritis. *Seminars in Immunopathology*, *36*(3), 313–325. doi:10.1007/s00281-014-0429-5 PMID:24763532

Bayat, A. (2002). Science, medicine and the future: Bioinformatics. *British Medical Journal*, *324*(7344), 1018–1022. doi:10.1136/bmj.324.7344.1018 PMID:11976246

Bazzano, L. A., He, J., Ogden, L. G., Loria, C., Vupputuri, S., Myers, L., & Whelton, P. K. (2002). Dietary intake of folate and risk of stroke in US men and women: NHANES I Epidemiologic Follow-up Study. National Health and Nutrition Examination Survey. *Stroke*, *33*(5), 1183–1188. doi:10.1161/01.STR.0000014607.90464.88 PMID:11938588

Bean, J., Brennan, C., Shih, J. Y., Riely, G., Viale, A., Wang, L., & Pao, W. et al. (2007). MET amplification occurs with or without T790M mutations in EGFR mutant lung tumors with acquired resistance to gefitinib or erlotinib. *Proceedings of the National Academy of Sciences of the United States of America*, *104*(52), 20932–20937. doi:10.1073/pnas.0710370104 PMID:18093943

Beer, C., Wood, S., & Veghte, R. H. (2014). A Clinical Trial to Investigate the Effect of Cynatine HNS on Hair and Nail Parameters. *TheScientificWorldJournal*, *2014*, 1–6. doi:10.1155/2014/641723 PMID:25386509

Begoun, P. (2003). *Don't Go to the Cosmetics Counter without Me*. Retrieved 13.6.2015, from www.paulas choice.com/expert-advice/sensitive-skin/fragrance-and-skin-care-smells-like-trouble

Behnke, K., Jensen, G., Graubaum, H., & Gruenwald, J. (2002). *Hypericum perforatum* Versus Fluoxetine in the Treatment of Mild to Moderate Depression. *Advances in Natural Therapy.*, *19*(1), 43–52. doi:10.1007/BF02850017 PMID:12008860

Benatti, U. (1987). Comparative Tissue Distribution and Metabolism of Free Versus Erythrocyte-Encapsulated Adriamycin in the Mouse. *Advanced Biosciences, 67*, 129-136.

Benatti, P., Peluso, G., Nicolai, R., & Calvani, M. (2004). Polyunsaturated fatty acids: Biochemical, nutritional and epigenetic properties. *Journal of the American College of Nutrition*, *23*(4), 281–302. doi:10.1080/07315724.2004.10719371 PMID:15310732

Benatti, U., Zocchi, E., Tonetti, M., Guida, L., Polvani, C., & De Flora, A. (1987). Enhanced antitumor activity of adriamycin by encapsulation in mouse erythrocytes targeted to liver and lungs. *Pharmacological Research*, *2*, 27–33. PMID:2631085

Benavides, G. A., Squadrito, G. L., Mills, R. W., Patel, H. D., Isbell, T. S., Patel, R. P., & Kraus, D. W. et al. (2007). Hydrogen sulfide mediates the vasoactivity of garlic. *Proceedings of the National Academy of Sciences of the United States of America*, *104*(46), 17977–17982. doi:10.1073/pnas.0705710104 PMID:17951430

Bender, D. A. (1992). *Nutritional biochemistry of the vitamins*. New York: Cambridge University Press.

Benelli, L., Cortés-Rojas, D., Souza, C., & Pereira-Oliveira, W. (2015). Fluid bed drying and agglomeration of phytopharmaceutical compositions. *Powder Technology*, *273*, 145–153. doi:10.1016/j.powtec.2014.12.022

Benjamin, J. (2015). *Surprising Facts About Dandruff*. Retrieved 22.6.2015, from http://www.everydayhealth.com/news

Bennouna, J., Sastre, J., Arnold, D., Osterlund, P., Greil, R., Van Cutsem, E., & Investigators, M. L. S. et al. (2013). Continuation of bevacizumab after first progression in metastatic colorectal cancer (ML18147): A randomised phase 3 trial. *The Lancet Oncology*, *14*(1), 29–37. doi:10.1016/S1470-2045(12)70477-1 PMID:23168366

Benoit, M. R., Mayer, D., Barak, Y., Chen, I. Y., Hu, W., Cheng, Z., & Matin, A. et al. (2009). Visualizing implanted tumors in mice with magnetic resonance imaging using magnetotactic bacteria. *Clinical Cancer Research*, *15*(16), 5170–5177. PMID:19671860

Bentley, R. (2006). From miso, sake and shoyu to cosmetics: A century of science for kojic acid. *Natural Product Reports*, *23*(6), 1046–1062. doi:10.1039/b603758p PMID:17119644

Beringhs, A., Fagner, M., Souza, F., Angela, M., de Campo, A., Ferraz, H., & Sonaglio, D. (2012). Technological development of Cecropia glaziovi extract pellets by extrusion-spheronization. *Brazilian Journal of Pharmacognosy*, *23*(1), 160–168.

Berkholtz, C. B., Lai, B. E., Woodruff, T. K., & Shea, L. D. (2006). Distribution of extracellular matrix proteins type I collagen, type IV collagen, fibronectin, and laminin in mouse folliculogenesis. *Histochemistry and Cell Biology*, *126*(5), 583–592. doi:10.1007/s00418-006-0194-1 PMID:16758163

Berman, J. D. (1987). Antileishmanial Activity of Red Cell Encapsulated Drugs.[series]. *Advances in the Biosciences*, *67*, 145–152.

Bernard, S., Neville, K. A., Nguyen, A. T., & Flockhart, D. A. (2006). Interethnic differences in genetic polymorphisms of CYP2D6 in the U.S. population: Clinical implications. *The Oncologist*, *11*(2), 126–135. doi:10.1634/theoncologist.11-2-126 PMID:16476833

Bertilsson, L., Dahl, M. L., Dalen, P., & Al-Shurbaji, A. (2002). Molecular genetics of CYP2D6: Clinical relevance with focus on psychotropic drugs. *British Journal of Clinical Pharmacology*, *53*(2), 111–122. doi:10.1046/j.0306-5251.2001.01548.x PMID:11851634

Bessis, N., Chiocchia, G., & Kollias, G. (1988). Modulation of pro-inflammatory cytokine production in tumour necrosis factor alpha (TNF-alpha)-transgenic mice by treatment with cells engineered to secrete IL-4, IL-10 or IL-13. *Clinical and Experimental Immunology*, *111*, 391–396. PMID:9486409

Beutler, E., Dale, G. L., Guinto, D. E., & Kuhl, W. (1977). Enzyme Replacement Therapy in Gaucher's Disease. Preliminary Clinical Trial of a New Enzyme Preparation. *Proceedings of the National Academy of Sciences of the United States of America*, *74*(10), 4620–4623. doi:10.1073/pnas.74.10.4620 PMID:200923

Bhabra, G., Sood, A., Fisher, B., Cartwright, L., Saunders, M., Evans, W. H., & Case, C. P. et al. (2009). Nanoparticles can cause DNA damage across a cellular barrier. *Nature Nanotechnology*, *4*(12), 876–883. doi:10.1038/nnano.2009.313 PMID:19893513

Bhaskaran, S., & Dhir, S. S. (1995). Resealed Erythrocytes as Carriers of Salbutamol Sulphate. *Indian Journal of Pharmaceutical Sciences*, *57*, 240–242.

Bhattacharyya, S., Deb, J., Patra, A. K., Thuy Pham, D. A., Chen, W., Vaeth, M., & Serfling, E. et al. (2011). NFATc1 affects mouse splenic B cell function by controlling the calcineurin--NFAT signaling network. *The Journal of Experimental Medicine*, *208*(4), 823–839. doi:10.1084/jem.20100945 PMID:21464221

Bhattacharyya, T. K., Pathria, M., Mathison, C., Vargas, M., & Thomas, J. R. (2014). Cosmeceutical effect on skin surface profiles and epidermis in UV-B-irradiated mice. *JAMA Facial Plastic Surgery*, *16*(4), 253–260. doi:10.1001/jamafacial.2013.2582 PMID:24874724

Bhattaram, V. A., Graefe, U., Kohlert, C., Veit, M., & Derendorf, H. (2002). Pharmacokinetics and bioavailability of herbal medicinal products. *Phytomedicine*, *9*, 1–33. doi:10.1078/1433-187X-00210 PMID:12222652

Bhunia, S. K., Dey, B., Maity, K. K., Patra, S., Mandal, S., Maiti, S., & Islam, S. S. et al. (2010). Structural characterization of an immunoenhancing heteroglycan isolated from an aqueous extract of an edible mushroom, *Lentinus squarrosulus* (Mont.) Singer. *Carbohydrate Research*, *345*(17), 2542–2549. doi:10.1016/j.carres.2010.09.015 PMID:20934687

Bianchi, S., Bigazzi, R., & Campese, V. M. (2006). Long-term effects of spironolactone on proteinuria and kidney function in patients with chronic kidney disease. *Kidney International*, *70*(12), 2116–2123. doi:10.1038/sj.ki.5001854 PMID:17035949

Biesalski, H. K. (2001). Nutraceuticals: the link between nutrition and medicine. In K. Kramer, P. P. Hoppe, & L. Packer (Eds.), *Nutraceuticals in health and disease prevention* (pp. 1–26). New York: Marcel Dekker. doi:10.1201/9780203908174.ch1

Billah, M. M., Finean, J. B., Coleman, R., & Michell, R. H. (1977). Permeability characteristics of erythrocyte ghosts prepared under isoionic conditions by a glycol-induced osmotic lysis. *Biochimica et Biophysica Acta*, *465*(3), 515–526. doi:10.1016/0005-2736(77)90269-3 PMID:13834

Bixby, D., & Talpaz, M. (2009). *Mechanisms of resistance to tyrosine kinase inhibitors in chronic myeloid leukemia and recent therapeutic strategies to overcome resistance*. Hematology American Society of Hematology Education Program.

Bloomer, J. C., Baldwin, S. J., Smith, G. J., Ayrton, A. D., Clarke, S. E., & Chenery, R. J. (1994). Characterisation of the cytochrome P450 enzymes involved in the in vitro metabolism of granisetron. *British Journal of Clinical Pharmacology*, *38*(6), 557–566. doi:10.1111/j.1365-2125.1994.tb04397.x PMID:7888294

Blower, P. R. (2002). 5-HT3-receptor antagonists and the cytochrome P450 system: Clinical implications. *Cancer Journal (Sudbury, Mass.)*, *8*(5), 405–414. doi:10.1097/00130404-200209000-00012 PMID:12416899

Blum, K., Ross, J., Reuben, C., Gastelu, D., & Miller, D. K. (2001). *Nutritional gene therapy: Natural Healing in Recovery*. Counselor Magazine.

Boggs, J. M. (2006). Myelin basic protein: A multifunctional protein. *Cellular and Molecular Life Sciences*, *63*(17), 1945–1961. doi:10.1007/s00018-006-6094-7 PMID:16794783

Bohlmann, J., & Keeling, C. I. (2008). Terpenoid biomaterials. *The Plant Journal*, *54*(4), 656–669. doi:10.1111/j.1365-313X.2008.03449.x PMID:18476870

Bongartz, T., Sutton, A. J., Sweeting, M. J., Buchan, I., Matteson, E. L., & Montori, V. (2006). Anti-TNF antibody therapy in rheumatoid arthritis and the risk of serious infections and malignancies: Systematic review and meta-analysis of rare harmful effects in randomized controlled trials. *Journal of the American Medical Association*, *295*(19), 2275–2285. doi:10.1001/jama.295.19.2275 PMID:16705109

Borodina, N., Rumsh, D., Kunizhev, M., Sukhorukov, B., Vorozhtsov, N., Feldman, M., & Markvicheva, E. A. et al. (2008). Entrapment of herbal extracts into biodegradable microcapsules. *Biochemistry (Moscow) Supplement Series B. Biomedical Chemistry*, *2*(2), 176–182. doi:10.1134/S199075080802008X

Boyle, J., & Kennedy, C. T. (1985). Leukoderma from hydroquinone. *Contact Dermatitis*, *13*(4), 287–288. doi:10.1111/j.1600-0536.1985.tb02578.x PMID:4085240

Bradford, L. D. (2002). CYP2D6 allele frequency in European Caucasians, Asians, Africans and their descendants. *Pharmacogenomics*, *3*(2), 229–243. doi:10.1517/14622416.3.2.229 PMID:11972444

Brady, K., Ho, C. T., Rosen, R. T., Sang, S., & Karwe, M. V. (2007). Effects of processing on the nutraceutical profile of quinoa. *Food Chemistry*, *100*(3), 1209–1216. doi:10.1016/j.foodchem.2005.12.001

Brain, L. (2007). *Nutraceuticals* (2nd ed.). London: Pharmaceutical press.

Brandes, N., Welzel, P. B., Werner, C., & Kroh, L. W. (2006). Adsorption-induced conformational changes of proteins onto ceramic particles: Differential scanning calorimetry and FTIR analysis. *Journal of Colloid and Interface Science*, *299*(1), 56–69. doi:10.1016/j.jcis.2006.01.065 PMID:16500671

Brauch, H., Schroth, W., Goetz, M. P., Murdter, T. E., Winter, S., Ingle, J. N., & Eichelbaum, M. et al. (2013). Tamoxifen use in postmenopausal breast cancer: CYP2D6 matters. *Journal of Clinical Oncology*, *31*(2), 176–180. doi:10.1200/JCO.2012.44.6625 PMID:23091108

Braun, L. (2010) Principles of herbal medicine. In General practice: the integrative approach. Sydney. Australia: Elsevier.

Brenner, B. M., Cooper, M. E., de Zeeuw, D., Keane, W. F., Mitch, W. E., Parving, H. H., & Shahinfar, S. et al. (2001). Effects of losartan on renal and cardiovascular outcomes in patients with type 2 diabetes and nephropathy. *The New England Journal of Medicine*, *345*(12), 861–869. doi:10.1056/NEJMoa011161 PMID:11565518

Broaders, K. E., Cohen, J. A., Beaudette, T. T., Bachelder, E. M., & Frechet, J. M. (2009). Acetalated dextran is a chemically and biologically tunable material for particulate immunotherapy. *Proceedings of the National Academy of Sciences of the United States of America*, *106*(14), 5497–5502. doi:10.1073/pnas.0901592106 PMID:19321415

Brower, V. (1998). Nutraceuticals: Poised for a healthy slice of the healthcare market. *Nature Biotechnology*, *16*(8), 728–731. doi:10.1038/nbt0898-728 PMID:9702769

Brownlee, M. (2001). Biochemistry and molecular cell biology of diabetic complications. *Nature*, *414*(6865), 813–820. doi:10.1038/414813a PMID:11742414

Bruce, A. (2008). Essentra® - A Patented Extract that Reduces Stress and Enhances Sleep. *NutraGenesis*, *LLC*, 1–4.

Bruss, M., Barann, M., Hayer-Zillgen, M., Eucker, T., Gothert, M., & Bonisch, H. (2000). Modified 5-HT3A receptor function by co-expression of alternatively spliced human 5-HT3A receptor isoforms. *Naunyn-Schmiedeberg's Archives of Pharmacology*, *362*(4-5), 392–401. doi:10.1007/s002100000342 PMID:11111833

Bryant, J., Hlavaty, K. A., Zhang, X., Yap, W. T., Zhang, L., Shea, L. D., & Luo, X. (2014). Nanoparticle delivery of donor antigens for transplant tolerance in allogeneic islet transplantation. *Biomaterials*, *35*(31), 8887–8894. doi:10.1016/j.biomaterials.2014.06.044 PMID:25066477

Bryson, P., & Wang, P. (2013). Lentivector vaccines. In *Gene Therapy of Cancer* (3rd ed.; pp. 345–361). San Diego, CA: Elsevier.

Bucar, F., Wube, A., & Schmid, M. (2013). Natural product isolation- how to get from biological material to pure compounds. *Natural Product Reports*, *30*(4), 525–545. doi:10.1039/c3np20106f PMID:23396532

Buchbauer, G., & Jirovetz, L. (1994). Aromatherapy-use of fragrances and essential oils as medicaments. *Flavour and Fragrance Journal*, *9*(5), 217–222. doi:10.1002/ffj.2730090503

Buchman, A. L. (2001). Side effects of corticosteroid therapy. *Journal of Clinical Gastroenterology*, *33*(4), 289–294. doi:10.1097/00004836-200110000-00006 PMID:11588541

Bucks, D. A., McMaster, J. R., Guy, R. H., & Maibach, H. I. (1988). Percutaneous absorption of hydroquinone in humans: Effect of 1-dodecylazacycloheptan-2-one (azone) and the 2-ethylhexyl ester of 4-(dimethylamino) benzoic acid (escalol 507). *Journal of Toxicology and Environmental Health*, *24*(3), 279–289. doi:10.1080/15287398809531162 PMID:3260963

Buijs, J., Costa Vera, C., Ayala, E., Steensma, E., Hakansson, P., & Oscarsson, S. (1999). Conformational stability of adsorbed insulin studied with mass spectrometry and hydrogen exchange. *Analytical Chemistry*, *71*(15), 3219–3225. doi:10.1021/ac9809433 PMID:10450163

Bunn, H. F. (1997). Pathogenesis and treatment of sickle cell disease. *The New England Journal of Medicine*, *337*(11), 762–769. doi:10.1056/NEJM199709113371107 PMID:9287233

Burchett, M., Mousine, R., &Tarran, J. (2002).Phytomonitoring for urban environmental management. *Air Pollution & Plant Biotechnology*, 61-91.

Burdulis, D., Sarkinas, A., Jasutiene, I., Stackeviciene, E., Nikolajevas, L., & Janulis, V. (2009). Comparative study of anthocyanin composition, antimicrobial and antioxidant activity in bilberry (*Vaccinium myrtillus* L.) and blueberry (*Vaccinium corymbosum* L.) fruits. *Acta Poloniae Pharmaceutica-Drug Research*, *66*, 399–408. PMID:19702172

Burg van der, L.J., Muller, I., & Sloet van Oldruitenborgh-Oosterbaan, M.M. (2011). Horse milking industry in The Netherlands and Flanders. *Tijdschrift voor Diergeneeskunde*, *136*, 257–261. PMID:21534278

Burkhardt, S., Tan, D. X., Manchester, L. C., Hardeland, R., & Reiter, R. J. (2001). Detection and quantification of the antioxidant melatonin in Montmorency and Balaton tart cherries (Prunus cerasus). *Journal of Agricultural and Food Chemistry*, *49*(10), 4898–4902. doi:10.1021/jf010321+ PMID:11600041

Burleson, J. (n.d.). *Horse Milk*. Retrieved 10.6.2015, from http://www.burleson-arabians.com/horse_milk

Burlingame, B. et al.. (2009). Fats and fatty acids in human nutrition. JointFAO/WHO. Expert Consultation. *Annals of Nutrition & Metabolism*, *55*, 1–3. doi:10.1159/000228993 PMID:20104000

Burn, P. (2010). Type 1 diabetes. *Nature Reviews. Drug Discovery*, *9*(3), 187–188. doi:10.1038/nrd3097 PMID:20190784

Butler, M. S. (2005). Natural products to drugs: Natural product derived compounds in clinical trials. *Natural Product Reports*, *22*(2), 162–195. doi:10.1039/b402985m PMID:15806196

Cai, Y., Chen, J., Jiang, J., Cao, W., & He, L. (2010). Zhen-wu-tang, a blended traditional Chinese herbal medicine, ameliorates proteinuria and renal damage of streptozotocin-induced diabetic nephropathy in rats. *Journal of Ethnopharmacology*, *131*(1), 88–94. doi:10.1016/j.jep.2010.06.004 PMID:20547220

Calixto, J. (2000). Efficacy, safety, quality control, marketing and regulatory guidelines for herbal medicines (phytotherapeutic agents). *Brazilian Journal of Medical and Biological Research*, *33*(2), 179–189. doi:10.1590/S0100-879X2000000200004 PMID:10657057

Campanella, L., Martini, E., Pintore, M., & Tomassetti, M. (2009). Determination of lactoferrin and immunoglobulin G in animal milks by new immunosensors. *Sensors (Basel, Switzerland)*, *9*(3), 2202–2221. doi:10.3390/s90302202 PMID:22574009

Campbell, B. (2008). *Nutritional Supplements in Sports and Exercise*. J. Humana Press. LLC.

Campisi, J., Andersen, J. K., Kapahi, P., & Melov, S. (2011). Cellular senescence: A link between cancer and age-related degenerative disease? *Seminars in Cancer Biology*, *21*(6), 354–359. PMID:21925603

Camussi, G., & Lupia, E. (1998). The future role of anti-tumor necrosis factor (TNF) products in the treatment of rheumatoid arthritis. *Drugs*, *55*(5), 613–620. PMID:9585859

Cannon, E. P., Leung, P., Hawkins, A., Petrikovics, I., DeLoach, J., & Way, J. L. (1994). Antagonism of Cyanide Intoxication with Murine Carrier Erythrocytes Containing Bovine Rhodanese and Sodium Thiosulfate. *Journal of Toxicology and Environmental Health*, *41*(3), 267–274. doi:10.1080/15287399409531842 PMID:8126749

Canter, P., Thomas, H., & Ernst, E. (2005). Bringing medicinal plants into cultivation: Opportunities and challenges for biotechnology. *Trends in Biotechnology*, *23*(4), 180–185. doi:10.1016/j.tibtech.2005.02.002 PMID:15780709

Capasso, R., Izzo, A., Pinto, L., Bifulco, T., Vitobello, C., & Mascolo, N. (2002). Phytotherapy and quality of herbal medicines. *Fitoterapia*, *71*, 58–65. doi:10.1016/S0367-326X(00)00173-8 PMID:10930714

Capini, C., Jaturanpinyo, M., Chang, H. I., Mutalik, S., McNally, A., Street, S., & Thomas, R. et al. (2009). Antigen-specific suppression of inflammatory arthritis using liposomes. *Journal of Immunology (Baltimore, MD.: 1950)*, *182*(6), 3556–3565. doi:10.4049/jimmunol.0802972 PMID:19265134

Cappellano, G., Woldetsadik, A. D., Orilieri, E., Shivakumar, Y., Rizzi, M., Carniato, F., & Dianzani, U. et al. (2014). Subcutaneous inverse vaccination with PLGA particles loaded with a MOG peptide and IL-10 decreases the severity of experimental autoimmune encephalomyelitis. *Vaccine*, *32*(43), 5681–5689. doi:10.1016/j.vaccine.2014.08.016 PMID:25149432

Carmona-Ribeiro, A. M., & de Melo Carrasco, L. D. (2014). Novel formulations for antimicrobial peptides. *International Journal of Molecular Sciences*, *15*(10), 18040–18083. doi:10.3390/ijms151018040 PMID:25302615

Carneiro, J. R., & Sato, E. I. (1999). Double blind, randomized, placebo controlled clinical trial of methotrexate in systemic lupus erythematosus. *The Journal of Rheumatology*, *26*(6), 1275–1279. PMID:10381042

Carolina, P. (2014). Proteomic Tools for Cancer Research: Updating the Oncoproteomics. *Journal of Proteomics &. Bioinformatics (Oxford, England)*, S3.

Carr, A. C., & Frei, B. (1999). Toward a new recommended dietary allowance for vitamin C based on antioxidant and health effects in humans. *The American Journal of Clinical Nutrition*, *69*, 1086–1107. PMID:10357726

Cartea, M. E., & Velasco, P. (2008). Glucosinolates in Brassica foods: Bioavailability in food and significance for human health. *Phytochemistry Reviews*, *7*(2), 213–229. doi:10.1007/s11101-007-9072-2

Casado, B., Affolter, M., & Kussmann, M. (2009). OMICS-rooted studies of milk proteins, oligosaccharides and lipids. *Journal of Proteomics*, *73*(2), 196–208. doi:10.1016/j.jprot.2009.09.018 PMID:19793547

Caudle, K. E., Thorn, C. F., Klein, T. E., Swen, J. J., McLeod, H. L., Diasio, R. B., & Schwab, M. (2013). Clinical Pharmacogenetics Implementation Consortium guidelines for dihydropyrimidine dehydrogenase genotype and fluoropyrimidine dosing. *Clinical Pharmacology and Therapeutics*, *94*(6), 640–645. doi:10.1038/clpt.2013.172 PMID:23988873

Cavagnaro, J., & Lewis, R. M. (1987). Toxicological evaluation of drugs. In M. Williams & J. B. Malick (Eds.), *Drug Discovery and Development* (pp. 259–298). Clifton, NJ: Humana Press. doi:10.1007/978-1-4612-4828-6_10

Cavasotto, C. N., & Phatak, S. S. (2009). Homology modeling in drug discovery: Current trends and applications. *Drug Discovery Today*, *14*(13-14), 676–683. doi:10.1016/j.drudis.2009.04.006 PMID:19422931

Cazarolli, L. H., Folador, P., Moresco, H. H., Brighente, I. M. C., Pizzolatti, M. G., & Silva, F. R. M. B. (2009). Stimulatory effect of apigenin-6-C-beta-L-fucopyranoside on insulin secretion and glycogen synthesis. *European Journal of Medicinal Chemistry*, *44*(11), 4668–4673. doi:10.1016/j.ejmech.2009.07.001 PMID:19625113

Ceciliani, F., Eckersall, D., Burchmore, R., & Lecchi, C. (2014). Proteomics in veterinary medicine: Applications and trends in disease pathogenesis and diagnostics. *Veterinary Pathology*, *51*(2), 351–362. PMID:24045891

Celle, T., Heeringa, P., Strzelecka, A. E., Bast, A., Smits, J. F., & Janssen, B. J. (2004). Sustained protective effects of 7-monohydroxyethylrutoside in an in vivo model of cardiac ischemia perfusion. *European Journal of Pharmacology*, *494*(2-3), 205–212. doi:10.1016/j.ejphar.2004.05.017 PMID:15212976

Centers for Disease Control & Prevention. (2007). National and state medical expenditures and lost earnings attributable to arthritis and other rheumatic conditions--United States, 2003. *MMWR. Morbidity and Mortality Weekly Report*, *56*(1), 4–7. PMID:17218935

Chakraborty, I., Mondal, S., Pramanik, M., Rout, D., & Islam, S. S. (2004). Structural investigation of a water-soluble glucan from an edible mushroom, *Astraeus hygrometricus*. *Carbohydrate Research*, *339*(13), 2249–2254. doi:10.1016/j.carres.2004.07.013 PMID:15337453

Champion, J. A., & Mitragotri, S. (2006). Role of target geometry in phagocytosis. *Proceedings of the National Academy of Sciences of the United States of America*, *103*(13), 4930–4934. doi:10.1073/pnas.0600997103 PMID:16549762

Champion, J. A., Walker, A., & Mitragotri, S. (2008). Role of particle size in phagocytosis of polymeric microspheres. *Pharmaceutical Research*, *25*(8), 1815–1821. doi:10.1007/s11095-008-9562-y PMID:18373181

Chang, H. I., & Yeh, M. K. (2012). Clinical development of liposome-based drugs: Formulation, characterization, and therapeutic efficacy. *International Journal of Nanomedicine*, *7*, 49–60. doi:10.2147/IJN.S26766 PMID:22275822

Chang, S. T., & Miles, P. G. (1992). Mushroom biology-A new decipline. *The Mycologist*, *6*(2), 64–65. doi:10.1016/S0269-915X(09)80449-7

Chapman, P. B., Hauschild, A., Robert, C., Haanen, J. B., Ascierto, P., Larkin, J., & McArthur, G. A. et al. (2011). Improved survival with vemurafenib in melanoma with BRAF V600E mutation. *The New England Journal of Medicine*, *364*(26), 2507–2516. doi:10.1056/NEJMoa1103782 PMID:21639808

Charkoudian, N. (2003). Skin blood flow in adult human thermoregulation: How it works, when it does not, and why. *Mayo Clinic Proceedings*, *78*(5), 603–612. doi:10.4065/78.5.603 PMID:12744548

Chassaigne, R. M., & Nicoulau, C. (1987). *Advances in the BioSciences*. Oxford, UK: Pergamon Press.

Chassis, J. A., Agre, P., & Mohandas, N. (1988). Decreased membrane mechanical stability and *in vivo* loss of surface area reflect spectrin deficiencies in hereditary spherocytosis. *The Journal of Clinical Investigation*, *2*(2), 617–623. doi:10.1172/JCI113640 PMID:3403720

Chempakam, B. (1993). Hypoglycemic activity of arecoline in betel nut *Areca catechu* L. *Indian Journal of Experimental Biology*, *31*, 474–475. PMID:8359856

Chen, Chen, & Pan. (2008). Proteomics in rheumatoid arthritis. *Formosan Journal of Rheumatology*, *22*, 4–11.

Chen, D. H., Liu, C. J., Ye, H. C., Li, G. F., Liu, B. Y., Meng, Y. L., & Chen, X. Y. (1999). Ri-mediated transformation of *Artemisia annua* with a recombinant farnesyl diphosphate synthase gene for artemisinin production. *Plant Cell, Tissue and Organ Culture*, *57*(3), 157–162. doi:10.1023/A:1006326818509

Chen, H., Langer, R., & Edwards, D. A. (1997). A Film Tension Theory of Phagocytosis. *Journal of Colloid and Interface Science*, *190*(1), 118–133. doi:10.1006/jcis.1997.4865 PMID:9241149

Chen, J. J., Lee, Y. C., Cheng, T. J., Hsiao, H. Y., & Chen, R. L. C. (2006). Determination of glucosamine content in nutraceuticals by capillary electrophoresis using in-capillary OPA labeling techniques. *J. Food Drug Anal*, *14*(2), 203–206.

Chen, L., Mehta, A., Berenvaum, M., Zangerl, A. R., & Engeseth, J. (2000). Honeys from different floral sources as inhibitors of enzymatic browning in fruit and vegetable homogenates. *Journal of Agricultural and Food Chemistry*, *48*(10), 4997–5000. doi:10.1021/jf000373j PMID:11052768

Chen, S., Hong, S. W., Cruz, I. M. C., Isono, M., Casaretto, A., & Ziyadeh, F. N. (2001). Proteins, growth factors, and progression of kidney disease the key role of the transforming growth factor-b system in the pathogenesis of diabetic nephropathy. *Renal Failure*, *23*, 471–481. doi:10.1081/JDI-100104730 PMID:11499562

Cherney, D. Z. I., Perkins, B. A., Soleymanlou, N., Maione, M., Lai, V., Lee, A., & von Eynatten, M. et al. (2014). Renal hemodynamic effect of sodium-glucose co-transporter 2 inhibition in patients with type 1 diabetes mellitus. *Circulation*, *129*(5), 587–597. doi:10.1161/CIRCULATIONAHA.113.005081 PMID:24334175

Chiarantini, L., Rossi, L., Fraternale, A., & Magnani, M. (1995). Modulated red blood cell survival by membrane protein clustering. *Molecular and Cellular Biochemistry*, *144*(1), 53–59. doi:10.1007/BF00926740 PMID:7791745

Cho, E. C., Zhang, Q., & Xia, Y. (2011). The effect of sedimentation and diffusion on cellular uptake of gold nanoparticles. *Nature Nanotechnology*, *6*(6), 385–391. doi:10.1038/nnano.2011.58 PMID:21516092

Choi, H. et al.. (2012). Comparative nutritional analysis for genetically modified rice, Iksan483 and Milyang204, and nontransgenic counterparts. *J. Korean soc. Appl. Biol. Chem.*, *55*, 19–26.

Choi, J.-H., Cho, C.-W., Kim, J.-H., Park, S. H., Chang, S., & Yu, Y.-B. (2015). Liquid crystal formulation and optimization of anti-microbial polyherbal ointment. *Journal of Nanoscience and Nanotechnology*, *15*(8), 5656–5659. doi:10.1166/jnn.2015.10461 PMID:26369133

Choi, Y. L., Park, E. J., Kim, E., Na, D. H., & Shin, Y. H. (2014). Dermal stability and in vitro skin permeation of collagen pentapeptides (KTTKS and palmitoyl-KTTKS). *Biomolecules & Therapeutics*, *22*(4), 321–327. doi:10.4062/biomolther.2014.053 PMID:25143811

Chono, S., Tanino, T., Seki, T., & Morimoto, K. (2007). Uptake characteristics of liposomes by rat alveolar macrophages: Influence of particle size and surface mannose modification. *The Journal of Pharmacy and Pharmacology*, *59*(1), 75–80. doi:10.1211/jpp.59.1.0010 PMID:17227623

Chotchoungchatchai, S., Saralamp, P., Jenjittikul, T., Pornsiripongse, S., & Prathanturarug, S. (2012). Medicinal plants used with Thai traditional medicine in modern healthcare services: A case study in Kabchoeng hospital, Surin Province, Thailand. *Journal of Ethnopharmacology*, *141*(1), 193–205. doi:10.1016/j.jep.2012.02.019 PMID:22366679

Chou, W. Y., Yang, L. C., Lu, H. F., Ko, J. Y., Wang, C. H., Lin, S. H., & Hsu, C. J. et al. (2006). Association of mu-opioid receptor gene polymorphism (A118G) with variations in morphine consumption for analgesia after total knee arthroplasty. *Acta Anaesthesiologica Scandinavica*, *50*(7), 787–792. doi:10.1111/j.1399-6576.2006.01058.x PMID:16879459

Chow, F. Y., Nikolic-Paterson, D. J., Ma, F. Y., Ozols, E., Rollins, B. J., & Tesch, G. H. (2007). Monocyte chemo-attractant protein-1-induced tissue inflammation is critical for the development of renal injury but not type 2 diabetes in obese db/db mice. *Diabetologia*, *50*(2), 471–480. doi:10.1007/s00125-006-0497-8 PMID:17160673

Chung, S. Y., & Subbiah, S. (1996). A structural explanationfor the twilight zone of protein sequence homology. *Structure (London, England)*, *4*(10), 1123–1127. doi:10.1016/S0969-2126(96)00119-0 PMID:8939745

Chun, J., & Hartung, H. P. (2010). Mechanism of action of oral fingolimod (FTY720) in multiple sclerosis. *Clinical Neuropharmacology*, *33*(2), 91–101. doi:10.1097/WNF.0b013e3181cbf825 PMID:20061941

Cicero, A. F. G., & Ertek, S. (2008). Natural Sources of Antidyslipidaemic Agents: Is There an Evidence-Based Approach for Their Prescription. *Medit. J. Nutri. Metab.*, *1*(2), 85–93. doi:10.1007/s12349-008-0011-6

Cieslik, E., Greda, A., & Adamus, W. (2006). Contents of polyphenols in fruits and vegetables. *Food Chemistry*, *94*(1), 135–142. doi:10.1016/j.foodchem.2004.11.015

Circu, M. L., & Aw, T. Y. (2012). Glutathione and modulation of cell apoptosis,*Biochimica et Biophysica Acta (BBA) -. Molecular Cell Research*, *1823*, 1767–1777.

Ciszkowski, C., Madadi, P., Phillips, M. S., Lauwers, A. E., & Koren, G. (2009). Codeine, ultrarapid-metabolism genotype, and postoperative death. *The New England Journal of Medicine*, *361*(8), 827–828. doi:10.1056/NEJMc0904266 PMID:19692698

Ciunab, R. R. (2012). Phytotherapeutic and naturopathic adjuvant therapies in otorhinolaryngology. *European Archives of Oto-Rhino-Laryngology*, *269*(2), 389–397. doi:10.1007/s00405-011-1755-z PMID:21922427

Claeson, P. (n.d.). *Assessment report on Melissa officinalis L.* London: European Medicines Agency.

Clark, D. E., & Pickett, S. D. (2000). Computational Methods for the Prediction of Drug-Likeness. *Drug Discovery Today*, *5*(2), 49–58. doi:10.1016/S1359-6446(99)01451-8 PMID:10652455

Clement, F., Pramod, S. N., & Venkatesh, Y. P. (2010). Identity of the immunomodulatory proteins from garlic (*Allium sativum*) with the major garlic lectins or agglutinins. *International Immunopharmacology*, *10*(3), 316–324. doi:10.1016/j.intimp.2009.12.002 PMID:20004743

Cohen, J. (2004). Bioinformatics an Introduction for Computer Scientists: Brandeis University. *ACM Computing Surveys*, *36*(2), 122–158. doi:10.1145/1031120.1031122

Cohen, J. A., & Chun, J. (2011). Mechanisms of fingolimod's efficacy and adverse effects in multiple sclerosis. *Annals of Neurology*, *69*(5), 759–777. doi:10.1002/ana.22426 PMID:21520239

Combs, T. (2015). *Animal Ingredients – What is Lactoferrin?* Retrieved 12.6.2015, from http://www.logicalharmony.net/animal-ingredients-what-is-lactoferrin

Comins, C., Simpson, G., Relph, K., Harrington, K., Melcher, A., & Pandha, H. (2013). Reoviral therapy for cancer: strategies for improving antitumor efficacy using radio- and chemotherapy. In *Gene Therapy of Cancer* (3rd ed.; pp. 185–198). San Diego, CA: Elsevier.

Committee on Herbal Medicinal Products. (2007). *Assessment report on Valeriana officinales L., Radix* (pp. 3–21). London, MD: European Medicines Agency.

Cooke, R. C. (1977). *Fungi, man and his environment*. London: Largman.

Cook, N. C., & Samman, S. (1996). Flavonoids-Chemistry, metabolism, cardioprotective effects, and dietary sources. *The Journal of Nutritional Biochemistry*, *7*(2), 66–76. doi:10.1016/0955-2863(95)00168-9

Cooper, Z. D., & Haney, M. (2009). Actions of delta-9-tetrahydrocannabinol in cannabis: Relation to use, abuse, dependence. *International Review of Psychiatry (Abingdon, England)*, *21*(2), 104–112. doi:10.1080/09540260902782752 PMID:19367504

Corbridge, D. E. C. (1995). Phosphorus: An outline of its chemistry, biochemistry, and technology (5th ed.). Amsterdam: Elsevier Science Pub Co.

Cortés-Rojas, D., Chagas-Paula, A., Da Costa, F., Souza, C., & Oliveira, W. (2013). *Bidens pilosa L.* populations: A key step in the standardization of phytopharmaceutical preparations. *Brazilian Journal of Pharmacognosy.*, *23*(1), 28–35.

Cortina, M. S., & Bazan, H. E. (2011). Docosahexaenoic acid, Protectins, and Dry Eye. *Current Opinion in Clinical Nutrition and Metabolic Care*, *14*(2), 132–137. doi:10.1097/MCO.0b013e328342bb1a PMID:21157308

Cote, R. A., & Robboy, S. (1980). Progress in medical information management. Systematized nomenclature of medicine. *Journal of the American Medical Association*, *243*(8), 756–762. doi:10.1001/jama.1980.03300340032015 PMID:6986000

Couto R., Martins F., Chaul L., Conceicao E., Alexandre L., Freitas P., Bara M., Paula J. (2013) Spray drying of *Eugenia dysenterica* extract: effects of in-process parameters on product quality. *Revista brasileira de Farmacognosia, 23*(1), 115-123.

Couto, D., Ribeiro, D., Freitas, M., Gomes, A., Lima, J. L., & Fernandes, E. (2010). Scavenging of reactive oxygen and nitrogen species by the prodrug sulfasalazine and its metabolites 5-aminosalicylic acid and sulfapyridine. *Redox Report*, *15*(6), 259–267. doi:10.1179/135100010X12826446921707 PMID:21208525

Cragg, G. M., & Newman, D. J. (2004). A tale of two tumor targets: Topoisomerase I and tubulin. The Wall and Wani contribution to cancer chemotherapy. *Journal of Natural Products*, *67*(2), 232–244. doi:10.1021/np030420c PMID:14987065

Cragg, G. M., & Newman, D. J. (2009). Nature: A vital source of leads for anticancer drug development. *Phytochemistry Reviews*, *8*(2), 313–331. doi:10.1007/s11101-009-9123-y

Cragg, G. M., & Newman, D. J. (2013). Natural products: A continuing source of novel drug leads. *Biochimica et Biophysica Acta, 1830*(6), 3670–3695. doi:10.1016/j.bbagen.2013.02.008 PMID:23428572

Cramer, R. D., Patterso, D. E., & Bunce, J. D. (1989). Recent advances incomparative molecular field analysis (CoMFA). *Progress in Clinical and Biological Research, 291*, 161–165. PMID:2726839

Cranney, A., Horsley, T., & O'Donnell, S. (2007). Effectiveness and Safety of Vitamin D in Relation to Bone Health. *Evid. Rep. Technol. Assess, 158*, 1–235. PMID:18088161

Craven, P. A., Davidson, C. M., & De-Rubertis, F. R. (1990). Increase in diacylglycerol mass in isolated glomeruli by glucose from de novo synthesis of glycerolipids. *Diabetes, 39*(6), 667–674. doi:10.2337/diab.39.6.667 PMID:2347431

Crews, K. R., Gaedigk, A., Dunnenberger, H. M., Leeder, J. S., Klein, T. E., Caudle, K. E., . . . Skaar, T. C. (2014). Clinical Pharmacogenetics Implementation Consortium Guidelines for Cytochrome P450 2D6 Genotype and Codeine Therapy: 2014 Update. *Clinical Pharmacology and Therapeutics.*

Crisan, E. W. S. (1978). A nutritional value. In The biology and cultivation of edible mushrooms. Academic Press.

Croan, S. C. (2004). Conversion of conifer wastes into edible and medicinal mushrooms. *Forest Products Journal, 54*, 68–76.

Crofford, L. J. (2013). Use of NSAIDs in treating patients with arthritis. *Arthritis Research & Therapy, 15*(Suppl 3), S2. doi:10.1186/ar4174 PMID:24267197

Crozier, A., Jaganath, I. B., & Clifford, M. N. (2009). Dietary phenolics: Chemistry, bioavailability and effects on health. *Natural Product Reports, 26*(8), 1001–1043. doi:10.1039/b802662a PMID:19636448

Crum -Brown, A., & Fraser, T.R. (1969). On the connection between chemical constitution and physiological action. Part 1. On the physiological action of the ammonium bases, derived from Strychia, Brucia, Thebaia, Codeia, Morphia and Nicotia. *Transactions of the Royal Society of Edinburgh, 25*, 257–274.

Crutchley, R. D., Miller, J., & Garey, K. W. (2010). Crofelemer, a novel agent for treatment of secretory diarrhea. *The Annals of Pharmacotherapy, 44*(5), 878–884. doi:10.1345/aph.1M658 PMID:20388859

Cunnane, G., Hummel, K. M., Muller-Ladner, U., Gay, R. E., & Gay, S. (1998). Mechanism of joint destruction in rheumatoid arthritis. *Archivum Immunologiae et Therapiae Experimentalis, 46*(1), 1–7. PMID:9510939

Cuppoletti, J., Mayhew, E., Zobel, C. R., & Jung, C. Y. (1981). Erythrosomes: Large Proteoliposomes Derived from Cross-Linked Human Erythrocyte Cytoskeletons and Exogenous Lipid. *Proceedings of the National Academy of Sciences of the United States of America, 78*(5), 2786–2790. doi:10.1073/pnas.78.5.2786 PMID:6789323

Curra, M., Martinis, M., Lauxen, I., Pellicioli, A., Filho, M., Pavesi, V., & Martinis, M. et al. (2013). Effect of topical chamomile on immunohistochemical levels of IL-1b and TNF-a in 5-fluorouracil-induced oral mucositis in hamsters. *Cancer Chemotherapy and Pharmacology, 71*(2), 293–299. doi:10.1007/s00280-012-2013-9 PMID:23096219

Current Procedural Terminology (CPT). (1970). Current Procedural Terminology (CPT). *Journal of the American Medical Association, 212*(5), 873–874. doi:10.1001/jama.1970.03170180149024

Cutolo, M., Sulli, A., Pizzorni, C., Seriolo, B., & Straub, R. H. (2001). Anti-inflammatory mechanisms of methotrexate in rheumatoid arthritis. *Annals of the Rheumatic Diseases, 60*(8), 729–735. doi:10.1136/ard.60.8.729 PMID:11454634

Czajkowsky, D. M., Hu, J., Shao, Z., & Pleass, R. J. (2012). Fc-fusion proteins: New developments and future perspectives. *EMBO Molecular Medicine, 4*(10), 1015–1028. doi:10.1002/emmm.201201379 PMID:22837174

D'Antuono, L. F., Elementi, S., & Neri, R. (2008). Glucosinolates in Diplotaxis and Eruca leaves: Diversity, taxonomic relations and applied aspects. *Phytochemistry*, *69*(1), 187–199. doi:10.1016/j.phytochem.2007.06.019 PMID:17669448

D'Archivio, M., Filesi, C., Vari, R., Scazzocchio, B., & Masella, R. (2010). Bioavailability of the polyphenols: Status and controversies. *International Journal of Molecular Sciences*, *11*(4), 1321–1342. doi:10.3390/ijms11041321 PMID:20480022

Daferera, D. J., Ziogas, B. N., & Polissiou, M. G. (2000). GC-MS analysis of essential oils from some Greek aromatic plants and their fungi toxicity on *Penicillium digitatum*. *Journal of Agricultural and Food Chemistry*, *48*(6), 2576–2581. doi:10.1021/jf990835x PMID:10888587

Dahiya, K. (2013). Nutraceuticals and Their Impact on Human Health. *J Plant Biochem Physiol*, *1*, 4.

Daleke, D. L., Hess, D. T., & Stamler, J. S. (2008). Hypoxic vasodilation by red blood cells: Evidence for an s-nitrosothiol-based signal. *Circulation Research*, *103*(5), 545–553. doi:10.1161/CIRCRESAHA.108.176867 PMID:18658051

Daleke, D. L., & Lyles, J. V. (2000). Identification and purification of aminophospholipid flippases. *Biochimica et Biophysica Acta*, *1486*(1), 108–127. doi:10.1016/S1388-1981(00)00052-4 PMID:10856717

Dall'Acqua, S., & Innocenti, G. (2007). Steroidal glycosides from Hoodia gordonii. *Steroids*, *72*(6-7), 559–568. doi:10.1016/j.steroids.2007.03.008 PMID:17485103

Dall, T. M., Mann, S. E., Zhang, Y., Quick, W. W., Seifert, R. F., Martin, J., & Zhang, S. et al. (2009). Distinguishing the economic costs associated with type 1 and type 2 diabetes. *Population Health Management*, *12*(2), 103–110. doi:10.1089/pop.2009.12203 PMID:19361253

Dalton, E. J., Rotondi, D., Levitan, R. D., Kennedy, S. H., & Brown, G. M. (2000). Use of slow-release melatonin in treatment-resistant depression. *Journal of Psychiatry & Neuroscience*, *25*(1), 48–52. PMID:10721684

Dams, E. T., Laverman, P., Oyen, W. J., Storm, G., Scherphof, G. L., van Der Meer, J. W., & Boerman, O. C. et al. (2000). Accelerated blood clearance and altered biodistribution of repeated injections of sterically stabilized liposomes. *The Journal of Pharmacology and Experimental Therapeutics*, *292*(3), 1071–1079. PMID:10688625

Das, A. V., Padayatti, P. S., & Paulose, C. S. (1996). Effect of leaf extract of *Aegle marmelos* (L.) Correa ex Roxb. on histological and ultra structural changes in tissues of streptozotocin induced diabetic rats. *Indian Journal of Experimental Biology*, *34*, 341–345. PMID:8698423

Dasilva, N., Diez, P., Matarraz, S., Gonzalez-Gonzalez, M., Paradinas, S., Orfao, A., & Fuentes, M. (2012). Biomarker Discovery by Novel Sensors Based on Nanoproteomics Approaches. *Sensors (Basel, Switzerland)*, *12*(2), 2284–2308. PMID:22438764

Das, K. (2010). Diversity and conservation of wild mushrooms in Sikkim with special reference to Barsey Rhododendron Sanctuary. *NeBIO*, *1*(2), 1–13.

Dasture, A. (2002). Global market potentials of ayuvedra drugs- some facts. *Ancient Science of Life*, *XXI*(4), 281–286. PMID:22557067

David, B., Woldenfer, J. L., & Dias, D. A. (2014). The pharmaceitucial industry and natural products: Historical status and new trends. *Phytochemistry Reviews*, *14*(2), 299–315. doi:10.1007/s11101-014-9367-z

Davies, S., Howard, J. M., Hunnisett, A., & Howard, M. (1997). Age-related decreases in chromium levels in 51,665 hair, sweat, and serum samples from 40,872 patients – implications for the prevention of cardiovascular disease and type II diabetes. *Metabolism: Clinical and Experimental*, *46*(5), 469–473. doi:10.1016/S0026-0495(97)90179-7 PMID:9160809

Davson, H., & Danielli, J. F. (1970). *Dannen Conn*. Hanfer Publishing Co.

de Galan, B. E., Zoungas, S., Chalmers, J., Dufouil, C., Pillai, A., & Cooper, M. (2009). …Woodward, M. Cognitive function and risks of cardiovascular disease and hypoglycaemia in patients with type 2 diabetes: the Action in Diabetes and Vascular Disease: Preterax and Diamicron Modified Release Controlled Evaluation (ADVANCE) trial. *Diabetologia*, *52*(11), 2328–2336. doi:10.1007/s00125-009-1484-7 PMID:19688336

De John, A. (2012). *Benefits of goat milk acknowledged by beauty industry*. Retrieved 13.6.2105, from http://www.cosmeticsdesign.com/Market-Trends/Benefits-of-goat-s-milk-acknowledged-by-beauty-industry

de Klein, A., van Kessel, A. G., Grosveld, G., Bartram, C. R., Hagemeijer, A., Bootsma, D., & Stephenson, J. R. et al. (1982). A cellular oncogene is translocated to the Philadelphia chromosome in chronic myelocytic leukaemia. *Nature*, *300*(5894), 765–767. doi:10.1038/300765a0 PMID:6960256

De Leersnyder, H., Bresson, J. L., de Blois, M. C., Souberbielle, J. C., Mogenet, A., Delhotal-Landes, B., & Munnich, A. et al. (2003). Beta 1-adrenergic antagonists and melatonin reset the clock and restore sleep in a circadian disorder, Smith-Magenis syndrome. *Journal of Medical Genetics*, *40*(1), 74–78. doi:10.1136/jmg.40.1.74 PMID:12525548

De Noon, D. J. (2009). Human Skin Alive With Bacteria. *WebMD News Archive*. Retrieved 12.6.2015, from http://www.webmd.com/skin-problems-and-treatments/news/

De Simone, C., Picariello, G., Mamone, G., Stiuso, P., Dicitore, A., Vanacore, D., & Ferranti, P. et al. (2009). Characterisation and cytomodulatory properties of peptides from Mozzarella di Bufala Campana cheese whey. *Journal of Peptide Science*, *15*(3), 251–258. doi:10.1002/psc.1093 PMID:19035578

De Vivo, M. (2013). The Benefits Of Raw Milk Cosmetics. *HelaD*. Retrieved 12.6.2015, from http://www.helladelicious.com/our-food/2013/03/the-benefits-of-raw-milk-cosmetics

de Wit, R., Aapro, M., & Blower, P. R. (2005). Is there a pharmacological basis for differences in 5-HT3-receptor antagonist efficacy in refractory patients?. *Cancer Chemotherapy and Pharmacology*, *56*(3), 231–238. doi:10.1007/s00280-005-1033-0 PMID:15838653

Decker, A., & Graber, E. M. (2012). Over-the-counter acne treatments: A review. *The Journal of Clinical and Aesthetic Dermatology*, *5*(5), 32–40. PMID:22808307

Deenen, M. J., Cats, A., Sechterberger, M. K., Severens, J. L., Smits, P. H. M., Bakker, R., … Schellens, J. H. M. (2011). Safety, pharmacokinetics (PK), and cost effectiveness of upfront genotyping of DPYD in fluoropyrimidine therapy. *Journal of Clinical Oncology, 29*.

Deenen, M. J., Cats, A., Beijnen, J. H., & Schellens, J. H. (2011). Part 1: Background, methodology, and clinical adoption of pharmacogenetics. *The Oncologist*, *16*(6), 811–819. doi:10.1634/theoncologist.2010-0258 PMID:21632456

Deloach, J. R. (1983). Encapsulation of Exogenous Agents in Erythrocytes and the Circulating Survival of Carrier Erythrocytes. *Journal of Applied Biochemistry*, *5*(3), 149–157. PMID:6438049

Deloach, J. R. (1987). Subcutaneous Administration of [35-S] r-IL-2 in Mice Carrier Erythrocytes: Alteration of IL-2 Pharmacokinetics. *Advances in the Biosciences*, *67*, 183–190.

Deloach, J. R., & Doleskey, R. (1987). Preparation and Properties of Microcytic Carrier Erythrocytes from Sheep and Goats. *Advances in the Biosciences*, *67*, 199–212.

Deloach, J. R., Harris, R. L., & Ihler, G. M. (1980). An Erythrocyte Encapsulator Dialyzer Used in Preparing Large Quantities of Erythrocyte Ghosts and Encapsulation of a Pesticide in Erythrocyte Ghosts. *Analytical Biochemistry*, *102*(1), 220–227. doi:10.1016/0003-2697(80)90342-5 PMID:6766688

Deloach, J. R., & Ihler, G. M. (1977). A Dialysis Procedure for Loading of Erythrocytes with Enzymes and Lipids. *Biochimica et Biophysica Acta*, *496*(1), 136–145. doi:10.1016/0304-4165(77)90121-0 PMID:836891

DeMan, J. (1999). *Principles of Food chemistry* (3rd ed.). Aspen Publication Inc. doi:10.1007/978-1-4614-6390-0_1

Demetri, G. D., Rankin, C.J., Benjamin, R. S., Boreden, E.C., Ryan, C.W., Priebat, D.A., . . . Blanke, C.D. (2014). Long-term disease control of advanced gastrointestinal stromal tumors (GIST) with imatinib (IM): 10-year outcomes from SWOG phase III intergroup trial S0033. *Journal of Clinical Oncology, 32*(5).

Demetri, G. D., Reichardt, P., Kang, Y. K., Blay, J. Y., Rutkowski, P., Gelderblom, H., & Casali, P. G et al.. (2013). Efficacy and safety of regorafenib for advanced gastrointestinal stromal tumours after failure of imatinib and sunitinib (GRID): An international, multicentre, randomised, placebo-controlled, phase 3 trial. *Lancet*, *381*(9863), 295–302. doi:10.1016/S0140-6736(12)61857-1 PMID:23177515

Demetri, G. D., van Oosterom, A. T., Garrett, C. R., Blackstein, M. E., Shah, M. H., Verweij, J., & Casali, P. G. et al. (2006). Efficacy and safety of sunitinib in patients with advanced gastrointestinal stromal tumour after failure of imatinib: A randomised controlled trial. *Lancet*, *368*(9544), 1329–1338. doi:10.1016/S0140-6736(06)69446-4 PMID:17046465

Deng, Z. J., Mortimer, G., Schiller, T., Musumeci, A., Martin, D., & Minchin, R. F. (2009). Differential plasma protein binding to metal oxide nanoparticles. *Nanotechnology*, *20*(45), 455101. doi:10.1088/0957-4484/20/45/455101 PMID:19822937

Derbyshire, D. (n.d.). How your wrinkle cream could destroy. *Mail Online*. Retrieved 12.6.2015, from http://www.dailymail.co.uk/femail/article-2359596/How-wrinkle-cream-destroy-skin-Chemicals-cosmetics-trigger-severe-allergies.html#ixzz3Zj8FRcMf

Dernovics, M., Giusti, P., Lobinski, R. (2007). *ICP-MS-assisted nanoHPLC-electrospray Q/time*. Academic Press.

Dernovics, M., Giusti, P., & Lobinski, R. (2007). of-flight MS/MS selenopeptide mapping in Brazil nuts. *Journal of Analytical Atomic Spectrometry*, *22*(1), 41–50. doi:10.1039/B608041C

Desjardins, D., Huret, C., & Dalba, C. (2009). Recombinant retrovirus-like particle forming DNA vaccines in prime-boost immunization and their use for hepatitis C virus vaccine development. *The Journal of Gene Medicine*, *11*, 313–325. PMID:19248137

Desreumaux, P., & Ghosh, S. (2006). Review article: Mode of action and delivery of 5-aminosalicylic acid - new evidence. *Alimentary Pharmacology & Therapeutics*, *24*(Suppl 1), 2–9. doi:10.1111/j.1365-2036.2006.03069.x PMID:16939423

DeVita, V. T. Jr, & Rosenberg, S. A. (2012). Two hundred years of cancer research. *The New England Journal of Medicine*, *366*(23), 2207–2214. PMID:22646510

Devi, V., Jain, N., & Vali, K. (2010). Importance of novel drug delivery systemps in herbal medicines. *Pharmagonogsy Review*, *4*(7), 27–31. PMID:22228938

Devon, T. K., & Scott, A. I. (1972). *Handbook of Naturally occurring Compounds: The Terpenes*. London: Academic Press.

DeVrese, M., & Schrezenmeir, J. (2008). Probiotics, prebiotics and synbiotics. *Advances in Biochemical Engineering/Biotechnology*, *111*, 1–66. doi:10.1007/10_2008_097 PMID:18461293

Dey, B., Bhunia, S. K., Maity, K. K., Patra, S., Mandal, S., Maiti, S., & Islam, S. S. et al. (2010). Chemical analysis of an immunoenhancing water-soluble polysaccharide of an edible mushroom, *Pleurotus florida* blue variant. *Carbohydrate Research*, *345*(18), 2736–2741. doi:10.1016/j.carres.2010.09.032 PMID:20971448

Dhami, N. (2013). Trends in Pharmacognosy: A modern science of natural medicines. *Journal of Herbal Medicine.*, *3*(4), 123–131. doi:10.1016/j.hermed.2013.06.001

Dhib-Jalbut, S., & Marks, S. (2010). Interferon-beta mechanisms of action in multiple sclerosis. *Neurology*, *74*(Suppl 1), S17–S24. doi:10.1212/WNL.0b013e3181c97d99 PMID:20038758

Di Marco, M., Shamsuddin, S., Razak, K. A., Aziz, A. A., Devaux, C., Borghi, E., & Sadun, C. et al. (2010). Overview of the main methods used to combine proteins with nanosystems: Absorption, bioconjugation, and encapsulation. *International Journal of Nanomedicine*, *5*, 37–49. PMID:20161986

Di Nicolantonio, F., Martini, M., Molinari, F., Sartore-Bianchi, A., Arena, S., Saletti, P., & Bardelli, A. et al. (2008). Wild-type BRAF is required for response to panitumumab or cetuximab in metastatic colorectal cancer. *Journal of Clinical Oncology*, *26*(35), 5705–5712. doi:10.1200/JCO.2008.18.0786 PMID:19001320

di Noia, J. (2014). *Defining powerhouse fruits and vegetables: a nutrient density approach. Preventing chronic disease*. National Center for Chronic Disease Prevention and Health Promotion.

Diamond, D. L., Jacobs, J. M., Paeper, B., Proll, S. C., Gritsenko, M. A., Carithers, R. L., & Katze, M. G. et al. (2007). Proteomic profiling of human liver biopsies: Hepatitis C virus-induced fibrosis and mitochondrial dysfunction. *Hepatology (Baltimore, Md.)*, *46*(3), 649–657. PMID:17654742

DiCesare, D., DuPont, H. L., Mathewson, J. J., Ashley, D., Martinez-Sandoval, F., Pennington, J. E., & Porter, S. B. (2002). A double blind, randomized, placebo-controlled study of SP-303 (Provir) in the symptomatic treatment of acute diarrhea among travelers to Jamaica and Mexico. *The American Journal of Gastroenterology*, *97*(10), 2585–2588. doi:10.1111/j.1572-0241.2002.06027.x PMID:12385443

Diedrich, T., Dybowska, A., Schott, J., Valsami-Jones, E., & Oelkers, E. H. (2012). The dissolution rates of SiO2 nanoparticles as a function of particle size. *Environmental Science & Technology*, *46*(9), 4909–4915. doi:10.1021/es2045053 PMID:22482930

Di, G. F., Del, C. F., Caenaro, G., Lante, I., & Muraca, M. (2012). Human serum proteome analysis: New source of markers in metabolic disorders. *Biomarkers in Medicine*, *6*, 759–773. PMID:23227840

Dillard, C. J., & German, J. B. (2000). Review Phytochemicals: Nutraceuticals and human health. *Journal of the Science of Food and Agriculture*, *80*(12), 1744–1756. doi:10.1002/1097-0010(20000915)80:12<1744::AID-JSFA725>3.0.CO;2-W

Dinda, S. C., & Pattnaik, G. (2013). Nanobiotechnology-based drug delivery in brain targeting. *Current Pharmaceutical Biotechnology*, *14*(15), 1264–1274. doi:10.2174/1389201015666140608143719 PMID:24910011

Dixon, S. L., Smondyrev, A. M., Knoll, E. H., Rao, S., Shaw, D. E., & Friesner, R. A. (2006). PHASE: A new engine for pharmacophore perception, 3D QSAR model development, and 3D database screening: 1. Methodology and preliminary results. *Journal of Computer-Aided Molecular Design*, *20*(10-11), 647–671. doi:10.1007/s10822-006-9087-6 PMID:17124629

do Carmo, F. A., Sathler, P. C., Zancan, P., Rodrigues, C. R., Castro, H. C., de Sousa, V. P., & Cabral, L. M. et al. (2014). Therapeutic nanosystems for oral administration of insulin. *Current Pharmaceutical Biotechnology*, *15*(7), 620–628. doi:10.2174/1389201015666140915150826 PMID:25219867

Dobrovolskaia, M. A., & McNeil, S. E. (2007). Immunological properties of engineered nanomaterials. *Nature Nanotechnology*, *2*(8), 469–478. doi:10.1038/nnano.2007.223 PMID:18654343

Dodick, D. W., & Capobianco, D. J. (2001). Treatment and management of cluster headache. *Current Pain and Headache Reports*, *5*(1), 83–91. doi:10.1007/s11916-001-0015-0 PMID:11252143

Dolberg, O. T., Hirschmann, S., & Grunhaus, L. (1998). Melatonin for the treatment of sleep disturbances in major depressive disorder. *The American Journal of Psychiatry*, *155*(8), 1119–1121. doi:10.1176/ajp.155.8.1119 PMID:9699707

Dompeipen, E. J., Srikandace, Y., Suharso, W. P., Cahyana, H., & Simanjuntak, P. (2009). Potential endophytic microbes selection for antidiabetic bioactive compounds production. *Asian Journal of Biochemistry*, *6*(6), 465–471. doi:10 3923/ajb.2011.465.471

Douillard, J. Y., Oliner, K. S., Siena, S., Tabernero, J., Burkes, R., Barugel, M., & Patterson, S. D. et al. (2013). Panitumumab-FOLFOX4 treatment and RAS mutations in colorectal cancer. *The New England Journal of Medicine*, *369*(11), 1023–1034. doi:10.1056/NEJMoa1305275 PMID:24024839

Draelos, Z. D. (2009). Cosmeceuticals: Undefined, unclassified, and unregulated. *Clinics in Dermatology*, *27*(5), 431–434. doi:10.1016/j.clindermatol.2009.05.005 PMID:19695473

Dreaden, E. C., Austin, L. A., Mackey, M. A., & El-Sayed, M. A. (2012). Size matters: Gold nanoparticles in targeted cancer drug delivery. *Ther Deliv*, *3*(4), 457–478. doi:10.4155/tde.12.21 PMID:22834077

Drewnowski, A. (2010). The Nutrient Rich Foods Index helps to identify healthy, affordable foods. *The American Journal of Clinical Nutrition*, *91*(4), 1095S–1101S. doi:10.3945/ajcn.2010.28450D PMID:20181811

Duad, A., Ribas, A., & Robert, C. (2015). Long-term efficacy of pembrolizumab (pembro; MK-3475) in a pooled analysis of 655 patients (pts) with advanced melanoma (MEL) enrolled in KEYNOTE-001. *Journal of Clinical Oncology*.

Duan, H., Struble, E., & Zhong, L. (2010). Hepatitis C virus with a naturally occurring single amino-acid substitution in the E2 envelope protein escapes neutralization by naturally-induced and vaccine-induced antibodies. *Vaccine*, *28*, 4138–4144. PMID:20433800

Duan, J., Dixon, S. L., Lowrie, J. F., & Sherman, W. (2010). Analysis and comparison of 2D fingerprints: Insights into database screening performance using eight fingerprints Methods. *Journal of Molecular Graphics & Modelling*, *29*(2), 157–170. doi:10.1016/j.jmgm.2010.05.008 PMID:20579912

Dubey, T., & Guerra, D. J. (2002). Use of biotechnology for growing medicinal plants. *Recent Progress in Medicinal Plants*, *5*, 47–61.

Duckworth, W., Abraira, C., Moritz, T., Reda, D., Emanuele, N., Reaven, P. D., & Huang, G. D. et al. (2009). Glucose control and vascular complications in veterans with type 2 diabetes. *The New England Journal of Medicine*, *360*(2), 129–139. doi:10.1056/NEJMoa0808431 PMID:19092145

Duell, E. A., Kang, S., & Voorhees, J. J. (1997). Unoccluded retinol penetrates human skin in vivo more effectively than unoccluded retinyl palmitate or retinoic acid. *The Journal of Investigative Dermatology*, *109*(3), 301–305. doi:10.1111/1523-1747.ep12335788 PMID:9284094

Duke, S. O., Dayan, F. E., Romagni, J. G., & Rimando, A. M. (2000). Natural products as sources of herbicides: Current status and future trends. *Weed Research*, *40*(1), 99–111. doi:10.1046/j.1365-3180.2000.00161.x

Duong, A. D., Sharma, S., Peine, K. J., Gupta, G., Satoskar, A. R., Bachelder, E. M., & Ainslie, K. M. et al. (2013). Electrospray encapsulation of toll-like receptor agonist resiquimod in polymer microparticles for the treatment of visceral leishmaniasis. *Molecular Pharmaceutics*, *10*(3), 1045–1055. doi:10.1021/mp3005098 PMID:23320733

Durbin, R., Eddy, S., Krogh, A., & Mitchison, G. (1998). *Biological Sequence Analysis*. Cambridge, UK: Cambridge University Press. doi:10.1017/CBO9780511790492

Dureja, H., Kaushik, D., & Kumar, V. (2003). Developments in nutraceuticals. *Indian Journal of Pharmacology*, *35*, 363–372.

Ebos, J. M., Lee, C. R., & Kerbel, R. S. (2009). Tumor and host-mediated pathways of resistance and disease progression in response to antiangiogenic therapy. *Clinical Cancer Research*, *15*(16), 5020–5025. doi:10.1158/1078-0432.CCR-09-0095 PMID:19671869

Eichhorn, T., Greten, H., & Efferth, T. (2011). Self-medication with nutritional supplements and herbal over-thecounter products. *Natural Products and Bioprospecting.*, *1*(2), 62–70. doi:10.1007/s13659-011-0029-1

Eichler, H. C., Gasic, S., Daum, B., Bacher, S., & Sreger, G. (1987). In Vitro Drug Release From Human Carrier Erythrocytes. *Advances in the Biosciences*, *67*, 11–15.

Eichler, H. G., Gasicm, S., Bauer, K., Korn, A., & Bacher, S. (1986). *In Vivo* Clearance of Antibody-Sensitized Human Drug Carrier Erythrocytes. *Clinical Pharmacology and Therapeutics*, *40*(3), 300–303. doi:10.1038/clpt.1986.180 PMID:3091309

Eichler, H. G., Raffesberg, W., Gasic, S., Korn, A., & Bauer, K. (1985). Release of Vitamin B 12 from Carrier Erythrocytes *In Vitro. Research in Experimental Medicine. Zeitschrift fur die Gesamte Experimentelle Medizin Einschliesslich Experimenteller Chirurgie*, *185*(4), 341–344. doi:10.1007/BF01851959 PMID:4048655

Eid, H. M., Martineau, L. C., Saleem, A., Muhammad, A., Vallerand, D., Benhaddou-Andaloussi, A., & Haddad, P. S. et al. (2010). Stimulation of AMP-activated protein kinase and enhancement of basal glucose uptake in muscle cells by quercetin and quercetin glycosides, active principles of the antidiabetic medicinal plant Vaccinium vitis-idaea. *Molecular Nutrition & Food Research*, *54*(7), 991–1003. doi:10.1002/mnfr.200900218 PMID:20087853

El-Abhar, H., & Schaalan, M. (2014). Phytotherapy in diabetes: Review on potential mechanistic perspectives. *World Journal of Diabetes*, *5*(2), 176–197. PMID:24748931

Elgart, A., Cherniakov, I., Aldouby, Y., Domb, A. J., & Hoffman, A. (2012). Lipospheres and pro-nano lipospheres for delivery of poorly water soluble compounds. *Chemistry and Physics of Lipids*, *165*(4), 438–453. doi:10.1016/j.chemphyslip.2012.01.007 PMID:22342324

Elizabeth, A. C. (2002). Over the counter products: Nonprescription medications, nutraceuticals, and herbal agents. *Clinical Obstetrics and Gynecology*, *45*(1), 89–98. doi:10.1097/00003081-200203000-00010 PMID:11862061

Eller, K., Kirsch, A., Wolf, A. M., Sopper, S., Tagwerker, A., Stanzl, U., & Eller, P. et al. (2011). Potential role of regulatory T cells in reversing obesity-linked insulin resistance and diabetic nephropathy. *Diabetes*, *60*(11), 2954–2962. doi:10.2337/db11-0358 PMID:21911743

Elsohly, M. A. (2002). Chemical constituents of Cannabis. In F. Grotenhermen & E. Russo (Eds.), *Cannabis and cannabinoids. Pharmacology, toxicology, and therapeutic potential*. Binghamton, New York: The Haworth Press.

Elsohly, M. A., & Slade, D. (2005). Chemical constituents of marijuana: The complex mixture of natural cannabinoids. *Life Sciences*, *78*(5), 539–548. doi:10.1016/j.lfs.2005.09.011 PMID:16199061

Emile, J. F., Theou, N., Tabone, S., Cortez, A., Terrier, P., Chaumette, M. T., & Lemoine, A. et al. (2004). Clinicopathologic, phenotypic, and genotypic characteristics of gastrointestinal mesenchymal tumors. *Clinical Gastroenterology and Hepatology*, *2*(7), 597–605. doi:10.1016/S1542-3565(04)00243-5 PMID:15224284

Engelen, M.P., Rutten, E.P., De Castro, C.L., Wouters, E.F., Schols, A.M., & Deutz, N.E. (2012) Casein protein results in higher prandial and exercise induced whole body protein anabolism than whey protein in chronic obstructive pulmonary disease. *Metabolism, 61*(9), 1289–1300.

Engelen, M. P., De De Castro, C. L., Rutten, E. P., Wouters, E. F., Schols, A. M., & Deutz, N. E. (2012). Enhanced anabolic response to milk protein sip feeding in elderly subjects with COPD is associated with a reduced splanchnic extraction of multiple amino acids. *Clinical Nutrition (Edinburgh, Lothian)*, *31*(5), 616–624. doi:10.1016/j.clnu.2012.04.006 PMID:22682082

English, C., & Aloi, J. J. (2015). New FDA-Approved Disease-Modifying Therapies for Multiple Sclerosis. *Clinical Therapeutics*, *37*(4), 691–715. doi:10.1016/j.clinthera.2015.03.001 PMID:25846320

Enrich, L. B., Scheuermann, M. L., Mohadjer, A., Matthias, K. R., Eller, C. F., Newman, M. S., & Poon, T. (2008). Liquidambar styraciflua: A renewable source of shikimic acid. *Tetrahedron Letters*, *49*(16), 2503–2505. doi:10.1016/j.tetlet.2008.02.140

Erickson, K. L., Medina, E. A., & Hubbard, N. E. (2000). Micronutrients and innate immunity. *The Journal of Infectious Diseases*, *182*(s1), S5–S10. doi:10.1086/315922 PMID:10944478

Erkucuk, A., Akgun, I. H., & Yesil-Celiktas, O. (2009). Supercritical CO2 extraction of glycosides from Stevia rebaudiana leaves: Identification and optimization. *The Journal of Supercritical Fluids*, *51*(1), 29–35. doi:10.1016/j.supflu.2009.07.002

Escott-Stump, S. (2008). Nutrition and Diagnosis-Related Care (8th ed.). Lippincott Williams & Wilkins.

Escott-Stump, S. (Ed.). (2008). *Nutrition and Diagnosis-Related Care* (6th ed.). Philadelphia: Wolters Kluwer Health Lippincott Williams & Wilkins.

Eswar, N., Eramian, D., Webb, B., Shen, M., & Sali, A. (2008). Protein structure modeling with MODELLER. *Methods in Molecular Biology (Clifton, N.J.)*, *426*, 145–159. doi:10.1007/978-1-60327-058-8_8 PMID:18542861

Eteng, M. U., Eyong, E. U., Akpanyung, E. C., Agiang, M. A., & Aremu, C. Y. (1997). Recent advances in caffeine and theobromine toxicities: A review. *Plant Foods for Human Nutrition (Dordrecht, Netherlands)*, *51*(3), 231–243. doi:10.1023/A:1007976831684 PMID:9629863

European Commission. (2015). *Cosmetics*. Retrieved October 13, 2015, from http://ec.europa.eu/growth/sectors/cosmetics/index_en.htm

European Medicines Agency. (2015). *Frequently asked questions*. Retrieved October 11, 2015, from http://www.ema.europa.eu/ema/index.jsp?curl=pages/about_us/q_and_a/q_and_a_detail_000114.jsp

Evers, D. L., Chao, C. F., Wang, X., Zhang, Z. G., Huong, S. M., & Huang, E. S. (2005). Human cytomegalo virus-inhibitory flavonoids: Studies on antiviral activity and mechanism of action. *Antiviral Research*, *68*(3), 124–134. doi:10.1016/j.antiviral.2005.08.002 PMID:16188329

Eyberger, A. L., Dondapati, R., & Porter, J. R. (2006). Endophyte fungal isolates from *Podophyllum peltatum* produce podophyllotoxin. *Journal of Natural Products*, *69*(8), 1121–1124. doi:10.1021/np060174f PMID:16933860

Fahey, J. W., Haristoy, X., Dolan, P. M., Kensler, T. W., Scholtus, I., Stephenson, K. K., & Lozniewski, A. et al. (2002). Sulforaphane inhibits extracellular, intracellular, and antibiotic-resistant strains of Helicobacter pylori and prevents benzopyrene-induced stomach tumors. *Proceedings of the National Academy of Sciences of the United States of America*, *99*(11), 7610–7615. doi:10.1073/pnas.112203099 PMID:12032331

Faria, A. M., & Weiner, H. L. (2005). Oral tolerance. *Immunological Reviews*, *206*(1), 232–259. doi:10.1111/j.0105-2896.2005.00280.x PMID:16048553

Farris, P. K. (2005). Topical vitamin C: A useful agent for treating photoaging and other dermatologic conditions. *Dermatologic Surgery*, *31*(7 Pt 2), 814–817. PMID:16029672

Farris, P. K., Edison, B. L., Brouda, I., Weinkauf, R. L., & Green, B. A. (2012). A high-potency, multimechanism skin care regimen provides significant antiaging effects: Results from a double-blind, vehicle-controlled clinical trial. *Journal of Drugs in Dermatology*, *11*(12), 1447–1454. PMID:23377515

Fasching, P. A., Kollmannsberger, B., Strissel, P. L., Niesler, B., Engel, J., Kreis, H., & Strick, R. et al. (2008). Polymorphisms in the novel serotonin receptor subunit gene HTR3C show different risks for acute chemotherapy-induced vomiting after anthracycline chemotherapy. *Journal of Cancer Research and Clinical Oncology*, *134*(10), 1079–1086. doi:10.1007/s00432-008-0387-1 PMID:18389280

Fassett, R. G., & Coombes, J. S. (2011). Astaxanthin: A potential therapeutic agent in cardiovascular disease. *Marine Drugs*, *9*(12), 447–465. doi:10.3390/md9030447 PMID:21556169

Fava, M., Rush, A. J., Trivedi, M. H., Nierenberg, A. A., Thase, M. E., Sackheim, H. A., & Kupfer, D. J. et al. (2003). Background and rationale for the sequenced treatment alternatives to relieve depression (STAR*D) study. *The Psychiatric Clinics of North America*, *26*(2), 457–494. doi:10.1016/S0193-953X(02)00107-7 PMID:12778843

FDA. (2015). Retrieved October 13, 2015, from http://www.fda.gov/RegulatoryInformation/Legislation/FederalFoodDrugandCosmeticActFDCAct/default.htm

FDA-U.S. Food and Drug Administration Protecting and Promoting Your Health. (2015). Retrieved 1.6.2015, from http://www.fda.gov/cosmetics/guidanceregulation/default.htm

Feldmann, M., & Maini, R. N. (2001). Anti-TNF alpha therapy of rheumatoid arthritis: What have we learned? *Annual Review of Immunology*, *19*(1), 163–196. doi:10.1146/annurev.immunol.19.1.163 PMID:11244034

Feng, Y., Carroll, A. R., Addepalli, R., Fechner, G., Avery, V. M., & Quinn, R. J. (2007). Vanillic acid derivatives from the green algae *Cladophora socialis* as potent protein tyrosine phosphatase 1B inhibitors. *Journal of Natural Products*, *70*(11), 1790–1792. doi:10.1021/np070225o PMID:17949055

Fennema, O. (2008). Fennema's Food Chemistry. CRC Press.

Fernandes, C., Mascarenhas, M., Zibetti, F., Lima, G., Oliveira, R., Rocha, L., & Falcão, D. (2013). HLB value, an important parameter for the development of essential oil PP. *Brazilian Journal of Pharmacognosy*, *23*(1), 108–114.

Ferrara, N., Gerber, H. P., & LeCouter, J. (2003). The biology of VEGF and its receptors. *Nature Medicine*, *9*(6), 669–676. doi:10.1038/nm0603-669 PMID:12778165

Fetrow, C. W., & Avila, K. R. (2001). Efficacy of the dietary supplement S-adenosyl-L-methionine. *The Annals of Pharmacotherapy*, *35*(11), 1414–1425. doi:10.1345/aph.1Z443 PMID:11724095

Feyer, P., & Jordan, K. (2011). Update and new trends in antiemetic therapy: The continuing need for novel therapies. *Annals of Oncology*, *22*(1), 30–38. doi:10.1093/annonc/mdq600 PMID:20947707

Fielding, A. K. (2011). Current treatment of Philadelphia chromosome-positive acute lymphoblastic leukemia. *Hematology*, *2011*(1), 231–237. doi:10.1182/asheducation-2011.1.231 PMID:22160039

Fiorelli, G., Fargion, S., Piperno, A., Cappellini, M. D., Rossi, F., Sabionedda, L., & Zanella, A. (1987). Transfusion of Thalasemic Patients with Desferrioxamine Loaded Standard Red Blood Cell Units. *Advanced Biosciences67*, 47-54.

Fiorina, P., Vergani, A., Bassi, R., Niewczas, M., Altintas, M. M., Pezzolesi, M. G., & Sayegh, M. H. et al. (2014). Role of Podocyte B7-1 in Diabetic Nephropathy. *Journal of the American Society of Nephrology*, *25*(7), 1415–1429. doi:10.1681/ASN.2013050518 PMID:24676639

Firenzuoli, F., & Gori, L. (2007). Herbal medicine today: Clinical and research issues. *Evidence-Based Complementary and Alternative Medicine*, *4*(s1), 37–40. doi:10.1093/ecam/nem096 PMID:18227931

Fischer, P. M. (2008). Computational chemistry approaches to drug discovery in signal transduction. *Biotechnology Journal*, *3*(4), 452–470. doi:10.1002/biot.200700259 PMID:18412174

Fisher, A. A. (1983). Current contact news. Hydroquinone uses and abnormal reactions. *Cutis*, *31*(3), 240–244, 250. PMID:6220868

Fisher, A. A. (1988). Tetracycline treatment for sarcoid-like ochronosis due to hydroquinone. *Cutis*, *42*(1), 19–20. PMID:3203531

Fisk, W. A., Agbai, O., Lev-Tov, H. A., & Sivamani, R. K. (2014). The use of botanically derived agents for hyperpigmentation: A systematic review. *Journal of the American Academy of Dermatology*, *70*(2), 352–365. doi:10.1016/j.jaad.2013.09.048 PMID:24280646

Fitch, W. M. (1970). Distinguishing homologous from analogous proteins. *Systematic Zoology*, *19*(2), 99–110. doi:10.2307/2412448 PMID:5449325

Fitton, A., & Goa, K. L. (1991). Azelaic acid. A review of its pharmacological properties and therapeutic efficacy in acne and hyperpigmentary skin disorders. *Drugs*, *41*(5), 780–798. doi:10.2165/00003495-199141050-00007 PMID:1712709

Flaherty, K. T., Infante, J. R., Daud, A., Gonzalez, R., Kefford, R. F., Sosman, J., & Weber, J. et al. (2012). Combined BRAF and MEK inhibition in melanoma with BRAF V600 mutations. *The New England Journal of Medicine*, *367*(18), 1694–1703. doi:10.1056/NEJMoa1210093 PMID:23020132

Fleck, A., Gupta, R. C., Goad, J. T., Lasher, M. A., Canerdy, T. D., & Kalidindi, S. R. (2014). Anti-arthritic efficacy and safety of crominex® 3+ (Trivalent chromium, phyllanthus emblica extract, and shilajit) in moderately arthritic dogs. *Journal of Veterinary Science & Animal Husbandry.*, *1*(4), 1–8.

Fleischer, D. M., Burks, A. W., Vickery, B. P., Scurlock, A. M., Wood, R. A., Jones, S. M., . . . Consortium of Food Allergy. (2013). Sublingual immunotherapy for peanut allergy: a randomized, double-blind, placebo-controlled multicenter trial. *J Allergy Clin Immunol, 131*(1), 119-127. doi: 10.1016/j.jaci.2012.11.011

Flo, T. H., Smith, K. D., Sato, S., Rodriguez, D. J., Holmes, M. A., Strong, R. K., & Aderem, A. et al. (2004). Lipocalin-2 Mediates an Innate Immune Response to Bacterial Infection by Sequestrating Iron. *Nature*, *432*(7019), 917–921. doi:10.1038/nature03104 PMID:15531878

Flynn, G., McHale, L., & McHale, A. P. (1994). Methotrexate-Loaded, Photosensitized Erythrocytes: A Photo-Activatable Carrier/Delivery System for Use in Cancer Therapy. *Cancer Letters*, *82*(2), 225–229. doi:10.1016/0304-3835(94)90016-7 PMID:8050095

Foley, P., Nixon, R., Marks, R., Frowen, K., & Thompson, S. (1993). The frequency of reactions to sunscreens: Results of a longitudinal population-based study on the regular use of sunscreens in Australia. *The British Journal of Dermatology*, *128*(5), 512–518. doi:10.1111/j.1365-2133.1993.tb00227.x PMID:8504041

Food & Drug Administration. (2011). Labeling and effectiveness testing; sunscreen drug products for over-the-counter human use. Final rule. *Federal Register, 76*(117), 35620.

Food and Drug Administration. (2010). *Caffeine intake by the U.S. population*. Retrieved from (http://www.fda.gov/downloads/AboutFDA/CentersOffices/OfficeofFoods/CFSAN/CFSANFOIAElectronicReadingRoom/UCM333191.pdf)

Food and Nutrition Board, Institute of Medicine. (2005). *Dietary Reference Intakes for Energy, Carbohydrates, Fiber, Fat, Fatty Acids, Cholesterol, Protein, and Amino Acids*. Washington, DC: National Academies Press.

Forbes, J. M., & Cooper, M. E. (2013). Mechanisms of diabetic complications. *Physiological Reviews*, *93*(1), 137–188. doi:10.1152/physrev.00045.2011 PMID:23303908

Forbes, J. M., Cooper, M. E., Oldfield, M. D., & Thomas, M. C. (2003). Role of advanced glycation end products in diabetic nephropathy. *Journal of the American Society of Nephrology*, *14*(90003), S254–S258. doi:10.1097/01.ASN.0000077413.41276.17 PMID:12874442

Foroozandeh, P., & Aziz, A. A. (2015). Merging worlds of nanomaterials and biological environment: Factors governing protein corona formation on nanoparticles and its biological consequences. *Nanoscale Research Letters*, *10*(1), 221. doi:10.1186/s11671-015-0922-3 PMID:25995715

Fort-Lacoste, L., Verscheure, Y., Tisne-Versailles, J., & Navarro, R. (1999). Comedolytic effect of topical retinaldehyde in the rhino mouse model. *Dermatology (Basel, Switzerland)*, *199*(Suppl 1), 33–35. doi:10.1159/000051376 PMID:10473958

Fox, H. M. (1984). Pantothenic acid. In L. J. Machlin (Ed.), *Handbook of Vitamins* (Vol. 437). New York: Marcel Dekker.

Fox, R. I., Herrmann, M. L., Frangou, C. G., Wahl, G. M., Morris, R. E., Strand, V., & Kirschbaum, B. J. (1999). Mechanism of action for leflunomide in rheumatoid arthritis. *Clinical Immunology (Orlando, Fla.)*, *93*(3), 198–208. doi:10.1006/clim.1999.4777 PMID:10600330

Fozzard, H.A., & Hanck, D.A. (1996). Structure and function of voltage-dependent sodium channels: comparison of brain II and cardiac isoforms. *American Physiological Society, 76*(3), 887-926.

Fraternale, A., Rossi, L., & Magnani, M. (1996). Encapsulation, Metabolism, and Release of 2-Fluoro-Ara-AMP from Human Erythrocytes. *Biochimica et Biophysica Acta*, *1291*(2), 149–154. doi:10.1016/0304-4165(96)00059-1 PMID:8898876

Frei, B., England, L., & Ames, B. N. (1989). Ascorbate is an outstanding antioxidant in human blood plasma. *Proceedings of the National Academy of Sciences of the United States of America*, *86*(16), 6377–6381. doi:10.1073/pnas.86.16.6377 PMID:2762330

Frenking, G., Antes, I., Böhme, M., Dapprich, S., Ehlers, A. W., Jonas, V., … Vyboishchikov, S.F. (1996). Reviews in Computational Chemistry. New York: VCH.

Friese, M. A., Schattling, B., & Fugger, L. (2014). Mechanisms of neurodegeneration and axonal dysfunction in multiple sclerosis. *Nat Rev Neurol*, *10*(4), 225–238. doi:10.1038/nrneurol.2014.37 PMID:24638138

Fuchs, C. S., Tomasek, J., Yong, C. J., Dumitru, F., Passalacqua, R., Goswami, C., & Investigators, R. T. et al. (2014). Ramucirumab monotherapy for previously treated advanced gastric or gastro-oesophageal junction adenocarcinoma (REGARD): An international, randomised, multicentre, placebo-controlled, phase 3 trial. *Lancet*, *383*(9911), 31–39. doi:10.1016/S0140-6736(13)61719-5 PMID:24094768

Fujita, H., Taniai, H., Murayama, H., Ohshiro, H., Hayashi, H., Sato, S., & Yamada, Y. et al. (2013). DPP-4 inhibition with alogliptin on top of angiotensin II type 1 receptor blockade ameliorates albuminuria via up-regulation of SDF-1α in type 2 diabetic patients with incipient nephropathy. *Endocrine Journal*, *61*(2), 159–166. doi:10.1507/endocrj.EJ13-0305 PMID:24225429

Fukami, K., Yamagishi, S. I., Ueda, S., & Okuda, S. (2008). Role of AGEs in diabetic nephropathy. *Current Pharmaceutical Design*, *14*(10), 946–952. doi:10.2174/138161208784139710 PMID:18473844

Furusawa, M., Nishimura, T., Yamaizumi, M., & Okada, Y. (1974). Injection of foreign substances into single cells by cell fusion. *Nature*, *249*(456), 449–450. doi:10.1038/249449a0 PMID:4365359

Gandara, D. R., Roila, F., Warr, D., Edelman, M. J., Perez, E. A., & Gralla, R. J. (1998). Consensus proposal for 5HT3 antagonists in the prevention of acute emesis related to highly emetogenic chemotherapy. Dose, schedule, and route of administration. *Supportive Care in Cancer*, *6*(3), 237–243. doi:10.1007/s005200050160 PMID:9629876

Gangadharan, B., Bapat, M., Rossa, J., & Antrobus, R. (2014). Discovery of novel biomarker candidates for liver fibrosis in hepatitis C patients using proteomics. *Journal of Molecular Biomarkers & Diagnosis*, *5*, 106.

Gao, X. H., Zhang, L., Wei, H. C., & Chen, H. D. (2008). Efficacy and safety of innovative cosmeceuticals. *Clinics in Dermatology*, *26*(4), 367–374. doi:10.1016/j.clindermatol.2008.01.013 PMID:18691517

García-Gavín, J., González-Vilas, D., Fernández-Redondo, V., & Toribio, J. (2010). Pigmented contact dermatitis due to kojic acid. A paradoxical side effect of a skin lightener. *Contact Dermatitis*, *62*(1), 63–64. doi:10.1111/j.1600-0536.2009.01673.x PMID:20136888

Gardos, G. (1956). Akkumulation de Kalium Onen Durch Menschiche Blutkorperchen. *Acta Physiologica Academiae Scientiarum Hungaricae*, *6*, 191–196.

Garín, M. I., López, R. M., Sanz, S., Pinilla, M., & Luque, J. (1996). Erythrocytes as carriers for recombinant human erythropoietin. *Pharmaceutical Research*, *13*(6), 869–874. doi:10.1023/A:1016049027661 PMID:8792424

Garon, E. B., Ciuleanu, T. E., Arrieta, O., Prabhash, K., Syrigos, K. N., Goksel, T., & Perol, M. et al. (2014). Ramucirumab plus docetaxel versus placebo plus docetaxel for second-line treatment of stage IV non-small-cell lung cancer after disease progression on platinum-based therapy (REVEL): A multicentre, double-blind, randomised phase 3 trial. *Lancet*, *384*(9944), 665–673. doi:10.1016/S0140-6736(14)60845-X PMID:24933332

Garris, C. S., Wu, L., Acharya, S., Arac, A., Blaho, V. A., Huang, Y., & Han, M. H. et al. (2013). Defective sphingosine 1-phosphate receptor 1 (S1P1) phosphorylation exacerbates TH17-mediated autoimmune neuroinflammation. *Nature Immunology*, *14*(11), 1166–1172. doi:10.1038/ni.2730 PMID:24076635

Gasche, Y., Daali, Y., Fathi, M., Chiappe, A., Cottini, S., Dayer, P., & Desmeules, J. (2004). Codeine intoxication associated with ultrarapid CYP2D6 metabolism. *The New England Journal of Medicine*, *351*(27), 2827–2831. doi:10.1056/NEJMoa041888 PMID:15625333

Gauss, D. (2012). *Breast Milk Lotion Recipe*. Retrieved 12.6.215, from http://www.justbreastfeeding.com/benefits-to-breastfeeding/breast-milk-lotion-recipe

Gaut, B. N., & Lopes, D. (Eds.). (2005). *The Routledge companion to aesthetics* (2nd ed.). London: Routledge.

Ge, D., Fellay, J., Thompson, A. J., Simon, J. S., Shianna, K. V., Urban, T. J., & Muir, A. J. et al. (2009). Genetic variation in il28b predicts Hepatitis C treatmentinduced viral clearance. *Nature*, *461*, 399–401. PMID:19684573

Geetha, M., & Wahi, A. K. (2001). Antidiabetic activity of *Barleria prionitis* Linn. *Journal of Natural Remedies*, *1*, 64–66.

Geng, J., Xiao, S., Zhang, S., Liu, C., Li, Y., Ji, J., & Xu, B. et al. (2014). Clinical effectiveness of recombinant adenovirus-p53 combined with radiotherapy in advanced soft tissue sarcoma: A report of 37 cases. *Journal of Clinical Oncology*, 32.

Gerger, A., LaBonte, M., & Lenz, H. J. (2011). Molecular predictors of response to antiangiogenesis therapies. *Cancer Journal (Sudbury, Mass.)*, *17*(2), 134–141. doi:10.1097/PPO.0b013e318212db3c PMID:21427557

Gerlinger, M., Rowan, A. J., Horswell, S., Larkin, J., Endesfelder, D., Gronroos, E., & Swanton, C. et al. (2012). Intratumor heterogeneity and branched evolution revealed by multiregion sequencing. *The New England Journal of Medicine*, *366*(10), 883–892. doi:10.1056/NEJMoa1113205 PMID:22397650

German, J. B., & Walzem, R. L. (2000). The health benefits of wine. *Annual Review of Nutrition*, *20*(1), 561–593. doi:10.1146/annurev.nutr.20.1.561 PMID:10940346

Gerstein, H. C., Miller, M. E., Byington, R. P., Goff, D. C., Bigger, J. T., Buse, J. B., & Friedewald, W. T. et al. (2008). Effects of intensive glucose lowering in type 2 diabetes. *The New England Journal of Medicine*, *358*(24), 2545–2559. doi:10.1056/NEJMoa0802743 PMID:18539917

Gerstein, M., & Hegyi, H. (1998). Comparing genomes in terms of protein structure: Surveys of a finite parts list. *FEMS Microbiology Reviews*, *22*(4), 277–304. doi:10.1111/j.1574-6976.1998.tb00371.x PMID:10357579

Getchell, J. P. (2013). Testing for HCV infection: An update of guidance for clinicians and laboratorians. *Morbidity and Mortality Weekly Report*, *62*, 362–365. PMID:23657112

Getts, D. R., Martin, A. J., McCarthy, D. P., Terry, R. L., Hunter, Z. N., Yap, W. T., & Miller, S. D. et al. (2012). Microparticles bearing encephalitogenic peptides induce T-cell tolerance and ameliorate experimental autoimmune encephalomyelitis. *Nature Biotechnology*, *30*(12), 1217–1224. doi:10.1038/nbt.2434 PMID:23159881

Geyer, C. E., Forster, J., Lindquist, D., Chan, S., Romieu, C. G., Pienkowski, T., & Cameron, D. et al. (2006). Lapatinib plus capecitabine for HER2-positive advanced breast cancer. *The New England Journal of Medicine*, *355*(26), 2733–2743. PMID:17192538

Ghebre, M. A., Hart, D. J., Hakim, A. J., Kato, B. S., Thompson, V., Arden, N. K., & Zhai, G. et al. (2011). Association between DHEAS and bone loss in postmenopausal women: A 15-year longitudinal population-based study. *Calcified Tissue International*, *89*(4), 295–302. doi:10.1007/s00223-011-9518-9 PMID:21789637

Ghosh, D., & Konishi, T. (2007). Anthocyanins and anthocyanin-rich extracts: Role in diabetes and eye function. *Asia Pacific Journal of Clinical Nutrition*, *16*, 200–208. PMID:17468073

Ghosh, S., & Bhattacharjee, P. (2014). Supercritical carbon dioxide extract of *Ocimum sanctum* improves nutraceutical properties of ice cream. *Nutrafood.*, *13*(2), 69–78. doi:10.1007/s13749-014-0004-7

Gibbs, W. (2005). Camel natural nanobodies. *Scientific American*, *293*(2), 78–83. doi:10.1038/scientificamerican0805-78 PMID:16053141

Gibofsky, A. (2012). Overview of epidemiology, pathophysiology, and diagnosis of rheumatoid arthritis. *The American Journal of Managed Care*, *18*(13Suppl), S295–S302. PMID:23327517

Gladstone, H. B., Nguyen, S. L., Williams, R., Ottomeyer, T., Wortzman, M., Jeffers, M., & Moy, R. L. (2000). Efficacy of hydroquinone cream (USP 4%) used alone or in combination with salicylic acid peels in improving photodamage on the neck and upper chest. *Dermatologic Surgery*, *26*(4), 333–337. doi:10.1046/j.1524-4725.2000.99233.x PMID:10759820

Gloor, M., Fluhr, J., Lehmann, L., Gehring, W., & Thieroff-Ekerdt, R. (2002). (20020. Do urea/ammonium lactate combinations achieve better skin protection and hydration than either component alone? *Skin Pharmacology and Applied Skin Physiology*, *15*(1), 35–43. doi:10.1159/000049387 PMID:11803256

Gobezie, R., Millett, P. J., Sarracino, D. S., Evans, C., & Thornhill, T. S. (2006). Proteomics: Applications to the study of rheumatoid arthritis and osteoarthritis. *The Journal of the American Academy of Orthopaedic Surgeons*, *14*(6), 325–332. PMID:16757672

Goetz, M. P., Sun, J. X., Suman, V. J., Silva, G. O., Perou, C. M., Nakamura, Y., & Yelensky, R. et al. (2015). Loss of heterozygosity at the CYP2D6 locus in breast cancer: Implications for germline pharmacogenetic studies. *Journal of the National Cancer Institute*, *107*(2). PMID:25490892

Goldfaben, G. (2009). *Revitalize Aging Skin with Topical Vitamin C*. Life Extension Magazine.

Goldstein, S. L. (2011). Acute kidney injury biomarkers: Renal angina and the need for a renal troponin I. *BMC Medicine*, *9*(1), 135. doi:10.1186/1741-7015-9-135 PMID:22189039

Golmakani, M. T., & Rezaei, K. (2008). Comparison of microwave-assisted hydrodistillation with the traditional hydrodistillation method in the extraction of essential oils from *Thymus vulgaris* L. *Food Chemistry*, *109*(4), 925–930. doi:10.1016/j.foodchem.2007.12.084 PMID:26050009

Goncalves, L. D. R., Campanhon, I. B., Domingues, R. R., Leme, A. F. P., & Dasilva, M. R. S. (2014). Comparative salivary proteome of hepatitis B- and C-infected patients. *PLoS ONE*, 1–13.

Goodman, G. J. (2011). Treatment of acne scarring. *International Journal of Dermatology*, *50*(10), 1179–1194. doi:10.1111/j.1365-4632.2011.05029.x PMID:21950285

Goodman, L. S., Wintrobe, M. M., Dameshek, W., Goodman, M. J., Gilman, A., & McLennan, M. T. (1984). Landmark article Sept. 21, 1946: nitrogen mustard therapy: use of methyl-bis(betachloroethyl)amine hydrochloride and tris(betachloroethyl)amine hydrochloride for Hodgkin's disease, lymphosarcoma, leukemia and certain allied and miscellaneous disorders by Louis S. Goodman, Maxwell M. Wintrobe, William Dameshek, Morton J. Goodman, Alfred Gilman and Margaret T. McLennan. *Journal of the American Medical Association*, *251*(17), 2255–2261. PMID:6368885

Gopan, A. (2014). *Sunheal*. Retrieved 15.6.2015, from http://goarticles.com/article/SUNHEAL-Best-for-Sun-Protection/9522049

Gornitsky, M., Shenouda, G., Sultanem, K., Katz, H., Hier, M., Black, M., & Velly, A. M. (2004). Double-blind randomized, placebo-controlled study of pilocarpine to salvage salivary gland function during radiotherapy of patients with head and neck cancer. *Oral Radiology & Endodontology*, *98*, 45–52.

Gorre, M. E., Mohammed, M., Ellwood, K., Hsu, N., Paquette, R., Rao, P. N., & Sawyers, C. L. (2001). Clinical resistance to STI-571 cancer therapy caused by BCR-ABL gene mutation or amplification. *Science*, *293*(5531), 876–880. doi:10.1126/science.1062538 PMID:11423618

Gothoskar, A. V. (2004). Resealed Erythrocytes: A Review. *Pharmaceutical Technology*, 140-158.

Gould, S. E. (2013). The bacteria in breast milk. *Scientific American*, 7.

Grace, E. (2013). *How to choose the best supplement*. Health Beacon.

Grasmader, K., Verwohlt, P. L., Rietschel, M., Dragicevic, A., Muller, M., Hiemke, C., & Rao, M. L. et al. (2004). Impact of polymorphisms of cytochrome-P450 isoenzymes 2C9, 2C19 and 2D6 on plasma concentrations and clinical effects of antidepressants in a naturalistic clinical setting. *European Journal of Clinical Pharmacology*, *60*(5), 329–336. doi:10.1007/s00228-004-0766-8 PMID:15168101

Gray, J. (2003). *Carbohydrates: Nutritional and Health Aspects*. Washington, DC: ILSI Press.

Green, R., & Widder, K. J. (1987). *Methods in Enzymology*. San Diego, CA: Academic Press.

Grimley, E. J., Malouf, R., Huppert, F., & van Niekerk, J. K. (2006). Malouf, Reem, ed. Dehydroepiandrosterone (DHEA) supplementation for cognitive function in healthy elderly people. Cochrane Database of Systematic Reviews, 4.

Grossman, E., Laudon, M., & Zisapel, N. (2011). Effect of melatonin on nocturnal blood pressure: Meta-analysis of randomized controlled trials. *Vascular Health and Risk Management*, *7*, 577–584. PMID:21966222

Grossman, R. (2005). The role of dimethylaminoethanol in cosmetic dermatology. *American Journal of Clinical Dermatology*, *6*(1), 39–47. doi:10.2165/00128071-200506010-00005 PMID:15675889

Grover, J. K., Vats, V., & Rathi, S. S. (2000). Anti-hyperglycemic effect of *Eugeniajambolanaand* *Tinosporacordifoliain* experimental diabetes and their effects on key metabolic enzymes involved in carbohydrate metabolism. *Journal of Ethnopharmacology*, *73*(3), 461–470. doi:10.1016/S0378-8741(00)00319-6 PMID:11091000

Gruen, V. E. C., & Wong, H. X. (1982). Immunomodulatory and antitumour activities of a polysaccharide-peptide complex from a mycelial culture of Trichoderma sp. *The Sciences*, *57*, 269–281.

Guclu-Ustundag, O., & Mazza, G. (2008). Extraction of saponins and cyclopeptides from cow cockle seed with pressurized low polarity water. *Food Science and Technology (Campinas.)*, *41*, 1600–1606.

Gujrati, M., & Lu, Z. (2013). Targeted systemic delivery of therapeutic siRNA. In *Gene Therapy of Cancer* (3rd ed.; pp. 47–65). San Diego, CA: Elsevier.

Gunasekara, T., Haile, T., Nigusse, T., & Dhanaraju, M. (2014). Nanotechnology: An effective tool for enhancing bioavailability and bioactivity of phytomedicine. *Asian Pacific Journal of Tropical Biomedicine*, *4*(1), S1–S7. doi:10.12980/APJTB.4.2014C980 PMID:25183064

Gund, P. (2000). Evolution of the pharmacophore Concept in Pharmaceutical Research. In O. F. Güner (Ed.), *Pharmacophore Perception, Development, and Use in Drug Design*. La Jolla, CA: International University Line.

Gupta, A. K., & Gupta, M. (2005). Synthesis and surface engineering of iron oxide nanoparticles for biomedical applications. *Biomaterials*, *26*(18), 3995–4021. doi:10.1016/j.biomaterials.2004.10.012 PMID:15626447

Gupta, C., & Prakash, D. (2014). Phytonutrients as therapeutic agents. *Journal of Complementary and Integrative Medicine*, *11*(3), 151–169. doi:10.1515/jcim-2013-0021 PMID:25051278

Gupta, R. K., Gupta, S., & Samuel, K. C. (1977). Blood sugar lowering effects of various fractions of onion. *Indian Journal of Experimental Biology*, *15*, 313–314. PMID:914348

Gurib-Fakim, A. (2006). Medicinal plants: Traditions of yesterday and drugs of tomorrow. *Molecular Aspects of Medicine*, *27*(1), 1–93. doi:10.1016/j.mam.2005.07.008 PMID:16105678

Guyton, A. C., & Hall, J. E. (1996). *Red Blood Cells, Anemia and Polycytemia. In Textbook of Medical Physiology* (pp. 425–433). Philadelphia, PA: W.B. Saunders.

Guyton, A. C., & Hall, J. E. (1996). *Transport of Oxygen and Carbon Dioxide in the Blood and Body Fluids. In Textbook of Medical Physiology* (pp. 513–523). Philadelphia, PA: W.B. Saunders.

Guyton, A. C., & Hall, J. E. (2006). *Textbook of Medical Physiology* (11th ed.). Elsevier Inc.

Haberlandt, G. (1902). Kulturversuche mit isolierten Pflanzenzellen.*S. B. Weisen Wien Naturwissenschaften*, *111*, 69–92.

Hajipour, M. J., Laurent, S., Aghaie, A., Rezaee, F., & Mahmoudi, M. (2014). Personalized protein coronas: A "key" factor at the nanobiointerface. *Biomaterials Science*, *2*(9), 1210–1221. doi:10.1039/C4BM00131A

Hajipour, M. J., Raheb, J., Akhavan, O., Arjmand, S., Mashinchian, O., Rahman, M., & Mahmoudi, M. et al. (2015). Personalized disease-specific protein corona influences the therapeutic impact of graphene oxide. *Nanoscale*, *7*(19), 8978–8994. doi:10.1039/C5NR00520E PMID:25920546

Hall, M. G., Wilks, M. F., Provan, W. M., Eksborg, S., & Lumholtz, B. (2001). Pharmacokinetics and pharmacodynamics of NTBC (2-(2-nitro-4-fluoromethylbenzoyl)-1,3-cyclohexanedione) and mesotrione, inhibitors of 4-hydroxyphenyl pyruvate dioxygenase (HPPD) following a single dose to healthy male volunteers. *British Journal of Clinical Pharmacology*, *52*(2), 169–177. doi:10.1046/j.0306-5251.2001.01421.x PMID:11488774

Hall, S. S., Mitragotri, S., & Daugherty, P. S. (2007). Identification of peptide ligands facilitating nanoparticle attachment to erythrocytes. *Biotechnology Progress*, *23*(3), 749–754. doi:10.1021/bp0603331 PMID:17469847

Hamada, Y., Seto, Y., Yago, K., & Kuroyama, M. (2012). Investigation and threshold of optimum blood concentration of voriconazole: A descriptive statistical meta-analysis. *Journal of Infection and Chemotherapy*, *18*(4), 501–507. doi:10.1007/s10156-011-0363-6 PMID:22231601

Hamburger, M. (2002). *Isatis tinctoria* – From the rediscovery of an ancient medicinal plant towards a novel anti-inflammatory phytopharmaceutical. *Phytochemistry Reviews*, *1*(3), 333–344. doi:10.1023/A:1026095608691

Hamers-Casterman, C., Atarouch, T., Muyldermans, S., Bendolman, N., & Hamers, R. (1993). Naturally occurring antibodies devoid of light chains. *Nature*, *363*(6428), 446–448. doi:10.1038/363446a0 PMID:8502296

Hamidi, M., & Tajerzadeh, H. (2003). Carrier erythrocytes: An overview. *Drug Delivery*, *10*(1), 9–20. doi:10.1080/713840329 PMID:12554359

Hamidi, M., Tajerzadeh, H., Dehpour, A. R., Rouini, M. R., & Ejtemaee-Mehr, S. (2001). *In vitro* characterization of human intact erythrocytes loaded by enalaprilat. *Drug Delivery*, *8*(4), 223–230. doi:10.1080/107175401317245903 PMID:11757780

Hamrick, I., & Counts, S. H. (2008). Vitamin and mineral supplements. *Wellness Prevent*, *35*(4), 729–747. PMID:18928827

Hamzawy, M., El-Denshary, E., Hassan, N., Mannaa, F., & Abdel-Wahhab, M. (2013). Dietary Supplementation of *Calendula officinalis* Counteracts the Oxidative Stress and Liver Damage Resulted from Aflatoxin. *ISRB Nutrition*, 538427-538436.

Hansch, C. (1969). A quantitative approach to biochemical structure-activity relationships. *Accounts of Chemical Research*, *2*(8), 232–239. doi:10.1021/ar50020a002

Haraoui, B., & Bykerk, V. (2007). Etanercept in the treatment of rheumatoid arthritis. *Ther Clin Risk Manag*, *3*(1), 99–105. doi:10.2147/tcrm.2007.3.1.99 PMID:18360618

Harborne, J. B., & Williams, C. A. (2000). Advances in flavonoid research since 1992. *Phytochemistry*, *55*(6), 481–504. doi:10.1016/S0031-9422(00)00235-1 PMID:11130659

Hardeland, R., Pandi-Perumal, S. R., & Cardinali, D. P. (2006). Melatonin. *The International Journal of Biochemistry & Cell Biology*, *38*(3), 313–316. doi:10.1016/j.biocel.2005.08.020 PMID:16219483

Harris, G. K., Qian, Y., Leonard, S. S., Sbarra, D. C., & Shi, X. L. (2006). Luteolin and chrysin differentially inhibit cyclooxygenase-2 expression and scavenge reactive oxygen species but similarly inhibit prostaglandin-E2 formation in RAW 264.7 cells. *The Journal of Nutrition*, *136*(6), 1517–1521. PMID:16702314

Harris, J. M., Martin, N. E., & Modi, M. (2001). Pegylation: A novel process for modifying pharmacokinetics. *Clinical Pharmacokinetics*, *40*(7), 539–551. doi:10.2165/00003088-200140070-00005 PMID:11510630

Harris, R. C. (1977). Enzyme Replacement in Red Cells. *The New England Journal of Medicine*, *296*(16), 942–943. doi:10.1056/NEJM197704212961618 PMID:846521

Hassan, A., Burhenne, J., Riedel, K. D., Weiss, J., Mikus, G., Haefeli, W. E., & Czock, D. (2011). Modulators of very low voriconazole concentrations in routine therapeutic drug monitoring. *Therapeutic Drug Monitoring*, *33*(1), 86–93. doi:10.1097/FTD.0b013e31820530cd PMID:21192313

Hathout, Y. (2007). Approaches to the study of the cell secretome. *Expert Review of Proteomics*, *4*(2), 239–248. PMID:17425459

Hattori, A., Migitaka, H., Iigo, M., Itoh, M., Yamamoto, K., Ohtani-Kaneko, R., & Reiter, R. J. et al. (1995). Identification of melatonin in plants and its effects on plasma melatonin levels and binding to melatonin receptors in vertebrates. *Biochemistry and Molecular Biology International*, *35*(3), 627–634. PMID:7773197

Hauschild, A., Grob, J. J., Demidov, L. V., Jouary, T., Gutzmer, R., Millward, M., & Chapman, P. B. et al. (2012). Dabrafenib in BRAF-mutated metastatic melanoma: A multicentre, open-label, phase 3 randomised controlled trial. *Lancet*, *380*(9839), 358–365. doi:10.1016/S0140-6736(12)60868-X PMID:22735384

Havrlentova, et al.. (2011). Cereal β-glucans and their significance for the preparation of functional foods-a review. *Czech Journal of Food Science*, *29*(1), 1–14.

Hawiger, D., Inaba, K., Dorsett, Y., Guo, M., Mahnke, K., Rivera, M., & Nussenzweig, M. C. et al. (2001). Dendritic cells induce peripheral T cell unresponsiveness under steady state conditions in vivo. *The Journal of Experimental Medicine*, *194*(6), 769–779. doi:10.1084/jem.194.6.769 PMID:11560993

Hawksworth, D. L. (2001). Mushrooms: The extent of the unexplored potential. *Int. J. Med. Mushr*, *3*(4), 333–337. doi:10.1615/IntJMedMushr.v3.i4.50

Hayat, M. A. (2013). Introduction to Autophagy: Cancer, Other Pathologies, Inflammation, Immunity, Infection, and Aging: Vol. 1-4. *Autophagy: Cancer, Other Pathologies, Inflammation, Immunity, Infection, and Aging*. Elsevier Inc.

Hayden, C. G., Roberts, M. S., & Benson, H. A. (1997). Systemic absorption of sunscreen after topical application. *Lancet*, *350*(9081), 863–864. doi:10.1016/S0140-6736(05)62032-6 PMID:9310609

Hayes, C. N., Imamura, M., Aikata, H., & Chayama, K. (2012). Genetics of IL28B and HCV response to infection and treatment. Nature Reviews. *Gastroenterologia y Hepatologia*, *9*, 406–417.

Hayes, J. D., Kelleher, M. O., & Eggleston, I. M. (2008). The cancer chemopreventive actions of phytochemicals derived from glucosinolates. *European Journal of Nutrition*, *47*(S2), 73–88. doi:10.1007/s00394-008-2009-8 PMID:18458837

He, H., Yin, J. Y., Xu, Y. J., Li, X., Zhang, Y., Liu, Z. G., . . . Liu, Z. Q. (2014). Association of ABCB1 polymorphisms with the efficacy of ondansetron in chemotherapy-induced nausea and vomiting. *Clinical Therapeutics, 36*(8), 1242-1252.

Heber, D., Berdanier, C. D., Dwyer, J. T., & Feldman, E. B. (2008). Plant Foods and Phytochemicals in human health. CRC Press.

Hebert, L. E., Weuve, J., Scherr, P. A., & Evans, D. A. (2013). Alzheimer disease in the United States (2010-2050) estimated using the 2010 census. *Neurology*, *80*(19), 1778–17783. doi:10.1212/WNL.0b013e31828726f5 PMID:23390181

Hehlgans, T., & Pfeffer, K. (2005). The intriguing biology of the tumour necrosis factor/tumour necrosis factor receptor superfamily: Players, rules and the games. *Immunology*, *115*, 1–20. PMID:15819693

Heinrich, M. C., Corless, C. L., Demetri, G. D., Blanke, C. D., von Mehren, M., Joensuu, H., & Fletcher, J. A. et al. (2003). Kinase mutations and imatinib response in patients with metastatic gastrointestinal stromal tumor. *Journal of Clinical Oncology*, *21*(23), 4342–4349. doi:10.1200/JCO.2003.04.190 PMID:14645423

Heinrich, M., & Teoh, H. L. (2004). Galanthamine from snowdrop-the development of a modern drug against Alzheimer's disease from local Caucasian knowledge. *Journal of Ethnopharmacology*, *92*(2-3), 147–162. doi:10.1016/j.jep.2004.02.012 PMID:15137996

Heisterkamp, N., Stam, K., Groffen, J., de Klein, A., & Grosveld, G. (1985). Structural organization of the bcr gene and its role in the Ph' translocation. *Nature*, *315*(6022), 758–761. doi:10.1038/315758a0 PMID:2989703

He, L. F., Wang, Y. G., Xiao, T., Zhang, K. J., Li, G. C., & Gu, J. F. (2009). Suppression of cancer growth in mice by adeno-associated virus vector-mediated IFN-beta expression driven by hTERT promoter. *Cancer Letters*, *286*, 196–205. PMID:19564073

Henke, J. M., & Bassler, B. L. (2004). Bacterial social engagements. *Trends in Cell Biology*, *14*(11), 648–656. doi:10.1016/j.tcb.2004.09.012 PMID:15519854

Henry, J. (2009). Processing, manufacturing, uses and labeling of fat in the food supply. *Annals of Nutrition & Metabolism*, *55*(1-3), 273–300. doi:10.1159/000229006 PMID:19752546

Herbst, R. S., Ansari, R., Bustin, F., Flynn, P., Hart, L., Otterson, G. A., & Hainsworth, J. et al. (2011). Efficacy of bevacizumab plus erlotinib versus erlotinib alone in advanced non-small-cell lung cancer after failure of standard first-line chemotherapy (BeTa): A double-blind, placebo-controlled, phase 3 trial. *Lancet*, *377*(9780), 1846–1854. doi:10.1016/S0140-6736(11)60545-X PMID:21621716

Hercberg, S., Ezzedine, K., Guinot, C., Preziosi, P., Galan, P., Bertrais, S., & Malvy, D. (2007). Antioxidant supplementation increases the risk of skin cancers in women but not in men. *The Journal of Nutrition*, *137*, 2098–2105. PMID:17709449

Herrero-Beaumont, G., Martinez Calatrava, M. J., & Castaneda, S. (2012). Abatacept mechanism of action: Concordance with its clinical profile. *Reumatol Clin*, *8*(2), 78–83. doi:10.1016/j.reuma.2011.08.002 PMID:22104048

Herrero, M., Ibáñez, E., Fanali, S., & Cifuentes, A. (2007). Quantitation of chiral amino acids from microalgae by MEKC and LIF detection. *Electrophoresis*, *28*(15), 2701–2709. doi:10.1002/elps.200600599 PMID:17592610

Herrero, M., Vicente, M. J., Cifuentes, A., & Ibanez, E. (2007). Characterization by high performance liquid chromatography/electrospray ionization quadrupole time-of-flight mass spectrometry of the lipid fraction of *Spirulina platensis* pressurized ethanol extract. *Rapid Communications in Mass Spectrometry*, *21*(11), 1729–1738. doi:10.1002/rcm.3017 PMID:17487827

Heyland, D. K. (2001). In search of the magic nutraceuticals: Problems with current approaches. *The Journal of Nutrition*, *131*(9), 2591–2595. PMID:11533319

Hicheri, Y., Cook, G., & Cordonnier, C. (2012). Antifungal prophylaxis in haematology patients: The role of voriconazole. *Clinical Microbiology and Infection*, *18*(Suppl 2), 1–15. doi:10.1111/j.1469-0691.2012.03772.x PMID:22409648

Hicks, J. K., Crews, K. R., Flynn, P., Haidar, C. E., Daniels, C. C., Yang, W., & Relling, M. V. et al. (2014). Voriconazole plasma concentrations in immunocompromised pediatric patients vary by CYP2C19 diplotypes. *Pharmacogenomics*, *15*(8), 1065–1078. doi:10.2217/pgs.14.53 PMID:25084200

Hicks, J. K., Swen, J. J., Thorn, C. F., Sangkuhl, K., Kharasch, E. D., Ellingrod, V. L., & Stingl, J. C. et al. (2013). Clinical Pharmacogenetics Implementation Consortium guideline for CYP2D6 and CYP2C19 genotypes and dosing of tricyclic antidepressants. *Clinical Pharmacology and Therapeutics*, *93*(5), 402–408. doi:10.1038/clpt.2013.2 PMID:23486447

Hidalgo, M., Oruna-Concha, M. J., Kolida, S., Walton, G. E., Kallithraka, S., Spencer, J. P., & de Pascual-Teresa, S. (2012). Metabolism of anthocyanins by human gut microflora and their influence on gut bacterial growth. *Journal of Agricultural and Food Chemistry*, *60*(15), 3882–3890. doi:10.1021/jf3002153 PMID:22439618

Hidehiko, S., Hooi-Ming, L., & Norihiro, N. (2010). DNA microarray analysis of rheumatoid arthritis susceptibility genes identified by genome-wide association studies. *Arthritis Research & Therapy*, *12*, 401. PMID:20346099

Higgins, S., & Wesley, N. (2015). Topical retinoids and cosmeceuticals: Where is the scientific evidence to recommend products to patients? *Current Dermatology Reports*, *4*(2), 56–62. doi:10.1007/s13671-015-0102-9

Hippocrates, . (1931). *Nature of man* (vol. 4). Cambridge, MA: Harward University Press.

Hirn, S., Semmler-Behnke, M., Schleh, C., Wenk, A., Lipka, J., Schaffler, M., & Kreyling, W. G. et al. (2011). Particle size-dependent and surface charge-dependent biodistribution of gold nanoparticles after intravenous administration. *European Journal of Pharmaceutics and Biopharmaceutics*, *77*(3), 407–416. doi:10.1016/j.ejpb.2010.12.029 PMID:21195759

Hodek, P., Trebil, P., & Stiborova, M. (2002). Flavonoids- potent and versatile biologically active compounds interacting with cytochromes. *Chemico-Biological Interactions*, *139*(1), 1–21. doi:10.1016/S0009-2797(01)00285-X PMID:11803026

Hodgson, J. M., Puddey, I. B., Burke, V., Beilin, L. J., & Jordan, N. (1999). Effect of blood pressure of drinking green and black tea. *Journal of Hypertension*, *17*(4), 457–463. doi:10.1097/00004872-199917040-00002 PMID:10404946

Hogquist, K. A., Baldwin, T. A., & Jameson, S. C. (2005). Central tolerance: Learning self-control in the thymus. *Nature Reviews. Immunology*, *5*(10), 772–782. doi:10.1038/nri1707 PMID:16200080

Holash, J., Davis, S., Papadopoulos, N., Croll, S. D., Ho, L., Russell, M., & Rudge, J. S. et al. (2002). VEGF-Trap: A VEGF blocker with potent antitumor effects. *Proceedings of the National Academy of Sciences of the United States of America*, *99*(17), 11393–11398. doi:10.1073/pnas.172398299 PMID:12177445

Holly, R., Ramage, G., Renuka, K., Erik, V., Jeffrey, R. J., John, V. D., & Billy, N. et al. (2015). A Combined Proteomics/Genomics Approach Links Hepatitis C Virus Infection with Nonsense-Mediated mRNA Decay. *Molecular Cell*, *57*(2), 329–340. PMID:25616068

Holman, R. R., Paul, S. K., Bethel, M. A., Matthews, D. R., & Neil, H. A. (2013). 10-year follow-up of intensive glucose control in type 2 diabetes. *The New England Journal of Medicine*, *359*(15), 1577–1589. doi:10.1056/NEJMoa0806470 PMID:18784090

Holodniy, M., Koch, J., Mistal, M., Schmidt, J. M., Khandwala, A., Pennington, J. E., & Porter, S. B. (1999). A double blind, randomized, placebo-controlled phase II study to assess the safety and efficacy of orally administered SP-303 for the symptomatic treatment of diarrhea in patients with AIDS. *The American Journal of Gastroenterology*, *94*(11), 3267–3273. doi:10.1111/j.1572-0241.1999.01535.x PMID:10566728

Holstege, F. C., Wyrick, J. E., Lee, T. I., Hengartner, C. J., Green, M. R., Golub, T. R., & Young, R. A. et al. (1998). Dissecting the regulatory circuitry of a eukaryotic genome. *Cell*, *95*(5), 717–728. doi:10.1016/S0092-8674(00)81641-4 PMID:9845373

Holtcamp, W. (2012). The emerging science of BMAA: Do cyanobacteria contribute to neurodegenerative disease? *Environmental Health Perspectives*, *120*(3), a110–a116. doi:10.1289/ehp.120-a110 PMID:22382274

Holton, R. A., Somoza, C., Kim, H. B., Liang, F., Biediger, R. J., Boatman, P. D., & Kim, S. (1994). First total synthesis of taxol. 1. Functionalization of the B ring. *Journal of the American Chemical Society*, *116*(4), 1597–1598. doi:10.1021/ja00083a066

Hondermarck, H. (2003). Breast cancer: When proteomics challenges biological complexity. *Molecular & Cellular Proteomics*, *2*, 281–291. PMID:12775769

Hooper, M., Kirby, G. C., Kulkarni, M. M., Kulkarni, S. N., Nagasampagi, B. A., O'Neill, M. J., & Warhurst, D. C. (1990). Antimalarial activity of parthenin and its derivatives. *European Journal of Medicinal Chemistry*, *25*(9), 717–723. doi:10.1016/0223-5234(90)90190-E

Hoshaw, R. A., Zimmerman, K. G., & Menter, A. (1985). Ochronosislike pigmentation from hydroquinone bleaching creams in American blacks. *Archives of Dermatology*, *121*(1), 105–108. doi:10.1001/archderm.1985.01660010109032 PMID:3966811

Hoskins, J. M., Goldberg, R. M., Qu, P., Ibrahim, J. G., & McLeod, H. L. (2007). UGT1A1*28 genotype and irinotecan-induced neutropenia: Dose matters. *Journal of the National Cancer Institute*, *99*(17), 1290–1295. doi:10.1093/jnci/djm115 PMID:17728214

Hossein, K., Mehdi, F., Seyed, H. R. M., & Hamid, R. M. (2012). Hepatitis C Virus - Proteins, Diagnosis, Treatment and New Approaches for Vaccine Development. *Asian Pacific Journal of Cancer Prevention*, *13*, 5917–5935. PMID:23464383

Huang, J. S., Guh, J. Y., Chen, J. C., Hung, W. C., Lai, Y. H., & Chuang, L. Y. (2001). Role of receptor for advanced glycation end-product (RAGE) and the JAK/STAT-signaling pathway in AGE-induced collagen production in NRK-49F cells. *Journal of Cellular Biochemistry*, *81*(1), 102–113. doi:10.1002/1097-4644(20010401)81:1<102::AID-JCB1027>3.0.CO;2-Y PMID:11180401

Hueber, W., & Robinson, W. (2006). Proteomic biomarkers for autoimmune disease. *Proteomics*, *6*(14), 4100–4105. PMID:16786488

Huezo-Diaz, P., Perroud, N., Spencer, E. P., Smith, R., Sim, S., Virding, S., & Aitchison, K. J. et al. (2012). CYP2C19 genotype predicts steady state escitalopram concentration in GENDEP. *Journal of Psychopharmacology (Oxford, England)*, *26*(3), 398–407. doi:10.1177/0269881111414451 PMID:21926427

Hunter, Z., McCarthy, D. P., Yap, W. T., Harp, C. T., Getts, D. R., Shea, L. D., & Miller, S. D. (2014). A biodegradable nanoparticle platform for the induction of antigen-specific immune tolerance for treatment of autoimmune disease. *ACS Nano*, *8*(3), 2148–2160. doi:10.1021/nn405033r PMID:24559284

Huppertz, B. (2011). Nanoparticles: Barrier thickness matters. *Nature Nanotechnology*, *6*(12), 758–759. doi:10.1038/nnano.2011.206 PMID:22056727

Hurakadle, P. J., Gadkar, S. S., & Pai, S. R. (2010). Callus culture studies on *Jasminum malabaricum*-An endemic medicinal plant. *Planta Medica, 77.*

Hurvitz, S. A., Dirix, L., Kocsis, J., Bianchi, G. V., Lu, J., Vinholes, J., & Perez, E. A. et al. (2013). Phase II randomized study of trastuzumab emtansine versus trastuzumab plus docetaxel in patients with human epidermal growth factor receptor 2-positive metastatic breast cancer. *Journal of Clinical Oncology*, *31*(9), 1157–1163. doi:10.1200/JCO.2012.44.9694 PMID:23382472

Hurwitz, H. I., Tebbutt, N. C., Kabbinavar, F., Giantonio, B. J., Guan, Z. Z., Mitchell, L., & Tabernero, J. et al. (2013). Efficacy and safety of bevacizumab in metastatic colorectal cancer: Pooled analysis from seven randomized controlled trials. *The Oncologist*, *18*(9), 1004–1012. doi:10.1634/theoncologist.2013-0107 PMID:23881938

Hu, S. X., Kyulo, N. L., Xia, V. W., Hillebrand, D. J., & Hu, K. Q. (2009). Factors associated with hepatic fibrosis in patients with chronic hepatitis C: A retrospective study of a large cohort of US patients. *Journal of Clinical Gastroenterology*, *43*, 758–764. PMID:19238091

Huseini, H. F., Larijani, B., Heshmat, R., Fakhrzadeh, H., Radjabipour, B., Toliat, T., & Raza, M. (2006). The efficacy of silybum marianum (L.) Gaertn. (silymarin) in the treatment of type II diabetes: A randomized, double-blind, placebo-controlled, clinical trial. *Phytotherapy Research*, *20*(12), 1036–1039. doi:10.1002/ptr.1988 PMID:17072885

Hussain, H., Krohn, K., Draeger, S., Meier, K., & Schulz, B. (2009). Bioactive chemical constituents of a sterile endophytic fungus from *Meliotus dentatus*. *Records of Natural Products*, *3*, 114–117.

Hutchinson, M., Fox, R. J., Havrdova, E., Kurukulasuriya, N. C., Sarda, S. P., Agarwal, S., & Deniz, B. et al. (2014). Efficacy and safety of BG-12 (dimethyl fumarate) and other disease-modifying therapies for the treatment of relapsing-remitting multiple sclerosis: A systematic review and mixed treatment comparison. *Current Medical Research and Opinion*, *30*(4), 613–627. doi:10.1185/03007995.2013.863755 PMID:24195574

Hüttenhain, R., Soste, M., Selevsek, N., Rãist, H., Sethi, A., Carapito, C., ... Moritz, R.L. (2012). Reproducible Quantification of Cancer-Associated Proteins in Body Fluids Using Targeted Proteomics. *Science Translational Medicine, 4*(142).

Iher, G. M., Glew, R. M., & Schnure, F. W. (1973). Enzyme Loading of Erythrocytes. *Proceedings of the National Academy of Sciences of the United States of America, 70*(9), 2663–2666. doi:10.1073/pnas.70.9.2663 PMID:4354859

Ihler, G. M. (1983). Erythrocyte Carriers. *Pharmacology & Therapeutics, 20*(2), 151–169. doi:10.1016/0163-7258(83)90037-2 PMID:6351110

Ihler, G. M., & Tsang, H. C. W. (1987). Hypotonic Hemolysis Methods For Entrapment of Agents in Resealed Erythrocytes.[series]. *Methods in Enzymology, 149*, 221–229. doi:10.1016/0076-6879(87)49059-9 PMID:3121983

Ihler, G., Lantzy, A., Purpura, J., & Glew, R. H. (1975). Enzymatic Degradation of Uricase-Loaded Human Erythrocytes. *The Journal of Clinical Investigation, 56*(3), 595–602. doi:10.1172/JCI108129 PMID:1159075

Ilan, Y., Maron, R., Tukpah, A.-M., Maioli, T. U., Murugaiyan, G., Yang, K., & Weiner, H. L. (2010). Induction of regulatory T cells decreases adipose inflammation and alleviates insulin resistance in ob/ob mice. *Proceedings of the National Academy of Sciences of the United States of America, 107*(21), 9765–9770. doi:10.1073/pnas.0908771107 PMID:20445103

Imura, K., & Okada, A. (1998). Amino acid metabolism in pediatric patients. *Nutrition (Burbank, Los Angeles County, Calif.), 14*(1), 143–148. doi:10.1016/S0899-9007(97)00230-X PMID:9437700

Ingelman-Sundberg, M. (2004). Pharmacogenetics of cytochrome P450 and its applications in drug therapy: The past, present and future. *Trends in Pharmacological Sciences, 25*(4), 193–200. doi:10.1016/j.tips.2004.02.007 PMID:15063083

Innocenti, F., Schilsky, R. L., Ramirez, J., Janisch, L., Undevia, S., House, L. K., & Ratain, M. J. et al. (2014). Dose-finding and pharmacokinetic study to optimize the dosing of irinotecan according to the UGT1A1 genotype of patients with cancer. *Journal of Clinical Oncology, 32*(22), 2328–2334. doi:10.1200/JCO.2014.55.2307 PMID:24958824

Institute of Medicine (IM). (1998). *Food and Nutrition Board. Dietary Reference Intakes for Thiamin, Riboflavin, Niacin, Vitamin B6, Folate, Vitamin B12, Pantothenic Acid, Biotin, and Choline*. Washington, DC: National Academy Press.

Iragavarapu, C., Mustafa, M., Akinleye, A., Furqan, M., Mittal, V., Cang, S., & Liu, D. (2015). Novel ALK inhibitors in clinical use and development. *Journal of Hematology and Oncology, 8*(1), 17. PMID:25888090

Iriti, M., Faoro, F. (2006). Grape phytochemicals: A bouquet of old and new nutraceuticals for human health. *Med Hypoth*, 833-838.

Iriti, M., & Faoro, F. (2009). Bioactivity of grape chemicals for human health. *Nat. Prod. Commun., 4*(5), 611–634. PMID:19445314

Irvin, W. J. Jr, Walko, C. M., Weck, K. E., Ibrahim, J. G., Chiu, W. K., Dees, E. C., & Carey, L. A. et al. (2011). Genotype-guided tamoxifen dosing increases active metabolite exposure in women with reduced CYP2D6 metabolism: A multicenter study. *Journal of Clinical Oncology, 29*(24), 3232–3239. doi:10.1200/JCO.2010.31.4427 PMID:21768473

Ishida, T., & Kiwada, H. (2008). Accelerated blood clearance (ABC) phenomenon upon repeated injection of PEGylated liposomes. *International Journal of Pharmaceutics, 354*(1-2), 56–62. doi:10.1016/j.ijpharm.2007.11.005 PMID:18083313

Ishikawa, T., Hirano, H., Onishi, Y., Sakurai, A., & Tarui, S. (2004). Functional evaluation of ABCB1 (P-glycoprotein) polymorphisms: High-speed screening and structure-activity relationship analyses. *Drug Metabolism and Pharmacokinetics, 19*(1), 1–14. doi:10.2133/dmpk.19.1 PMID:15499164

Ismail-Beigi, F., Craven, T., Banerji, M. A., Basile, J., Calles, J., Cohen, R. M., & Hamilton, B. et al. (2010). Effect of intensive treatment of hyperglycaemia on microvascular outcomes in type 2 diabetes: An analysis of the ACCORD randomised trial. *Lancet*, *376*(9739), 419–430. doi:10.1016/S0140-6736(10)60576-4 PMID:20594588

Ito, K., Lim, S., Caramori, G., Cosio, B., Chung, K. F., Adcock, I. M., & Barnes, P. J. (2002). A molecular mechanism of action of theophylline: Induction of histone deacetylase activity to decrease inflammatory gene expression. *Proceedings of the National Academy of Sciences of the United States of America*, *99*(13), 8921–8926. doi:10.1073/pnas.132556899 PMID:12070353

Ivanovic, J., Meyer, F., Stamenic, M., Jaeger, P., Zizovic, I., & Eggers, R. (2014). Pretreatment of natural materials used for supercritical fluid extraction of commercial phytopharmaceticals. *Chemical Engineering & Technology*, *9*(9), 1606–1611. doi:10.1002/ceat.201300715

Iwu, M. M., Igboko, A. O., Onwubiko, H., & Ndu, U. E. (1988). Effect of cajaminose from Cajanus cajan on gelation and oxygen affinity of sickle cell haemoglobin. *Journal of Ethnopharmacology*, *23*(1), 99–104. doi:10.1016/0378-8741(88)90118-3 PMID:3419206

Jabbour, E., Kantarjian, H., O'Brien, S., Shan, J., Quintas-Cardama, A., Faderl, S., & Cortes, J. et al. (2011). The achievement of an early complete cytogenetic response is a major determinant for outcome in patients with early chronic phase chronic myeloid leukemia treated with tyrosine kinase inhibitors. *Blood*, *118*(17), 4541–4546, quiz 4759. doi:10.1182/blood-2011-04-348110 PMID:21803854

Jackson, H., Braun, C. L., & Ernst, H. (2008). The chemistry of novel xanthophyll carotenoids. *The American Journal of Cardiology*, *101*(10), S50–S57. doi:10.1016/j.amjcard.2008.02.008 PMID:18474275

Jacob, R. A., & Sotoudeh, G. (2002). Vitamin C function and status in chronic disease. *Nutrition in Clinical Care*, *5*(2), 66–74. doi:10.1046/j.1523-5408.2002.00005.x PMID:12134712

Jagadeesh, R., Raaman, N., Periyasamy, K., Hariprasath, L., Thangaraj, R., Srikumar, R., & Ayyappan, S. R. (2010). Proximate analysis and antibacterial activity of edible mushroom *Volvariella Bombycina*. *Int. J. Microbiol. Res*, *1*(3), 110–113.

Jagadish, L. K., Krishnan, V. V., Shenbhagaraman, R., & Kaviyarasan, V. (2009). Comparative study on the antioxidant, anticancer and antimicrobial property of *Agaricus bisporus* (J. E. Lange) Imbach before and after boiling. *African Journal of Biotechnology*, *8*, 654–661.

Jain, R. K., & Stylianopoulos, T. (n.d.). Delivering nanomedicine to solid tumors. *Nature Reviews Clinical Oncology*, *7*(11), 653-664.

Jain, K. K. (2008). Innovations, challenges and future prospects of oncoproteomics. *Molecular Oncology*, *2*, 153–160. PMID:19383334

Jain, S., & Jain, N. K. (1997). Engineered Erythrocytes as a Drug Delivery System. *Indian Journal of Pharmaceutical Sciences*, *59*, 275–281.

Jain, S., Jain, S. K., & Dixit, V. K. (1995). Erythrocytes Based Delivery of Isoniazid: Preparation and *In Vitro* Characterization. *Indian Drugs*, *32*, 471–476.

Jain, S., Jain, S. K., & Dixit, V. K. (1997). Magnetically Guided Rat Erythrocytes Bearing Isoniazid: Preparation, Characterization, and Evaluation. *Drug Development and Industrial Pharmacy*, *23*(10), 999–1006. doi:10.3109/03639049709149153

Jaitely, V., Kanaujia, P., Venkatesan, N., Jain, S., & Vyas, S. P. (1996). Resealed Erythrocytes: Drug Carrier Potentials and Biomedical Applications. *Indian Drugs*, *33*, 589–594.

Jancik, S., Drabek, J., Radzioch, D., & Hajduch, M. (2010). Clinical relevance of KRAS in human cancers. *Journal of Biomedicine & Biotechnology*, *2010*, 150960. doi:10.1155/2010/150960 PMID:20617134

Jan, J. E., Hamilton, D., Seward, N., Fast, D. K., Freeman, R. D., & Laudon, M. (2000). Clinical trials of controlled-release melatonin in children with sleep-wake cycle disorders. *Journal of Pineal Research*, *29*(1), 34–39. doi:10.1034/j.1600-079X.2000.290105.x PMID:10949538

Jankun, J., Selman, S. H., Aniola, J., & Skrzypczak-Jankun, E. (2006). Nutraceutical inhibitors of urokinase: Potential applications in prostate cancer prevention and treatment. *Oncology Reports*, *16*, 341–346. PMID:16820913

Jarad, G., & Miner, J. H. (2009). Update on the glomerular filtration barrier. *Current Opinion in Nephrology and Hypertension*, *18*(3), 226–232. doi:10.1097/MNH.0b013e3283296044 PMID:19374010

Jaswir, I., Noviendri, D., Hasrini, R. F., & Octavianti, F. (2011). Carotenoids: Sources, medicinal properties and their application in food and nutraceutical industry. *Journal of Medicinal Plants Research*, *5*(33), 7119–7131.

Javier, C., Emiliano, C., Ana, V., Jose, P. G., Juan, A. R., & Joan, S. (2014). New Approach to Cancer Therapy Based on a Molecularly Defined Cancer Classification. *CA: a Cancer Journal for Clinicians*, *64*, 70–74. PMID:24249308

Jellin, J. M. (2009). *Natural medicines comprehensive database*. Retrieved from http://www.naturaldatabase.com

Jemal, A., Siegel, R., Xu, J., & Ward, E. (2010). Cancer statistics 2010. *CA: a Cancer Journal for Clinicians*, *60*, 277–300. PMID:20610543

Jenner, D. J., Lewis, D. A., Pitt, E., & Offord, R. A. (1981). The Effect of the Intravenous Administration of Corticosteroids Encapsulated in Intact Erythrocytes on Adjuvant Arthritis in the Rat. *British Journal of Pharmacology*, *73*, 212P–213P.

Jessell, T. M., & Sanes, J. R. (2000). The generation and survival of new cell. In E. R. Kandel, J. Schwartz, & T. M. Jessell (Eds.), *In principal of neural science* (pp. 41–62). New York, NY: McGraw-Hill.

Jiménez-Sousa, M., Fernández-Rodríguez, A., & Guzmán-Fulgencio, M., García-Álvarez, M., & Resino, S. (2013). Meta-analysis: Implications of interleukin-28B polymorphisms in spontaneous and treatment-related clearance for patients with hepatitis C. *BMC Medicine*, *11*, 6. PMID:23298311

Jin, Y., Desta, Z., Stearns, V., Ward, B., Ho, H., Lee, K. H., & Flockhart, D. A. et al. (2005). CYP2D6 genotype, antidepressant use, and tamoxifen metabolism during adjuvant breast cancer treatment. *Journal of the National Cancer Institute*, *97*(1), 30–39. doi:10.1093/jnci/dji005 PMID:15632378

Jin, Y., Pollock, B. G., Frank, E., Cassano, G. B., Rucci, P., Muller, D. J., & Bies, R. R. et al. (2010). Effect of age, weight, and CYP2C19 genotype on escitalopram exposure. *Journal of Clinical Pharmacology*, *50*(1), 62–72. doi:10.1177/0091270009337946 PMID:19841156

John, S., Sorokin, A. V., & Thompson, P. D. (2007). Phytosterols and vascular disease. *Current Opinion in Lipidology*, *18*(1), 35–40. doi:10.1097/MOL.0b013e328011e9e3 PMID:17218830

Johnson, J. T., Ferretti, G. A., Nethery, W. J., Valdez, I. H., Fox, P. C., Ng, D., & Gallagher, S. C. et al. (1993). Oral pilocarpine for post-irradiation xerostomia in patients with head and neck cancer. *The New England Journal of Medicine*, *329*(6), 390–305. doi:10.1056/NEJM199308053290603 PMID:8326972

Johnson, K. P., Brooks, B. R., Ford, C. C., Goodman, A., Guarnaccia, J., Lisak, R. P., & Wolinsky, J. S. et al. (2000). Sustained clinical benefits of glatiramer acetate in relapsing multiple sclerosis patients observed for 6 years. Copolymer 1 Multiple Sclerosis Study Group. *Multiple Sclerosis*, *6*(4), 255–266. doi:10.1177/135245850000600407 PMID:10962546

Jomana. (2015). *Welcome to the World of Nature*. Retrieved 12.6.2015, fromhttp://www.s-jomana.com/eng

Jones, S., & Janardhanan, K. K. (2000). Antioxidant and antitumor activity of *Ganoderma lucidum (*curt ex Fr.). P. Karst-Reshi (Aphyllophoromycetieae) from south India. *Int. J. Med. Mushr, 2*(3), 195–200. doi:10.1615/IntJMedMushr.v2.i3.20

Jong, A., Plat, J., & Mensink, R. P. (2003). Metabolic effects of plant sterols and stanols. *The Journal of Nutritional Biochemistry, 14*(7), 362–369. doi:10.1016/S0955-2863(03)00002-0 PMID:12915216

Jose, N., Ajith, T. A., & Janardhanan, K. K. (2002). Antioxidant, anti-inflammatory and antitumor activities of culinarymedicinal mushroom *Pleurotus pulmonarius* (Fr.) Quel. (Agaricomycetideae). *Int. J. Med. Mushr, 4*(4), 329–335. doi:10.1615/IntJMedMushr.v4.i4.60

Jose, N., & Janardhanan, K. K. (2000). Antioxidant and antitumor activity of *Pleurotus florida. Current Science, 79*, 941–943.

Joshi, R. K. (2010). In vitro antimicrobial and antioxidant activity of the essential oil of *Craniotome furcata. Journal of Applied and Natural Science, 2*, 57–62.

Joshi, R. K. (2012a). In vitro antimicrobial activity of the essential oil of the endemic plant *Senecio belgaumensis. Journal of Biologically Active Products from Nature, 2*(6), 382–386. doi:10.1080/22311866.2012.10719147

Joshi, R. K. (2012b). Comparative analysis by GC-MS and *in vitro* antimicrobial activity of the essential oils of noxious weed (*Lantana camara* L.) from Western Ghats region of North West Karnataka, India. *Journal of Biologically Active Products from Nature, 2*(3), 135–143. doi:10.1080/22311866.2012.10719120

Joshi, R. K. (2013a). Volatile composition and antimicrobial activity of the essential oil of *Artemisia absinthium* growing in Western Ghats region of North West Karnataka, India. *Pharmaceutical Biology, 51*(7), 888–892. doi:10.3109/13880209.2013.768676 PMID:23570523

Joshi, R. K. (2013b). Chemical composition, *in vitro* antimicrobial and antioxidant activities of the essential oils of *Ocimum gratissimum, O. sanctum* and their major constituents. *Indian Journal of Pharmaceutical Sciences, 75*(4), 457–462. doi:10.4103/0250-474X.119834 PMID:24302801

Joshi, R. K. (2013c). Chemical constituents and antibacterial property of the essential oil of the roots of *Cyathocline purpurea. Journal of Ethnopharmacology, 145*(2), 621–625. doi:10.1016/j.jep.2012.11.045 PMID:23220198

Joshi, R. K. (2013d). Pulegone and menthone chemotypes of *Mentha spicata* Linn.from Western Ghats region of North West Karnataka, India. *National Academy Science Letters, 36*(3), 349–352. doi:10.1007/s40009-013-0141-3

Joshi, R. K. (2014a). Chemical composition and antimicrobial activity of the essential oil of *Plectranthus mollis* (Lamiaceae) from Western Ghats region, Karnataka, India. *Revista de Biologia Tropical, 62*, 423–431. doi:10.15517/rbt.v62i2.9396 PMID:25102628

Joshi, R. K. (2014b). Chemical composition and antimicrobial activity of the essential oil of *Ocimum basilicum* L. (sweet basil) from Western Ghats of North West Karnataka, India. *Ancient Science of Life, 33*(3), 149–154. doi:10.4103/0257-7941.144618 PMID:25538349

Joshi, R. K. (2014c). 2,4,6-Trimethoxy-styrene new chemotype from the essential oil of *Zanthoxylum ovalifolium* Wight from India. *National Academy Science Letters, 37*(4), 331–333. doi:10.1007/s40009-014-0243-6

Joshi, R. K., & Badakar, V. (2012). Chemical composition and *in vitro* antimicrobial activity of the essential oil of the flowers of *Tridax procumbens* L. *Natural Product Communications, 7*, 941–942. PMID:22908588

Joshi, R. K., Badakar, V. M., Kholkute, S. D., & Khatib, N. (2011). Chemical composition and antimicrobial activity of the essential oil of the leaves of *Feronia elephantum* (Rutaceae) from North West Karnataka. *Natural Product Communications, 6*, 141–143. PMID:21366066

Joshi, R. K., Mujawar, M. H. K., Badakar, V., & Khatib, N. A. (2011). *In vitro* antimicrobial activity of the essential oil of *Erigeron floribundus*. *International Journal of Research in Ayurveda and Pharmacy*, *2*, 236–238.

Joshi, R. K., Pande, C., Mujawar, M. H. K., & Kholkute, S. D. (2009). Chemical composition and antimicrobial activity of the essential oil of *Anaphalis nubigena* var. *monocephala*. *Natural Product Communications*, *4*, 993–996. PMID:19731610

Joshi, R. K., Pande, V., & Thakuri, B. C. (2011). Antimicrobial activity of the essential oil of *Phlomis bracteosa*. *Scientific World*, *9*(9), 63–65. doi:10.3126/sw.v9i9.5521

Joshi, R. K., Patil, P. A., Mujawar, M. H. K., Kumar, D., & Kholkute, S. D. (2009a). Hypoglycemic activity of aqueous leaf extract of *Feronia elephantum* in normal and streptozotocin- induced diabetic rats. *Pharmacologyonline*, *3*, 815–821.

Joshi, R. K., Patil, P. A., Mujawar, M. H. K., Kumar, D., & Kholkute, S. D. (2009b). Hypoglycemic activity of *Bambusa arundinacea* leaf aqueous extract in euglycemic and hyperglycemic Wistar rats. *Pharmacologyonline*, *3*, 789–795.

Jrade, M., Villereal, M. C., Boynard, M., & Ropars, C. (1987). Rheological Approach to Human Red Blood Cell Carriers Desferrioxamine Encapsulation. *Advances in the Biosciences*, *67*, 29–36.

Juan, J., & Yan, C., & Wei, W. (2010). Clinical application and evaluation of anti-TNF-alpha agents for the treatment of rheumatoid arthritis. *Acta Pharmacologica Sinica*, *31*, 1133–1140. PMID:20711219

Jung, H., Yoo, D., Kin, W., Nam, S., Kim, H., Choi, J., & Yoon, Y. et al. (2014). *Valeriana officinalis* root extract suppresses physical stress by electric shock and psychological stress by nociceptive stimulation-evoked responses by decreasing the ratio of monoamine neurotransmitters to their metabolites. *Complementary and Alternative Medicine.*, *14*(1), 476–483. doi:10.1186/1472-6882-14-476 PMID:25495725

Kador, P. F., Guo, C., Kawada, H., Randazzo, J., & Blessing, K. (2014). Topical Nutraceutical Optixcare EH Ameliorates Experimental Ocular Oxidative Stress in Rats. *Journal of Ocular Pharmacology and Therapeutics*, *30*(7), 593–602. doi:10.1089/jop.2014.0016 PMID:25188009

Kagan, V., Khan, S., Swanson, C., Shvedova, A., Serbinova, E., & Packer, L. (1990). Antioxidant action of thioctic acid and dihydrolipoic acid. *Free Radical Biology & Medicine*, *9S*, 15. doi:10.1016/0891-5849(90)90220-D

Kahalid, H., Zhari, I., Amirin, S., & Pazilah, I. (2011). Accelerated stability and chemical kinetics of ethanol extracts of fruit of *Piper sarmestosum* using high performance liquid chromatography. *Iranian Journal of Pharmaceutical Research*, *10*(3), 403–413. PMID:24250372

Kaiser, R., Sezer, O., Papies, A., Bauer, S., Schelenz, C., Tremblay, P. B., & Brockmoller, J. et al. (2002). Patient-tailored antiemetic treatment with 5-hydroxytryptamine type 3 receptor antagonists according to cytochrome P-450 2D6 genotypes. *Journal of Clinical Oncology*, *20*(12), 2805–2811. doi:10.1200/JCO.2002.09.064 PMID:12065557

Kalac, P., & Moudry, J. (2000). Chemical composition and nutritional value of amaranth grains[in Czech]. *Czech Food Scienc*, *18*, 201–206.

Kalra, E. K. (2003). Nutraceutical Definition and Introduction. *AAPS PharmSci*, *5*(3), 25. doi:10.1208/ps050325 PMID:14621960

Kanchan, S. D. (1975). Growth inhibitors from *Parthenium hysterophorus* Linn. *Current Science*, *44*, 358–359.

Kang, K. S., Yamabe, N., Kim, H. Y., Park, J. H., & Yokozawa, T. (2010). Effects of heat-processed ginseng and its active component ginsenoside 20(S)-Rg3 on the progression of renal damage and dysfunction in type 2 diabetic Otsuka Long- Evans Tokushima Fatty rats. *Biological & Pharmaceutical Bulletin*, *33*(6), 1077–1081. doi:10.1248/bpb.33.1077 PMID:20522983

Kang, S. Y., Kim, M. H., & Lee, W. I. (2010). Measurement of inflammatory cytokines in patients with rheumatoid arthritis. *The Korean Journal of Laboratory Medicine*, *30*, 301–306. PMID:20603592

Kang, S., Duell, E. A., Fisher, G. J., Datta, S. C., Wang, Z. Q., Reddy, A. P., & Voorhees, J. J. et al. (1995). Application of retinol to human skin in vivo induces epidermal hyperplasia and cellular retinoid binding proteins characteristic of retinoic acid but without measurable retinoic acid levels or irritation. *The Journal of Investigative Dermatology*, *105*(4), 549–556. doi:10.1111/1523-1747.ep12323445 PMID:7561157

Kanodia, S., Fahey, L., Kast, W., & Martin-Kast, W. (2007). Mechanisms Used by Human Papillomaviruses to Escape the Host Immune Response. *Current Cancer Drug Targets*, *7*(1), 79–89. doi:10.2174/156800907780006869 PMID:17305480

Kanter, M., Coskun, O., & Budancamanak, M. (2005). Hepatoprotective effects of Nigella sativa L. and Urtica dioica L. on lipid peroxidation, antioxidant enzyme systems and liver enzymes in carbon tetrachloride-treated rats. *World Journal of Gastroenterology*, *11*(42), 6684–6688. doi:10 3748/wjg.v11.i42.6684 PMID:16425366

Karen, N., & Eggleston, W. H. S. (2011). Prescribing institutions: Explaining the evolution of physician dispensing. *Journal of Institutional Economics*, *8*(02), 247–270.

Karim, M. Y., Alba, P., Cuadrado, M. J., Abbs, I. C., D'Cruz, D. P., Khamashta, M. A., & Hughes, G. R. (2002). Mycophenolate mofetil for systemic lupus erythematosus refractory to other immunosuppressive agents. *Rheumatology (Oxford, England)*, *41*(8), 876–882. doi:10.1093/rheumatology/41.8.876 PMID:12154204

Katchamart, W., Trudeau, J., Phumethum, V., & Bombardier, C. (2009). Efficacy and toxicity of methotrexate (MTX) monotherapy versus MTX combination therapy with nonbiological disease-modifying antirheumatic drugs in rheumatoid arthritis: A systematic review and meta-analysis. *Annals of the Rheumatic Diseases*, *68*, 1105–1112. PMID:19054823

Katiyar, S., Elmets, C. A., & Katiyar, S. K. (2007). Green tea and skin cancer: Photoimmunology, angiogenesis and DNA repair. *The Journal of Nutritional Biochemistry*, *18*(5), 287–296. doi:10.1016/j.jnutbio.2006.08 004 PMID:17049833

Kay, J., & Calabrese, L. (2004). The role of interleukin-1 in the pathogenesis of rheumatoid arthritis. *Rheumatology (Oxford, England)*, *43*(Suppl 3), iii2–iii9. doi:10.1093/rheumatology/keh201 PMID:15150426

Kelber, O., Nieber, K., & Kraft, K. (2014). Valerian: No evidence for clinically relevant interactions. *Evidence-Based Complementary and Alternative Medicine*, *2014*, 1–8. doi:10.1155/2014/879396 PMID:25093031

Kelly, E., & Russell, S. J. (2007). History of oncolytic viruses: Genesis to genetic engineering. *Molecular Therapy*, *15*(4), 651–659. PMID:17299401

Kendall, M., Hodges, N. J., Whitwell, H., Tyrrell, J., & Cangul, H. (2015). Nanoparticle growth and surface chemistry changes in cell-conditioned culture medium. *Philosophical Transactions of the Royal Society B: Biological Sciences*, *370*(1661), 20140100.

Kerem, Z., Chetrit, D., Shoseyov, O., & Regev-Shoshani, G. (2006). Protection of lipids from oxidation by epicatechin, trans-resveratrol, and gallic and caffeic acids in intestinal model systems. *Journal of Agricultural and Food Chemistry*, *54*(26), 10288–10293. doi:10.1021/jf0621828 PMID:17177572

Kerns, E. H., & Carte, G. T. (2009). Drug-like property concepts in Pharmaceutical design. *Current Pharmaceutical Design*, *15*(19), 2184–2194. doi:10.2174/138161209788682479 PMID:19601822

Kerwin, S. M. (2004). Soy saponins and the anticancer effects of soybeans and soy-based foods. *Current Medicinal Chemistry*, *4*, 263–272. PMID:15134504

Keselowsky, B. G., Xia, C. Q., & Clare-Salzler, M. (2011). Multifunctional dendritic cell-targeting polymeric microparticles: Engineering new vaccines for type 1 diabetes. *Human Vaccines*, *7*(1), 37–44. doi:10.4161/hv.7.1.12916 PMID:21157186

Keservani, R. K., Kesharwani, R. K., Sharma, A. K., & Jarouliya, U. (2015d). Dietary Supplements, Nutraceutical and Functional Foods in Immune Response (Immunomodulators). CRC Press, Taylor and Francis.

Keservani, R. K., Singh, S., Singh, V., Kesharwani, R.K., & Sharma, A. K. (2015b). Nutraceuticals and Functional Foods in the Prevention of Mental Disorder. CRC Press, Taylor and Francis.

Keservani, R. K., Kesharwani, R. K., & Sharma, A. K. (2015c). *Pulmonary and Respiratory Health: Antioxidants and Nutraceuticals*. CRC Press, Taylor and Francis.

Keservani, R. K., Kesharwani, R. K., Sharma, A. K., & Ahmad, M. F. (2015a). *Stress, Parkinson's,Alzemer's disease: Role of Dietary Supplements*. CRC Press, Taylor and Francis.

Keservani, R. K., Kesharwani, R. K., Sharma, A. K., Vyas, N., & Chadoker, A. (2010b). Nutritional Supplements: An Overview.[IJCPR]. *Int. J. Curr. Pharm. Rev. Res.*, *1*, 59–75.

Keservani, R. K., Kesharwani, R. K., Vyas, N., Jain, S., Raghuvanshi, R., & Sharma, A. K. (2010a). Nutraceutical and functional food as future food: A Review. *Der Pharmacia. Lett*, *2*, 106–116.

Keservani, R. K., & Sharma, A. K. (2014). Flavonoids: Emerging trends and potential health benefits. *J Chin. Pharm. Sci.*, *23*(12), 815–822.

Ketkar, P. M., Nayak, S. U., Pai, S. R., & Joshi, R. K. (2015). Monitoring seasonal variation of epicatechin and gallic acid in the bark of *Saraca asoca* using reverse phase high performance liquid chromatography (RP-HPLC) method. *Journal of Ayurveda and Integrative Medicine*, *6*(1), 29–34. doi:10.4103/0975-9476.146568 PMID:25878461

Khadra, A., Tsai, S., Santamaria, P., & Edelstein-Keshet, L. (2010). On how monospecific memory-like autoregulatory CD8+ T cells can blunt diabetogenic autoimmunity: A computational approach. *Journal of Immunology (Baltimore, MD.: 1950)*, *185*(10), 5962–5972. doi:10.4049/jimmunol.1001306 PMID:20962260

Khan, B. A., Abraham, A., & Leelamma, S. (1995). Hypoglycemic action of *Murraya Koeingii* (curry leaf) and *Brassica juncea* (mustard): Mechanism of action. *Indian Journal of Biochemistry & Biophysics*, *32*, 106–108. PMID:7642200

Khan, M. M. (1974). Sahihal_Bukhari.The translation of the Meanings of the Koran. *Sahih Bukhari Book*, *7*, 582–590.

Kharkwal, H., Panthari, P., Pant, M. K., Kharkwal, H., Kharkwal, A. C., & Joshi, D. D. (2012). Foaming Glycosides: A review. *IOSR Journal of Pharmacy*, *2*(5), 23–28. doi:10.9790/3013-25202328

Khodaie, L., & Sadeghpoor, O. (2015). Ginger form acient times to the new outlook. *Jundishapur Journal of Natural Pharmaceutical Products.*, *10*(1), 1–5. doi:10.17795/jjnpp-18402 PMID:25866718

Khorasani, G., Hosseinimerh, S., Azadbakht, M., Zamani, A., & Mahdavi, M. (2009). Aloe Versus Silver Sulfadiazine Creams for Second-Degree Burns: A Randomized Controlled Study. *Surgery Today*, *39*(7), 587–591. doi:10.1007/s00595-008-3944-y PMID:19562446

Kiefer, C. R., & Snyder, L. M. (2000). Oxidation and erythrocyte senescence. *Current Opinion in Hematology*, *7*(2), 113–116. doi:10.1097/00062752-200003000-00007 PMID:10698298

Kim, D. M., & Zolinev, C. (1973). The Influence of Amphotericin-B on the Permeability of Mammalian Erythrocytes to Nonelectrolytes, anions and Cations. *Biochimica et Biophysica Acta*, *318*(3), 345–359. doi:10.1016/0005-2736(73)90199-5

Kim, M. S., Song, H. J., Lee, S. H., & Lee, C. K. (2014). Comparative study of various growth factors and cytokines on type I collagen and hyaluronan production in human dermal fibroblasts. *Journal of Cosmetic Dermatology*, *13*(1), 44–51. doi:10.1111/jocd.12073 PMID:24641605

Kim, S. H., Kim, S., & Oligino, T. J. (2002). Effective treatment of established mouse collagen-induced arthritis by systemic administration of dendritic cells genetically modified to express FasL. *Molecular Therapy*, *6*, 584–590. PMID:12409256

Kim, S. J., Kawaharada, C., Suzuki, T., Saito, K., Hashimoto, N., Takigawa, S., & Yamauchi, H. et al. (2005). Effect of natural light periods on rutin, free amino acid and vitamin C contents in the sprouts of common (Fagopyrum esculentum Moench) and tartary (F. tataricum Gaertn.) buckwheats. *Food Science and Technology Research*, *12*(3), 199–205. doi:10.3136/fstr.12.199

Kim, S. Y., & Hahn, W. C. (2007). Cancer genomics: Integrating form and function. *Carcinogenesis*, *28*(7), 1387–1392. PMID:17434922

Kim, T. H., Lee, S., & Chen, X. (2013). Nanotheranostics for personalized medicine. *Expert Review of Molecular Diagnostics*, *13*(3), 257–269. doi:10.1586/erm.13.15 PMID:23570404

Kim, W., Fan, Y. Y., Smith, R., Patil, B., Jayaprakasha, G. K., McMurray, D. N., & Chapkin, R. S. (2009). Dietary curcumin and limonin suppress CD4+ T-cell proliferation and interleukin-2 production in mice. *The Journal of Nutrition*, *139*(5), 1042–1048. doi:10.3945/jn.108.102772 PMID:19321585

Kim, Y. S., Sohn, E., Lee, Y. M., Kim, C.-S., & Kim, J. S. (2014). Extract of *Cassiae semen* attenuates diabetic nephropathy via inhibition of advanced glycation end products accumulation in streptozotocin-induced diabetic rats. *Phytomedicine*, *21*(5), 734–739. doi:10.1016/j.phymed.2013.11.002 PMID:24374123

Kinghorn, A. D. (1987). Biologically active compounds from plants with reputed medicinal and sweetening properties. *Journal of Natural Products*, *50*(6), 1009–1024. doi:10.1021/np50054a002 PMID:3327919

Kinosita, K., & Tsong, T. Y. (1977a). Hemolysis of Human Erythrocytes by a Transient Electric Field. *Proceedings of the National Academy of Sciences of the United States of America*, *74*(5), 1923–1927. doi:10.1073/pnas.74.5.1923 PMID:266714

Kinosita, K., & Tsong, T. Y. (1977b). Formation and Resealing of Pores of Controlled Sizes in Human Erythrocyte Membrane. *Nature*, *268*(5619), 438–441. doi:10.1038/268438a0 PMID:895849

Kintzios, S., & Michaelakis, A. (1999). Induction of somatic embryogenesis and in vitro flowering from inflorescences of chamomile (*Chamomilla recutita* L.). *Plant Cell Reports*, *8*(7-8), 684–690. doi:10.1007/s002990050643

Kipen, Y., Littlejohn, G. O., & Morand, E. F. (1997). Methotrexate use in systemic lupus erythematosus. *Lupus*, *6*(4), 385–389. doi:10.1177/096120339700600407 PMID:9175024

Kirchmair, J., Markt, P., Distinto, S., Wolber, G., & Langer, T. (2008). Evaluation of the performance of 3D virtual screening protocols: RMSD comparisons, enrichment assessments, and decoy selection--what can we learn from earlier mistakes. *Journal of Computer-Aided Molecular Design*, *22*(3-4), 213–228. doi:10.1007/s10822-007-9163-6 PMID:18196462

Kitao, T., Hattori, K., & Takeshita, M. (1978). Agglutination of Leukemic Cells and Daunomycin Entrapped Erythrocytes with Lectin *In Vitro* and *In Vivo*. *Experimentia*, *341*(1), 94–95. doi:10.1007/BF01921924 PMID:620752

Kittler, S. G. C., Diendorf, J., Köller, M., & Epple, M. (2010). Toxicity of Silver Nanoparticles Increases during Storage Because of Slow Dissolution under Release of Silver Ions. *Chemistry of Materials*, *22*(16), 4548–4554. doi:10.1021/cm100023p

Kjeldsen, L., Johnsen, A. H., Sengeløv, H., & Borregaard, N. (1993). Isolation and primary structure of NGAL, a novel protein associated with human neutrophil gelatinase. *The Journal of Biological Chemistry*, *268*(14), 10425–10432. PMID:7683678

Kladney, R. D., Cui, X., Bulla, G. A., Brunt, E. M., & Fimmel, C. J. (2002). Expression of GP73, a resident Golgi membrane protein, in viral and nonviral liver disease. *Hepatology (Baltimore, Md.)*, *35*, 1431–1440. PMID:12029628

Klebe, G. (2000). Recent developments in structure-based drug design. *Journal of Molecular Medicine*, *78*(5), 269–281. doi:10.1007/s001090000084 PMID:10954199

Klebe, G., & Abraham, U. (1999). Comparative molecular similarity index analysis (CoMSIA) to study hydrogen-bonding properties and to score combinatorial libraries. *Journal of Computer-Aided Molecular Design*, *13*(1), 1–10. doi:10.1023/A:1008047919606 PMID:10087495

Kleinbongard, P., Schulz, R., Rassaf, T., Lauer, T., Dejam, A., Jax, T., & Kelm, M. et al. (2006). Red blood cells express a functional endothelial nitric oxide synthase. *Blood*, *107*(7), 2943–2951. doi:10.1182/blood-2005-10-3992 PMID:16368881

Klepstad, P., Rakvag, T. T., Kaasa, S., Holthe, M., Dale, O., Borchgrevink, P. C., & Skorpen, F. et al. (2004). The 118 A > G polymorphism in the human mu-opioid receptor gene may increase morphine requirements in patients with pain caused by malignant disease. *Acta Anaesthesiologica Scandinavica*, *48*(10), 1232–1239. doi:10.1111/j.1399-6576.2004.00517.x PMID:15504181

Kleywegt, G. J., Harris, M. R., Zou, J. Y., Taylor, T. C., Wahlby, A., & Jones, T. A. (2004). The uppsala electron-density server. *Acta Crystallographica. Section D, Biological Crystallography*, *60*(12), 2240–2249. doi:10.1107/S0907444904013253 PMID:15572777

Kligman, A. (2005). The future of cosmeceuticals: An interview with Albert Kligman, MD, PhD. Interview by Zoe Diana Draelos. *Dermatologic Surgery*, *31*(7 Pt 2), 890–891. PMID:16029684

Klopfleisch, R., & Gruber, A. D. (2009). Increased expression of BRCA2 and RAD51 in lymph node metastases of canine mammary adenocarcinomas. *Veterinary Pathology*, *46*(3), 416–422. PMID:19176491

Klopfleisch, R., Klose, P., Weise, C., Bondzio, A., Multhaup, G., Einspanier, R., & Gruber, A. D. (2010). Proteome of metastatic canine mammary carcinomas: Similarities to and differences from human breast cancer. *Journal of Proteome Research*, *9*(12), 6380–6391. PMID:20932060

Kobayashi, S., Takeana, M., Kanke, M., Itoh, S., & Ogata, E. (1998). Postadministration protective effect of magnesium-L-ascorbyl-phosphate on the development of UVB-induced cutaneous damage in mice. *Photochemistry and Photobiology*, *67*(6), 669–675. doi:10.1111/j.1751-1097.1998.tb09111.x PMID:9648533

Kodera, R., Shikata, K., Takatsuka, T., Oda, K., Miyamoto, S., Kajitani, N., & Makino, H. et al. (2014). Dipeptidyl peptidase-4 inhibitor ameliorates early renal injury through its anti-inflammatory action in a rat model of type 1 diabetes. *Biochemical and Biophysical Research Communications*, *443*(3), 828–833. doi:10.1016/j.bbrc.2013.12.049 PMID:24342619

Kolch, W., & Pitt, A. (2010). Functional proteomics to dissect tyrosine kinase signalling pathways in cancer. *Nature Reviews. Cancer*, *10*, 618–629. PMID:20720570

Kondratyuk, T. P., & Pezzuto, J. M. (2004). Natural Product Polyphenols of Relevance to Human Health. *Pharmaceutical Biology*, *42*(sup1), 46–63. doi:10.3109/13880200490893519

Kong, W. S. (2004). Descriptions of commercially important Pleurotus species. In Oyster mushroom cultivation. Part II. Oyster mushrooms. Seoul: Heineart Incorporation.

Kontos, S., Kourtis, I. C., Dane, K. Y., & Hubbell, J. A. (2013). Engineering antigens for in situ erythrocyte binding induces T-cell deletion. *Proceedings of the National Academy of Sciences of the United States of America*, *110*(1), E60–E68. doi:10.1073/pnas.1216353110 PMID:23248266

Koren, G., Cairns, J., Chitayat, D., Gaedigk, A., & Leeder, S. J. (2006). Pharmacogenetics of morphine poisoning in a breastfed neonate of a codeine-prescribed mother. *Lancet*, *368*(9536), 704. doi:10.1016/S0140-6736(06)69255-6 PMID:16920476

Korkina, L. G., Pastore, S., Dellambra, E., & De Luca, C. (2013). New molecular and cellular targets for chemoprevention and treatment of skin tumors by plant polyphenols: A critical review. *Current Medicinal Chemistry*, *20*(7), 852–868. PMID:23210776

Kornhauser, A., Coelho, S. G., & Hearing, V. J. (2010). Applications of hydroxy acids: Classification, mechanisms, and photoactivity. *Journal of Clinical. Cosmetic and Investigational Dermatology*, *3*, 135–142. doi:10.2147/CCID.S9042

Koshihara, Y., & Hoshi, K. (1996). Vitamin K2 promotes 1α,25(oh)2 vitamin D3-induced mineralization in human periosteal osteoblasts. *Calcified Tissue International*, *59*, 466–473. PMID:8939773

Kosugi, T., Heinig, M., Nakayama, T., Matsuo, S., & Nakagawa, T. (2010). eNOS Knockout Mice with Advanced Diabetic Nephropathy Have Less Benefit from Renin-Angiotensin Blockade than from Aldosterone Receptor Antagonists. *American Journal of Pathology*, *176*(2), 619–629. doi:10.2353/ajpath.2010.090578 PMID:20042665

Kovacs, B. (2008). *Sources of caffeine*. Retrieved from http://www.Medicinenet.Com

Krause, I., Blank, M., & Shoenfeld, Y. (2000). Immunomodulation of experimental autoimmune diseases via oral tolerance. *Critical Reviews in Immunology*, *20*(1), 1–16. PMID:10770268

Krieger, E., Nabuurs, S. B., & Vriend, G. (2003). Homology modeling. *Structural Bioinformatics*, *5*, 507–521. PMID:12647402

Kris, M. G., Johnson, B. E., Kwiatkowski, D. J., & Iafrate, A. J. (2011). Identification of driver mutations in tumor specimens from 1000 patients with lung adenocarcinoma: The NCI's lung cancer mutation consortium (LCMC). *Journal of Clinical Oncology*, 29.

Kruse, C. A., James, G. T., Cederbaum, S. D., et al., (1987). Arginase-Loaded Erythrocyte Carriers: Their Fusion to Host Cells with Viral Fusogenic Proteins and Subcellular Localization of Arginase. *Advanced Biosciences, 67*, 113-122

Kruse, C. A., Spector, E. B., Cederbaum, S. D., Wisnieski, B. J., & Popják, G. (1981). Microinjection of Arginase into Enzyme-Deficient Cells with the Isolated Glycoprotein of Sendai Virus as Fusogen. *Biochimica et Biophysica Acta*, *645*(2), 339–345. doi:10.1016/0005-2736(81)90205-4 PMID:6268159

Krzywkowski, K., Jensen, A. A., Connolly, C. N., & Brauner-Osborne, H. (2007). Naturally occurring variations in the human 5-HT3A gene profoundly impact 5-HT3 receptor function and expression. *Pharmacogenetics and Genomics*, *17*(4), 255–266. doi:10.1097/FPC.0b013e3280117269 PMID:17496724

Kuang, Q. T., Zhao, J. J., Ye, C. L., Wang, J. R., Ye, K. H., Zhang, X. Q., & Ye, W. C. et al. (2012). Nephro-protective effects of total triterpenoids from *Psidium guajava* leaves on type 2 diabetic rats. *Journal of Chinese Medicinal Materials*, *35*, 94–97. PMID:22734419

Kucuk, O., Sarkar, F. H., Sak, W., Djuric, Z., Pollak, M. N., & Khachik, F. (2002). Phase II randomized clinical trial of lycopene supplementation before radical prostatectomy. *Cancer Epidemiology, Biomarkers & Prevention*, *10*, 861–868. PMID:11489752

Kugelman, A., & Durand, M. (2011). A comprehensive approach to the prevention of bronchopulmonary dysplasia. *Pediatric Pulmonology*, *46*(12), 1153–1165. doi:10.1002/ppul.21508 PMID:21815280

Kukreja, A. K., & Dhawan, O. P. (2000). Somaclonal breeding for improvement of herb and essential oil yield in mints: A case study. *Journal of Medicinal & Aromatic Plant Sciences*, *22*, 431–442.

Kullavanijaya, P., & Lim, H. W. (2005). Photoprotection. *Journal of the American Academy of Dermatology*, *52*(6), 937–958. doi:10.1016/j.jaad.2004.07.063 PMID:15928611

Kumari, K., Mathew, B. C., & Augusti, K. T. (1995). Antidiabetic and hypolipidemic effects of S-methyl cysteine sulphoxide isolated from *Allium cepa* Linn. *Indian Journal of Biochemistry & Biophysics*, *32*, 49–54. PMID:7665195

Kumar, S., & Andy, A. (2012). Health promoting bioactive chemicals from *Brassica*. *International Food Research Journal*, *19*, 141–152.

Kuroyanagi, K., Kang, M. S., Goto, T., Hirai, S., Ohyama, K., Kusudo, T., & Kawada, T. et al. (2008). *Citrus auraptene* acts as an agonist for PPARs and enhances adiponectin production and MCP-1 reduction in 3T3-L1 adipocytes. *Biochemical and Biophysical Research Communications*, *366*(1), 219–225. doi:10.1016/j.bbrc.2007.11.119 PMID:18060855

Kyungsoo, C., Tianyi, W., & Guangxiang, L. (2009). Proteomics Study of the Hepatitis C Virus Replication Complex. *Methods in Molecular Biology (Clifton, N.J.)*, *510*, 185–193. PMID:19009262

Labet, M., & Thielemans, W. (2009). Synthesis of polycaprolactone: A review. *Chemical Society Reviews*, *38*(12), 3484–3504. doi:10.1039/b820162p PMID:20449064

Lacomba, R., Salcedo, J., Alegria, A., & Lagarda, M. J. (2010). Determination of sialic acid and gangliosides in biological samples and dairy products: A review. *J. Pharmaceut. Biomed*, *51*(2), 346–357. doi:10.1016/j.jpba.2009.04.023 PMID:19481897

Lago, J. H. G., Toledo-Arruda, A. C., Mernak, M., Barrosa, K., Martins, M., Tibério, I., & Prado, C. (2014). Structure-Activity Association of Flavonoids in Lung Diseases. *Molecules (Basel, Switzerland)*, *19*(3), 3570–3595. doi:10.3390/molecules19033570 PMID:24662074

Lakshmanan, P., Danesh, M., & Taji, A. (2002). Production of four commercially cultivated *Echinacea* species by different methods of *in vitro* regeneration. *The Journal of Horticultural Science & Biotechnology*, *77*(2), 158–163. doi:10.1080/14620316.2002.11511473

Lakshmi, B., Ajith, T.A., & Sheena, M., NidhI, G., & Janardhanan, K.K. (2003). Antiperoxidative, anti-inflammatory and antimutagenic activities of ethanol extract of the mycelium of *Ganoderma lucidum* occurring in South India. *Teratogenesis, Carcinogenesis, and Mutagenesis*, *22*, 1–13. PMID:12616600

Lammers, T., Rizzo, L. Y., Storm, G., & Kiessling, F. (2012). Personalized nanomedicine. *Clinical Cancer Research*, *18*(18), 4889–4894. doi:10.1158/1078-0432.CCR-12-1414 PMID:22829203

Lammers, T., Subr, V., Ulbrich, K., Peschke, P., Huber, P. E., Hennink, W. E., & Storm, G. (2009). Simultaneous delivery of doxorubicin and gemcitabine to tumors in vivo using prototypic polymeric drug carriers. *Biomaterials*, *30*(20), 3466–3475. doi:10.1016/j.biomaterials.2009.02.040 PMID:19304320

Lamont, K. T., Somers, S., Lacerda, L., Opie, L. H., & Lecour, S. (2011). Is red wine a SAFE sip away from cardioprotection? Mechanisms involved in resveratrol- and melatonin-induced cardioprotection. *Journal of Pineal Research*, *50*(4), 374–380. doi:10.1111/j.1600-079X.2010.00853.x PMID:21342247

Lamottke, K., Ripoll, C., & Walzack, R. (2011). The roots of innovation. *European Biopharmaceutical Review*, *15*, 52–56.

Lang, F., Hoerr, R., Noeldner, M., & Koch, E. (2013). Ginkgo biloba Extract EGb 761®: From an Ancient Asian Plant to a Modern European Herbal Medicinal Product. In Evidence and Rational Based Research on Chinese Drugs (pp. 431-470). Wien, Austria: Wiley-VCH Verlag GmbH & Co. KGaA.

Langham, R. G., Kelly, D. J., Gow, R. M., Zhang, Y., Cox, A. J., Qi, W., & Gilbert, R. E. et al. (2008). Increased renal gene transcription of protein kinase C-beta in human diabetic nephropathy: Relationship to long-term glycaemic control. *Diabetologia*, *51*(4), 668–674. doi:10.1007/s00125-008-0927-x PMID:18278479

Langridge, R. (1974). Interactive three-dimensional computer graphics in molecular biology. *Federation Proceedings*, *33*(12), 2332–2335. PMID:4435233

Lansky, E. P., & Newman, R. A. (2007). *Punica granatum* (pomegranate) and its potential for prevention and treatment of inflammation and cancer. *Journal of Ethnopharmacology*, *19*(2), 177–206. doi:10.1016/j.jep.2006.09.006 PMID:17157465

Laouini, A., Charcosset, C., Fessi, H., Holdich, R. G., & Vladisavljevic, G. T. (2013). Preparation of liposomes: A novel application of microengineered membranes--from laboratory scale to large scale. *Colloids and Surfaces. B, Biointerfaces*, *112*, 272–278. doi:10.1016/j.colsurfb.2013.07.066 PMID:23999143

Larochelle, C., Alvarez, J. I., & Prat, A. (2011). How do immune cells overcome the blood-brain barrier in multiple sclerosis? *FEBS Letters*, *585*(23), 3770–3780. doi:10.1016/j.febslet.2011.04.066 PMID:21550344

Larsson, S. C., Hakansson, N., Giovannucci, E., & Wolk, A. (2006). Folate intake and pancreatic cancer incidence: A prospective study of Swedish women and men. *Journal of the National Cancer Institute*, *98*(6), 407–413. doi:10.1093/jnci/djj094 PMID:16537833

Laukens, D., Peeters, H., Cruyssen, B.V., Boonefaes, T., & Elewaut, D., De, K. F., … Rottiers, P. (2006). Altered gut transcriptome in spondyloarthropathy. *Annals of the Rheumatic Diseases*, *65*, 1293–1300. PMID:16476712

Laverman, P., Boerman, O. C., Oyen, W. J. G., Corstens, F. H. M., & Storm, G. (2001). In vivo applications of PEG liposomes: Unexpected observations. *Critical Reviews in Therapeutic Drug Carrier Systems*, *18*(6), 551–566. doi:10.1615/CritRevTherDrugCarrierSyst.v18.i6.40 PMID:11789675

Leach, A. R., & Gillet, V. J. (2003). An introduction to chemoinformatics. Springer.

Leach, A. R., Gillet, V. J., Lewis, R. A., & Taylor, R. (2010). Three-dimensional pharmacophore methods in drug discovery. *Journal of Medicinal Chemistry*, *53*(2), 539–558. doi:10.1021/jm900817u PMID:19831387

Ledda, A., Bottari, A., Luzzi, R., Belcaro, G., Hu, S., Dugall, M., & Togni, S. et al. (2015). Cranberry supplementation in the prevention of non-severe lower urinary tract infections: A pilot study. *European Review for Medical and Pharmacological Sciences*, *19*, 77–80. PMID:25635978

Lee, C. K., Brown, C., Gralla, R. J., Hirsh, V., Thongprasert, S., Tsai, C. M., & Yang, J. C. et al. (2013). Impact of EGFR inhibitor in non-small cell lung cancer on progression-free and overall survival: A meta-analysis. *Journal of the National Cancer Institute*, *105*(9), 595–605. doi:10.1093/jnci/djt072 PMID:23594426

Lee, H. S., Kim, J. Y., Lee, W. I., Kim, S. J., Ko, M. J., & Jeong, S. (2011). Acquisition of selective antitumoral effects of recombinant adeno-associated virus by genetically inserting tumor-targeting peptides into capsid proteins. *Oncology Letters*, *2*, 1113–1119. PMID:22848276

Lee, J. J., Yang, S. Y., Kim, D. H., Hur, S. J., Lee, J. D., Yum, M. J., & Song, M. D. (2014). Liver fibrosis protective effect of hovenia dulcis fruit. *Current Topics in Nutraceutical Research*, *12*(1/2), 43–50.

Lee, L. (1999). Introducing herbal medicine into conventional health care settings. *Journal of Nurse-Midwifery*, *44*(3), 253–266. doi:10.1016/S0091-2182(99)00042-7 PMID:10380444

Lee, M. H., Yoon, E. S., Jeong, J. H., & Choi, Y. E. (2004). *Agrobacterium rhizogenes*-mediated transformation of *Taraxacum platycarpum* and changes of morphological characters. *Plant Cell Reports*, *22*(11), 822–827. doi:10.1007/s00299-004-0763-5 PMID:14986056

Lee, M. S., Lee, K. H., Sin, H. S., Um, S. J., Kim, J. W., & Koh, B. K. (2006). A newly synthesized photostable retinol derivative (retinyl N-formyl aspartamate) for photodamaged skin: Profilometric evaluation of 24-week study. *Journal of the American Academy of Dermatology*, *55*(2), 220–224. doi:10.1016/j.jaad.2006.01.013 PMID:16844502

Leiro, J., Alvarez, E., Arranz, J. A., Laguna, R., Uriarte, E., & Orallo, F. (2004). Effects of cis-resveratrol on inflammatory murine macrophages: Antioxidant activity and down regulation of inflammatory genes. *Journal of Leukocyte Biology*, *75*(6), 1156–1165. doi:10.1189/jlb.1103561 PMID:14982945

Lejeune, A., Poyet, P., Gaudreault, R. C., & Gicquaud, C. (1997). Nanoerythrosomes, A New Derivative of Erythrocyte Ghost: III. Is Phagocytosis Involved in the Mechanism of Action? *Anticancer Research*, *17*, 5A. PMID:9413209

Leonard, T. K., Waison, R. R., & Mohs, M. S. (1987). The effect of caffeine on various body systems: A review. *Journal of the American Dietetic Association*, *87*, 1048–1053. PMID:3301987

Lesk, A. M., & Chothia, C. (1980). How different amino acid sequences determine similar protein structures: The structure and evolutionary dynamics of the globins. *Journal of Molecular Biology*, *136*(3), 225–270. doi:10.1016/0022-2836(80)90373-3 PMID:7373651

Leung, W. K., Ching, A. K., & Wong, N. (2010). Phosphorylation of caldesmon by PFTAIRE1 kinase promotes actin binding and formation of stress fibers. *Molecular and Cellular Biochemistry*, *350*, 201–206. PMID:21184254

LeVeque, F. G., Montgomery, M., Potter, D., Zimmer, M. B., Rieke, J. W., Steiger, B. W., & Muscoplat, C. C. (1993). A multicenter, randomized, double-blind, placebo-controlled, dose-titration study of oral pilocarpine for treatment of radiation-induced xerostomia in head and neck cancer patients. *Journal of Clinical Oncology*, *11*, 1124–1131. PMID:8501499

Lewandowska, U., Szewczyk, K., Hrabec, E., Janecka, A., & Gorlach, S. (2013). Overview of metabolism and bioavailability enhancement of polyphenols. *Journal of Agricultural and Food Chemistry*, *61*(50), 12183–12199. doi:10.1021/jf404439b PMID:24295170

Lewis, A. (1999). *Melatonin and the Biological Clock*. McGraw-Hill.

Lewis, D. A. (1984). Red Blood Cells for Drug Delivery. *Pharmaceutics Journal*, *233*, 384–385.

Lewis, D. A., & Alpar, H. O. (1984). Therapeutic Possibilities of Drugs Encapsulated in Erythrocytes. *International Journal of Pharmaceutics*, *22*(2-3), 137–146. doi:10.1016/0378-5173(84)90017-6

Lewis, D. A., & Desai, J. (1987). The Use of Animal Models in the Encapsulation of Drugs in Erythrocytes.[series]. *Advances in the Biosciences*, *67*, 213–222.

Li, G., Weizhen, L., & Zhengxiang, L. (2002). Effect of Ginsenoside-Rb on cardiomyocyte Apoptosis after Ischemia and Reperfusion in Rats. *Journal of Huazjong Univerity of Science and Technology, 22*(3), 212-215.

Li, D., Ng, A., Mann, N., & Sinclair, A. J. (1998). Meat fat can make a significant contribution to dietary arachidonic acid. *Lipids*, *33*, 437–440. doi:10.1007/s11745-998-0225-7 PMID:9590632

Lievre, A., Bachet, J. B., Boige, V., Cayre, A., Le Corre, D., Buc, E., & Laurent-Puig, P. et al. (2008). KRAS mutations as an independent prognostic factor in patients with advanced colorectal cancer treated with cetuximab. *Journal of Clinical Oncology*, *26*(3), 374–379. doi:10.1200/JCO.2007.12.5906 PMID:18202412

Li, H., Li, Q., Wang, Y., Xu, X., Fan, W., Wang, M., & Xie, X. et al. (2004). An intervention study to prevent gastric cancer by micro-selenium and large dose of allitridum. *Chinese Medical Journal*, *117*(8), 1155–1160. PMID:15361287

Lilienfeld, S. (2002). Galantamine-a novel cholinergic drug with a unique dual mode of action for the treatment of patients with Alzheimer's disease. *CNS Drug Reviews*, *8*(2), 159–176. doi:10.1111/j.1527-3458.2002.tb00221.x PMID:12177686

Lill, M. A. (2007). Multi-dimensional QSAR in drug discovery. *Drug Discovery Today, 12*(23-24), 1013–1017. doi:10.1016/j.drudis.2007.08.004 PMID:18061879

Lim, A. K. H. (2014). Diabetic nephropathy- complications and treatment. *International Journal of Nephrology and Renovascular Disease, 7*, 361–381. doi:10.2147/IJNRD.S40172 PMID:25342915

Lim, A. K., Ma, F. Y., Nikolic-Paterson, D. J., Kitching, A. R., Thomas, M. C., & Tesch, G. H. (2010). Lymphocytes promote albuminuria, but not renal dysfunction or histological damage in a mouse model of diabetic renal injury. *Diabetologia, 53*(8), 1772–1782. doi:10.1007/s00125-010-1757-1 PMID:20422398

Lim, A. K., Ma, F. Y., Nikolic-Paterson, D. J., Thomas, M. C., Hurst, L. A., & Tesch, G. H. (2009). Antibody blockade of c-fms suppresses the progression of inflammation and injury in early diabetic nephropathy in obese db/db mice. *Diabetologia, 52*(8), 1669–1679. doi:10.1007/s00125-009-1399-3 PMID:19466391

Lim, A. K., & Tesch, G. H. (2012). Inflammation in diabetic nephropathy. *Mediators of Inflammation*. PMID:22969168

Limberger, R. P., Jacques, A. L. B., Schmitt, G. C., & Arbo, M. D. (2013). Pharmacological effects of ephedrine. In K. G. Ramawar & J. M. Merillon (Eds.), *Natural Products*. Heidelberg, Germany: Springer-Verlag Berlin. doi:10.1007/978-3-642-22144-6_41

Lim, J. T. E., Frcpi, , & Fams, . (1999). Treatment of melasma using kojic acid in a gel containing hydroquinone and glycolic acid. *Dermatologic Surgery, 25*(4), 282–284. doi:10.1046/j.1524-4725.1999.08236.x PMID:10417583

Lin, C. Y., & Yin, M. C. (2012). Renal Protective Effects of Extracts from Guava Fruit (Psidium guajava L.) in Diabetic Mice. *Plant Foods for Human Nutrition (Dordrecht, Netherlands), 67*(3), 303–308. doi:10.1007/s11130-012-0294-0 PMID:22581156

Linker, R. A., & Gold, R. (2013). Dimethyl fumarate for treatment of multiple sclerosis: Mechanism of action, effectiveness, and side effects. *Current Neurology and Neuroscience Reports, 13*(11), 394. doi:10.1007/s11910-013-0394-8 PMID:24061646

Lin, W., Mota de Freitas, D., Zhang, Q., & Olsen, K. W. (1999). Nuclear magnetic resonance and oxygen affinity study of cesium binding in human erythrocytes. *Archives of Biochemistry and Biophysics, 369*(1), 78–88. doi:10.1006/abbi.1999.1285 PMID:10462442

Liotta, L., & Petricoin, E. (2000). Molecular profiling of human cancer. *Nature Reviews. Genetics, 1*(1), 48–56. doi:10.1038/35049567 PMID:11262874

Lipinski, C. A., Lombardo, F., Dominy, B. W., & Feeny, P. J. (2001). Experimental and computational approaches to estimate solubility and permeability in drug discovery and development settings. *Advanced Drug Delivery Reviews, 46*(1-3), 3–26. doi:10.1016/S0169-409X(00)00129-0 PMID:11259830

Lipkowitz, K. B., & Boyed, D. B. (1996). Reviews in Computational Chemistry. New York, NY: VCH Publishers.

Lippi, G., Aloe, R., Storelli, A., Cervellin, G., & Trenti, T. (2012). Evaluation of NGAL Test™, a fully-automated neutrophil gelatinase-associated lipocalin (NGAL) immunoassay on Beckman Coulter AU 5822. *Clinical Chemistry and Laboratory Medicine, 50*(9), 1581–1584. doi:10.1515/cclm.2011.839 PMID:22962213

Liu, H. Y., Fang, M., & Zhang, Y. Q. (2014). *In Vivo Hypoglycaemic Effect and Inhibitory Mechanism of the Branch Bark Extract of the Mulberry on STZ-Induced Diabetic Mice*. The Scientific World Journal.

Liu, J., & Henkel, T. (2002). Traditional Chineese medicine (TCM): Are polyphenols and saponins the key ingredients triggering biological activities? *Current Medicinal Chemistry, 9*(15), 1483–1485. doi:10.2174/0929867023369709 PMID:12173978

Liu, K., Xu, H., Lv, G., Liu, B., Lee, M. K. K., Lu, C., & Wu, Y. et al. (2015). Loganin attenuates diabetic nephropathy in C57BL/6J mice with diabetes induced by streptozotocin and fed with diets containing high level of advanced glycation end products. *Life Sciences*, *123*, 78–85. doi:10.1016/j.lfs.2014.12.028 PMID:25623853

Liu, X., Kelm, R. J., & Strauch, A. R. (2009). Transforming Growth Factor β1-mediated Activation of the Smooth Muscle α-Actin Gene in Human Pulmonary Myofibroblasts Is Inhibited by Tumor Necrosis Factor-α via Mitogen-activated Protein Kinase 1-dependent Induction of the Egr-1 Transcriptional Repressor. *Molecular Biology of the Cell*, *20*, 2174–2185. doi:10.1091/mbc.E08-10-0994 PMID:19261809

Li, X., Xiao, Y., Gao, H., Li, B., Xu, L., Cheng, M., & Ma, Y. et al. (2009). Grape seed proanthocyanidins ameliorate diabetic nephropathy via modulation of levels of AGE, RAGE and CTGF. *Nephron. Experimental Nephrology*, *111*(2), e31–e41. doi:10.1159/000191103 PMID:19142024

Li, Y., & Schellhorn, H. E. (2007). New developments and novel therapeutic perspectives for vitamin C. *The Journal of Nutrition*, *137*, 2171–2184. PMID:17884994

Lloyd, J. U. (1897). *Physostigma by venenosum (Calabar)*. Chicago: The Western Druggist.

Lobello, K. W., Preskorn, S. H., Guico-Pabia, C. J., Jiang, Q., Paul, J., Nichols, A. I., & Ninan, P. T. et al. (2010). Cytochrome P450 2D6 phenotype predicts antidepressant efficacy of venlafaxine: A secondary analysis of 4 studies in major depressive disorder. *The Journal of Clinical Psychiatry*, *71*(11), 1482–1487. doi:10.4088/JCP.08m04773blu PMID:20441720

Longmire, M., Choyke, P. L., & Kobayashi, H. (2008). Clearance properties of nano-sized particles and molecules as imaging agents: Considerations and caveats. *Nanomedicine (London)*, *3*(5), 703–717. doi:10.2217/17435889.3.5.703 PMID:18817471

Lopez, J.L. (2007). Use of *Opuntia* Cactus as a Hypoglycemic. *Nutrition Bytes, 12*, Article 2.

Lopez-Olivo, M. A., Siddhanamatha, H. R., Shea, B., Tugwell, P., Wells, G. A., & Suarez-Almazor, M. E. (2014). Methotrexate for treating rheumatoid arthritis. *Cochrane Database of Systematic Reviews*, *6*, CD000957. doi:10.1002/14651858.CD000957.pub2 PMID:24916606

Loria, R. M. (2002). Immune up-regulation and tumor apoptosis by androstene steroids. *Steroids*, *67*(12), 953–966. doi:10.1016/S0039-128X(02)00043-0 PMID:12398992

Lotta, T., Vidgren, J., Tilgmann, C., Ulmanen, I., Melen, K., Julkunen, I., & Taskinen, J. (1995). Kinetics of human soluble and membrane-bound catechol O-methyltransferase: A revised mechanism and description of the thermolabile variant of the enzyme. *Biochemistry*, *34*(13), 4202–4210. doi:10.1021/bi00013a008 PMID:7703232

Lourenço, R., & Camilo, M. E. (2002). Taurine: A conditionally essential amino acid in humans? An overview in health and disease. *Nutricion Hospitalaria*, *17*(6), 262–270. PMID:12514918

Lowe, F., Dreikorn, K., Borkowski, A., Braechman, J., Denis, L., Ferrari, P., & Senge, T. et al. (1998). Review of Recent Placebo-Controlled Trials Utilizing Phytotherapeutic Agents for Treatment of BPH. *The Prostate*, *37*(3), 187–193. doi:10.1002/(SICI)1097-0045(19981101)37:3<187::AID-PROS8>3.0.CO;2-T PMID:9792136

Lubbe, A., & Verpoorte, R. (2011). Cultivation of medicinal and aromatic plants for specialty industrial materials. *Industrial Crops and Products*, *34*(1), 785–801. doi:10.1016/j.indcrop.2011.01.019

Lugović, L., Šitum, M., Ožanić-Bulić, S., & Sjerobabski-Masnec, I. (2007). Phototoxic and photoallergic skin reactions. *Collegium Antropologicum*, *31*(1), 63–67. PMID:17469754

Lu, H., Li, W., Noble, W. S., Payan, D., & Anderson, D. C. (2004). Riboproteomics of the Hepatitis C Virus Internal Ribosomal Entry Site. *Journal of Proteome Research*, 1–9. PMID:15473682

Lu, L., Luo, S. T., Shi, S. H., Li, M., Zhang, H. L., & He, S. S. (2012). AAV2-mediated gene transfer of VEGF-Trap with potent suppression of primary breast tumor growth and spontaneous pulmonary metastases by long-term expression. *Oncology Reports*, *28*, 1332–1338. PMID:22824831

Lu, L., Peter, S. J., Lyman, M. D., Lai, H. L., Leite, S. M., Tamada, J. A., & Mikos, A. G. et al. (2000). In vitro and in vivo degradation of porous poly(DL-lactic-co-glycolic acid) foams. *Biomaterials*, *21*(18), 1837–1845. doi:10.1016/S0142-9612(00)00047-8 PMID:10919687

Lu, M. K., Cheng, J. J., Lin, C.-Y., & Chang, C. C. (2010). Purification, structural elucidation, and Lukaski, H.C. (1999). Chromium as a supplement. *Annual Review of Nutrition*, *19*(1), 279–302.

Lu, M.-K., Cheng, J.-J., Lin, C.-Y., & Chang, C.-C. (2010, January). anti-inflammatory effect of a water-soluble 1,6-branched 1,3-α-D-galactan from cultured mycelia of *Poria cocos*. *Food Chemistry*, *118*(2), 349–356. doi:10.1016/j.foodchem.2009.04.126

Luo, X. D., & Shen, C. C. (1987). The chemistry, pharmacology, and clinical applications of qinghaosu (Artemisinin) and its derivatives. *Medicinal Research Reviews*, *7*(1), 29–52. doi:10.1002/med.2610070103 PMID:3550324

Lupo, M. P., & Cole, A. L. (2007). Cosmeceutical peptides. *Dermatologic Therapy*, *20*(5), 343–349. doi:10.1111/j.1529-8019.2007.00148.x PMID:18045359

Luscombe, N. M., Greenbaum, D., & Gerstein, M. (2001). What is Bioinformatics? An Introduction and Overview. *Yearbook of Medical Informatics*, 83–99. Retrieved from http://www.ebi.ac.uk/luscombe/publications.html

Lutterotti, A., Yousef, S., Sputtek, A., Sturner, K. H., Stellmann, J. P., Breiden, P., & Martin, R. et al. (2013). Antigen-specific tolerance by autologous myelin peptide-coupled cells: A phase 1 trial in multiple sclerosis. *Science Translational Medicine*, *5*(188), 188ra175. doi:10.1126/scitranslmed.3006168 PMID:23740901

Lux, S. E., & Palek, J. (1995). Disorders of the red cell membrane. In *Blood: Principles and Practice of Hematology*. Academic Press.

Lv, F., Qiu, Y., Zhang, Y., Liu, S., Shi, J., & Liu, Y. (2011). Adeno-associated virus-mediated anti-DR5 chimeric antibody expression suppresses human tumor growth in nude mice. *Cancer Letters*, *302*, 119–127. PMID:21306822

Lv, J., Perkovic, V., Foote, C. V., Craig, M. E., Craig, J. C., & Strippoli, G. F. (2012). Antihypertensive agents for preventing diabetic kidney disease. *Cochrane Database of Systematic Reviews*, *12*, CD004136. PMID:23235603

Lynch, T. J., Bell, D. W., Sordella, R., Gurubhagavatula, S., Okimoto, R. A., Brannigan, B. W., & Haber, D. A. et al. (2004). Activating mutations in the epidermal growth factor receptor underlying responsiveness of non-small-cell lung cancer to gefitinib. *The New England Journal of Medicine*, *350*(21), 2129–2139. doi:10.1056/NEJMoa040938 PMID:15118073

Maassen, C. B., Laman, J. D., van Holten-Neelen, C., Hoogteijling, L., Groenewegen, L., Visser, L., & Claassen, E. et al. (2003). Reduced experimental autoimmune encephalomyelitis after intranasal and oral administration of recombinant lactobacilli expressing myelin antigens. *Vaccine*, *21*(32), 4685–4693. doi:10.1016/S0264-410X(03)00522-X PMID:14585676

Ma, B., Duan, X., & Wang, Z. (2000). Clinical and experimental study on Shuanghua aerosol in treating infantile upper respiratory tract infection. *Zhongguo Zhong Xi Yi Jie He Za Zhi.*, *20*, 653–655. PMID:11789167

Mabberly, D. J. (1997). *A Portable Dictionary of the Vascular Plants* (2nd ed.). Cambridge, UK: Cambridge University Press.

Macconaill, L. E., Van Hummelen, P., Meyerson, M., & Hahn, W. C. (2011). Clinical implementation of comprehensive strategies to characterize cancer genomes: Opportunities and challenges. *Cancer Discovery*, *1*(4), 297–311. doi:10.1158/2159-8290.CD-11-0110 PMID:21935500

Machu, T. K. (2011). Therapeutics of 5-HT3 receptor antagonists: Current uses and future directions. *Pharmacology & Therapeutics*, *130*(3), 338–347. doi:10.1016/j.pharmthera.2011.02.003 PMID:21356241

Macisaac, R. J., Ekinci, E. I., & Jerums, G. (2014). Markers of and risk factors for the development and progression of diabetic kidney disease. *American Journal of Kidney Diseases*, *63*(2), S39–S62. doi:10.1053/j.ajkd.2013.10.048 PMID:24461729

Madadi, P., Ciszkowski, C., Gaedigk, A., Leeder, J. S., Teitelbaum, R., Chitayat, D., & Koren, G. (2011). Genetic transmission of cytochrome P450 2D6 (CYP2D6) ultrarapid metabolism: Implications for breastfeeding women taking codeine. *Current Drug Safety*, *6*(1), 36–39. doi:10.2174/157488611794479991 PMID:21241245

Madadi, P., Joly, Y., Avard, D., Chitayat, D. C., Smith, M. A., Ross, C. J., & Koren, G. et al. (2010). Communicating pharmacogenetic research results to breastfeeding mothers taking codeine: A pilot study of perceptions and benefits. *Clinical Pharmacology and Therapeutics*, *88*(6), 792–795. doi:10.1038/clpt.2010.125 PMID:20739920

Madadi, P., & Koren, G. (2008). Pharmacogenetic insights into codeine analgesia: Implications to pediatric codeine use. *Pharmacogenomics*, *9*(9), 1267–1284. doi:10.2217/14622416.9.9.1267 PMID:18781855

Madlensky, L., Natarajan, L., Tchu, S., Pu, M., Mortimer, J., Flatt, S. W., & Pierce, J. P. et al. (2011). Tamoxifen metabolite concentrations, CYP2D6 genotype, and breast cancer outcomes. *Clinical Pharmacology and Therapeutics*, *89*(5), 718–725. doi:10.1038/clpt.2011.32 PMID:21430657

Maetzel, A., Wong, A., Strand, V., Tugwell, P., Wells, G., & Bombardier, C. (2000). Meta-analysis of treatment termination rates among rheumatoid arthritis patients receiving disease-modifying anti-rheumatic drugs. *Rheumatology (Oxford, England)*, *39*(9), 975–981. doi:10.1093/rheumatology/39.9.975 PMID:10986302

Magnani, M., Laguerre, M., Rossi, L., Bianchi, M., Ninfali, P., Mangani, F., & Ropars, C. (1989). Acetaldehyde dehydrogenase-loaded erythrocytes as bioreactors for the removal of blood acetaldehyde. *Alcoholism, Clinical and Experimental Research*, *13*(6), 849–859. doi:10.1111/j.1530-0277.1989.tb00436.x PMID:2690672

Magnani, M., Rossi, L., D'ascenzo, M., Panzani, I., Bigi, L., & Zanella, A. (1998). Erythrocyte engineering for drug delivery and targeting. *Biotechnology and Applied Biochemistry*, *28*(Pt 1), 1–6. PMID:9693082

Ma, H., Liu, Y., Liu, S., Xu, R., & Zheng, D. (2005). Oral adeno-associated virus-sTRAIL gene therapy suppresses human hepatocellular carcinoma growth in mice. *Hepatology (Baltimore, Md.)*, *42*, 1355–1363. PMID:16317690

Maheshwari, R. A., Balaraman, R., Sen, A. K., & Seth, A. K. (2014). Effect of coenzyme Q10 alone and its combination with metformin on streptozotocin-nicotinamide-induced diabetic nephropathy in rats. *Indian Journal of Pharmacology*, *46*(6), 627–632. doi:10.4103/0253-7613.144924 PMID:25538335

Mahmmoud, Y. A. (2011). Curcumin is a lipid dependent inhibitor of the Na, K-ATPase that likely interacts at the protein-lipid interface. *Biochimica et Biophysica Acta*, *1808*(1), 466–473. doi:10.1016/j.bbamem.2010.09.021 PMID:20888791

Maity, K. K., Patra, S., Dey, B., Bhunia, S. K., Mandal, S., Das, D., & Islam, S. S. et al. (2011). A heteropolysaccharide from aqueous extract of an edible mushroom, *Pleurotus ostreatus* cultivar: Structural and biological studies. *Carbohydrate Research*, *346*(2), 366–372. doi:10.1016/j.carres.2010.10.026 PMID:21129732

Majithia, V., & Geraci, S. A. (2007). Rheumatoid arthritis: Diagnosis and management. *The American Journal of Medicine*, *120*(11), 936–939. PMID:17976416

Ma, L., Reinhardt, F., Pan, E., Soutschek, J., Bhat, B., Marcusson, E. G., & Weinberg, R. A. et al. (2010). Therapeutic silencing of miR-10b inhibits metastasis in a mouse mammary tumor model. *Nature Biotechnology*, *28*, 341–347. PMID:20351690

Ma, L., Teruya-Feldstein, J., & Weinberg, R. A. (2007). Tumour invasion and metastasis initiated by microRNA-10b in breast cancer. *Nature*, *449*, 682–688. PMID:17898713

Malavaki, C. J., Asimakopoulou, A. P., Lamari, F. N., Theocharis, A. D., Tzanakakis, G. N., & Karamanos, N. K. (2008). Capillary electrophoresis for the quality control of chondroitin sulfates in raw materials and formulations. *Analytical Biochemistry*, *374*(1), 213–220. doi:10.1016/j.ab.2007.11.006 PMID:18054774

Maldonado, R. A., LaMothe, R. A., Ferrari, J. D., Zhang, A. H., Rossi, R. J., Kolte, P. N., & Kishimoto, T. K. et al. (2015). Polymeric synthetic nanoparticles for the induction of antigen-specific immunological tolerance. *Proceedings of the National Academy of Sciences of the United States of America*, *112*(2), E156–E165. doi:10.1073/pnas.1408686111 PMID:25548186

Maliepaard, M., Nofziger, C., Papaluca, M., Zineh, I., Uyama, Y., Prasad, K., & Paulmichl, M. et al. (2013). Pharmacogenetics in the evaluation of new drugs: A multiregional regulatory perspective. *Nature Reviews. Drug Discovery*, *12*(2), 103–115. doi:10.1038/nrd3931 PMID:23370249

Maltzman, J. S., & Koretzky, G. A. (2003). Azathioprine: Old drug, new actions. *The Journal of Clinical Investigation*, *111*(8), 1122–1124. doi:10.1172/JCI200318384 PMID:12697731

Manach, C., Williamson, G., Morand, C., Scalbert, A., & Remesy, C. (2005). Bioavailability and bioefficacy of polyphenols in humans: Review of 97 bioavailability studies. *The American Journal of Clinical Nutrition*, *81*(supplement 1), 230S–242S. PMID:15640486

Mancone, C., Steindler, C., Santangelo, L., Simonte, G., Vlassi, C., Longo, M. A., & Alonzi, T. et al. (2011). Hepatitis C virus production requires apolipoprotein A-I and affects its association with nascent low-density lipoproteins. *Gut*, *60*, 378–386. PMID:20940285

Mandel, S., Packer, L., Youdim, M. B. H., & Weinreb, O. (2005). Proceedings from the Third Int. Conf. Mechanism of Action of Nutraceuticals. *The Journal of Nutritional Biochemistry*, *16*, 513–520. doi:10.1016/j.jnutbio.2005.03.001 PMID:16115539

Mandrekar, S. J., & Sargent, D. J. (2009). Clinical trial designs for predictive biomarker validation: Theoretical considerations and practical challenges. *Journal of Clinical Oncology*, *27*(24), 4027–4034. doi:10.1200/JCO.2009.22.3701 PMID:19597023

Manikowski, S. T., & Atta, M. G. (2013). Diabetic Kidney Disease: Pathophysiology and Therapeutic Targets. Journal of Diabetes Research.

Manikowski, S.T., & Atta, M.G. (2015) Diabetic Kidney Disease: Pathophysiology and Therapeutic Targets. *Journal of Diabetes Research.*

Mann, R., & Harman, R. (1983). Nail staining due to hydroquinone skin-lightening creams. *The British Journal of Dermatology*, *108*(3), 363–365. doi:10.1111/j.1365-2133.1983.tb03976.x PMID:6219692

Manolova, V., Flace, A., Bauer, M., Schwarz, K., Saudan, P., & Bachmann, M. F. (2008). Nanoparticles target distinct dendritic cell populations according to their size. *European Journal of Immunology*, *38*(5), 1404–1413. doi:10.1002/eji.200737984 PMID:18389478

Manson, M. M., Farmer, P. B., Gescher, A., & Steward, W. P. (2005). Innovative agents in cancer prevention. *Recent Results in Cancer Research. Fortschritte der Krebsforschung. Progres Dans les Recherches Sur le Cancer*, *166*, 257–275. doi:10.1007/3-540-26980-0_17 PMID:15648195

Ma, Q., & Lu, A. Y. (2011). Pharmacogenetics, pharmacogenomics, and individualized medicine. *Pharmacological Reviews*, *63*(2), 437–459. doi:10.1124/pr.110.003533 PMID:21436344

Marcuello, E., Paez, D., Pare, L., Salazar, J., Sebio, A., del Rio, E., & Baiget, M. (2011). A genotype-directed phase I-IV dose-finding study of irinotecan in combination with fluorouracil/leucovorin as first-line treatment in advanced colorectal cancer. *British Journal of Cancer*, *105*(1), 53–57. doi:10.1038/bjc.2011.206 PMID:21654688

Margaret, A., & Hamburg, M. D. (2013). *Paving the Way for Personalized Medicine*. U.S. Food and Drug Administration.

Marín, L., Miguélez, E. M., Villar, C. J., & Lombó, F. (2015). Bioavailability of Dietary Polyphenols and Gut Microbiota Metabolism: Antimicrobial Properties. BioMed Research International.

Marinova, K., Kleinschmidt, K., Weissenbock, G., & Klein, M. (2007). Flavonoid biosynthesis in barley primary leaves requires the presence of the vacuole and controls the activity of vacuolar flavonoid transport. *Plant Physiology*, *144*(1), 432–444. doi:10.1104/pp.106.094748 PMID:17369433

Markowitz, V. M., & Ritter, O. (1995). Characterizing heterogeneous molecular biology database systems. *Journal of Computational Biology*, *2*(4), 547–556. doi:10.1089/cmb.1995.2.547 PMID:8634907

Markt, P., Schuster, D., Kirchmair, J., Laggner, C., & Langer, T. (2007). Pharmacophore modeling and parallel screening for PPAR ligands. *Journal of Computer-Aided Molecular Design*, *21*(10-11), 575–590. doi:10.1007/s10822-007-9140-0 PMID:17960326

Marrero, J. A. (2005). GP73, a resident Golgi glycoprotein, is a novel serum marker for hepatocellular carcinoma. *Journal of Hepatology*, *43*, 1007–1012. PMID:16137783

Martino, F., Puddu, R. E., Pannarale, G., & Barilla, F. (2013). Dietary Fibers and Nutraceuticals for Primary Cardiovascular Prevention in Children and Adolescents: A Critical Review. *Food and Nutrition Sciences*, *4*(07), 39–47. doi:10.4236/fns.2013.47A006

Maruotti, N., Cantatore, F. P., Crivellato, E., Vacca, A., & Ribatti, D. (2007). Macrophages in rheumatoid arthritis. *Journal of Histology &. Histopathology*, *22*(5), 581–586.

Maslow, A. H., & Frager, R. (Eds.). (1987). *Motivation and Personality*. New York, London: Harper & Row.

Mason, J. B. (2011). Vitamins, trace minerals, and other micronutrients. In L. Goldman & D. Ausiello (Eds.), *Cecil Medicine. Saunders* (p. 225). Philadelphia, Pa.: Elsevier.

Mason, R. M. (2009). Connective tissue growth factor (CCN2), a pathogenic factor in diabetic nephropathy. What does it do? How does it do it? *Journal of Cell Communication and Signaling*, *3*(2), 95–104. doi:10.1007/s12079-009-0038-6 PMID:19214781

Massarelli, E., Varella-Garcia, M., Tang, X., Xavier, A. C., Ozburn, N. C., Liu, D. D., & Wistuba, I. I. et al. (2007). KRAS mutation is an important predictor of resistance to therapy with epidermal growth factor receptor tyrosine kinase inhibitors in non-small-cell lung cancer. *Clinical Cancer Research*, *13*(10), 2890–2896. doi:10.1158/1078-0432.CCR-06-3043 PMID:17504988

Mateos, J., Lourido, L., Patricia, F. P., Valentina, C., Carlos, F. L., Natividad, O., & Blanco, F. J. et al. (2012). Differential protein profiling of synovial fluid from rheumatoid arthritis and osteoarthritis patients using LC–MALDI TOF/TOF. *Journal of Proteomics*, *75*(10), 2869–2878. PMID:22245418

Mathela, D. K., Mathela, C. S., & Taskinen, J. (1986). Polyacetylenes and terpenoids from *Erigeron karwinskyanus. Journal of the Indian Chemical Society*, *63*, 603–604.

Mathela, D. K., Pant, A. K., & Mathela, C. S. (1984). A pyrone glycoside from *Erigeron karwinskyanus. Phytochemistry*, *23*(9), 2090–2091. doi:10.1016/S0031-9422(00)84988-2

Mathew, P. T., & Augusti, K. T. (1973). Studies on the effect of allicin (diallyl disulphide-oxide) on alloxan diabetes. Hypoglycemic action and enhancement of serum insulin effect and glycogen synthesis. *Indian Journal of Biochemistry & Biophysics*, *10*, 209–212. PMID:4792931

Mathew, P., & Augusti, K. T. (1975). Hypoglycaemic effects of onion, *Allium cepa* Linn.on diabetes mellitus-a preliminary report. *Indian Journal of Physiology and Pharmacology*, *19*, 213–217. PMID:1223000

Matissek, R. (1997). Evaluation of xanthine derivatives in chocolate-nutritional and chemical aspects. *Zeitschrift für Lebensmitteluntersuchung und -Forschung A, 205*, 175-184.

Matsuura, H. (2001). Saponins in garlic as modifiers of the risk of cardiovascular disease. *The Journal of Nutrition*, *131*, 1000S–1005S. PMID:11238805

Mattila, P., Konko, K., Eurola, M., Pihlawa, J. M., & Astola, J. (2001). Contents of vitamins, mineral elements, and some phenolic compounds in cultivated mushrooms. *Journal of Agricultural and Food Chemistry*, *49*(5), 2343–2348. doi:10.1021/jf001525d PMID:11368601

Mauro, M. J. (2006). Defining and managing imatinib resistance. Hematology American Society of Hematology Education Program.

McArthur, G. A., Chapman, P. B., Robert, C., Larkin, J., Haanen, J. B., Dummer, R., & Hauschild, A. et al. (2014). Safety and efficacy of vemurafenib in BRAF(V600E) and BRAF(V600K) mutation-positive melanoma (BRIM-3): Extended follow-up of a phase 3, randomised, open-label study. *The Lancet Oncology*, *15*(3), 323–332. doi:10.1016/S1470-2045(14)70012-9 PMID:24508103

McCarthy, D. P., Bryant, J., Galvin, J. P., Miller, S. D., & Luo, X. (2015). Tempering allorecognition to induce transplant tolerance with chemically modified apoptotic donor cells. *American Journal of Transplantation*, *15*(6), 1475–1483. doi:10.1111/ajt.13237 PMID:25807873

McChesney, J. D. (1999). Quality of botanical preparations: environmental issues and methodology for detecting environmental contaminants. In M. A. Liebert (Ed.), *Botanical Medicine: Efficacy, quality assurance and regulation* (pp. 127–131). New Rochelle Inc. Publishers.

McDougall, A. (2011). *Sustainable beauty the main theme at in-cosmetics*. Cosmetics design-Europe.com.

McGaha, T. L., Chen, Y., Ravishankar, B., van Rooijen, N., & Karlsson, M. C. (2011). Marginal zone macrophages suppress innate and adaptive immunity to apoptotic cells in the spleen. *Blood*, *117*(20), 5403–5412. doi:10.1182/blood-2010-11-320028 PMID:21444914

McGeough, C.M., & Bjourson, A.J. (2012). Diagnostic, Prognostic and Theranostic Genetic Biomarkers for Rheumatoid Arthritis. *Journal of* Clinical *& Cellular Immunology, S6*.

McKiernan, P. J. (2006). Nitisinone in the treatment of hereditary tyrosinaemia type 1. *Drugs*, *66*(6), 743–750. doi:10.2165/00003495-200666060-00002 PMID:16706549

McLeod, H. L., Krynetski, E. Y., Relling, M. V., & Evans, W. E. (2000). Genetic polymorphism of thiopurine methyltransferase and its clinical relevance for childhood acute lymphoblastic leukemia. *Leukemia*, *14*(4), 567–572. doi:10.1038/sj.leu.2401723 PMID:10764140

McLeod, H. L., Lin, J. S., Scott, E. P., Pui, C. H., & Evans, W. E. (1994). Thiopurine methyltransferase activity in American white subjects and black subjects. *Clinical Pharmacology and Therapeutics*, *55*(1), 15–20. doi:10.1038/clpt.1994.4 PMID:8299312

McNaught, A. D., & Wilkinson, A. (1997). *IUPAC Flavonoids (isoflavonoids and neoflavonoids) IUPAC Compendium of Chemical Terminology* (2nd ed.). Oxford, UK: Blackwell Scientific.

Md Yusof, M. Y., & Emery, P. (2013). Targeting interleukin-6 in rheumatoid arthritis. *Drugs*, *73*(4), 341–356. doi:10.1007/s40265-013-0018-2 PMID:23456676

Meena, A. J., Singh, A., Sharma, K., Kumari, S., & Rao, M. M. (2010). Physicochemical and preliminary phytochemical studies on the Rhizomes of *Glycyrrhiza glabra* Linn. *International Journal of Pharmacy and Pharmaceutical Sciences*, *2*, 48–50.

Meghwal, M., & Sahu, C. K. (2015). Soy Isoflavonoids as Nutraceutical for Human Health: An Update. *Journal of Cell Science and Therapy*, *6*, 194. doi:10.4172/2157-7013.1000194

Mehdi, M. M., & Rizvi, S. I. (2013). Plasma protein hydroperoxides during aging in humans: Correlation with paraoxonase 1 (PON1) arylesterase activity and plasma total thiols. *Archives of Medical Research*, *44*(2), 136–141. doi:10.1016/j.arcmed.2013.01.003 PMID:23376056

Mehdi, M. M., Singh, P., & Rizvi, S. I. (2012). Erythrocyte sialic acid content during aging in humans: Correlation with markers of oxidative stress. *Disease Markers*, *32*(3), 179–186. doi:10.1155/2012/293429 PMID:22377734

Mehdi, U., & Toto, R. D. (2009). Anemia, Diabetes, and Chronic Kidney Disease. *Diabetes Care*, *32*(7), 1320–1326. doi:10.2337/dc08-0779 PMID:19564475

Mehnert, W., & Mader, K. (2001). Solid lipid nanoparticles: Production, characterization and applications. *Advanced Drug Delivery Reviews*, *47*(2-3), 165–196. doi:10.1016/S0169-409X(01)00105-3 PMID:11311991

Meier, B. (2001). Comparing phytopharmaceuticlas: The example of St. John's wort. *Advances in Natural Therapy*, *18*(1), 35–46. doi:10.1007/BF02850249 PMID:11512531

Meiyanto, E., Hermawan, A., & Anindyajati, A. (2012). Natural products for cancer-targeted therapy:citrus flavonoids as potent chemopreventive agents. *Asian Pacific Journal of Cancer Prevention*, *13*(2), 427–436. doi:10.7314/APJCP.2012.13.2.427 PMID:22524801

Meltretter, J., Schmidt, A., Humeny, A., Becker, C. M., & Pischetsrieder, M. (2008). Analysis of the peptide profile of milk and its changes during thermal treatment and storage. *Journal of Agricultural and Food Chemistry*, *56*(9), 2899–2906. doi:10.1021/jf073479o PMID:18419126

Mendiola, J. A., Torres, C. F., Martín-Álvarez, P. J., & Santoyo, S. (2007). Use of supercritical CO2 to obtain extracts with antimicrobial activity from *Chaetoceros muelleri* microalga. A correlation with their lipidic content. *European Food Research and Technology*, *224*(4), 505–510. doi:10.1007/s00217-006-0353-6

Mendiola, J., Torres-Cantero, A. M., Vioque, J., Moreno-Grau, J. M., Ten, J., Roca, M., & Bernabeu, R. et al. (2010). A low intake of antioxidant nutrients is associated with poor semen quality in patients attending fertility clinics. *Fertility and Sterility*, *93*(4), 1128–1133. doi:10.1016/j.fertnstert.2008.10.075 PMID:19147135

Menne, J., Park, J. K., Boehne, M., Elger, M., Lindschau, C., Kirsch, T., & Haller, H. et al. (2004). Diminished loss of proteoglycans and lack of albuminuria in protein kinase C-??-deficient diabetic mice. *Diabetes*, *53*(8), 2101–2109. doi:10.2337/diabetes.53.8.2101 PMID:15277392

Meragelman, K. M., Mckee, T. C., & Boyd, M. R. (2001). Anti-HIV prenylated flavonoids from *Monotes africanus*. *Journal of Natural Products*, *64*(4), 546–548. doi:10.1021/np0005457 PMID:11325248

Mercenier, A., Pavan, S., & Pot, B. (2002). Probiotics as biotherapeutic agents: Present knowledge and future prospects. *Current Pharmaceutical Design*, *8*, 99–110. PMID:11812252

Mercola. (2009). *Top 12 Foods for Healthy Immune Response*. Retrieved 4.6.2015, from http://articles.mercola.com/sites/articles

Meshnick, S. R., & Dobson, M. J. (2001). The history of antimalarial drugs. In P. J. Posenthal (Ed.), *Antimalarial chemotherapy mechanism of action, resistance and new drug directions in drug discovery*. Humana Press. doi:10.1385/1-59259-111-6:15

Meyer, A. (1998). The 1998 top 100® R&D survey. *Food Processing.*, *58*(8), 32–40.

Meyer, H. (1899). Zur Theorie der Alkoholnarkose. *Arch. Exp Pathol. Pharmakol*, *42*(2-4), 109–118. doi:10.1007/BF01834479

Michaely, P., & Bennett, V. (1995). The ANK repeats of erythrocyte ankyrin form two distinct but cooperative binding sites for the erythrocyte anion exchanger. *The Journal of Biological Chemistry*, *270*(37), 22050–22057. doi:10.1074/jbc.270.37.22050 PMID:7665627

Mignat, C., Wille, U., & Ziegler, A. (1995). Affinity profiles of morphine, codeine, dihydrocodeine and their glucuronides at opioid receptor subtypes. *Life Sciences*, *56*(10), 793–799. doi:10.1016/0024-3205(95)00010-4 PMID:7885194

Miguet, L., Zhang, Z., Barbier, M., & Grigorov, M. G. (2006). Comparison of a homology model and the crystallographic structure of human 11beta-hydroxysteroid dehydrogenase type 1 (11betaHSD1) in a structure-based identification of inhibitors. *Journal of Computer-Aided Molecular Design*, *20*(2), 67–81. doi:10.1007/s10822-006-9037-3 PMID:16783599

Mikus, G., Scholz, I. M., & Weiss, J. (2011). Pharmacogenomics of the triazole antifungal agent voriconazole. *Pharmacogenomics*, *12*(6), 861–872. doi:10.2217/pgs.11.18 PMID:21692616

Miladinovic, B., Kostic, M., Savikin, K., Đorđević, B., Mihajilov-Krstev, T., Živanović, S., & Kitić, D. (2014). Chemical Profile and Antioxidative and Antimicrobial Activity of Juices and Extracts of 4 Black Currants Varieties (*Ribes nigrum* L.). *Journal of Food Science*, *79*(3), C301–C309. doi:10.1111/1750-3841.12364 PMID:24506271

Miller, S. D., & Karpus, W. J. (2007). Experimental autoimmune encephalomyelitis in the mouse. Curr Protoc Immunol. doi:10.1002/0471142735.im1501s77

Miller, K. I., Qing, C., Sze, D. M., Roufogalis, B. D., & Neilan, B. A. (2012). Culturable endophytes of medicinal plants and the genetic basis for their bioactivity. *Microbial Ecology*, *64*(2), 431–449. doi:10.1007/s00248-012-0044-8 PMID:22430508

Miller, V. A., Hirsh, V., Cadranel, J., Chen, Y. M., Park, K., Kim, S. W., & Yang, J. C. et al. (2012). Afatinib versus placebo for patients with advanced, metastatic non-small-cell lung cancer after failure of erlotinib, gefitinib, or both, and one or two lines of chemotherapy (LUX-Lung 1): A phase 2b/3 randomised trial. *The Lancet Oncology*, *13*(5), 528–538. doi:10.1016/S1470-2045(12)70087-6 PMID:22452896

Mindful Minerals. (n.d.). Retrieved 13.6.2015, from https://mindfulminerals.com

Mischoulon, D., Fava, M., & Stahl, S. (2009). Folate Supplementation. *The Journal of Clinical Psychiatry*, *70*(5), 767–769. doi:10.4088/JCP.08lr04824a PMID:19552872

Mishra, A., Bhatti, R., Singh, A., & Singh Ishar, M. P. (2010). Ameliorative effect of the cinnamon oil from *Cinnamomum zeylanicum* upon early stage diabetic nephropathy. *Planta Medica*, *76*(5), 412–417. doi:10.1055/s-0029-1186237 PMID:19876811

Misra, S. K., Dybowska, A., Berhanu, D., Luoma, S. N., & Valsami-Jones, E. (2012). The complexity of nanoparticle dissolution and its importance in nanotoxicological studies. *The Science of the Total Environment*, *438*, 225–232. doi:10.1016/j.scitotenv.2012.08.066 PMID:23000548

Miyakis, S., van Hal, S. J., Ray, J., & Marriott, D. (2010). Voriconazole concentrations and outcome of invasive fungal infections. *Clinical Microbiology and Infection*, *16*(7), 927–933. doi:10.1111/j.1469-0691.2009.02990.x PMID:19845698

Mobh, S. (1938). Research for Vitamin P. *Journal of Biochemistry*, *29*(3), 487–501.

Moerman, D. (1988). *Native American Ethnobotany*. Timber Press.

Moghimi, S. M., Hunter, A. C., & Andresen, T. L. (2012). Factors controlling nanoparticle pharmacokinetics: An integrated analysis and perspective. *Annual Review of Pharmacology and Toxicology*, *52*(1), 481–503. doi:10.1146/annurev-pharmtox-010611-134623 PMID:22035254

Mohamed, I., Shuid, A., Borhanuddin, B., & Fozi, N. (2012). The Application of Phytomedicine in Modern Drug Development. *The Internet Journal of Herbal and Plant Medicine*, *1*(2), 16–22.

Mohan, C., & Putterman, C. (2015). Genetics and pathogenesis of systemic lupus erythematosus and lupus nephritis. *Nature Reviews. Nephrology*, *11*(6), 329–341. doi:10.1038/nrneph.2015.33 PMID:25825084

Mohandas, N., & Gallagher, P. G. (2008). Red cell membrane: Past, present, and future. *Blood*, *112*(10), 3939–3948. doi:10.1182/blood-2008-07-161166 PMID:18988878

Mohan, V., Sandeep, S., Deepa, R., Shah, B., & Varghese, C. (2007). Epidemiology of type 2 diabetes: Indian scenario. *The Indian Journal of Medical Research*, *125*, 217–230. PMID:17496352

Moja, L., Tagliabue, L., Balduzzi, S., Parmelli, E., Pistotti, V., Guarneri, V., & D'Amico, R. (2012). Trastuzumab containing regimens for early breast cancer. *Cochrane Database of Systematic Reviews*, *4*, CD006243. PMID:22513938

Mok, C. C., & Lau, C. S. (2003). Pathogenesis of systemic lupus erythematosus. *Journal of Clinical Pathology*, *56*(7), 481–490. doi:10.1136/jcp.56.7.481 PMID:12835292

Moller, P., Jacobsen, N. R., Folkmann, J. K., Danielsen, P. H., Mikkelsen, L., Hemmingsen, J. G., & Loft, S. et al. (2010). Role of oxidative damage in toxicity of particulates. *Free Radical Research*, *44*(1), 1–46. doi:10.3109/10715760903300691 PMID:19886744

Molloy, M. P. (2000). Two-dimensional electrophoresis of membrane proteins using immobilized pH gradients. *Analytical Biochemistry*, *280*, 1–10. PMID:10805514

Monopoli, M. P., Aberg, C., Salvati, A., & Dawson, K. A. (2012). Biomolecular coronas provide the biological identity of nanosized materials. *Nature Nanotechnology*, *7*(12), 779–786. doi:10.1038/nnano.2012.207 PMID:23212421

Moon, S., Cho, G., Jung, S., Gal, S., Kwon, T. K., Lee, Y.-C., & Kim, C.-H. et al. (2003). Quercetin exerts multiple inhibitory effects on vascular smooth muscle cells: Roleof ERK1/2, cell-cycle regulation, and matrix metalloproteinase-9. *Biochemical and Biophysical Research Communications*, *301*(4), 1069–1078. doi:10.1016/S0006-291X(03)00091-3 PMID:12589822

Moorjani, M., Lejeune, A., Gicquaud, C., Lacroix, J., Poyet, P., & Gaudreault, R. C. (1996). Nanoerythrosomes, a new derivative of erythrocyte ghost II: Identification of the mechanism of action. *Anticancer Research*, *16*(5A), 2831–2836. PMID:8917393

Mooyaart, A. L., Valk, E. J. J., & Van, E. S. (2011). Genetic associations in diabetic nephropathy: A meta-analysis. *Diabetologia*, *54*(3), 544–553. doi:10.1007/s00125-010-1996-1 PMID:21127830

Morgan, S. L., & Baggott, J. E. (2006). Medical foods: Products for the management of chronic diseases. *Nutrition Reviews*, *64*(11), 495–501. doi:10.1111/j.1753-4887.2006.tb00182.x PMID:17131945

Mori, H., Okada, Y., Arao, T., & Tanaka, Y. (2014). Sitagliptin improves albuminuria in patients with type 2 diabetes mellitus. *Journal of Diabetes and Investigation*, *5*(3), 313–319. doi:10.1111/jdi.12142 PMID:24843780

Mori, T. A., Bao, D. Q., Burke, V., Puddey, I. B., & Beilin, L. J. (1999). Docohexanoic acid but not eicasapentanoic acid lowers ambulatory blood pressure and heart rate in humans. *Hypertension*, *34*(2), 253–260. doi:10.1161/01.HYP.34.2.253 PMID:10454450

Morita, Y., Yang, J., & Gupta, R. (2001). Dendritic cells genetically engineered to express IL-4 inhibit murine collagen-induced arthritis. *The Journal of Clinical Investigation*, *107*, 1275–1284. PMID:11375417

Motavaf, M., Safari, S., & Alavian, S. M. (2012). Therapeutic potential of RNA interference: A new molecular approach to antiviral treatment for hepatitis C. *Journal of Viral Hepatitis*, *19*, 757–765. PMID:23043382

Moyano, E., Fornale, S., Palazon, J., Cusido, R. M., Bonfill, M., Morales, C., & Pinol, M. T. (1999). Effect of *Agrobacterium rhizogenes* T-DNA on alkaloid production in Solanaceae plants. *Phytochemistry*, *52*(7), 1287–1292. doi:10.1016/S0031-9422(99)00421-5

Mudaliar, H., Pollock, C., Komala, M. G., Chadban, S., Wu, H., & Panchapakesan, U. (2013). The role of Toll-like receptor proteins (TLR) 2 and 4 in mediatinginflammation in proximal tubules. *American Journal of Physiology. Renal Physiology*, *305*(2), F143–F154. doi:10.1152/ajprenal.00398.2012 PMID:23576640

Muir, A. D., Paton, D., Ballantyne, K., & Aubin., A. A. (2002). *US Patent, 6,355,249*. US Patent Office.

Mukherjee, K., Ghosh, N. C., & Datta, T. (1972). *Coccinia indica* Linn.As potential hypoglycemic agent. *Indian Journal of Experimental Biology*, *10*, 347–349. PMID:4658184

Mulhall, J. P., Daller, M., Traish, A. M., Gupta, S., Park, K., Salimpour, P., & Goldstein, I. et al. (1997). Intracavernosal forskolin: Role in management of pharmacotherapy vasculogenic impotence resistant to standard 3-agent. *The Journal of Urology*, *158*, 1752–1759. doi:10.1016/S0022-5347(01)64118-1 PMID:9334594

Muller-Ladner, U., Pap, T., Gay, R. E., Neidhart, M., & Gay, S. (2005). Mechanisms of disease: The molecular and cellular basis of joint destruction in rheumatoid arthritis. *Nature Clinical Practice. Rheumatology*, *1*(2), 102–110. PMID:16932639

Muniba, S. (2010). *Application of Bioinformatics in medicine*. Retrieved from http://www.biotecharticles.com/Bioinformatics-Article/Application-of-Bioinformatics-in-Medicine-222.html

Musshoff, F., Madea, B., Stuber, F., & Stamer, U. M. (2006). Enantiomeric determination of tramadol and O-desmethyltramadol by liquid chromatography- mass spectrometry and application to postoperative patients receiving tramadol. *Journal of Analytical Toxicology*, *30*(7), 463–467. doi:10.1093/jat/30.7.463 PMID:16959140

Muyldermans, S., Cambilla, C., & Wyns, L. (2001). Recognition of antigens by single-domain antibody, fractions: The superfluous luxury of paired domains. *Trends in Biochemical Sciences*, *26*(4), 230–235. doi:10.1016/S0968-0004(01)01790-X PMID:11295555

Nagahama, T., Hayashi, K., Ozawa, Y., Takenaka, T., & Saruta, T. (2000). Role of protein kinase C in angiotensin II-induced constriction of renal microvessels. *Kidney International*, *57*(1), 215–223. doi:10.1046/j.1523-1755.2000.00822.x PMID:10620202

Nagwani, S., & Tripathi, Y. B. (2010). Amelioration of cisplatin induced nephrotoxicity by PTY: A herbal preparation. *Food and Chemical Toxicology*, *48*(8-9), 2253–2258. doi:10.1016/j.fct.2010.05.057 PMID:20510324

Nair, K. S., Rizza, R. A., O'Brien, P., Dhatariya, K., Short, K. R., Nehra, A., & Jensen, M. D. et al. (2006). DHEA in elderly women and DHEA or testosterone in elderly men. *The New England Journal of Medicine*, *355*(16), 1647–1659. doi:10.1056/NEJMoa054629 PMID:17050889

Nakamura, Y., Ratain, M. J., Cox, N. J., McLeod, H. L., Kroetz, D. L., & Flockhart, D. A. (2012). Re: CYP2D6 genotype and tamoxifen response in postmenopausal women with endocrine-responsive breast cancer: the Breast International Group 1-98 trial. *Journal of the National Cancer Institute*, *104*(16), 1264, author reply 1266–1268. doi:10.1093/jnci/djs304 PMID:22851270

Narasimhan, S., & Lohoff, F. W. (2012). Pharmacogenetics of antidepressant drugs: Current clinical practice and future directions. *Pharmacogenomics*, *13*(4), 441–464. doi:10.2217/pgs.12.1 PMID:22380000

Narasinga Rao, B. S. (2003). Bioactive phytochemicals in Indian foods and their potential in health promotion and disease prevention. *Asia Pacific Journal of Clinical Nutrition*, *12*, 9–22. PMID:12737006

National Institute of Neurological Disorders and Stroke. (2013). *Dementia: hope through research*. Bethesda, MD: Office of Communications and Public Liaison, National Institute of Neurological Disorders and Stroke, US National Institutes of Health.

National Institute on Drug Abuse. (2015). *Is Marijuana Medicine?* National Institute on Drug Abuse, Drug Facts.

National Medicinal Plans Board, Government of India, Ministry of Ayush. (n.d.). Retrieved from http://www.nmpb.nic.in

National Organization for Rare Disorders. (2012). *Physician's Guide to Tyrosinemia Type 1*. The National Organization for Rare Disorders.

NCBI (National Center for Biotechnology Information). Retrieved from http://www.ncbi.nlm.nih.gov

Ncube, B., Finnie, J. F., & Van Staden, J. (2012). Quality from the field: The impact of environmental factors as quality determinants in medicinal plants. *South African Journal of Botany*, *82*, 11–20. doi:10.1016/j.sajb.2012.05.009

Nehlig, A., Daval, J. L., & Debry, G. (1992). Caffeine and the central nervous system: Mechanisms of action, biochemical, metabolic and psychostimulant effects. *Brain Research. Brain Research Reviews*, *17*(2), 139–170. doi:10.1016/0165-0173(92)90012-B PMID:1356551

Nel, A. E., Madler, L., Velegol, D., Xia, T., Hoek, E. M., Somasundaran, P., & Thompson, M. (2009). Understanding biophysicochemical interactions at the nano-bio interface. *Nature Materials*, *8*(7), 543–557. doi:10.1038/nmat2442 PMID:19525947

Nelson, D. L., & Cox, M. M. (2000). Lehninger Principles of Biochemistry (3rd ed.). W. H. Freeman.

Newman, D. J., & Cragg, G. M. (2007). Natural products as sources of new drugs over the last 25 Years. *Journal of Natural Products*, *70*(3), 461–477. doi:10.1021/np068054v PMID:17309302

Niacin Compound Summary (NCS). (n.d.). PubChem. National Center for Biotechnology Information, U.S. National Library of Medicine.

Nichenametla, S. N., Taruscio, T. G., Barney, D. L., & Exon, J. H. (2006). A review of the effects and mechanism of polyphenolics in cancer. *Critical Reviews in Food Science and Nutrition*, *46*(2), 161–183. doi:10.1080/10408390591000541 PMID:16431408

Nichols, A. I., Focht, K., Jiang, Q., Preskorn, S. H., & Kane, C. P. (2011). Pharmacokinetics of venlafaxine extended release 75 mg and desvenlafaxine 50 mg in healthy CYP2D6 extensive and poor metabolizers: A randomized, open-label, two-period, parallel-group, crossover study. *Clinical Drug Investigation*, *31*(3), 155–167. doi:10.2165/11586630-000000000-00000 PMID:21288052

Nichols, J. A., & Katiyar, S. K. (2010). Skin photoprotection by natural polyphenols: Anti-inflammatory, anti-oxidant and DNA repair mechanisms. *Archives of Dermatological Research*, *302*(2), 71–83. doi:10.1007/s00403-009-1001-3 PMID:19898857

Nicholson, L. B., Murtaza, A., Hafler, B. P., Sette, A., & Kuchroo, V. K. (1997). A T cell receptor antagonist peptide induces T cells that mediate bystander suppression and prevent autoimmune encephalomyelitis induced with multiple myelin antigens. *Proceedings of the National Academy of Sciences of the United States of America*, *94*(17), 9279–9284. doi:10.1073/pnas.94.17.9279 PMID:9256473

Nicolaou, K. C., Yang, Z., Liu, J. J., Ueno, H., Nantermet, P. G., Guy, R. K., & Sorensen, E. J. (1994). Total synthesis of taxol. *Nature*, *367*(6464), 630–634. doi:10.1038/367630a0 PMID:7906395

Nicolau, C., & Gersonde, K. (1979). Incorporation of Inositol Hexaphosphate into Intact Red Blood Cells, I: Fusion of Effector-Containing Lipid Vesicles with Erythrocytes. *Naturwissenschaften*, *66*(11), 563–566. doi:10.1007/BF00368810 PMID:514370

Nittynen, L., Nurminen, M. L., Korpela, I., & Vapaatalo, H. (1999). Role of arginine, taurine and homocysteine in cardiovascular disease. *Annals of Medicine*, *31*(5), 318–326. doi:10.3109/07853899908995898 PMID:10574504

Nobili, S., Lippi, D., Witort, E., Donnini, M., Bausi, L., Mini, E., & Capaccioli, S. (2009). Natural compounds for cancer treatment and prevention. *Pharmacological Research*, *59*(6), 365–378. doi:10.1016/j.phrs.2009.01.017 PMID:19429468

Noehr-Jensen, L., Zwisler, S. T., Larsen, F., Sindrup, S. H., Damkier, P., Nielsen, F., & Brosen, K. (2009). Impact of CYP2C19 phenotypes on escitalopram metabolism and an evaluation of pupillometry as a serotonergic biomarker. *European Journal of Clinical Pharmacology*, *65*(9), 887–894. doi:10.1007/s00228-009-0657-0 PMID:19404631

Noh, H., & King, G. L. (2007). The role of protein kinase C activation in diabetic nephropathy. *Kidney International*, *106*, S49–S53. doi:10.1038/sj.ki.5002386 PMID:17653211

Nohynek, G. J., Antignac, E., Re, T., & Toutain, H. (2010). Safety assessment of personal care products/cosmetics and their ingredients. *Toxicology and Applied Pharmacology*, *243*(2), 239–259. doi:10.1016/j.taap.2009.12.001 PMID:20005888

Nordeen, S. K., Bona, B. J., Jones, D. N., Lambert, J. R., & Jackson, T. A. (2013). Endocrine disrupting activities of the flavonoid nutraceuticals luteolin and quercetin. *Horm. Canc.*, *4*(5), 293–300. doi:10.1007/s12672-013-0150-1 PMID:23836117

Norman, A. W., & Henry, H. L. (2012). *Hormones* (3rd ed.). Oxford, UK: Academic Press.

Nounou, M. M., El-Khordagui, L. K., & Khalafallah, N. (2005). Release stability of 5-fluorouracil liposomal concentrates, gels and lyophilized powder. *Acta Poloniae Pharmaceutica*, *62*(5), 381–391. PMID:16459487

Nugroho, A. E., Andrie, M., Warditiani, N. K., Siswanto, E., Pramono, S., & Lukitaningsih, E. (2012). Antidiabetic and antihiperlipidemic effect of Andrographis paniculata (Burm. f.) Nees and andrographolide in high-fructose-fat-fed rats. *Indian Journal of Pharmacology*, *44*(3), 377–381. doi:10.4103/0253-7613.96343 PMID:22701250

Nusgens, B. V., Humbert, P., Rougier, A., Colige, A. C., Haftek, M., Lambert, C. A., & Lapiere, C. M. et al. (2001). Topically applied vitamin C enhances the mRNA level of collagens I and III, their processing enzymes and tissue inhibitor of matrix metalloproteinase 1 in the human dermis. *The Journal of Investigative Dermatology*, *116*(6), 853–859. doi:10.1046/j.0022-202x.2001.01362.x PMID:11407971

Nutraceutical World. (n.d.). Retrieved from http://www.nutraceuticalsworld.com/

Nutrition, H. (2009). *Iodine*. George Mateljan Foundation.

Nutrition, H. (2009). *Iron*. George Mateljan Foundation.

Nutrition, H. (2009). *Magnesium*. George Mateljan Foundation.

Nutrition, H. (2009). *Selenium*. George Mateljan Foundation.

Nutrition, H. (2009). *Zinc*. George Mateljan Foundation.

Oblong, J. E., & Bisset, D. L. (2005). Retinoids. In Z. D. Draelos (Ed.), *Cosmeceuticals* (pp. 35–45). Philadelphia: Elsevier Saunders.

Ohga, S., Shikata, K., Yozai, K., Okada, S., Ogawa, D., Usui, H., & Makino, H. et al. (2007). Thiazolidinedione ameliorates renal injury in experimental diabetic rats through anti-inflammatory effects mediated by inhibition of NF-kB activation. *American Journal of Physiology. Renal Physiology*, *292*(4), F1141–F1150. doi:10.1152/ajprenal.00288.2005 PMID:17190910

Oh, J. U., Jang, H., & Kim, S. J. (2014). Inhibition of inducible nitric oxide synthase and cyclooxygenase-2 by methanolic extract of *Crataegi Fructus. Current Topics in Nutraceutical Research.*, *12*(1/2), 35–42.

Oh, J., & O'Connor, P. W. (2014). Teriflunomide in the treatment of multiple sclerosis: Current evidence and future prospects. *Ther Adv Neurol Disord*, *7*(5), 239–252. doi:10.1177/1756285614546855 PMID:25342978

Oh, N., & Park, J. H. (2014). Endocytosis and exocytosis of nanoparticles in mammalian cells. *International Journal of Nanomedicine*, *9*(Suppl 1), 51–63. doi:10.2147/IJN.S26592 PMID:24872703

Okanoto, M. et al.. (2000). Effects of perilla seed oil supplementation on leukotriene generation by leucocytes in patients with asthma associated with lipometabolism. *International Archives of Allergy and Immunology*, *122*(2), 137–142. doi:10.1159/000024369 PMID:10878492

Okuda, H. (2001). Comparison of clinicopathological features of patients with hepatocellular carcinoma seropositive for alphafetoprotein alone and those seropositive for des-gamma-carboxy prothrombin alone. *Journal of Gastroenterology and Hepatology*, *16*, 1290–1296. PMID:11903749

Onifade, A. K. (2007). Research trends: Bioactive metabolites of fungal origin. *Research Journal of Biological Sciences*, *2*, 81–84.

Oomah, B. D., Ladet, S., Godfrey, D. V., Liang, J., & Girard, B. (2000). Characteristics of raspberry (Rubus idaeus L.) seed oil. *Food Chemistry*, *69*(2), 187–193. doi:10.1016/S0308-8146(99)00260-5

Orban, T., Bundy, B., Becker, D. J., DiMeglio, L. A., Gitelman, S. E., Goland, R., & Skyler, J. S. et al. (2011). Co-stimulation modulation with abatacept in patients with recent-onset type 1 diabetes: A randomised, double-blind, placebo-controlled trial. *Lancet*, *378*(9789), 412–419. doi:10.1016/S0140-6736(11)60886-6 PMID:21719096

Oricha, B. S. (2010). Cosmeceuticals: A review. *African Journal of Pharmacy and Pharmacology*, *4*(4), 127–129.

Orozco-Topete, R., Sierra-Madero, J., Cano-Dominguez, C., Kershenovich, J., Ortiz-Pedroza, G., Vazquez-Valls, E., & Rozhon, E. J. (1997). Safety and efficacy of Virend for topical treatment of genital and anal herpes simplex lesions in patients with AIDS. *Antiviral Research*, *35*(2), 91–103. doi:10.1016/S0166-3542(97)00015-6 PMID:9217246

Ospelt, C., & Gay, S. (2007). Antirheumatic drugs and gene signatures. *Current Opinion in Investigational Drugs (London, England)*, *8*, 385–389. PMID:17520867

Oumeish, O. Y. (2001). The cultural and philosophical concepts of cosmetics in beauty and art through the medical history of mankind. *Clinics in Dermatology*, *19*(4), 375–386. doi:10.1016/S0738-081X(01)00194-8 PMID:11535377

Overton, E. (1901). *Studien uber die Narkose, zugleich ein Beitrag zur allgemeiner Pharmakologie*. Jena, Switzerland: Gustav Fischer.

Owusu Obeng, A., Egelund, E. F., Alsultan, A., Peloquin, C. A., & Johnson, J. A. (2014). CYP2C19 polymorphisms and therapeutic drug monitoring of voriconazole: Are we ready for clinical implementation of pharmacogenomics? *Pharmacotherapy*, *34*(7), 703–718. doi:10.1002/phar.1400 PMID:24510446

P450 Drug interaction Table. (2010). *Indiana University Division of Clinical Pharmacology*. Retrieved from http://medicine.iupui.edu/clinpharm/ddis/table.asp

Pacholczyk, R., & Kern, J. (2008). The T-cell receptor repertoire of regulatory T cells. *Immunology*, *125*(4), 450–458. doi:10.1111/j.1365-2567.2008.02992.x PMID:19128356

Packaged Facts. (2012). *Cosmeceuticals in the U.S.* (6th ed.). Retrieved October 11, 2015, from http://www.marketresearch.com/Packaged-Facts-v768/Cosmeceuticals-Edition-6281775/

Paduch, R., Kandefer-Szerszen, M., Trytek, M., & Fiedurek, J. (2007). Terpenes: Substances useful in human healthcare. *Archivum Immunologiae et Therapiae Experimentalis*, *55*(5), 315–327. doi:10.1007/s00005-007-0039-1 PMID:18219762

Page, T. H., Brown, A. C., Timms, E. M., Brennan, F. M., Ray, K. P., & Foxwell, B. M. J. (2007). Treatment with Non-steroidal Anti-inflammatory Drugs Increases TNF Production in Rheumatoid Arthritis. *Cytokine*, *39*(1), 32–32. PMID:17544674

Pai, S. R., Nimbalkar, M. S., Pawar, N. V., Kedage, V. V., & Dixit, G. B. (2008). *In vitro* embryo culture and ex situ regeneration studies in *Ancistrocladus heyneanus* Wall. Ex Grah. *Plant Cell Biotechnology & Molecular Biology*, *9*, 95–100.

Palanisamy, U. D., Ling, L. T., Manaharan, T., & Appleton, D. (2011). Rapid isolation of geraniin from *Nephelium lappaceum* rind waste and its hyperglycemic activity. *Food Chemistry*, *127*(1), 21–27. doi:10.1016/j.foodchem.2010.12.070

Pandey, K. B., & Rizvi, S. I. (2010). Markers of oxidative stress in erythrocytes and plasma during aging in humans. *Oxidative Medicine and Cellular Longevity*, *3*(1), 2–12. doi:10.4161/oxim.3.1.10476 PMID:20716923

Pandey, K. B., & Rizvi, S. I. (2014a). Resveratrol *in vitro* ameliorates tert-butyl hydroperoxide-induced alterations in erythrocyte membranes from young and older humans. *Applied Physiology, Nutrition, and Metabolism*, *31*, 1–5. PMID:24914573

Pandey, K. B., & Rizvi, S. I. (2014b). Role of resveratrol in regulation of membrane transporters and integrity of human erythrocytes. *Biochemical and Biophysical Research Communications*, *453*(3), 521–526. doi:10.1016/j.bbrc.2014.09.117 PMID:25285638

Pandey, M. M., Rastogi, S., & Rawat, A. K. S. (2013). Indian traditional Ayurvedic system of medicine and nutritional supplementation. *Evidence-Based Complementary and Alternative Medicine*, *2013*, 1–12. PMID:23864888

Pandey, N., Meena, R. P., Rai, S. K., & Pandey-Rai, S. (2011). Medicinal plants derived nutraceuticals: A re-emerging health aid. *International Journal of Pharma and Bio Sciences*, *2*(4), 419–441.

Pan, Q. W., Henry, S. D., Scholte, B. J., Tilanus, H. W., Janssen, H. L., & van der Laan, L. J. (2007). New therapeutic opportunities for hepatitis C based on small RNA. *World Journal of Gastroenterology*, *13*(33), 4431–4436. PMID:17724797

Pardoll, D. M. (2012). The blockade of immune checkpoints in cancer immunotherapy. *Nature Reviews. Cancer*, *12*(4), 252–264. doi:10.1038/nrc3239 PMID:22437870

Paredes, S. D., Korkmaz, A., Manchester, L. C., Tan, D. X., & Reiter, R. J. (2009). Phytomelatonin: A review. *Journal of Experimental Botany*, *60*(1), 57–69. doi:10.1093/jxb/ern284 PMID:19033551

Park, M. (2013). *Half of Americans use supplements*. CNN.

Park, S. U., & Facchini, P. J. (2000). *Agrobacterium rhizogenes* mediated transformation of opium poppy, *Papaver somniferum* L., and *California poppy, Eschscholzia californica*Cham., root cultures. *Journal of Experimental Botany*, *51*(347), 1005–1016. doi:10.1093/jexbot/51.347.1005 PMID:10948228

Park, W. B., Kim, N. H., Kim, K. H., Lee, S. H., Nam, W. S., Yoon, S. H., & Yu, K. S. et al. (2012). The effect of therapeutic drug monitoring on safety and efficacy of voriconazole in invasive fungal infections: A randomized controlled trial. *Clinical Infectious Diseases*, *55*(8), 1080–1087. doi:10.1093/cid/cis599 PMID:22761409

Patel, J. N. (2014). Application of genotype-guided cancer therapy in solid tumors. *Pharmacogenomics*, *15*(1), 79–93. doi:10.2217/pgs.13.227 PMID:24329193

Patel, J. N., Fuchs, C. S., Owzar, K., Chen, Z., & McLeod, H. L. (2013). Gastric cancer pharmacogenetics: Progress or old tripe? *Pharmacogenomics*, *14*(9), 1053–1064. doi:10.2217/pgs.13.88 PMID:23837480

Patel, J. N., Mandock, K., & McLeod, H. L. (2014). Clinically relevant cancer biomarkers and pharmacogenetic assays. *Journal of Oncology Pharmacy Practice*, *20*(1), 65–72. doi:10.1177/1078155212473862 PMID:23353710

Pathak, R., & Bridgeman, M. B. (2010). Dipeptidyl Peptidase-4 (DPP-4) Inhibitors in the Management of Diabetes. *Pharmacy and Therapeutics*, *35*, 509–513. PMID:20975810

Patil, T. M., & Hegde, B. A. (1988). Isolation and purification of a sesquiterpene lactone from the leaves of *Parthenium hysterophorus*-Its allelopathic and cytotoxic effects. *Current Science*, *57*, 1178–1181.

Pattanaik, B., & Lindberg, P. (2015). Terpenoids and Their Biosynthesis in Cyanobacteria. *Life (Chicago, Ill.)*, *5*, 269–293. PMID:25615610

Paul, J. C., Alex, J. T., & John, G. McHutchison. (2011). IL28B Genomic-Based Treatment Paradigms for Patients with Chronic Hepatitis C Infection: The Future of Personalized HCV Therapies. *The American Journal of Gastroenterology*, *106*, 38–45. PMID:20924369

Peakman, M., & Dayan, C. M. (2001). Antigen-specific immunotherapy for autoimmune disease: Fighting fire with fire? *Immunology*, *104*(4), 361–366. doi:10.1046/j.1365-2567.2001.01335.x PMID:11899420

Pechere, M., Pechere, J. C., Siegenthaler, G., Germanier, L., & Saurat, J. H. (1999). Antibacterial activity of retinaldehyde against Propionibacterium acnes. *Dermatology (Basel, Switzerland)*, *199*(Suppl 1), 29–31. doi:10.1159/000051375 PMID:10473957

Pedersen, A. G., Jensen, L. J., Brunak, S., Staerfeldt, H. H., & Ussery, D. W. (2000). A DNA structural atlas for Escherichia coli. *Journal of Molecular Biology*, *299*(4), 907–930. doi:10.1006/jmbi.2000.3787 PMID:10843847

Peet, M. (2004). International variations in the outcome of schizophrenia and the prevalence of depression in relation to national dietary practices: An ecological analysis. *The British Journal of Psychiatry*, *184*(5), 404–408. doi:10.1192/bjp.184.5.404 PMID:15123503

Pei, L., Omburo, G., McGuinn, W. D., Petrikovics, I., Dave, K., Raushel, F. M., & Way, J. L. et al. (1994). Encapsulation of phosphotriesterase within murine erythrocytes. *Toxicology and Applied Pharmacology*, *124*(2), 296–301. doi:10.1006/taap.1994.1035 PMID:8122276

Peine, K. J., Guerau-de-Arellano, M., Lee, P., Kanthamneni, N., Severin, M., Probst, G. D., & Ainslie, K. M. et al. (2014). Treatment of experimental autoimmune encephalomyelitis by codelivery of disease associated Peptide and dexamethasone in acetalated dextran microparticles. *Molecular Pharmaceutics*, *11*(3), 828–835. doi:10.1021/mp4005172 PMID:24433027

Peng, H. J., Chang, Z. N., Lin, S. Y., Han, S. H., & Chang, C. H. (1998). Chemical denaturation of ovalbumin abrogates the induction of oral tolerance of mouse reaginic antibody responses. *Scandinavian Journal of Immunology*, *47*(5), 475–480. doi:10.1046/j.1365-3083.1998.00333.x PMID:9627132

Peng, H. J., Chang, Z. N., Tsai, L. C., Su, S. N., Shen, H. D., & Chang, C. H. (1998). Heat denaturation of egg-white proteins abrogates the induction of oral tolerance of specific Th2 immune responses in mice. *Scandinavian Journal of Immunology*, *48*(5), 491–496. doi:10.1046/j.1365-3083.1998.00432.x PMID:9822257

Peng, H., Guerau-de-Arellano, M., Mehta, V. B., Yang, Y., Huss, D. J., Papenfuss, T. L., & Racke, M. K. et al. (2012). Dimethyl fumarate inhibits dendritic cell maturation via nuclear factor kappaB (NF-kappaB) and extracellular signal-regulated kinase 1 and 2 (ERK1/2) and mitogen stress-activated kinase 1 (MSK1) signaling. *The Journal of Biological Chemistry*, *287*(33), 28017–28026. doi:10.1074/jbc.M112.383380 PMID:22733812

Peng, X., Guo, W., Liu, T., Wang, X., Tu, X., Xiong, D., & Zou, X. et al. (2011). Identification of miRs-143 and -145 that is associated with bone metastasis of prostate cancer and involved in the regulation of EMT. *PLoS ONE*, *6*(5), e20341. PMID:21647377

Perdue, R. E., Smith, R. L., Wall, M. E., Hartwell, J. L., & Abbott, B. J. (1970). *Camptotheca acuminata Decaisne (Nyssaceae). Source of camptothecin, an antileukemic alkaloid.US department of agriculture agricultural research service.* Technical Bulletin No.1415.

Perera, M. A., Innocenti, F., & Ratain, M. J. (2008). Pharmacogenetic testing for uridine diphosphate glucuronosyltransferase 1A1 polymorphisms: Are we there yet? *Pharmacotherapy*, *28*(6), 755–768. doi:10.1592/phco.28.6 755 PMID:18503403

Perez-Fons, L., Aranda, F. J., Guillén, J., Villalaín, J., & Micol, V. (2006). Rosemary (*Rosmarinus officinalis*) diterpenes affect lipid polymorphism and fluidity in phospholipid membranes. *Archives of Biochemistry and Biophysics*, *453*(2), 224–236. doi:10.1016/j.abb.2006.07.004 PMID:16949545

Perkin, B.A., Ficociello, L.H., Ostrander, B.E., Silva, K.H., Weinberg, J., Warram, J. H.& Krolewski, A.S. (2007). Microalbuminuria and the risk for early progressive renal function decline in type 1 diabetes. *Journal ofthe American Society of Nephrology*, *18*, 1353-1361.

Perkins, M. R., Ryschkewitsch, C., Liebner, J. C., Monaco, M. C., Himelfarb, D., Ireland, S., & Douek, D. C. et al. (2012). Changes in JC virus-specific T cell responses during natalizumab treatment and in natalizumab-associated progressive multifocal leukoencephalopathy. *PLoS Pathogens*, *8*(11), e1003014. doi:10.1371/journal.ppat.1003014 PMID:23144619

Perkins, R., Fang, H., Tong, W., & Welsh, W. J. (2003). Quantitative structure-activity relationship methods: Perspectives on drug discovery and toxicology. *Environmental Toxicology and Chemistry*, *22*(8), 1666–1679. doi:10.1897/01-171 PMID:12924569

Perkovic, V., Heerspink, H. L., Chalmers, J., Woodward, M., Jun, M., Li, Q., & Zoungas, S. et al. (2013). Intensive glucose control improves kidney outcomes in patients with type 2 diabetes. *Kidney International*, *83*(3), 517–523. doi:10.1038/ki.2012.401 PMID:23302714

Persaud, S. J., Al-Majed, H., Raman, A., & Jones, P. M. (1999). *Gymnema sylvestre* stimulates insulin release in vitro by increased membrane permeability. *The Journal of Endocrinology*, *163*(2), 207–212. doi:10.1677/joe.0.1630207 PMID:10556769

Peters, S., Michielin, O., & Zimmermann, S. (2013). Dramatic response induced by vemurafenib in a BRAF V600E-mutated lung adenocarcinoma. *Journal of Clinical Oncology*, *31*(20), e341–e344. doi:10.1200/JCO.2012.47.6143 PMID:23733758

Petricoin, E. F., Ardekani, A. M., & Hitt, B. A. (2002). 'Use of proteomic patterns in serum to identify ovarian cancer'. *Lancet*, *359*, 572–577. PMID:11867112

Petri, M. (2004). Cyclophosphamide: New approaches for systemic lupus erythematosus. *Lupus*, *13*(5), 366–371. doi:10.1191/0961203303lu1028oa PMID:15230294

Petrovska B.B. (2012). Historical review of medicinal plants´s usage. *Pharmacognosy Review, 6*(11), 1-5.

Piceno, J. (2011). *Smooth as silk skin. Cleopatra bathing in camel milk*. Retrieved 5.6.2015, from https://jenpiceno.wordpress.com/tag/cleopatras-beauty-secrets

Pieper, S., Kolve, H., Gumbinger, H. G., Goletz, G., Wurthwein, G., & Groll, A. H. (2012). Monitoring of voriconazole plasma concentrations in immunocompromised paediatric patients. *The Journal of Antimicrobial Chemotherapy*, *67*(11), 2717–2724. doi:10.1093/jac/dks258 PMID:22796890

Pietroiusti, A., Campagnolo, L., & Fadeel, B. (2013). Interactions of engineered nanoparticles with organs protected by internal biological barriers. *Small*, *9*(9-10), 1557–1572. doi:10.1002/smll.201201463 PMID:23097249

Pinazo-Duran, M. D., Galbis-Estrada, C., Pons-Vázquez, , Cantu-Dibildox, J., Marco-Ramirez, C., & Benitez-del-castillo, F. (2013). Effects of a nutraceutical formulation based on the combination of antioxidants and ω-3 essential fatty acids in the expression of inflammation and immune response mediators in tears from patients with dry eye disorders. *Clinical Interventions in Aging*, *8*, 139–148. doi:10.2147/CIA.S40640 PMID:23430672

Pinheiro, C. U. B. (1997). Jaborandi (*Pilocarpus* sp., Tutaceae): A wild species and its rapid transformation into a crop. *Economic Botany*, *51*, 49–58. doi:10.1007/BF02910403

Piriou, Y., Sirvent, A., Natalizio, A., & Girad-ory, F. (2014). Skin-lightening and anti-ageing effect of a food supplement containing *Pinus pinaster* extract. *Naturafood*, *13*(3), 123–131. doi:10.1007/s13749-014-0036-z

Pisoni, C. N., & D'Cruz, D. P. (2008). The safety of mycophenolate mofetil in pregnancy. *Expert Opinion on Drug Safety*, *7*(3), 219–222. doi:10.1517/14740338.7.3.219 PMID:18462179

Pitt, E., Lewis, D. A., & Offord, R. (1983). The Use of Corticosteroids Encapsulated in Erythrocytes in the Treatment of Adjuvant Induced Arthritis in the Rat. *Biochemical Pharmacology*, *132*(22), 3355–3358. doi:10.1016/0006-2952(83)90362-3 PMID:6651860

Planchard, D., Mazieres, J., Riely, G. J., Rudin, C. M., Barlesi, F., Quoix, E. A., & Souquet, M. A. (2013). Interim results of phase II study BRF113928 of dabrafenib in BRAF V600E mutation–positive non-small cell lung cancer (NSCLC) patients. *Journal of Clinical Oncology*.

Porchezhian, E., & Dobriyal, R. M. (2003). An overview on the advances of *Gymnema sylvestre*: Chemistry, pharmacology and patents. *Die Pharmazie*, *58*, 5–12. PMID:12622244

Postow, M. A., Chesney, J., Pavlick, A. C., Robert, C., Grossmann, K., McDermott, D., & Hodi, F. S. et al. (2015). Nivolumab and ipilimumab versus ipilimumab in untreated melanoma. *The New England Journal of Medicine*, *372*(21), 2006–2017. doi:10.1056/NEJMoa1414428 PMID:25891304

Prahallad, A., Sun, C., Huang, S., Di Nicolantonio, F., Salazar, R., Zecchin, D., & Bernards, R. et al. (2012). Unresponsiveness of colon cancer to BRAF(V600E) inhibition through feedback activation of EGFR. *Nature*, *483*(7387), 100–103. doi:10.1038/nature10868 PMID:22281684

Prakash, D., Dhakarey, R., & Mishra, A. (2004). Carotenoids: The phytochemicals of nutraceutical importance. *Indian Journal of Agricultural Biochemistry*, *17*, 1–8.

Prakash, D., & Gupta, C. (2014a). Role of Phytoestrogens as Nutraceuticals in Human Health. In D. Prakash & G. Sharma (Eds.), *Phytochemicals of Nutraceutical Importance* (pp. 148–172). CABI International Publishers. doi:10.1079/9781780643632.0000

Prakash, D., Gupta, C., & Sharma, G. (2012). Importance of Phytochemicals in Nutraceuticals. *Journal of Chinese Medicine Research and Development*, *1*(3), 70–78.

Prakash, D., & Gupta, K. R. (2009). The antioxidant phytochemicals of nutraceutical importance. *The Open Nutraceuticals Journal*, *2*(1), 20–35. doi:10.2174/1876396000902010020

Prakash, D., & Kumar, N. (2011). Cost Effective Natural Antioxidants. In R. R. Watson, J. K. Gerald, & V. R. Preedy (Eds.), *Nutrients, Dietary Supplements and Nutraceuticals* (pp. 163–188). Humana Press, Springer. doi:10.1007/978-1-60761-308-4_12

Pribitkin E. (2005). Herbal medicine and surgery. *Seminar in Integrative Medicine, 3*, 17-23.

Price, R. J., Skyba, D. M., Kaul, S., & Skalak, T. C. (1998). Delivery of Colloidal Particles and Red Blood Cells to Tissue through Microvessel Ruptures Created by Targeted Microbubble Destruction with Ultrasound. *Circulation*, *98*(13), 1264–1267. doi:10.1161/01.CIR.98.13.1264 PMID:9751673

Prieto, J. M., Iacopini, P., Cioni, P., & Chericoni, S. (2007). In vitro activity of the essential oils of *Origanum vulgare*, *Satureja montana* and their main constituents in peroxynitrite-induced oxidative processes. *Food Chemistry*, *104*(3), 889–895. doi:10.1016/j.foodchem.2006.10.064

Probiotics in food: health and nutritional properties and guidelines for evaluation. (2002). Food and Agricultural Organization of the United Nations and World Health Organization (FAO-UN-WHO).

Puri, D., & Baral, N. (1998). Hypoglycemic effect of *Biophytum sensitivum* in the alloxan diabetic rabbits. *Indian Journal of Physiology and Pharmacology*, *42*, 401–406. PMID:9741656

Qa'dan, F., Verspohl, E. J., Nahrstedt, A., Petereit, F., & Matalka, K. Z. (2009). Cinchonain Ib isolated from *Eriobotrya japonica* induces insulin secretion in vitro and in vivo. *Journal of Ethnopharmacology*, *124*(2), 224-227.

Qin, Y., Xia, M., Ma, J., Hao, Y., Liu, J., Mou, H., & Ling, W. et al. (2009). Anthocyanin supplementation improves serum LDL- and HDL-cholesterol concentrations associated with the inhibition of cholesteryl ester transfer protein in dyslipidemic subjects. *The American Journal of Clinical Nutrition*, *90*(3), 485–492. doi:10.3945/ajcn.2009.27814 PMID:19640950

Quan, L. D., Thiele, G. M., Tian, J., & Wang, D. (2008). The Development of Novel Therapies for Rheumatoid Arthritis. *Expert Opin Ther Pat*, *18*(7), 723–738. doi:10.1517/13543776.18.7.723 PMID:19578469

Racca, A., Biondi, C., Cotorruelo, C., Galizzi, S., Rasia, R. J., Stoltz, J. F., & Valverde, J. (1999). Senescent erythrocytes: Modification of rheologic properties, antigenic expression and interaction with monocytes. *Medicina*, *59*(1), 33–37. PMID:10349116

Radha, M., & Laxmipriya, N. (2015). Evaluation of biological properties and clinical effectiveness of Aloe vera: A systematic review. *Journal of Traditional and Complementary Medicine*, *5*(1), 21–26. doi:10.1016/j.jtcme.2014.10.006 PMID:26151005

Rae, J. M., Drury, S., Hayes, D. F., Stearns, V., Thibert, J. N., Haynes, B. P., & Dowsett, M. et al. (2012). CYP2D6 and UGT2B7 genotype and risk of recurrence in tamoxifen-treated breast cancer patients. *Journal of the National Cancer Institute*, *104*(6), 452–460. doi:10.1093/jnci/djs126 PMID:22395643

Rae, J. M., Regan, M. M., Thibert, J. N., Gersch, C., Thomas, D., Leyland-Jones, B., & Van Poznak, C. et al. (2013). Concordance between CYP2D6 genotypes obtained from tumor-derived and germline DNA. *Journal of the National Cancer Institute*, *105*(17), 1332–1334. doi:10.1093/jnci/djt204 PMID:23958736

Rafraf, M., Zemestani, M., & Asghari-Jifaaradi, M. (2015). Effectiveness of *chamomile* tea on glycemic control and serum lipid profile in patients with type 2 diabetes. *Journal of Endocrinological Investigation*, *38*(2), 163–170. doi:10.1007/s40618-014-0170-x PMID:25194428

Rahman, A. (2000). *Studies in Natural Product Chemistry*. Elsevier Science B.V.

Rahman, I., Biswas, S. K., & Kirkham, P. A. (2006). Regulation of inflammation and redox signaling by dietary polyphenols. *Biochemical Pharmacology*, *72*(11), 1439–1452. doi:10.1016/j.bcp.2006.07.004 PMID:16920072

Rajani, M., & Kanaki, S. (2008). Phytochemical Standardization of Herbal Drugs and Polyherbal Formulations. In Bioactive Molecules and Medicinal Plants (pp 349-369). Berlin, Germany: Springer-Verlag Berlin Heidelberg. doi:doi:10.1007/978-3-540-74603-4_19 doi:10.1007/978-3-540-74603-4_19

Rajasekar, P., & Anuradha, C. V. (2007). Effect of L-carnitine on skeletal muscle lipids and oxidative stress in rats fed high-fructose diet. *Experimental Diabetes Research*, *2007*, 72741. doi:10.1155/2007/72741 PMID:17641743

Raj, M. V., Selvakumar, K., Krishnamoorthy, G., Revathy, S., Elumalai, P., & Arunakaran, J. (2014). Impact of lycopene on epididymal androgen and estrogen receptors' expression in polychlorinated biphenyls-exposed rat. *Reproductive Sciences (Thousand Oaks, Calif.)*, *21*(1), 89–101. doi:10.1177/1933719113492213 PMID:23749762

Rakvag, T. T., Klepstad, P., Baar, C., Kvam, T. M., Dale, O., Kaasa, S., & Skorpen, F. et al. (2005). The Val158Met polymorphism of the human catechol-O-methyltransferase (COMT) gene may influence morphine requirements in cancer pain patients. *Pain*, *116*(1-2), 73–78. doi:10.1016/j.pain.2005.03.032 PMID:15927391

Ramaa, C. S., Shirode, A. R., Mundada, A. S., & Kadam, V. J. (2006). Nutraceuticals--an emerging era in the treatment and prevention of cardiovascular diseases. *Current Pharmaceutical Biotechnology*, *7*(1), 15–23. doi:10.2174/138920106775789647 PMID:16472130

Ramesh, C., & Pattar, M. G. (2010). Antimicrobial properties, antioxidant activity and bioactive compounds from six wild edible mushrooms of Western Ghats of Karnataka, India. *Pharmacognosy Res*, *2*(2), 107–112. doi:10.4103/0974-8490.62953 PMID:21808550

Ramshini, H., & Ayoubi, F. (2014). Inhibitory Effect of *Cinnamomum Zeylanicum* and *Camellia sinensis* Extracts on the Hen Egg-White Lysozyme Fibrillation. *Journal of Kerman University of Medical Sciences*, *21*(4), 3–9.

Ranasinghe, P., Pigera, S., Premakumara, G., Galappaththy, P., Constantine, G. R., & Katulanda, P. (2013). Medicinal properties of "true" cinnamon (Cinnamomum zeylanicum): A systematic review. *BMC Complementary and Alternative Medicine*, *13*(1), 275. doi:10.1186/1472-6882-13-275 PMID:24148965

Rao. (2013). *Maintaining good skin.* Retrieved 13.6.2015, from http://www.mindbodygreen.com/0-8355/15-natural-ways-to-maintain-beautiful-youthful-skin.html

Rao, A. V., & Gurfinkel, D. M. (2000). The bioactivity of saponins: Triterpenoid and steroidal glycosides. *Drug Metabolism and Drug Interactions*, *17*(1-4), 211–235. doi:10 1515/DMDI.2000.17.1-4.211 PMID:11201296

Rao, A. V., & Shen, H. (2002). Effect of low dose lycopene intake on lycopene bioavailability and oxidative stress. *Nutrition Research (New York, N.Y.)*, *22*(10), 1125–1131. doi:10.1016/S0271-5317(02)00430-X

Rasineni, K., Bellamkonda, R., Singareddy, S. R., & Desireddy, S. (2010). Antihyperglycemic activity of *Catharanthus roseus* leaf powder in streptozotocin-induced diabetic rats. *Pharmacognosy Research*, *2*(3), 195–201. doi:10.4103/0974-8490.65523 PMID:21808566

Ravi Subbiah, M. T. (2007). Nutrigenetics and nutraceuticals: The next wave riding on personalized medicine. *Translational Research; the Journal of Laboratory and Clinical Medicine*, *149*(2), 55–61. doi:10.1016/j.trsl.2006.09.003 PMID:17240315

Rechsteiner, M. C. (1975). Uptake of Protein by Red Cells. *Experimental Cell Research*, *43*(2), 487–492. doi:10.1016/0014-4827(75)90478-4 PMID:1098917

Regan, M. M., Leyland-Jones, B., Bouzyk, M., Pagani, O., Tang, W., Kammler, R., & Viale, G. et al. (2012). CYP2D6 genotype and tamoxifen response in postmenopausal women with endocrine-responsive breast cancer: The breast international group 1-98 trial. *Journal of the National Cancer Institute*, *104*(6), 441–451. doi:10.1093/jnci/djs125 PMID:22395644

Reichardt, P., Blay, J. Y., Gelderblom, H., Schlemmer, M., Demetri, G. D., Bui-Nguyen, B., & Rutkowski, P. et al. (2012). Phase III study of nilotinib versus best supportive care with or without a TKI in patients with gastrointestinal stromal tumors resistant to or intolerant of imatinib and sunitinib. *Annals of Oncology*, *23*(7), 1680–1687. doi:10.1093/annonc/mdr598 PMID:22357255

Reindl, M., Di Pauli, F., Rostasy, K., & Berger, T. (2013). The spectrum of MOG autoantibody-associated demyelinating diseases. *Nat Rev Neurol*, *9*(8), 455–461. doi:10.1038/nrneurol.2013.118 PMID:23797245

Reis, L. C., & Hibbeln, J. R. (2006). Cultural symbolism of fish and the psychotropic properties of omega-3 fatty acids. *Prostaglandins, Leukotrienes, and Essential Fatty Acids*, *75*(4-5), 227–236. doi:10.1016/j.plefa.2006.07.014 PMID:16962306

Relling, M. V., Gardner, E. E., Sandborn, W. J., Schmiegelow, K., Pui, C. H., Yee, S. W., & Klein, T. E. et al. (2011). Clinical Pharmacogenetics Implementation Consortium guidelines for thiopurine methyltransferase genotype and thiopurine dosing. *Clinical Pharmacology and Therapeutics*, *89*(3), 387–391. doi:10.1038/clpt.2010.320 PMID:21270794

Relling, M. V., Gardner, E. E., Sandborn, W. J., Schmiegelow, K., Pui, C. H., Yee, S. W., & Klein, T. E. et al. (2013). Clinical pharmacogenetics implementation consortium guidelines for thiopurine methyltransferase genotype and thiopurine dosing: 2013 update. *Clinical Pharmacology and Therapeutics*, *93*(4), 324–325. doi:10.1038/clpt.2013.4 PMID:23422873

Relling, M. V., Hancock, M. L., Rivera, G. K., Sandlund, J. T., Ribeiro, R. C., Krynetski, E. Y., & Evans, W. E. et al. (1999). Mercaptopurine therapy intolerance and heterozygosity at the thiopurine S-methyltransferase gene locus. *Journal of the National Cancer Institute*, *91*(23), 2001–2008. doi:10.1093/jnci/91.23.2001 PMID:10580024

Remuzzi, G., Perico, N., Macia, M., & Ruggenenti, P. (2005). The role of renin-angiotensin-aldosterone system in the progression of chronic kidney disease. *Kidney International. Supplement*, *99*, S57–S65. doi:10.1111/j.1523-1755.2005.09911.x PMID:16336578

Rendon, M. I., Vazquez, Y., & Micciantuono, S. (2013). Cosmeceutical Skin Lighteners. In P. K. Farris (Ed.), *Cosmeceuticals and Cosmetic Practice* (pp. 218–225). New Orleans, LA: Wiley-Blackwell. doi:10.1002/9781118384824.ch22

Ren, W., Qiao, Z., Wang, H., Zhu, L., & Zhang, L. (2003). Flavonoids: Promising anti-cancer agents. *Medicinal Research Reviews*, *23*(4), 519–534. doi:10.1002/med.10033 PMID:12710022

Reshetnikov, S. V., Wasser, S. P., Duckman, I., & Tsukor, K. (2000). Medicinal value of the genus Tremella Pers. (Heterobasidiomycetes) (review). *International Journal of Medicinal Mushrooms*, *2*(3), 345–367. doi:10.1615/IntJMedMushr.v2.i3.10

Rettig, M. P., Low, P. S., Gimm, J. A., Mohandas, N., Wang, J., & Christian, J. A. (1999). Evaluation of biochemical changes during in vivo erythrocyte senescence in the dog. *Blood*, *93*(1), 376–384. PMID:9864184

Ricciotti, E., & FitzGerald, G. A. (2011). Prostaglandins and inflammation. *Arteriosclerosis, Thrombosis, and Vascular Biology*, *31*(5), 986–1000. doi:10.1161/ATVBAHA.110.207449 PMID:21508345

Richards, W. G. (1994). Computer-Aided Drug Design. *Pure and Applied Chemistry*, *66*(8), 1589–1596. doi:10.1351/pac199466081589

Richet, M. C. (1893). Compt. *Rend. Soc. Biol.*, *45*, 775–776.

Rickert, D. A., Meyer, M. A., Hu, J., & Murphy, P. A. (2004). Effect of extraction pH and temperature on Isoflavone and saponin partitioning and profile during soy protein isolate production. *Journal of Food Science*, *69*(8), C623–C631. doi:10.1111/j.1365-2621.2004.tb09910.x

Rietveld, A., & Wiseman, S. (2003). Antioxidant Effects of Tea: Evidence from Human Clinical Trials. *The Journal of Nutrition*, *133*(10), 3285S–3292S. PMID:14519827

Rijkers, G. T., de Vos, W. M., Brummer, R. J., Morelli, L., Corthier, G., & Marteau, P. et al.. (2011). Health benefits and health claims of probiotics: Bridging science and marketing. *The British Journal of Nutrition*, *106*(9), 1291–1296. doi:10.1017/S000711451100287X PMID:21861940

Rios, J. L., & Recio, M. C. (2005). Medicinal plants and antimicrobial activity. *Journal of Ethnopharmacology*, *100*(1-2), 80–84. doi:10.1016/j.jep.2005.04.025 PMID:15964727

Rischer, H., & Oksman-Caldentey, K. M. (2005). Biotechnological utilization of plant genetic resources for the production of PP. *Plant Genetic Resources*, *3*(2), 83–89. doi:10.1079/PGR200564

Ritz, E., & Zeng, X. (2011). Diabetic nephropathy – Epidemiology in Asia and the current state of treatment. *Indian Journal of Nephrology*, *21*(2), 75–84. doi:10.4103/0971-4065.82122 PMID:21769168

Rivera-Chavez, J., Gonzalez-Andrade, M., Gonzalez, M. C., Glenn, A. E., & Mata, R. (2013). Thielavins A, J and K: α-Glucosidase inhibitors from MEXU 27095, an endophytic fungus from *Hintonia latiflora*. *Phytochemistry*, *94*, 198–205. doi:10.1016/j.phytochem.2013.05.021 PMID:23809634

Rizvi, N. A., Mazieres, J., Planchard, D., Stinchcombe, T. E., Dy, G. K., Antonia, S. J., & Ramalingam, S. S. et al. (2015). Activity and safety of nivolumab, an anti-PD-1 immune checkpoint inhibitor, for patients with advanced, refractory squamous non-small-cell lung cancer (CheckMate 063): A phase 2, single-arm trial. *The Lancet Oncology*, *16*(3), 257–265. doi:10.1016/S1470-2045(15)70054-9 PMID:25704439

Rizvi, S. I., & Pandey, K. B. (2011). Activation of the erythrocyte plasma membrane redox system by resveratrol: A possible mechanism for antioxidant properties. *Pharmacological Reports*, *62*(4), 726–732. doi:10.1016/S1734-1140(10)70330-3 PMID:20885013

Robert, C., Karaszewska, B., Schachter, J., Rutkowski, P., Mackiewicz, A., Stroiakovski, D., & Schadendorf, D. et al. (2015). Improved overall survival in melanoma with combined dabrafenib and trametinib. *The New England Journal of Medicine*, *372*(1), 30–39. doi:10.1056/NEJMoa1412690 PMID:25399551

Robert, C., Long, G. V., Brady, B., Dutriaux, C., Maio, M., Mortier, L., & Ascierto, P. A. et al. (2015). Nivolumab in previously untreated melanoma without BRAF mutation. *The New England Journal of Medicine*, *372*(4), 320–330. doi:10.1056/NEJMoa1412082 PMID:25399552

Robert, C., Schachter, J., Long, G. V., Arance, A., Grob, J. J., Mortier, L., & Ribas, A. et al. (2015). Pembrolizumab versus Ipilimumab in Advanced Melanoma. *The New England Journal of Medicine*, *372*(26), 2521–2532. doi:10.1056/NEJMoa1503093 PMID:25891173

Roe, M. R., & Griffin, T. J. (2006). Gel-freemass spectrometry-based high throughput proteomics: Tools for studying biological response of proteins and proteomes. *Proteomics*, *6*(17), 4678–4687. PMID:16888762

Roila, F., Herrstedt, J., Aapro, M., Gralla, R. J., Einhorn, L. H., Ballatori, E., & Group, E. M. C. W. et al. (2010). Guideline update for MASCC and ESMO in the prevention of chemotherapy- and radiotherapy-induced nausea and vomiting: Results of the Perugia consensus conference. *Annals of Oncology*, *21*(Suppl 5), v232–v243. doi:10.1093/annonc/mdq194 PMID:20555089

Rojas, C., & Slusher, B. S. (2012). Pharmacological mechanisms of 5-HT(3) and tachykinin NK(1) receptor antagonism to prevent chemotherapy-induced nausea and vomiting. *European Journal of Pharmacology*, *684*(1-3), 1–7. doi:10.1016/j.ejphar.2012.01.046 PMID:22425650

Rong, X. Y., Xiang, L. M., & Gui, G. J. (2014). Dietary supplements and insomnia. *Current Topics in Nutraceutical Research*, *12*(1/2), 51–56.

Rosell, R., Carcereny, E., Gervais, R., Vergnenegre, A., Massuti, B., Felip, E., & Associazione Italiana Oncologia, T. et al. (2012). Erlotinib versus standard chemotherapy as first-line treatment for European patients with advanced EGFR mutation-positive non-small-cell lung cancer (EURTAC): A multicentre, open-label, randomised phase 3 trial. *The Lancet Oncology*, *13*(3), 239–246. doi:10.1016/S1470-2045(11)70393-X PMID:22285168

Rosmarin, D., Palles, C., Church, D., Domingo, E., Jones, A., Johnstone, E., & Tomlinson, I. et al. (2014). Genetic markers of toxicity from capecitabine and other fluorouracil-based regimens: Investigation in the QUASAR2 study, systematic review, and meta-analysis. *Journal of Clinical Oncology*, *32*(10), 1031–1039. doi:10.1200/JCO.2013.51.1857 PMID:24590654

Rossi, L., Serafini, S., Pierigé, F., Antonelli, A., Cerasi, A., Fraternale, A., & Magnani, M. et al. (2005). Erythrocyte-based drug delivery. *Expert Opinion on Drug Delivery*, *2*(2), 311–322. doi:10.1517/17425247.2.2.311 PMID:16296756

Rotimi, E. A. (2012). Functional foods and nutraceuticals. Springer.

Roy, P., & Shukla, Y. (2008). Applications of proteomic techniques in cancer research. *Cancer Therapy*, *6*, 841–856.

Roy, S. K., Das, D., Mondal, S., Maiti, D., Bhunia, B., Maiti, T. K., & Islam, S. S. (2009). Structural studies of an immunoenhancing water-soluble glucan isolated from hot water extract of an edible mushroom, *Pleurotus florida*, cultivar Assam Florida. *Carbohydrate Research*, *344*(18), 2596–2601. doi:10.1016/j.carres.2009.09.010 PMID:19836727

Ruan, X., & Arendshorst, W. J. (1996). Role of protein kinase C in angiotensin II-induced renal vasoconstriction in genetically hypertensive rats. *The American Journal of Physiology*, *270*, F945–F952. PMID:8764313

Rubin, B. P., Fletcher, J. A., & Fletcher, C. D. (2000). Molecular Insights into the Histogenesis and Pathogenesis of Gastrointestinal Stromal Tumors. *International Journal of Surgical Pathology*, *8*(1), 5–10. doi:10.1177/106689690000800105 PMID:11493959

Ruckemann, K., Fairbanks, L. D., Carrey, E. A., Hawrylowicz, C. M., Richards, D. F., Kirschbaum, B., & Simmonds, H. A. (1998). Leflunomide inhibits pyrimidine de novo synthesis in mitogen-stimulated T-lymphocytes from healthy humans. *The Journal of Biological Chemistry*, *273*(34), 21682–21691. doi:10.1074/jbc.273.34.21682 PMID:9705303

Ruggieri, R. M., Settipani, N., Viviano, L., Attanasio, M., Giglia, L., Almasio, P., & Piccoli, F. et al. (2003). Long-term interferon-beta treatment for multiple sclerosis. *Neurological Sciences*, *24*(5), 361–364. doi:10.1007/s10072-003-0190-3 PMID:14716534

Ruiz-Romero, & Blanco, F.J. (2013). Achievements and challenges of proteomics in the study of rheumatoid arthritis. *Current Topics in Medicinal Chemistry*, *13*(6), 732–742. PMID:23574522

Rush, A. J., Trivedi, M. H., Wisniewski, S. R., Nierenberg, A. A., Stewart, J. W., Warden, D., & Fava, M. et al. (2006). Acute and longer-term outcomes in depressed outpatients requiring one or several treatment steps: A STAR*D report. *The American Journal of Psychiatry*, *163*(11), 1905–1917. PMID:17074942

Russell, N. C., Hoelscher, D. M., & Lowenstein, N. (2007). Patients previously treated for lymphoma consume inadequate or excessive amounts of five key nutrients. *Journal of the Society for Integrative Oncology*, *5*(03), 118–124. doi:10.2310/7200.2007.009 PMID:17761131

Russell, R. B., Saqi, M. A., Bates, P. A., Sayle, R. A., & Sternberg, M. J. (1998). Recognition of analogous and homologous protein folds—assessment of prediction success and associated alignment accuracy using empirical substitution matrices. *Protein Engineering*, *11*(1), 1–9. doi:10.1093/protein/11.1.1 PMID:9579654

Russell, R. B., Saqi, M. A., Sayle, R. A., Bates, P. A., & Sternberg, M. J. (1997). Recognition of analogous and homologous protein folds: Analysis of sequence and structure conservation. *Journal of Molecular Biology*, *269*(3), 423–439. doi:10.1006/jmbi.1997.1019 PMID:9199410

Russo, E. (2000). Proteomics Factories. *Scientist (Philadelphia, Pa.)*, *14*(3), 1.

Russo, E. B. (2001). Hemp for headache: An in-depth historical and scientific review of cannabis in migraine treatment. *Journal of Cannabis Therapeutics*, *1*(2), 21–92. doi:10.1300/J175v01n02_04

Russo, E. B. (2002). Cannabis treatments in obstetrics and gynecology: A historical review. *Journal of Cannabis Therapeutics*, *2*(3-4), 5–34. doi:10.1300/J175v02n03_02

Rybicki, A. C., Schwartz, R. S., Hustedt, E. J., & Cobb, C. E. (1996). Increased rotational mobility and extractability of band 3 from protein 4.2-deficient erythrocyte membranes: Evidence of a role for protein 4.2 in strengthening the band 3-cytoskeleton linkage. *Blood*, *88*, 2745–2753. PMID:8839871

Sachs, D. L., Rittie, L., Chubb, H. A., Orringer, J., Fisher, G., & Voorhees, J. J. (2013). Hypo-collagenesis in photoaged skin predicts response to anti-aging cosmeceuticals. *Journal of Cosmetic Dermatology*, *12*(2), 108–115. doi:10.1111/jocd.12037 PMID:23725304

Sadee, W., & Dai, Z. (2005). Pharmacogenetics/genomics and personalized medicine. *Human Molecular Genetics*, *14*(2), R207-214.

Sae-Teaw, M., Johns, J., Johns, N. P., & Subongkot, S. (2012). Serum melatonin levels and antioxidant capacities after consumption of pineapple, orange, or banana by healthy male volunteers. *Journal of Pineal Research*, *55*(1), 58–64. doi:10.1111/jpi.12025 PMID:23137025

Saha, S., Sparks, A. B., Rago, C., Akmaev, V., Wang, C. J., Vogelstein, B., & Velculescu, V. E. et al. (2002). Using the transcriptome to annotate the genome. *Nature Biotechnology*, *20*, 508–512. PMID:11981567

Saif, M. W., Ezzeldin, H., Vance, K., Sellers, S., & Diasio, R. B. (2007). DPYD*2A mutation: The most common mutation associated with DPD deficiency. *Cancer Chemotherapy and Pharmacology*, *60*(4), 503–507. doi:10.1007/s00280-006-0392-5 PMID:17165084

Sakai, N., Wada, T., Furuichi, K., Iwata, Y., Yoshimoto, K., Kitagawa, K., & Yokoyama, H. et al. (2005). Involvement of extracellular signal-regulated kinase and p38 in human diabetic nephropathy. *American Journal of Kidney Diseases*, *45*(1), 54–65. doi:10.1053/j.ajkd.2004.08.039 PMID:15696444

Saklayen, M. G., Pesce, A. J., Pollak, V. E., & Michael, J. G. (1984). Kinetics of oral tolerance: Study of variables affecting tolerance induced by oral administration of antigen. *International Archives of Allergy and Applied Immunology*, *73*(1), 5–9. doi:10.1159/000233428 PMID:6693181

Saladores, P., Murdter, T., Eccles, D., Chowbay, B., Zgheib, N. K., Winter, S., & Brauch, H. et al. (2014). Tamoxifen metabolism predicts drug concentrations and outcome in premenopausal patients with early breast cancer. *The Pharmacogenomics Journal*. PMID:25091503

Salam, N. K., Nuti, R., & Sherman, W. (2009). Novel method for generating structure based pharmacophores using energetic analysis. *Journal of Chemical Information and Modeling*, *49*(10), 2356–2368. doi:10.1021/ci900212v PMID:19761201

Saleem, R., Ahmad, M., Hussain, S. A., Qazi, A. M., Ahmad, S. I., Qazi, M. H., & Hussein, S. N. (1999). Hypotensive, hypoglycemic and toxicological studies on the flavonol C-glycosides shamimim from *Bombax ceiba*. *Planta Medica*, *65*(4), 331–334. doi:10.1055/s-1999-14060 PMID:10364838

Saltarelli, R., Ceccaroli, P., Iotti, M., Zambonelli, A., Buffalini, M., Casadei, L., & Stocchi, V. et al. (2009). Biochemical characterisation and antioxidant activity of mycelium of *Ganoderma lucidum* from Central Italy. *Food Chemistry*, *116*(1), 143–151. doi:10.1016/j.foodchem.2009.02.023

Samer, C. F., Daali, Y., Wagner, M., Hopfgartner, G., Eap, C. B., Rebsamen, M. C., & Desmeules, J. A. et al. (2010). Genetic polymorphisms and drug interactions modulating CYP2D6 and CYP3A activities have a major effect on oxycodone analgesic efficacy and safety. *British Journal of Pharmacology*, *160*(4), 919–930. doi:10.1111/j.1476-5381.2010.00709.x PMID:20590588

Samer, C. F., Lorenzini, K. I., Rollason, V., Daali, Y., & Desmeules, J. A. (2013). Applications of CYP450 testing in the clinical setting. *Molecular Diagnosis & Therapy*, *17*(3), 165–184. doi:10.1007/s40291-013-0028-5 PMID:23588782

Samorini, G. (2001). *Fungi Hallucinogeni. Studi etnomicologici*. Bologna, Italy: Telesterion. Dozza.

Sandeep, S., Priyadarshini, V., Pradhan, D., Munikumar, M., & Umamaheswari, A. (2012). Docking and molecular dynamics simulations studies of human protein kinase catalytic subunit alpha with antagonist. *Journal of Clinical & Scientific Research*, *1*, 15–23.

Sanders, M.E. (2000). Considerations for use of probiotic bacteria to modulate human health. *The Journal of Nutrition*, *130*(Suppl 2), 384S–390S.

Sandhu, S. S., Abreu, I. N., Colombo, C. A., & Mazzafera, P. (2006). Pilocarpine content and molecular diversity in jaborandi. *Scientia Agricola*, *63*(5), 478–482. doi:10.1590/S0103-90162006000500010

Sandler, R. S., Halabi, S., Kaplan, E. B., Baron, J. A., Paskett, E., & Petrelli, N. J. (2001). Use of vitamins, minerals, and nutritional supplements by participants in a chemoprevention trial. *Cancer*, *91*(5), 1040–1045. doi:10.1002/1097-0142(20010301)91:5<1040::AID-CNCR1095>3.0.CO;2-N PMID:11251957

Sansonetti, P. J. (2004). War and peace at mucosal surfaces. *Nature Reviews. Immunology*, *4*(12), 953–964. doi:10.1038/nri1499 PMID:15573130

Santos, L., Marin, S., Sanchis, V., & Ramos, A. J. (2013). Mycotoxin in medicinal/aromatic herbs-a review. *Boletín Latinoamericanos y del Caribe de Plantas Medicinales y Aromáticas*, *12*(2), 119–142.

Santos, R., Limas, E., Sousa, M., da Conceição Castilho, M., Ramos, F., & da Silveira, M. I. N. (2007). Optimization of analytical procedures for GC-MS determination of phytosterols and phytostanols in enriched milk and yoghurt. *Food Chemistry*, *102*(1), 113–117. doi:10.1016/j.foodchem.2006.05.001

Saraf, A. (2010). Applications of novel drug delivery system for herbal formulations. *Fitoterapia*, *81*(7), 680–689. doi:10.1016/j.fitote.2010.05.001 PMID:20471457

Sarkar, S. (2007). Functional foods as self-care and complementary medicine. *Nutrition & Food Science*, *37*(3), 160–167. doi:10.1108/00346650710749053

Sato, Y., Murase, K., Kato, J., Kobune, M., Sato, T., Kawano, Y., & Niitsu, Y. et al. (2008). Resolution of liver cirrhosis using vitamin A-coupled liposomes to deliver siRNA against a collagen-specific chaperone. *Nature Biotechnology*, *26*(4), 431–442. PMID:18376398

Savjani, K. T., Gajjar, A. K., & Savjani, J. K. (2012). Drug solubility: Importance and enhancement techniques. *ISRN Pharm*, *195727*. doi:10.5402/2012/195727 PMID:22830056

Sawyers, C. L. (2008). The cancer biomarker problem. *Nature*, *452*(7187), 548–552. doi:10.1038/nature06913 PMID:18385728

Schacky, C. V. (2003). The role of Omega-3 fatty acids in cardiovascular disease. *Current Atherosclerosis Reports*, *5*(2), 139–145. doi:10.1007/s11883-003-0086-y PMID:12573200

Schaeffeler, E., Fischer, C., Brockmeier, D., Wernet, D., Moerike, K., Eichelbaum, M., & Schwab, M. et al. (2004). Comprehensive analysis of thiopurine S-methyltransferase phenotype-genotype correlation in a large population of German-Caucasians and identification of novel TPMT variants. *Pharmacogenetics*, *14*(7), 407–417. doi:10.1097/01.fpc.0000114745.08559.db PMID:15226673

Schalka, S., Steiner, D., Ravelli, F. N., Steiner, T., Terena, A. C., Marçon, C. R., & Ponzio, H. et al. (2014). Brazilian consensus on photoprotection. *Anais Brasileiros de Dermatologia*, *89*(6), 1–74. doi:10.1590/abd1806-4841.20143971 PMID:25761256

Scheindlin, S. (2010). Episodes in the story of physostigmine. *Molecular Interventions*, *10*(1), 5–10. doi:10.1124/mi.10.1.1 PMID:20124558

Schetter, A. J., & Harris, C. C. (2011). Alterations of microRNAs contribute to colon carcinogenesis. *Seminars in Oncology*, *38*, 734–742. PMID:22082759

Schiller, R. N., Barranger, E., Schauss, A. G., & Nichols, E. (2001). Life style management of Obesity. *Journal of the American Medical Association*, *4*, 34–41.

Schlegel, R. A., & McEvoy L. (1987). Red Cell-Mediated Microinjection. *Methods in Enzymology, 149*, 293-301.

Schleh, C., Semmler-Behnke, M., Lipka, J., Wenk, A., Hirn, S., Schaffler, M., & Kreyling, W. G. et al. (2012). Size and surface charge of gold nanoparticles determine absorption across intestinal barriers and accumulation in secondary target organs after oral administration. *Nanotoxicology*, *6*(1), 36–46. doi:10.3109/17435390.2011.552811 PMID:21309618

Schloss, P. D. (2014). Microbiology: An integrated view of the skin microbiome. *Nature*, *514*(7520), 44–45. doi:10.1038/514044a PMID:25279916

Schmid, H., Boucherot, A., Yasuda, Y., Henger, A., Brunner, B., Eichinger, F., & Kretzler, M. et al. (2006). Modular activation of nuclear factor-kappa B transcriptional programs in humandiabetic nephropathy. *Diabetes*, *55*(11), 2993–3003. doi:10.2337/db06-0477 PMID:17065335

Schmidt, B. (2005). Methylxanthine therapy for apnea of prematurity: Evaluation of treatment benefits and risks at age 5 years in the international caffeine for apnea of prematurity (CAP) trial. *Biology of the Neonate*, *88*(3), 208–213. doi:10.1159/000087584 PMID:16210843

Schmidt, B., Roberts, R. S., Davis, P., Doyle, L. W., Barrington, K. J., Ohlsson, A., & Tin, W. et al. (2006). Caffeine therapy for apnea of prematurity. *The New England Journal of Medicine*, *354*(20), 2112–2121. doi:10.1056/NEJMoa054065 PMID:16707748

Schmidt, B., Roberts, R. S., Davis, P., Doyle, L. W., Barrington, K. J., Ohlsson, A., & Tin, W. et al. (2007). Long-term effects of caffeine therapy for apnea of prematurity. *The New England Journal of Medicine*, *357*(19), 1893–1902. doi:10.1056/NEJMoa073679 PMID:17989382

Schmidt-Ott, K. M., Mori, K., Li, J. Y., Kalandadze, A., Cohen, D. J., Devarajan, P., & Barasch, J. (2007). Dual action of neutrophil gelatinase-associated lipocalin. *Journal of the American Society of Nephrology*, *18*(2), 407–413. doi:10.1681/ASN.2006080882 PMID:17229907

Schmitt, J., Seidler, A., Diepgen, T. L., & Bauer, A. (2011). Occupational ultraviolet light exposure increases the risk for the development of cutaneous squamous cell carcinoma: A systematic review and meta-analysis. *The British Journal of Dermatology*, *164*(2), 291–307. doi:10.1111/j.1365-2133.2010.10118.x PMID:21054335

Schneider, B. P., Radovich, M., & Miller, K. D. (2009). The role of vascular endothelial growth factor genetic variability in cancer. *Clinical Cancer Research*, *15*(17), 5297–5302. doi:10.1158/1078-0432.CCR-08-2575 PMID:19706811

Schriei, S. L., Bensch, K. G., Johnson, M., & Junga, I. (1975). Energized endocytosis in human erythrocyte ghosts. *The Journal of Clinical Investigation*, *56*(1), 8–22. doi:10.1172/JCI108083 PMID:124748

Schrier, S. L. (1987). Shape Changes and Deformability in Human Erythrocyte Membranes. *The Journal of Laboratory and Clinical Medicine*, *110*(6), 791–797. PMID:3500247

Schroth, W., Goetz, M. P., Hamann, U., Fasching, P. A., Schmidt, M., Winter, S., & Brauch, H. et al. (2009). Association between CYP2D6 polymorphisms and outcomes among women with early stage breast cancer treated with tamoxifen. *Journal of the American Medical Association*, *302*(13), 1429–1436. doi:10.1001/jama.2009.1420 PMID:19809024

Schueler, F. W. (1960). *Chemobiodynamics and Drug Design*. New York, NY: McGraw-Hill.

Schulz, S., Klann, R. C., Schönfeld, S., & Nyce, J. W. (1992). Mechanisms of cell growth inhibition and cell cycle arrest in human colonic adenocarcinoma cells by dehydroepiandrosterone: Role of isoprenoid biosynthesis. *Cancer Research*, *52*(5), 1372–1376. PMID:1531325

Schwab, M., Zanger, U. M., Marx, C., Schaeffeler, E., Klein, K., Dippon, J., & German, F. U. T. S. G. et al. (2008). Role of genetic and nongenetic factors for fluorouracil treatment-related severe toxicity: A prospective clinical trial by the German 5-FU Toxicity Study Group. *Journal of Clinical Oncology*, *26*(13), 2131–2138. doi:10.1200/JCO.2006.10.4182 PMID:18299612

Schweim, J., & Schweim, H. (2014). Status quo and future developments of combinations of medicinal products. *Synergy*, *1*(1), 70–75. doi:10.1016/j.synres.2014.07.007

Scott, K. A., Shah, S., Dalgleish, A. G., & Liu, W. M. (2013). Enhancing the activity of cannabidiol and other cannabinoids in vitro through modifications to drug combinations and treatment schedules. *Anticancer Research*, *33*, 4373–4480. PMID:24123005

Seema, P. V., Sudha, B., Padayatti, P. S., Abraham, A., Raghu, K. G., & Paulose, C. S. (1996). Kinetic studies of purified malate dehydrogenase in liver of streptozotocin-diabetic rats and the effect of leaf extract of *Aegle marmelos* (L.) Correa ex Roxb. *Indian Journal of Experimental Biology*, *34*, 600–602. PMID:8792652

Selewski, Segal, Rajdev, & Mukherji. (2010). Natalizumab (Tysabri). *American Journal of Neuroradiology*.

Selvamani, P., Latha, S., Elayaraja, K., Babu, P. S., Gupta, J. K., Pal, K., & Sen, D. J. (2008). Antidiabetic activity of the ethanol extract of *Capparis sepiaria* L leaves. *Indian Journal of Pharmaceutical Sciences*, *70*(3), 378–380. doi:10.4103/0250-474X.43008 PMID:20046752

Semsei, I., & Zs-Nagy, I. (1985). Superoxide radical scavenging ability of centrophenoxine and its salt dependence in vitro. *Journal of Free Radicals in Biology & Medicine*, *1*(5-6), 403–408. doi:10.1016/0748-5514(85)90153-9 PMID:3018064

Sequist, L. V., Soria, J. C., Goldman, J. W., Wakelee, H. A., Gadgeel, S. M., Varga, A., & Camidge, D. R. et al. (2015). Rociletinib in EGFR-mutated non-small-cell lung cancer. *The New England Journal of Medicine*, *372*(18), 1700–1709. doi:10.1056/NEJMoa1413654 PMID:25923550

Serretti, A., Calati, R., Massat, I., Linotte, S., Kasper, S., Lecrubier, Y., & Souery, D. et al. (2009). Cytochrome P450 CYP1A2, CYP2C9, CYP2C19 and CYP2D6 genes are not associated with response and remission in a sample of depressive patients. *International Clinical Psychopharmacology*, *24*(5), 250–256. doi:10.1097/YIC.0b013e32832e5b0d PMID:19593158

Seto, T., Kiura, K., Nishio, M., Nakagawa, K., Maemondo, M., Inoue, A., & Tamura, T. et al. (2013). CH5424802 (RO5424802) for patients with ALK-rearranged advanced non-small-cell lung cancer (AF-001JP study): A single-arm, open-label, phase 1-2 study. *The Lancet Oncology*, *14*(7), 590–598. doi:10.1016/S1470-2045(13)70142-6 PMID:23639470

Sevon, N., & Oksman-Caldentey, K. M. (2002). *Agrobacterium rhizogenes*-mediated transformation: Root cultures as a source of alkaloids. *Planta Medica*, *68*(10), 859–868. doi:10.1055/s-2002-34924 PMID:12391546

Shafie, A. A., Hassali, M. A., Azhar, S., & See, O. G. (2012). Separation of prescribing and dispensing in Malaysia: A summary of arguments. *Research in Social & Administrative Pharmacy*, *8*(3), 258–262. doi:10.1016/j.sapharm.2011.06.002 PMID:21824823

Shah, N. O., & Nickerson, T. A. (1978). Functional properties of hydrolyzed lactose: Solubility, viscosity and humectant properties. *Journal of Food Science*, *43*(4), 1081–1084. doi:10.1111/j.1365-2621.1978.tb15238.x

Shamir, E., Laudon, M., Barak, Y., Anis, Y., Rotenberg, V., Elizur, A., & Zisapel, N. (2000). Melatonin improves sleep quality of patients with chronic schizophrenia. *The Journal of Clinical Psychiatry*, *61*(5), 373–377. doi:10.4088/JCP.v61n0509 PMID:10847313

Sharma, P.L., & Sharma V. (2013). Role of Different Molecular Pathways in the Development of Diabetes Induced Nephropathy. *Journal of Diabetes & Metabolism, S9.*

Sharma, A. K., Kumar, R., Mishra, A., & Gupta, R. (2010). Problems associated with clinical trials of Ayurvedic medicines. *Brazilian Journal of Pharmacognosy*, *20*, 276–281.

Sharma, G. L., & Bhutani, M. M. (1988). Plant based antiamoebic drugs; Part II. Amoebicidal activity of parthenin isolated from *Parthenium hysterophorus*. *Planta Medica*, *54*(02), 120–122. doi:10.1055/s-2006-962366 PMID:2900531

Sharma, G., & Prakash, D. (2013). Nutraceuticals: Defense against Diseases? *Scientific Reports*, *50*(09), 32–33.

Sharma, G., Prakash, D., & Gupta, C. (2014). Phytochemicals of Nutraceutical Importance: Do they Defend against diseases? In D. Prakash & G. Sharma (Eds.), *Phytochemicals of Nutraceutical Importance* (pp. 1–19). CABI International Publishers.

Sharma, R. (2009). Nutraceuticals and nutraceutical supplementation criteria in cancer: A literature survey. *Open Nutraceuticals Journal*, *2*(1), 92–106. doi:10.2174/1876396000902010092

Sharma, S. R., Dwivedi, S. K., & Swarup, D. (1997). Hypoglycemic, antihyperglycemic and hypolipidemic activities of *Caesalpinia bonducella* seeds in rats. *Journal of Ethnopharmacology*, *58*(1), 39–44. doi:10.1016/S0378-8741(97)00079-2 PMID:9324003

Sharma, S., Kulkarni, S. K., & Chopra, K. (2006). Curcumin, the active principle of turmeric (Curcuma longa), ameliorates diabetic nephropathy in rats. *Clinical and Experimental Pharmacology & Physiology*, *33*(10), 940–945. doi:10.1111/j.1440-1681.2006.04468.x PMID:17002671

Shaw, A. T., Kim, D. W., Mehra, R., Tan, D. S., Felip, E., Chow, L. Q., & Engelman, J. A. et al. (2014). Ceritinib in ALK-rearranged non-small-cell lung cancer. *The New England Journal of Medicine*, *370*(13), 1189–1197. doi:10.1056/NEJMoa1311107 PMID:24670165

Shaw, A. T., Kim, D. W., Nakagawa, K., Seto, T., Crino, L., Ahn, M. J., & Janne, P. A. et al. (2013). Crizotinib versus chemotherapy in advanced ALK-positive lung cancer. *The New England Journal of Medicine*, *368*(25), 2385–2394. doi:10.1056/NEJMoa1214886 PMID:23724913

Sheela, C. G., & Augusti, K. T. (1992). Antidiabetic effects of S-allyl cysteine sulphoxide isolated from garlic *Allium sativum* Linn. *Indian Journal of Experimental Biology*, *30*, 523–526. PMID:1506036

Sheetz, M. J., & King, G. L. (2002). Molecular understanding of hyperglycemia's adverse effects for diabetic complications. *Journal of the American Medical Association*, *288*(20), 2579–2588. doi:10.1001/jama.288.20.2579 PMID:12444865

Shen, Y. J., Zhang, Z. W., Luo, X. G., Wang, X. F., & Wang, H. L. (2008). Nanoparticles of traditional chinese herbs inhibit thrombosis in vivo. *Haematologica*, *93*, J1457.

Shepherd, F. A., Rodrigues Pereira, J., Ciuleanu, T., Tan, E. H., Hirsh, V., Thongprasert, S., & Seymour, L. et al. (2005). Erlotinib in previously treated non-small-cell lung cancer. *The New England Journal of Medicine*, *353*(2), 123–132. doi:10.1056/NEJMoa050753 PMID:16014882

Sheridan, C. (2011). Gene therapy finds its niche. *Nature Biotechnology*, *29*(2), 121–128. PMID:21301435

Shim, J. S., Kang, M. H., Kim, Y. H., Roh, J. K., Roberts, C., & Lee, I. P. (1995). Chemopreventive effect of green tea (Camellia sinensis) among cigarette smokers. *Cancer Epidemiology, Biomarkers & Prevention*, *4*, 387–391. PMID:7655335

Shiojima, K., Suzuki, H., Kodera, N., Ageta, H., Chang, H. C., & Chen, Y. P. (1996). Composite constituents: Thirty-nine triterpenoids including two novel compounds from *Ixeris chinensis*. *Chemical & Pharmaceutical Bulletin*, *44*(3), 509–514. doi:10.1248/cpb.44.509

Shirani, A., Zhao, Y., Karim, M. E., Evans, C., Kingwell, E., van der Kop, M. L., & Tremlett, H. et al. (2012). Association between use of interferon beta and progression of disability in patients with relapsing-remitting multiple sclerosis. *Journal of the American Medical Association*, *308*(3), 247–256. doi:10.1001/jama.2012.7625 PMID:22797642

Shirley, S., Heller, R., & Heller, L. (2013). Electroporation gene therapy. In E. C. Lattime & S. L. Gerson (Eds.), *Gene Therapy of Cancer* (3rd ed.; pp. 93–106). San Diego, CA: Elsevier.

Shi, X. B., Tepper, C. G., White, R. W., Krichevsky, A. M., & Gabriely, G. (2008). MicroRNAs and prostate cancer. *Journal of Cellular and Molecular Medicine*, *5A*, 1456–1465. PMID:18624768

Shortliffe, E. H., & Blois, M. S. (2000). The Computer meets medicine and biology: Emergence of a discipline. In E. H. Shortliffe & L. E. Perreault (Eds.), *Medical Informatics: Computer Applications in Health Care and Biomedicine* (2nd ed.; pp. 3–40). New York, NY: Springer Verlag.

Shriharsh, V. et al.. (2014). Effect of nutraceutical and psychological interventions on cognitive functions of healthy human subjects. *Indian Journal of Traditional Knowledge.*, *13*(1), 95–102.

Shukla, M., Gupta, K., Rasheed, Z., Khan, K. A., & Haqqi, T. M. (2008). Bioavailable constituents/ metabolites of pomegranate (*Punicagranatum* L) preferentially inhibit COX2 activity *ex vivo* and IL-1beta-induced PGE_2 production in human chondrocytes in vitro. *Journal of Inflammation*, *5*(9), 1–10. PMID:18261214

Shukla, S., & Shukla, B. (1997). Aromatherapy in India: Yesterdays and Tomorrow. *Proceeding South Asian Countries Seminar on Medicinal Plants.*

Sicree, R., Shaw, J., & Zimmet, P. (2006). Diabetes and impaired glucose tolerance. In Diabetes Atlas. Gan D. International Diabetes Federation.

Sim, J. S., Im, A. R., Cho, S. M., Jang, H. J., Jo, J. H., & Kim, Y. S. (2007). Evaluation of chondroitin sulfate in shark cartilage powder as a dietary supplement: Raw materials and finished products. *Food Chemistry*, *101*(2), 532–539. doi:10.1016/j.foodchem.2006.02.011

Singh, L. W. (2011). Traditional medicinal plants of Manipur as anti-diabetics. *Journal of Medicinal Plants Research*, *5*, 677–687.

Singh, P., Kesharwani, R. K., Misra, K., & Rizvi, S. I. (2015). (in press). The modulation effects of curcumin on erythrocyte Na^+/K^+-ATPase activity. *Journal of Advanced Research*. doi:10.1016/j.jare.2014.12.007

Singh, P., & Rizvi, S. I. (2015). Role of curcumin in modulating plasma PON1 arylesterase activity and susceptibility to LDL oxidation in oxidatively challenged wistar rats. *Letters in Drug Design & Discovery*, *12*(4), 319–323. doi:10.2174/1570180811666141016000539

Singh, R. G., Rajak, M., & Ghosh, B. (2013). Comparative evaluation of fosinopril and herbal drug Dioscorea bulbifera in patients of diabetic nephropathy. *Saudi Journal of Kidney Diseases and Transplantation*, *24*(4), 737–742. doi:10.4103/1319-2442.113866 PMID:23816723

Singh, S. N., Vats, P., Suri, S., Shyam, R., Kumria, M. M. L., Ranganathan, S., & Sridharan, K. (2001). Effect of an antidiabetic extract of *Catharanthus roseus* on enzymic activities in streptozotocin induced diabetic rats. *Journal of Ethnopharmacology*, *76*(3), 269–277. doi:10.1016/S0378-8741(01)00254-9 PMID:11448549

Singh, V. P., Bali, A., Singh, N., & Jaggi, A. S. (2014). Advanced Glycation End Products and Diabetic Complications. *TheKorean Journal of Physiology and Pharmacology*, *18*(1), 1–14. doi:10.4196/kjpp.2014.18.1.1 PMID:24634591

Sivam, A. S., Sun-Waterhouse, G. I., Waterhouse, S., Quek, S. Y., & Perera, C. O. (2011). Physicochemical properties of bread dough and finished bread with added pectin fiber and phenolic antioxidants. *Journal of Food Science*, *76*(3), 97–107. doi:10.1111/j.1750-3841.2011.02086.x PMID:21535837

Sivilotti, M. L. (2004). Oxidant stress and haemolysis of the human erythrocyte. *Toxicological Reviews*, *23*(3), 169–188. doi:10.2165/00139709-200423030-00004 PMID:15862084

Skolnick, J., & Fetrow, J. S. (2000). From genes to protein structure and function: Novel applications of computational approaches in the genomic era. *Trends in Biotechnology*, *18*(1), 34–39. doi:10.1016/S0167-7799(99)01398-0 PMID:10631780

Slee, V. N. (1978). The International Classification of Diseases: Ninth revision (ICD-9). *Annals of Internal Medicine*, *88*(3), 424–426. doi:10.7326/0003-4819-88-3-424 PMID:629506

Sliwoski, G., Kothiwale, S., Meiler, J., & Lowe, E. W. (2014). Computational Methods in Drug Discovery. *Pharmacological Reviews*, *66*(1), 334–395. doi:10.1124/pr.112.007336 PMID:24381236

Smaji, S., Soetaredja, F. E., & Ayeitra, A. (2015). Green chemistry for sustainability. In S. K. Sharma (Ed.), *SpringerBriefs in molecular science*. Springer SBM.

Smith, K. J., & McDonald, W. I. (1999). The pathophysiology of multiple sclerosis: The mechanisms underlying the production of symptoms and the natural history of the disease. *Philosophical Transactions of the Royal Society of London. Series B, Biological Sciences*, *354*(1390), 1649–1673. doi:10.1098/rstb.1999.0510 PMID:10603618

Smith, S. R., Svetkey, L. P., & Dennis, V. W. (1991). Racial differences in the incidence and progression of renal diseases. *Kidney International*, *40*(5), 815–822. doi:10.1038/ki.1991.281 PMID:1762285

Soberman, R. J., & Christmas, P. (2003). The organization and consequences of eicosanoid signaling. *The Journal of Clinical Investigation*, *111*(8), 1107–1113. doi:10.1172/JCI200318338 PMID:12697726

Sohn, H. Y., Son, K. H., Kwon, C. S., Kwon, G. S., & Kang, S. S. (2004). Antimicrobial and cytotoxic activity of 18 prenylated flavonoids isolated from medicinal plants: *Morus alba* L., *Morus mongolica* Schneider, *Broussnetia papyrifera* (L.) Vent,*Sophora flavescens* Ait and *Echinosophora koreensis* Nakai. *Phytomedicine*, *11*(7-8), 666–672. doi:10.1016/j.phymed.2003.09.005 PMID:15636183

Solomon, B. J., Mok, T., Kim, D. W., Wu, Y. L., Nakagawa, K., Mekhail, T., & Investigators, P. et al. (2014). First-line crizotinib versus chemotherapy in ALK-positive lung cancer. *The New England Journal of Medicine*, *371*(23), 2167–2177. doi:10.1056/NEJMoa1408440 PMID:25470694

Solomon, P. R., Adams, F., Silver, A., Zimmer, J., & DeVeaux, R. (2002). Ginkgo for memory enhancement: A randomized controlled trial. *Journal of the American Medical Association*, *288*(7), 835–840. doi:10.1001/jama.288.7.835 PMID:12186600

Sommerfeld, B. (2007). Randomised, placebo-controlled, double-blind, split-face study on the clinical efficacy of Tricutan on skin firmness. *Phytomedicine*, *14*(11), 711–715. doi:10.1016/j.phymed.2007.09.015 PMID:17923398

Song, C. E. (Ed.). (2009). Cinchona alkaloids in synthesis and catalysis, ligands, immobilization and organocatalysis. Wiley-Vch Verlag GmbH & Co. KGaA. doi:doi:10.1002/9783527628179 doi:10.1002/9783527628179

Song, C. M., Lim, S. J., & Tong, J. C. (2009). Recent advances in computer-aided drug Design. *Briefings in Bioinformatics*, *10*(5), 579–591. doi:10.1093/bib/bbp023 PMID:19433475

Sood, A., Salih, S., Roh, D., Lacharme-Lora, L., Parry, M., Hardiman, B., & Keehan, R. C. P. (2011). Signalling of DNA damage and cytokines across cell barriers exposed to nanoparticles depends on barrier thickness. *Nature Nanotechnology*, *6*(12), 824–833. PMID:22056725

Sotaniemi, E. A., Haapakoski, E., & Rautio, A. (1995). Ginseng therapy in non-insulin dependent diabetic patients. *Diabetes Care*, *18*(10), 1373–1375. doi:10.2337/diacare.18.10.1373 PMID:8721940

Spatz, D. L. (2014). Changing Institutional Culture to Value Human Milk. *Advances in Neonatal Care*, *14*(4), 234–235. doi:10.1097/ANC.0000000000000128 PMID:25075920

Spencer, J. P., Abd El Mohsen, M. M., Minihane, A. M., & Mathers, J. C. (2008). Biomarkers of the intake of dietary polyphenols: Strengths, limitations and application in nutrition research. *The British Journal of Nutrition*, *99*(01), 12–22. doi:10.1017/S0007114507798938 PMID:17666146

Spigel, D.R., Reckamp, K.L., Rizvi, N.A., Poddubskaya, E., West, H.J, Eberhardt, W.E.E, . . . Brahmer, J.R. (2015). A phase III study (CheckMate 017) of nivolumab (NIVO, anti-programmed death-1 [PD-1]) versus docetaxel (DOC) in previously treated advanced or metastatic squamous cell non-small cell lung cancer. *Journal of Clinical Oncology.*

Staddon, S., Arranz, M. J., Mancama, D., Mata, I., & Kerwin, R. W. (2002). Clinical applications of pharmacogenetics in psychiatry. *Psychopharmacology*, *162*(1), 18–23. doi:10.1007/s00213-002-1084-4 PMID:12107612

Stamer, U. M., Lehnen, K., Hothker, F., Bayerer, B., Wolf, S., Hoeft, A., & Stuber, F. (2003). Impact of CYP2D6 genotype on postoperative tramadol analgesia. *Pain*, *105*(1-2), 231–238. doi:10.1016/S0304-3959(03)00212-4 PMID:14499440

Stamer, U. M., Musshoff, F., Kobilay, M., Madea, B., Hoeft, A., & Stuber, F. (2007). Concentrations of tramadol and O-desmethyltramadol enantiomers in different CYP2D6 genotypes. *Clinical Pharmacology and Therapeutics*, *82*(1), 41–47. doi:10.1038/sj.clpt.6100152 PMID:17361124

Stamer, U. M., Stuber, F., Muders, T., & Musshoff, F. (2008). Respiratory depression with tramadol in a patient with renal impairment and CYP2D6 gene duplication. *Anesthesia and Analgesia*, *107*(3), 926–929. doi:10.1213/ane.0b013e31817b796e PMID:18713907

Stamer, U. M., Zhang, L., Book, M., Lehmann, L. E., Stuber, F., & Musshoff, F. (2013). CYP2D6 genotype dependent oxycodone metabolism in postoperative patients. *PLoS ONE*, *8*(3), e60239. doi:10.1371/journal.pone.0060239 PMID:23555934

Staniek, A., Woerdenbag, H. J., & Kayser, O. (2008). Endophytes: Exploiting biodiversity for the improvement of natural product-based drug discovery. *Journal of Plant Interactions*, *3*(2), 75–93. doi:10.1080/17429140801886293

Stanulla, M., Schaeffeler, E., Flohr, T., Cario, G., Schrauder, A., Zimmermann, M., & Schwab, M. et al. (2005). Thiopurine methyltransferase (TPMT) genotype and early treatment response to mercaptopurine in childhood acute lymphoblastic leukemia. *Journal of the American Medical Association*, *293*(12), 1485–1489. doi:10.1001/jama.293.12.1485 PMID:15784872

Stauble, M. E., Moore, A. W., Langman, L. J., Boswell, M. V., Baumgartner, R., McGee, S., & Jortani, S. A. et al. (2014). Hydrocodone in postoperative personalized pain management: Pro-drug or drug? *Clinica Chimica Acta*, *429*, 26–29. doi:10.1016/j.cca.2013.11.015 PMID:24269714

Stevenson, R. (2004). Chemical harvest. *Chemistry & Industry*.

Stierle, A. A., & Stierle, D. B. (2000). Bioactive compounds from four endophytic Penicillium sp. of a Northwest Pacific yew tree. In A. R. Rahman (Ed.), *Studies in Natural Products Chemistry*. Elsevier Science B.V. doi:10.1016/S1572-5995(00)80058-7

Stierle, A., Strobel, G., Stierle, D., Grothaus, P., & Bignami, G. (1995). The Search for a taxol-producing microorganism among the endophytic fungi of the pacific yew, *Taxus brevifolia*. *Journal of Natural Products*, *58*(9), 1315–1324. doi:10.1021/np50123a002 PMID:7494141

Stocco, G., Cheok, M. H., Crews, K. R., Dervieux, T., French, D., Pei, D., & Evans, W. E. et al. (2009). Genetic polymorphism of inosine triphosphate pyrophosphatase is a determinant of mercaptopurine metabolism and toxicity during treatment for acute lymphoblastic leukemia. *Clinical Pharmacology and Therapeutics*, *85*(2), 164–172. doi:10.1038/clpt.2008.154 PMID:18685564

Street, A. (2015). Food as pharma: Marketing nutraceuticals to India's rural poor. *Critical Public Health*, *25*(3), 361–372. doi:10.1080/09581596.2014.966652 PMID:25865449

Strobel, C., Jahreis, G., & Kuhnt, K. (2012). Survey of n-3 and n-6 polyunsaturated fatty acids in fish and fish products. *Lipids in Health and Disease*, *11*(1), 144. doi:10.1186/1476-511X-11-144 PMID:23110317

Strobel, G., Daisy, B., Castillo, U., & Harper, J. (2004). Natural products from endophytic microorganisms. *Journal of Natural Products*, *67*(2), 257–268. doi:10.1021/np030397v PMID:14987067

Stuhlmüller, B., Häupl, T., Hernandez, M. M., Grützkau, A., Kuban, R. J., Tandon, N., & Burmester, G. R. et al. (2010). CD11c as a transcriptional biomarker to predict response to anti-TNF monotherapy with adalimumab in patients with rheumatoid arthritis. *Clinical Pharmacology and Therapeutics*, *87*, 311–321. PMID:20032971

Suba, V., Murugesan, T., Arunachalam, G., Mandal, S. C., & Saha, B. P. (2004). Anti-diabetic potential of *Barleria lupulina* extract in rats. *Phytomedicine*, *11*(2-3), 202–205. doi:10.1078/0944-7113-00316 PMID:15070173

Subramonium, A., Pushpangadan, P., Rajasekharan, S., Evans, D. A., Latha, P. G., & Valsaraj, R. (1996). Effects of *Artemisia pallens* Wall.on blood glucose levels in normal and alooxan-induced diabetic rats. *Journal of Ethnopharmacology*, *50*(1), 13–17. doi:10.1016/0378-8741(95)01329-6 PMID:8778502

Su, F., Viros, A., Milagre, C., Trunzer, K., Bollag, G., Spleiss, O., & Marais, R. et al. (2012). RAS mutations in cutaneous squamous-cell carcinomas in patients treated with BRAF inhibitors. *The New England Journal of Medicine*, *366*(3), 207–215. doi:10.1056/NEJMoa1105358 PMID:22256804

Summers, M. P. (1983). Recent Advances in Drug Delivery. *The Pharmaceutical Journal*, *230*, 643–645.

Tabata, Y., & Ikada, Y. (1988). Effect of the size and surface charge of polymer microspheres on their phagocytosis by macrophage. *Biomaterials*, *9*(4), 356–362. doi:10.1016/0142-9612(88)90033-6 PMID:3214660

Tabernero, J., Yoshino, T., Cohn, A. L., Obermannova, R., Bodoky, G., Garcia-Carbonero, R., & Investigators, R. S. et al. (2015). Ramucirumab versus placebo in combination with second-line FOLFIRI in patients with metastatic colorectal carcinoma that progressed during or after first-line therapy with bevacizumab, oxaliplatin, and a fluoropyrimidine (RAISE): A randomised, double-blind, multicentre, phase 3 study. *The Lancet Oncology*, *16*(5), 499–508. doi:10.1016/S1470-2045(15)70127-0 PMID:25877855

Tadicherla, S., Ross, K., Shenefelt, P. D., & Fenske, N. A. (2009). Article. *Journal of Drugs in Dermatology*, *8*, 1093–1105. PMID:20027937

Tak, P. P., & Bresnihan, B. (2000). The pathogenesis and prevention of joint damage in rheumatoid arthritis: Advances from synovial biopsy and tissue analysis. *Arthritis &. Rheumatology*, *43*, 2619–2633. PMID:11145019

Talaei, M., & Pan, A. (2015). Role of phytoestrogens in prevention and management of type 2 diabetes. *World Journal of Diabetes*, *6*(2), 271–283. doi:10.4239/wjd.v6.i2.271 PMID:25789108

Talwar, N., & Jain, N. K. (1992). Erythrocytes as Carriers of Metronidazole: *In-Vitro* Characterization. *Drug Development and Industrial Pharmacy*, *18*(16), 1799–1812. doi:10.3109/03639049209040903

Talwar, N., & Jain, N. K. (1992). Erythrocytes as Carriers of Primaquin Preparation: Characterization and Evaluation. *Journal of Controlled Release*, *20*(2), 133–142. doi:10.1016/0168-3659(92)90159-O

Tambeker, D. H., Sonar, T. P., Khodke, M. V., & Khante, B. S. (2006). The novel antimicrobials from two edible mushrooms: *Agaricus bisporus* and *Pleurotus sajor caju*. *Int. J. Pharmacol*, *2*(5), 584–587. doi:10.3923/ijp.2006.584.587

Tan, A. L. Y., Forbes, J. M., & Cooper, M. E. (2007). AGE, RAGE, and ROS in Diabetic Nephropathy. *Seminars in Nephrology*, *27*(2), 130–143. doi:10.1016/j.semnephrol.2007.01.006 PMID:17418682

Tanaka, S., Haruma, K., Kunihiro, M., Nagata, S., Kitada, Y., Manabe, N., & Chayama, K. et al. (2004). Effects of aged garlic extract (AGE) on colorectal adenomas: A double-blinded study. *Hiroshima Journal of Medical Sciences*, *53*(3–4), 39–45. PMID:15726891

Tan, B. R., Thomas, F., Myerson, R. J., Zehnbauer, B., Trinkaus, K., Malyapa, R. S., & McLeod, H. L. et al. (2011). Thymidylate synthase genotype-directed neoadjuvant chemoradiation for patients with rectal adenocarcinoma. *Journal of Clinical Oncology*, *29*(7), 875–883. doi:10.1200/JCO.2010.32.3212 PMID:21205745

Tan, C. (1972). L-Asparaginase in Leukemia. *Hospital Practice*, *7*, 99–103.

Tan, D. X., Chen, L. D., Poeggeler, B., Manchester, L. C., & Reiter, R. J. (1993). Melatonin: A potent, endogenous hydroxyl radical scavenger. *Endocrine Journal*, *1*, 57–60.

Tan, D. X., Hardeland, R., Manchester, L. C., Korkmaz, A., Ma, S., Rosales-Corral, S., & Reiter, R. J. (2012). Functional roles of melatonin in plants, and perspectives in nutritional and agricultural science. *Journal of Experimental Botany*, *63*(2), 577–597. doi:10.1093/jxb/err256 PMID:22016420

Tan, D. X., Hardeland, R., Manchester, L. C., Paredes, S. D., Korkmaz, A., Sainz, R. M., & Reiter, R. J. et al. (2010). The changing biological roles of melatonin during evolution: From an antioxidant to signals of darkness, sexual selection and fitness. *Biological Reviews of the Cambridge Philosophical Society*, *85*(3), 607–623. PMID:20039865

Tan, D. X., Zheng, X., Kong, J., Manchester, L., Hardeland, R., Kim, S., & Reiter, R. et al. (2014). Fundamental Issues Related to the Origin of Melatonin and Melatonin Isomers during Evolution: Relation to Their Biological Functions. *International Journal of Molecular Sciences*, *15*(9), 15858–15890. doi:10.3390/ijms150915858 PMID:25207599

Tang, D., Yu, Y., Zheng, X., Wu, J., Li, Y., Wu, X., & Yin, X. et al. (2014). Comparative investigation of in vitro biotransformation of 14 components in Ginkgo biloba extract in normal, diabetes and diabetic nephropathy rat intestinal bacteria matrix. *Journal of Pharmaceutical and Biomedical Analysis*, *100*, 1–10. doi:10.1016/j.jpba.2014.07.022 PMID:25117949

Tan, M. J., Ye, J. M., Turner, N., Hohnen-Behrens, C., Ke, C. Q., Tang, C. P., & Ye, Y. et al. (2008). Antidiabetic Activities of Triterpenoids Isolated from Bitter Melon Associated with Activation of the AMPK Pathway. *Chemistry & Biology*, *15*(3), 263–273. doi:10.1016/j.chembiol.2008.01.013 PMID:18355726

Tanumihardjo, S. A. (2011). Vitamin A: Biomarkers of nutrition for development. *The American Journal of Clinical Nutrition*, *94*(2), 658S–665S. doi:10.3945/ajcn.110.005777 PMID:21715511

Tan, Y., Wang, B., Keum, J.-S., & Jaffa, A. A. (2005). Mechanisms through which bradykinin promotes glomerular injury in diabetes. *American Journal of Physiology. Renal Physiology*, *288*(3), F483–F492. doi:10.1152/ajprenal.00165.2004 PMID:15692059

Tapas, A. R., Sakarkar, D. M., & Kakde, R. B. (2008). Flavonoids as Nutraceuticals: A Review. *Tropical Journal of Pharmaceutical Research*, *7*(3), 1089–1099. doi:10.4314/tjpr.v7i3.14693

Tarek, K. M., Manal, A. H., Manal, H. S., Reem, M. H., & Asmaa, F. A. N. (2011). Zingiber officinale acts as a nutraceutical agent against liver fibrosis. *Nutrition and Metabolism*, *8*(40), 1–11. PMID:21241467

Tarnow, L., Rossing, P., Carstensen, B., & Parving, H. H. (2004). Improved survival in patients obtaining remission of nephrotic range albuminuria in diabetic nephropathy. *Kidney International*, *66*(3), 1180–1186. doi:10.1111/j.1523-1755.2004.00870.x PMID:15327415

Tatusov, R. L., Koonin, E. V., & Lipman, D. J. (1997). A genomic perspective on protein families. *Science*, *278*(5338), 631–637. doi:10.1126/science.278.5338.631 PMID:9381173

Taylor, P. A., Friedman, T. M., Korngold, R., Noelle, R. J., & Blazar, B. R. (2002). Tolerance induction of alloreactive T cells via ex vivo blockade of the CD40:CD40L costimulatory pathway results in the generation of a potent immune regulatory cell. *Blood*, *99*(12), 4601–4609. doi:10.1182/blood.V99.12.4601 PMID:12036894

Teisseire, B. (1987). In Vivo Consequences of Rightward Shift of the Hemoglobin Dissociation Curve. Advanced Biosciences, 67, 89-94.

Telen, M. J. (1993). The mature erythrocyte. In Wintrobe's Clinical Hematology (9th Ed.). Lea & Febiger.

Tenore, G. C., Daglia, M., Ciampaglia, R., & Novellino, E. (2015). Exploring the nutraceutical potential of polyphenols from black, green and white tea infusions - an overview. *Current Pharmaceutical Biotechnology*, *16*(3), 265–271. doi:10.2174/1389201016666150118133604 PMID:25601602

Tenzer, S., Docter, D., Kuharev, J., Musyanovych, A., Fetz, V., Hecht, R., & Stauber, R. H. et al. (2013). Rapid formation of plasma protein corona critically affects nanoparticle pathophysiology. *Nature Nanotechnology*, *8*(10), 772–781. doi:10.1038/nnano.2013.181 PMID:24056901

Tenzer, S., Docter, D., Rosfa, S., Wlodarski, A., Kuharev, J., Rekik, A., & Stauber, R. H. et al. (2011). Nanoparticle size is a critical physicochemical determinant of the human blood plasma corona: A comprehensive quantitative proteomic analysis. *ACS Nano*, *5*(9), 7155–7167. doi:10.1021/nn201950e PMID:21866933

Terra, V. A., Souza-Neto, F. P., Frade, M. A., Ramalho, L. N., Andrade, T. A., Pasta, A. A., & Cecchini, A. L. et al. (2015). Genistein prevents ultraviolet B radiation-induced nitrosative skin injury and promotes cell proliferation. *Journal of Photochemistry and Photobiology. B, Biology*, *144*, 20–27. PMID:25668145

Thakur, G. S., Sharma, R., Sanodiya, B. S., Pandey, M., Prasad, G. B. K. S., & Bisen, P. S. (2012). *Gymnema sylvestre*: An alternative therapeutic agent for management of diabetes. *Journal of Applied Pharmaceutical Science*, *2*, 1–6.

Thatcher, N., Chang, A., Parikh, P., Rodrigues Pereira, J., Ciuleanu, T., von Pawel, J., & Carroll, K. et al. (2005). Gefitinib plus best supportive care in previously treated patients with refractory advanced non-small-cell lung cancer: Results from a randomised, placebo-controlled, multicentre study (Iressa Survival Evaluation in Lung Cancer). *Lancet*, *366*(9496), 1527–1537. doi:10.1016/S0140-6736(05)67625-8 PMID:16257339

The Freedonia Group. (2015). *Cosmeceuticals to 2015 - demand and sales forecasts, market share, market size, market leaders*. Retrieved September 18 2015, from http://www.freedoniagroup.com/Cosmeceuticals.html

Theodori, R., Karioti, A., Rancic, A., & Skaltsa, H. (2006). Linear sesquiterpene lactones from Anthemis auriculata and their antibacterial activity. *Journal of Natural Products*, *69*(4), 662–664. doi:10.1021/np058084i PMID:16643047

Theodori, R., Karioti, A., Racnic, A., & Skaltsa, H. (2006). Linear sesquiterpene lactones from Thijs, L., Fagard, R., Forette, F., Nawrot, T., Staessen, J.A. (2003). Are low dehydroepiandrosterone sulphate levels predictive for cardiovascular diseases? A review of prospective and retrospective studies. *Acta Cardiologica*, *58*(5), 403–410.

Theuns, H. G., Theuns, H. L., & Lousberg, R. J. J. (1986). Search for new natural sources of morphinans. *Economic Botany*, *40*(4), 485–497. doi:10.1007/BF02859662

Tian, Q., Miller, E. G., Jayaprakasha, G. K., & Patil, B. S. (2007). An improved HPLC method for the analysis of citrus limonoids in culture media. *Journal of Chromatography B. Analytical Technolology & Biomedical Life Sciences*, *846*(1-2), 385–390. doi:10.1016/j.jchromb.2006.09.012

Tibor, T. G., Katalin, M., & Tibor, A. R. (2014). Epigenetics in the pathogenesis of rheumatoid arthritis. *BMC Medicine*, *12*, 35. PMID:24568138

Tilleman, K., Van Beneden, K., Dhondt, A., Hoffman, I., De Keyser, F., Veys, E., & Deforce, D. et al. (2005). Chronically inflamed synovium from spondyloarthropathy and rheumatoid arthritis investigated by protein expression profiling followed by tandem mass spectrometry. *Proteomics. Clinical Applications*, *5*(8), 2247–2257. PMID:15846842

Toffoli, G., & Cecchin, E. (2007). Pharmacogenetics and stomach cancer: An update. *Pharmacogenomics*, *8*(5), 497–505. doi:10.2217/14622416.8.5.497 PMID:17465714

Toffoli, G., Cecchin, E., Gasparini, G., D'Andrea, M., Azzarello, G., Basso, U., & Innocenti, F. et al. (2010). Genotype-driven phase I study of irinotecan administered in combination with fluorouracil/leucovorin in patients with metastatic colorectal cancer. *Journal of Clinical Oncology*, *28*(5), 866–871. doi:10.1200/JCO.2009.23.6125 PMID:20038727

Torotra, G. J., & Grabowski, S. R. (1993). *The Cardiovascular System: The Blood. Principles of Anatomy and Physiology* (7th ed.). New York: Harper Collins College Publishers.

Traber, M. G. (2006). Vitamin E. In M. E. Shils, M. Shike, A. C. Ross, B. Caballero, & R. Cousins (Eds.), *Modern Nutrition in Health and Disease* (10th ed.). MD: Lippincott Williams & Wilkins, Baltimore.

Trachootham, D., Lu, W., Ogasawara, M. A., Valle, N. R. D., & Huang, P. (2008). Redox Regulation of Cell Survival. *Antioxidants & Redox Signalling*, *10*(8), 1343–1374. doi:10.1089/ars.2007.1957 PMID:18522489

Traka, M., & Mithen, R. (2009). Glucosinolates, isothiocyanates and human health. *Phytochemistry Reviews*, *8*(1), 269–282. doi:10.1007/s11101-008-9103-7

Tran, B., Dancey, J. E., Kamel-Reid, S., McPherson, J. D., Bedard, P. L., Brown, A. M., & Siu, L. L. et al. (2012). Cancer genomics: Technology, discovery, and translation. *Journal of Clinical Oncology*, *30*(6), 647–660. doi:10.1200/JCO.2011.39.2316 PMID:22271477

Tremblay, P. B., Kaiser, R., Sezer, O., Rosler, N., Schelenz, C., Possinger, K., & Brockmoller, J. et al. (2003). Variations in the 5-hydroxytryptamine type 3B receptor gene as predictors of the efficacy of antiemetic treatment in cancer patients. *Journal of Clinical Oncology*, *21*(11), 2147–2155. doi:10.1200/JCO.2003.05.164 PMID:12775740

Treuel, L., Docter, D., Maskos, M., & Stauber, R. H. (2015). Protein corona - from molecular adsorption to physiological complexity. *Beilstein Journal of Nanotechnology*, *6*, 857–873. doi:10.3762/bjnano.6.88 PMID:25977856

Treuel, L., Jiang, X., & Nienhaus, G. U. (2013). New views on cellular uptake and trafficking of manufactured nanoparticles. *Journal of the Royal Society, Interface*, *10*(82), 20120939. doi:10.1098/rsif.2012.0939 PMID:23427093

Trifilio, S., Pennick, G., Pi, J., Zook, J., Golf, M., Kaniecki, K., & Mehta, J. et al. (2007). Monitoring plasma voriconazole levels may be necessary to avoid subtherapeutic levels in hematopoietic stem cell transplant recipients. *Cancer*, *109*(8), 1532–1535. doi:10.1002/cncr.22568 PMID:17351937

Trinh, V. A., Davis, J. E., Anderson, J. E., & Kim, K. B. (2014). Dabrafenib therapy for advanced melanoma. *The Annals of Pharmacotherapy*, *48*(4), 519–529. doi:10.1177/1060028013513009 PMID:24259661

Tripathi, Y. B., Nagwani, S., Mishra, P., Jha, A., & Rai, S. P. (2012). Protective effect of Pueraria tuberosa DC Embedded biscuit on cisplatin-induced nephrotoxicity in mice. *Journal of Natural Medicines*, *66*(1), 109–118. doi:10.1007/s11418-011-0559-1 PMID:21717089

Tripathi, Y. B., & Yadav, D. (2013). Diabetic Nephropathy: Causes and Managements Recent Patents on Endocrine. *Metabolic & Immune Drug Discovery*, *7*, 57–64.

Trock, B. J., Hilakivi-Clarke, L., & Clarke, R. (2006). Meta-analysis of soy intake and breast cancer risk. *Journal of the National Cancer Institute*, *98*(7), 459–471. doi:10.1093/jnci/djj102 PMID:16595782

Troke, P. F., Hockey, H. P., & Hope, W. W. (2011). Observational study of the clinical efficacy of voriconazole and its relationship to plasma concentrations in patients. *Antimicrobial Agents and Chemotherapy*, *55*(10), 4782–4788. doi:10.1128/AAC.01083-10 PMID:21768513

Tsai, S., Shameli, A., Yamanouchi, J., Clemente-Casares, X., Wang, J., Serra, P., & Santamaria, P. et al. (2010). Reversal of autoimmunity by boosting memory-like autoregulatory T cells. *Immunity*, *32*(4), 568–580. doi:10 1016/j.immuni.2010.03.015 PMID:20381385

Tseng, H. H., Chang, J. G., Hwang, Y. H., Yeh, K. T., Chen, Y. L., & Yu, H. S. (2009). Expression of hepcidin and other iron-regulatory genes in human hepatocellular carcinoma and its clinical implication. *Journal of Cancer Research and Clinical Oncology*, *135*, 1413–1420. PMID:19387685

Tsong, T. Y., & Kinosita, K. Jr. (1985). Use of Voltage Pulses for the Pore, Opening and Drug Loading, and the Subsequent Resealing of Red, Blood Cells. *Bibliotheca Haematologica*, *51*, 108–114. PMID:4004753

Tsuchihashi, N., Watanabe, T., & Takai, Y. (1987). Effect of Spirulina platensis on caecum content in rats. *Bull Chiba Hygiene Coll*, *5*, 27–30.

Tufro, A., & Veron, D. (2012). VEGF and Podocytes in Diabetic Nephropathy. *Seminars in Nephrology*, *32*(4), 385–393. doi:10.1016/j.semnephrol.2012.06.010 PMID:22958493

Tundis, R., Loizzo, M. R., & Menichini, F. (2014). An Overview on Chemical Aspects and Potential Health Benefits of Limonoids and Their Derivatives. *Critical Reviews in Food Science and Nutrition*, *54*(2), 225–250. doi:10.1080/10408398.2011.581400 PMID:24188270

Turnbull, F. M., Abraira, C., Anderson, R. J., Byington, R. P., Chalmers, J. P., Duckworth, W. C., & Woodward, M. et al. (2009). Intensive glucose control and macrovascular outcomes in type 2 diabetes. *Diabetologia*, *52*(11), 2288–2298. doi:10.1007/s00125-009-1470-0 PMID:19655124

Tu, X., Liu, F., Jordan, J. B., Ye, X. F., Fu, P., Wang, F., & Zhong, S. (2013). *'Huang Qi Elixir'* for proteinuria in patients with diabetic nephropathy: A study protocol for a randomized controlled pilot trial. *Trials*, *14*(1), 223. doi:10.1186/1745-6215-14-223 PMID:23866835

Tzvetkov, M. V., Saadatmand, A. R., Bokelmann, K., Meineke, I., Kaiser, R., & Brockmoller, J. (2012). Effects of OCT1 polymorphisms on the cellular uptake, plasma concentrations and efficacy of the 5-HT(3) antagonists tropisetron and ondansetron. *The Pharmacogenomics Journal*, *12*(1), 22–29. doi:10.1038/tpj.2010.75 PMID:20921968

U.S Food and Drug Administration. (2013). *Table of Pharmacogenomic Biomarkers in Drug Labels*. Retrieved from http://www.fda.gov/drugs/scienceresearch/researchareas/ph

Udgata, J. R., & Naik, S. N. (2007). Soybean Isoflavones: Remedial nutraceuticals in Indian perspective. *Journal of Scientific and Industrial Research*, *66*, 11–18.

Uehara, S., Gotoh, K., Handa, H., Tomita, H., & Senshuu, M. (2005). Distribution of the heterogeneity of des-gamma-carboxyprothrombin in patients with hepatocellular carcinoma. *Journal of Gastroenterology and Hepatology*, *20*, 1545–1552. PMID:16174072

Ueno, H., Wang, J., Kaji, N., Tokeshi, M., & Baba, Y. (2008). Quantitative determination of amino acids in functional foods by microchip electrophoresis. *Journal of Separation Science*, *31*(5), 898–903. doi:10.1002/jssc.200700517 PMID:18266297

Ulker, P., Sati, L., Celik-Ozenci, C., Meiselman, H. J., & Baskurt, O. K. (2009). Mechanical stimulation of nitric oxide synthesizing mechanisms in erythrocytes. *Biorheology*, *46*(2), 121–132. PMID:19458415

Updike, S. J., & Wakamiya, R. T. (1983). Infusion of Red Blood Cell-Loaded Asparaginase in Monkey. *The Journal of Laboratory and Clinical Medicine*, *101*, 679–691. PMID:6187874

US Government Publishing Office. (2015). *Subpart B—Requirements for Specific Cosmetic Products*. Retrieved September 18 2015, from http://www.ecfr.gov/cgi-bin/text-idx?c=ecfr&sid=c108128827d21f2d274e894731665ef4&rgn=div6&view=text&node=21:7.0.1.2.10.2&idno=21

Vaidyanathan, G. (2012). Redefining clinical trials: The age of personalized medicine. *Cell*, *148*(6), 1079–1080. PMID:22424218

Vallittu, A. M., Peltoniemi, J., Elovaara, I., Kuusisto, H., Farkkila, M., Multanen, J., & Eralinna, J. P. (2005). The efficacy of glatiramer acetate in beta-interferon-intolerant MS patients. *Acta Neurologica Scandinavica*, *112*(4), 234–237. doi:10.1111/j.1600-0404.2005.00464.x PMID:16146492

Van Beek, T., & Montoro, P. (2009). Chemical analysis and quality control of Ginkgo biloba leaves, extracts, and PP. *Journal of Chromatography. A*, *1216*, 2002–2032. doi:10.1016/j.chroma.2009.01.013 PMID:19195661

Van Belle, T. L., Taylor, P., & von Herrath, M. G. (2009). Mouse Models for Type 1 Diabetes. *Drug Discovery Today. Disease Models*, *6*(2), 41–45. doi:10.1016/j.ddmod.2009.03.008 PMID:20407588

Van Cutsem, E., Kohne, C. H., Hitre, E., Zaluski, J., Chang Chien, C. R., Makhson, A., & Rougier, P. et al. (2009). Cetuximab and chemotherapy as initial treatment for metastatic colorectal cancer. *The New England Journal of Medicine*, *360*(14), 1408–1417. doi:10.1056/NEJMoa0805019 PMID:19339720

Van Cutsem, E., Tabernero, J., Lakomy, R., Prenen, H., Prausova, J., Macarulla, T., & Allegra, C. et al. (2012). Addition of aflibercept to fluorouracil, leucovorin, and irinotecan improves survival in a phase III randomized trial in patients with metastatic colorectal cancer previously treated with an oxaliplatin-based regimen. *Journal of Clinical Oncology*, *30*(28), 3499–3506. doi:10.1200/JCO.2012.42.8201 PMID:22949147

Van der Pouw Kraan, T. C. T. M., Van Gaalen, F. A., Huizinga, T. W. J., Pieterman, E., Breedveld, F. C., & Verweij, C. L. (2003). Discovery of distinctive gene expression profiles in rheumatoid synovium using cDNA microarray technology: Evidence for the existence of multiple pathways of tissue destruction and repair. *Genes and Immunity*, *4*, 187–196. PMID:12700593

Van Kuilenburg, A. B., Meinsma, R., Zoetekouw, L., & Van Gennip, A. H. (2002). High prevalence of the IVS14 + 1G>A mutation in the dihydropyrimidine dehydrogenase gene of patients with severe 5-fluorouracil-associated toxicity. *Pharmacogenetics*, *12*(7), 555–558. doi:10.1097/00008571-200210000-00007 PMID:12360106

Vazquez, L., Torres, C. F., Fornari, T., Senorans, F. J., & Reglero, G. (2007). Recovery of squalene from vegetable oil sources using countercurrent supercritical carbon dioxide extraction. *The Journal of Supercritical Fluids*, *40*(1), 59–66. doi:10.1016/j.supflu.2006.04.012

Veerkamp, J. H., van Kuppevelt, T. H., Maatman, R. G., & Prinsen, C. F. (1993). Structural and functional aspects of cytosolic fatty acid-binding proteins. *Prostaglandins, Leukotrienes, and Essential Fatty Acids*, *49*(6), 887–906. doi:10.1016/0952-3278(93)90174-U PMID:8140117

Verallo-Rowell, V. M., Verallo, V., Graupe, K., Lopez-Villafuerte, L., & Garcia-Lopez, M. (1989). Double-blind comparison of azelaic acid and hydroquinone in the treatment of melasma. *Acta Dermato-Venereologica*, *143*, 58–61. PMID:2528260

Verardo, V., Bendini, A., Cerretani, L., Malaguti, D., Cozzolino, E., & Caboni, M. F. (2009). Capillary gas chromatography analysis of lipid composition and evaluation of phenolic compounds by micellar electrokinetic chromatography in Italian walnut (*Juglans Regia l.*): Irrigation and fertilization influence. *Journal of Food Quality*, *32*(2), 262–281. doi:10.1111/j.1745-4557.2009.00249.x

Verma, J., Khedkar, V. M., & Coutinho, E. C. (2010). 3D-QSAR in drug design--a review. *Current Topics in Medicinal Chemistry*, *10*(1), 95–115. doi:10.2174/156802610790232260 PMID:19929826

Veronese, P., Li, X., Niu, X., Weller, S. C., Bressan, R. A., & Hasegawa, P. M. (2001). Bioengineering mint crop improvement. *Plant Cell, Tissue and Organ Culture*, *64*(2/3), 133–144. doi:10.1023/A:1010649207445

Verspohl, E. J. (2012). Novel pharmacological approaches to the treatment of type 2 diabetes. *Pharmacological Reviews*, *64*(2), 188–237. doi:10.1124/pr.110.003319 PMID:22407617

Veselovsky, A. V., & Ivanov, A. S. (2003). Strategy of computer-aided drug design. *Current Drug Targets. Infectious Disorders*, *3*(1), 33–40. doi:10.2174/1568005033342145 PMID:12570731

Vesterinen, H. M., Sena, E. S., ffrench-Constant, C., Williams, A., Chandran, S., & Macleod, M. R. (2010). Improving the translational hit of experimental treatments in multiple sclerosis. *Multiple Sclerosis*, *16*(9), 1044–1055. doi:10.1177/1352458510379612 PMID:20685763

Vienken, J., Jeltsch, E., & Zimmermann, U. (1978). Penetration and Entrapment of Large Particles in Erythrocytes by Electrical Breakdown Techniques. *Cytobiologie*, *17*, 182–186. PMID:689250

Vig, A. P., Rampal, G., Singh, T. S., & Arora, S. (2009). Bioprotective effects of glucosinolates- A review. *LWT Food Science and Technology*, *42*(10), 1561–1572. doi:10.1016/j.lwt.2009.05.023

Vilar, G., Tulla-Puche, J., & Albericio, F. (2012). Polymers and drug delivery systems. *Current Drug Delivery*, *9*(4), 367–394. doi:10.2174/156720112801323053 PMID:22640038

Villafranca, E., Okruzhnov, Y., Dominguez, M. A., Garcia-Foncillas, J., Azinovic, I., Martinez, E., & Brugarolas, A. et al. (2001). Polymorphisms of the repeated sequences in the enhancer region of the thymidylate synthase gene promoter may predict downstaging after preoperative chemoradiation in rectal cancer. *Journal of Clinical Oncology*, *19*(6), 1779–1786. PMID:11251009

Villareal, M. C. (1987). Modification of Cardiac Parameters in Piglets After Infusion of IHP-Loaded Red Blood Cells. [series]. *Advances in the Biosciences*, *67*, 81–88.

Virtanen, S. (2013). *Virtual Screening Development of a Novel Structure-Based Method.* Jyvaskyla.

Vlasova, M. A., Rytkonen, J., Riikonen, J., Tarasova, O. S., Monkare, J., Kovalainen, M., & Jarvinen, K. et al. (2014). Nanocarriers and the delivered drug: Effect interference due to intravenous administration. *European Journal of Pharmaceutical Sciences*, *63*, 96–102. doi:10.1016/j.ejps.2014.06.011 PMID:24964293

Vlasova, M. A., Tarasova, O. S., Riikonen, J., Raula, J., Lobach, A. S., Borzykh, A. A., & Järvinen, K. et al. (2014). Injected nanoparticles: The combination of experimental systems to assess cardiovascular adverse effects. *European Journal of Pharmaceutics and Biopharmaceutics*, *87*(1), 64–72. doi:10.1016/j.ejpb.2014.02.001 PMID:24530427

Vlietinck, A. J., De Bruyne, T., Apers, S., & Pieters, L. A. (1998). Plant-derived leading compounds for chemotherapy of human immunodeficiency virus (HIV) infection. *Planta Medica*, *64*(02), 97–109. doi:10.1055/s-2006-957384 PMID:9525100

Volpi, N. (2009). Capillary electrophoresis determination of glucosamine in nutraceutical formulations after labeling with anthranilic acid and UV detection. *Journal of Pharmaceutical and Biomedical Analysis*, *49*(3), 868–871. doi:10.1016/j.jpba.2009.01.006 PMID:19200685

Volpi, N., & Maccari, F. (2008). Quantitative and qualitative evaluation of chondroitin sulfate in dietary supplements. *Food Anal. Methods*, *1*(3), 195–204. doi:10.1007/s12161-008-9020-9

Von Bergmann, K., Sudhop, T., & Lutjohann, D. (2005). Cholesterol and plant sterol absorption: Recent insights. *The American Journal of Cardiology*, *96*(1), 10D–14D. doi:10.1016/j.amjcard.2005.03.014 PMID:15992510

Vroman, L. (1962). Effect of absorbed proteins on the wettability of hydrophilic and hydrophobic solids. *Nature*, *196*(4853), 476–477. doi:10.1038/196476a0 PMID:13998030

Vyas, S. P., & Dixit, V. K. (1999). Pharmaceutical Biotechnology 1. CBS Publishers & Distributors.

Vyas, S. P., & Khar, R. K. (2002). *Resealed Erythrocytes in Targeted and Controlled Drug Delivery: Novel Carrier Systems*. CBS Publishers and Distributors.

Wagner, E., Plank, C., Zatloukal, K., Cotton, M., & Birnstiel, M. L. (1992). Influenza virus hemagglutinin HA-2 N-terminal fusogenic peptides augment gene transfer by transferrin-polylysine-DNA complexes: Toward a synthetic virus-like gene-transfer vehicle. *Proceedings of the National Academy of Sciences of the United States of America*, *89*(17), 7934–7938. PMID:1518816

Wagner, H. (2011). Synergy research: Approaching a new generation of PP. *Fitoterapia*, *82*, 34–37. doi:10.1016/j.fitote.2010.11.016 PMID:21075177

Wagner, I., & Musso, H. (1983). New naturally occurring amino acids. *Angewandte Chemie International Edition in English*, *22*(22), 816–828. doi:10.1002/anie.198308161

Walkey, C. D., Olsen, J. B., Song, F., Liu, R., Guo, H., Olsen, D. W., & Chan, W. C. et al. (2014). Protein corona fingerprinting predicts the cellular interaction of gold and silver nanoparticles. *ACS Nano*, *8*(3), 2439–2455. doi:10.1021/nn406018q PMID:24517450

Walsh. (1982). *Calcium and Cell Function.* New York, NY: Academic Press,

Walsh, N. C., & Gravallese, E. M. (2004). Bone loss in inflammatory arthritis: Mechanisms and treatment strategies. *Current Opinion in Rheumatology*, *16*, 419–427. PMID:15201606

Walter, K., Harald, M., & Andrew, R. P. (2005). The molecular make-up of a tumour: Proteomics in cancer research. *Clinical Science*, *108*, 369–383. PMID:15831087

Wang, H., Mu, W., Zhai, J., Xing, D. S., Wang, J., Deng, Y., … Shang, H. (2013). *The key role of Shenyan Kangfu tablets, a Chinese patent medicine for diabetic nephropathy: study protocol for a randomized, double-blind and placebo-controlled clinical trial.* Academic Press.

Wang, Q.-S., Gao, T., Cui, Y.-L., Gao, L.-N., & Jiang, H.-L. (2014). Comparative studies of paeoniflorin and albiflorin from Paeonia lactiflora on anti-inflammatory activities. *Pharmaceutical Biology, 52*(9), 1189-1195.

Wang, G., Gong, Y., Anderson, J., Sun, D., Minuk, G., Roberts, M. S., & Burczynski, F. J. (2005). Antioxidative function of L-FABP in L-FABP stably transfected Chang liver cells. *Hepatology (Baltimore, Md.)*, *42*(4), 871–879. doi:10.1002/hep.20857 PMID:16175609

Wang, S., Zhang, X., Zhang, L., Bryant, J., Kheradmand, T., Hering, B. J., & Luo, X. et al. (2014). Preemptive Tolerogenic Delivery of Donor Antigens for Permanent Allogeneic Islet Graft Protection. *Cell Transplantation*. doi:10.3727/096368914X681027 PMID:24759564

Wang, T. Z., Chen, Y., He, Y. M., Fu, X. D., Wang, Y., Xu, Y. Q., & Wang, W. J. et al. (2013). Effects of Chinese herbal medicine Yiqi Huaju Qingli Formula in metabolic syndrome patients with microalbuminuria: A randomized placebo-controlled trial. *Journal of Internal Medicine*, *11*, 175–183. PMID:23743161

Wang, T., Zhu, H., Sun, J., Cheng, X., Xie, J., Dong, H., & Dong, Y. et al. (2014). Efficacy and safety of voriconazole and CYP2C19 polymorphism for optimised dosage regimens in patients with invasive fungal infections. *International Journal of Antimicrobial Agents*, *44*(5), 436–442. doi:10.1016/j.ijantimicag.2014.07.013 PMID:25239277

Wang, Y. D., Tao, M. F., Cheng, W. W., Liu, X. H., Wan, X. P., & Cui, K. (2012). Dehydroepiandrosterone indirectly inhibits human osteoclastic resorption via activating osteoblastic viability by the MAPK pathway. *Chinese Medical Journal*, *125*, 1230–1235. PMID:22613593

Wang, Y. H., Dhariwal, K. R., & Levine, M. (1992). Ascorbic acid bioavailability in humans. Ascorbic acid in plasma, serum, and urine. *Annals of the New York Academy of Sciences*, *669*(1), 383–386. doi:10.1111/j.1749-6632.1992.tb17130.x PMID:1444054

Wang, Y., Huang, F., Cai, H., Zhong, S., Liu, X., & Tan, W. S. (2008). Potent antitumor effect of TRAIL mediated by a novel adeno-associated viral vector targeting to telomerase activity for human hepatocellular carcinoma. *The Journal of Gene Medicine*, *10*, 518–526. PMID:18338833

Wan, J., Ristenpart, W. D., & Stone, H. A. (2008). Dynamics of shear-induced ATP release from red blood cells. *Proceedings of the National Academy of Sciences of the United States of America*, *105*(43), 16432–16437. doi:10.1073/pnas.0805779105 PMID:18922780

Wan, J., Wilcock, A., & Coventry, M. J. (1998). The effect of essential oils of basil on the growth of Aeromonas hydrophila and Pseudomonas fluorescens. *Journal of Applied Microbiology*, *84*(2), 152–158. doi:10.1046/j.1365-2672.1998.00338.x PMID:9633630

Wan, P., Chen, H., Guo, Y., & Bai, A. (2014). Advances in treatment of ulcerative colitis with herbs: From bench to bedside. *World Journal of Gastroenterology*, *20*(39), 14099–14104. doi:10.3748/wjg.v20.i39.14099 PMID:25339799

Ward, M. B., Kotasek, D., & McKinnon, R. A. (2008). Investigation of HTR3C mutations for association with 5HT(3) receptor antagonist anti-emetic efficacy. *Pharmacogenomics*, *9*(8), 1027–1033. doi:10.2217/14622416.9.8.1027 PMID:18681779

Waszkowycz, B. (2008). Towards improving compound selection in structure based virtual screening. *Drug Discovery Today*, *13*(5-6), 219–226 doi:10.1016/j.drudis.2007.12.002 PMID:18342797

Watkins, J. W., Schwarz, E. S., Arroyo-Plasencia, A. M., & Mullins, M. E. (2014). The use of physostigmine by toxicologists in anticholinergic toxicity. *Journal of Medical Toxicology; Official Journal of the American College of Medical Toxicology*, *11*(2), 179–184. doi:10.1007/s13181-014-0452-x PMID:25510306

Weber, J. S., D'Angelo, S. P., Minor, D., Hodi, F. S., Gutzmer, R., Neyns, B., & Larkin, J. et al. (2015). Nivolumab versus chemotherapy in patients with advanced melanoma who progressed after anti-CTLA-4 treatment (CheckMate 037): A randomised, controlled, open-label, phase 3 trial. *The Lancet Oncology*, *16*(4), 375–384. doi:10.1016/S1470-2045(15)70076-8 PMID:25795410

Wei-Jun, K., Yan-Ling, Z., Xiao-He, X., Cheng, J., & Zu-Lun, L. (2009). Quantitative and chemical fingerprint analysis for quality control of Rhizoma Coptidischinensis based on UPLC-PAD combined with chemometrics methods. *Phytomedicine*, *16*(10), 950–959. doi:10.1016/j.phymed.2009.03.016 PMID:19553096

Wei-Jun, K., Yan-Ling, Z., Xiao-He, X., Jia-Bo, W., Han-Bing, L., & Zu-Lun, L. (2009). Spectrum–effect relationships between ultra performance liquid chromatography fingerprints and anti-bacterial activities of *Rhizoma coptidis*. *Analytica Chimica Acta*, *634*(2), 279–285. doi:10.1016/j.aca.2009.01.005 PMID:19185133

Weiner, H. L. (2000). Oral tolerance, an active immunologic process mediated by multiple mechanisms. *The Journal of Clinical Investigation*, *106*(8), 935–937. doi:10.1172/JCI11348 PMID:11032852

Wermuth, C. G., Ganellin, C. R., Lindberg, P., & Mitscher, L. A. (1998). Glossary of terms used in medicinal chemistry. *Pure and Applied Chemistry*, *70*(5), 1129–1143. doi:10.1351/pac199870051129

Wesnes, K., Ward, T., McGinty, A., & Petrini, O. (2000). The memory enhancing effects of a Ginkgo biloba/Panax ginseng combination in healthy middle-aged volunteers. *Psychopharmacology*, *152*(4), 353–361. doi:10.1007/s002130000533 PMID:11140327

Wesseling, C., & Crowe, J. (2013). The Epidemic of Chronic Kidney Disease of Unknown Etiology in Mesoamerica: A Call for Interdisciplinary Research and Action. *American Journal of Public Health*, 1-4. Retrieved from http://www.ncbi.nlm.nih.gov/pubmed/24028232

Wheeler, G. S. (2005). Maintenance of a narrow host range by *Oxyops vitiosa*; a biological control agent of *Melaleuca quinquenervia*. *Biochemical Systematics and Ecology*, *33*(4), 365–383. doi:10.1016/j.bse.2004.10.010

Whelan, A. M., Jurgens, T. M., & Bowles, S. K. (2006). Natural health products in the prevention and treatment of osteoporosis: Systemic review of randomized controlled trials. *The Annals of Pharmacotherapy*, *40*(5), 836–849. doi:10.1345/aph.1G226 PMID:16670364

Whitman, M. (2001). Understanding the perceived need for complementary and alternative nutraceuticals: Lifestyle issues. *Clinical Journal of Oncology Nursing*, *5*, 190–194. PMID:11899764

WHO. (1990) Global programme on aids and traditional medicine programme. Report of a WHO consultation on traditional medicine and AIDS: Clinical evaluation of traditional medicines and natural products.

WHO. (1996). Expert committee on specifications for pharmaceutical preparations-WHO technical report series, No. 863, Annex 11. In *WHO Guidelines for the Assessmet of Herbal Medicines, Thirty-fourth report* (pp. 1–8). Munich, Germany: World Health Organization.

WHO. (2003). *WHO guidelines on good agricultural and collection practices (GACP) for medicinal plants*. Geneva, Switzerland: World Health Organization.

Wichtl, M. (2004). *Herbal drugs and PP: A handbook for practice on a scientific basis*. Stuttgart, Germany: CRC Press.

Widyawaruyanti, A., Asrory, M., Wiwied, E., Setiawan, D., Radjaram, A., Tumewu, L., & Hafid, A. (2014) In vivo Antimalarial Activity of *Andrographis paniculata* Tablets. *Procedia Chemistry, 13*, 101-104.

Wildman, R. E. C., & Medeiros, D. M. (2000). Food in relation to the human body. In Advance Human Nutrition. CRC Press.

Wild, S., Roglic, G., Green, A., Sicree, R., & King, H. (2004). Global prevalence of diabetes: Estimates for the year 2000 and projections for 2030. *Diabetes Care*, *27*(5), 1047–1053. doi:10.2337/diacare.27.5.1047 PMID:15111519

Wiley's Global Research. (2013). *Breast is best: Good bacteria arrive from mum's gut via breast milk*. Retrieved from www.sciencedaily.com

Wilke, H., Muro, K., Van Cutsem, E., Oh, S. C., Bodoky, G., Shimada, Y., & Group, R. S. et al. (2014). Ramucirumab plus paclitaxel versus placebo plus paclitaxel in patients with previously treated advanced gastric or gastro-oesophageal junction adenocarcinoma (RAINBOW): A double-blind, randomised phase 3 trial. *The Lancet Oncology*, *15*(11), 1224–1235. doi:10.1016/S1470-2045(14)70420-6 PMID:25240821

Wille, W., & Willecke, K. (1976). Retention of Purified Proteins in Resealed Human Erythrocyte Ghosts and Transfer by Fusion into Cultured Murine Cells. *FEBS Letters*, *65*(1), 59–62. doi:10.1016/0014-5793(76)80621-7 PMID:1278411

William, A. C. (2000). Structure and regulation of voltage –gated Ca channels. *Annual Review of Cell and Developmental Biology*, *16*(1), 521–555. doi:10.1146/annurev.cellbio.16.1.521 PMID:11031246

William, A. C., Goldin, A. L., & Stephen, G. W. (2005). International Union of Pharmacology. XLVII. Nomenclature and Structure-Function Relationships of Voltage-Gated Sodium Channels. *Pharmacological Reviews*, *57*(4), 397–409. doi:10.1124/pr.57.4.4 PMID:16382098

Wills, R., Bone, K., & Morgan, M. (2000). Herbal products: Active constituents, modes of action and quality control. *Nutrition Research Reviews*, *13*(01), 47–77. doi:10.1079/095442200108729007 PMID:19087433

Wilson, R., Whitelock, J. M., & Bateman, J. F. (2009). Proteomics makes progress in cartilage and arthritis research. *Matrix Biology*, *28*(3), 121–128. PMID:19379666

Windholz, M. (Ed.). (1983). The Merck Index (10th ed.). Rahway, NJ: Merck & Co.

Wolber, G., & Langer, T. (2005). Ligand Scout: 3-D pharmacophores derived from protein-bound ligands and their use as virtual screening filters. *Journal of Chemical Information and Modeling*, *45*(1), 160–169. doi:10.1021/ci049885e PMID:15667141

Wolever, T. M. S., & Jenkins, D. J. A. (1986). The use of the glycemic index in predicting the blood glucose response to mixed meals. *The American Journal of Clinical Nutrition*, *43*, 167–172. PMID:3942088

Wolf, G., Chen, S., & Ziyadeh, F. N. (2005). From the periphery of the glomerular capillary wall toward the center of disease: Podocyte injury comes of age in diabetic nephropathy. *Diabetes*, *54*(6), 1626–1634. doi:10.2337/diabetes.54.6.1626 PMID:15919782

Wong, D. W., Oudit, G. Y., Reich, H., Kassiri, J., Zhou, J., Liu, Q. C., & Scholey, J. W. et al. (2007). Loss of Angiotensin-Converting Enzyme-2 (*Ace2*) Accelerates Diabetic Kidney Injury. *American Journal of Pathology*, *171*(2), 438–451. doi:10.2353/ajpath.2007.060977 PMID:17600118

Wooley, J. C. (1999). Trends in Computational Biology: A Summary based on a RECOMB Plenary lecture. *Journal of Computational Biology*, *6*(3/4), 459–474. doi:10.1089/106652799318391 PMID:10582579

World Health Organization WHO. (1996b). *Guidelines for the Assessment of Herbal Medicines. WHO Technical Report Series*. Geneva: World Health Organization.

World Health Organization WHO. (2006). *Guidelines for the treatment of malaria*. World Health Organization.

World Health Organization. (1992). *Quality Control Methods for Medicinal Plant Materials*. Geneva: World Health Organization.

World Health Organization. (1996a). *Quality Assurance of Pharmaceuticals: A Compendum of Guidelines and Related Materials, Good Manufacturing Practices and Inspection*. Geneva: World Health Organization.

Woroniecka, K. I., Park, A. S., Mohtat, D., Thomas, D. B., Pullman, J. M., & Susztak, K. (2011). Transcriptome analysis of human diabetic kidney disease. *Diabetes*, *60*(9), 2354–2369. doi:10.2337/db10-1181 PMID:21752957

Woyengo, T. A., Ramprasath, V. R., & Jones, P. J. H. (2009). Anticancer effects of phytosterols. *European Journal of Clinical Nutrition*, *63*(7), 813–820. doi:10.1038/ejcn.2009.29 PMID:19491917

Wu, C. C., & Yates, J. R. III. (2003). The application of mass spectrometry to membrane proteomics. *Nature Biotechnology*, *21*, 262–267. PMID:12610573

Wu, G. C., Xu, X. D., Huang, Q., & Wu, H. (2013). Leflunomide: Friend or foe for systemic lupus erythematosus? *Rheumatology International*, *33*(2), 273–276. doi:10.1007/s00296-012-2508-z PMID:22961090

Wu, J.-S., Liu, Y., Shi, R., Lu, X., Ma, Y.-M., & Cheng, N.-N. (2014). Effects of combinations of Xiexin decoction constituents on diabetic nephropathy in rats. *Journal of Ethnopharmacology*, *157*, 126–133. PMID:25278183

Wulfkuhle, J. D., Liotta, L. A., & Petricoin, E. F. (2003). proteomic applications for the early detection of cancer. *National Review*, *3*, 267–275. PMID:12671665

Wu, Y. H., Zhou, C. X., Li, X. P., Song, L., Wu, X., Lin, W., & Zhao, Y. et al. (2006). Evaluation of antiinflammatory activity of the total flavonoids of aggerapterodonta on acute and chronic inflammation models. *Phytotherapy Research*, *20*(7), 585–590. doi:10.1002/ptr.1918 PMID:16673449

Xiao, H., Zhang, L., Zhou, H., Lee, J. M., Garon, E. B., & Wong, D. T. W. (2012). Proteomic analysis of human saliva from lung cancer patients using two-dimensional difference gel electrophoresis and mass spectrometry. *Molecular & Cellular Proteomics*, *11*(2), 1–12. PMID:22096114

Xiao, J. (2015). Phytochemicals in medicine and food. *Phytochemistry Reviews*, *14*(3), 317–320. doi:10.1007/s11101-015-9407-3

Xiaojiang, T., Jinsong, Z., Jiansheng, W., Chengen, P., Guangxiao, Y., & Quanying, W. (2010). Adeno-associated virus harboring fusion gene NT4-ant-shepherdin induce cell death in human lung cancer cells. *Cancer Investigation*, *28*, 465–471. PMID:19968500

Xia, X., Ling, W., Ma, J., Xia, M., Hou, M., Wang, Q., & Tang, Z. et al. (2006). An anthocyanin-rich extract from black rice enhances atherosclerotic plaque stabilization in apolipoprotein E-deficient mice. *The Journal of Nutrition*, *136*, 2220–2225. PMID:16857844

Xing, Y., & Hogquist, K. A. (2012). T-cell tolerance: Central and peripheral. *Cold Spring Harbor Perspectives in Biology*, *4*(6), a006957. doi:10.1101/cshperspect.a006957 PMID:22661634

Xue, J., Zhao, S., Liang, Y., Hou, C., & Wang, J. (2008). IFIP International Federation for Information Processing. In Computer and Computing Technologies in Agriculture (vol. 2, pp. 977–982). Boston: Springer.

Xue, K. X., Wang, S., Ma, G. J., Zhou, P., Wu, P. Q., Zhang, R. F., & Wang, Y. Q. et al. (1992). Micronucleus formation in peripheral-blood lymphocytes from smokers and the influence of alcohol- and tea-drinking habits. *International Journal of Cancer*, *50*(5), 702–705. doi:10.1002/ijc.2910500506 PMID:1544703

Xu, J., Su, H. L., Wang, J. H., & Zhang, C. H. (2009). Role of CD4+CD25+Foxp3+ regulatory T cells in type 2 diabetic nephropathy. *Journal of the Southern Medical University*, *29*, 137–139. PMID:19218134

Yaakob, N., Malone, D. T., Exintaris, B., & Irving, H. R. (2011). Heterogeneity amongst 5-HT(3) receptor subunits: Is this significant? *Current Molecular Medicine*, *11*(1), 57–68. doi:10.2174/156652411794474392 PMID:21189117

Yagil, R. (2000). Lactation in Camels. In T. K. Gahlot (Ed.), *Selected Topics on Camelids* (pp. 61–72). Bikaner, India: The Camel Publishers.

Yagil, R. (2013). Comparative Alternative Medicinal (CAM) Properties in Camel Milk for Treatment of Epidemic' Diseases. *Journal of Agricultural Science and Technology.*, *A3*, 575–580.

Yamaguchi, M. (2008). β-cryptoxanthin and Bone Metabolism: The Preventive Role in Osteoporosis. *Journal of Health Science*, *54*(4), 356–369. doi:10.1248/jhs.54.356

Yamakaqe, M. & Namiki, A. (2002). Calcium channels--basic aspects of their structure, function and gene encoding; anesthetic action on the channels--a review. *Canadian Journal of Anesthesia/Journal canadien d'anesthésie, 49*, 151-164.

Yamano, T., Watanabe, S., Hasegawa, H., Suzuki, T., Abe, R., Tahara, H., & Kishimoto, H. et al. (2011). Ex vivo-expanded DCs induce donor-specific central and peripheral tolerance and prolong the acceptance of donor skin grafts. *Blood*, *117*(9), 2640–2648. doi:10.1182/blood-2010-07-293860 PMID:21220748

Yang, J. C., Wu, Y. L., Schuler, M., Sebastian, M., Popat, S., Yamamoto, N., & Sequist, L. V. et al. (2015). Afatinib versus cisplatin-based chemotherapy for EGFR mutation-positive lung adenocarcinoma (LUX-Lung 3 and LUX-Lung 6): Analysis of overall survival data from two randomised, phase 3 trials. *The Lancet Oncology*, *16*(2), 141–151. doi:10.1016/S1470-2045(14)71173-8 PMID:25589191

Yang, K., Hu, L., Ma, X., Ye, S., Cheng, L., Shi, X., & Liu, Z. et al. (2012). Multimodal imaging guided photothermal therapy using functionalized graphene nanosheets anchored with magnetic nanoparticles. *Advanced Materials*, *24*(14), 1868–1872. doi:10.1002/adma.201104964 PMID:22378564

Yang, L., Belaguli, N., & Berger, D. H. (2009). MicroRNA and colorectal cancer. *World Journal of Surgery*, *33*, 638–646. PMID:19123024

Yang, N. C., Jeng, K. C., Ho, W. M., & Hu, M. L. (2002). ATP depletion is an important factor in DHEA-induced growth inhibition and apoptosis in BV-2 cells. *Life Sciences*, *70*(17), 1979–1988. doi:10.1016/S0024-3205(01)01542-9 PMID:12148690

Yan, Y. M., Fang, P., Yang, M. T., Li, N., Lu, Q., & Cheng, Y. X. (2015). Anti-diabetic nephropathy compounds from *Cinnamomum cassia*. *Journal of Ethnopharmacology*, *13*(165), 141–147. doi:10.1016/j.jep.2015.01.049 PMID:25725434

Yarden, Y., & Shilo, B. Z. (2007). SnapShot: EGFR signaling pathway. *Cell*, *131*(5), 1018. doi:10.1016/j.cell.2007.11.013 PMID:18045542

Yasuda, A., Sawai, H., Takahashi, H., Ochi, N., Matsuo, Y., Funahashi, H., & Manabe, T. et al. (2007). Stem cell factor/c-kit receptor signaling enhances the proliferation and invasion of colorectal cancer cells through the PI3K/Akt pathway. *Digestive Diseases and Sciences*, *52*(9), 2292–2300. doi:10.1007/s10620-007-9759-7 PMID:17410437

Yen, J. L., & McLeod, H. L. (2007). Should DPD analysis be required prior to prescribing fluoropyrimidines? *European Journal of Cancer*, *43*(6), 1011–1016. doi:10.1016/j.ejca.2007.01.030 PMID:17350823

Yeomans, M. (2015). *Donkey milk cosmetics*. Retrieved 13.6.2015, from http://www.cosmeticsdesign-asia.com/Market-Trends/Donkey-milk-cosmetics-creme-de-la-creme-for-Asian-consumers

Yeste, A., Nadeau, M., Burns, E. J., Weiner, H. L., & Quintana, F. J. (2012). Nanoparticle-mediated codelivery of myelin antigen and a tolerogenic small molecule suppresses experimental autoimmune encephalomyelitis. *Proceedings of the National Academy of Sciences of the United States of America*, *109*(28), 11270–11275. doi:10.1073/pnas.1120611109 PMID:22745170

Yeum, K. J., Aldini, G., Russell, R. M., & Krinsky, N. I. (2009). Antioxidant/Prooxidant Actions of Carotenoids. In Carotenoids: Nutrition and Health. Birkhauser Verlag Basel.

Yi, C., Shang-Bin, Z., Ming-Yong, X., Shao-Ping, N., Wei, L., Chang, L., & Yuan-Xing, W. et al. (2008). Quality control and original discrimination of Ganoderma lucidum based on high-performance liquid chromatographic fingerprints and combined chemometrics methods. *Analytica Chimica Acta*, *623*(2), 146–156. doi:10.1016/j.aca.2008.06.018 PMID:18620918

Yoshikawa, M., Murakami, T., Kadoya, M., Matsuda, H., Muraoka, O., Yamahara, J., & Murakami, N. (1996). Medicinal foodstuff. III. Sugar beet. (1): Hypoglycemic oleanolic acid oligoglycosides, betavulgarosides I, II, III, and IV, from the root of *Beta vulgaris* L. (Chenopodiaceae). *Chemical & Pharmaceutical Bulletin*, *44*(6), 1212–1217. doi:10.1248/cpb.44.1212 PMID:8814952

Young, B. A., Maynard, C., & Boyko, E. J. (2003). Racial differences in diabetic nephropathy, cardiovascular disease, and mortality in a national population of veterans. *Diabetes Care*, *26*(8), 2392–2399. doi:10.2337/diacare.26.8.2392 PMID:12882868

Young, V. R. (1994). Adult amino acid requirements: The case for a major revision in current recommendations. *The Journal of Nutrition*, *124*(8), 1517S–1523S. PMID:8064412

You, S. J., Udenigwe, C. C., Aluko, R. E., & Wu, J. (2010). Multifunctional peptides from egg white lysozyme. *Food Research International*, *43*(3), 848–855. doi:10.1016/j.foodres.2009.12.004

Yuan, Z., Pastoriza, J., Quinn, T., & Libutti, S. (2013). Targeting tumor vasculature using adenoassociated virus page vector coding tumor necrosis factor-a. In E. C. Lattime & S. L. Gerson (Eds.), *Gene Therapy of Cancer* (3rd ed.; pp. 19–33). San Diego, CA: Elsevier.

Yücekutlu, A. N., & Bildacı, I. (2008). Determination of plant saponins and some of Gypsophila species: A review of the literature. *Hacettepe Journal of Biololgy & Chemistry*, *36*, 129–135.

Yurystyn, E., Etzion, Z., van Creveld, C., & Yagil, R. (2014). Camel milk cosmeceuticals for comparative alternative medicine. *J Med. and Med. Res*, *2*, 8–12.

Zafra-Stone, S., Yasmin, T., Bagchi, M., Chatterjee, A., Vinson, J. A., & Bagchi, D. (2007). Berry anthocyanins as novel antioxidants in human health and disease prevention. *Molecular Nutrition & Food Research*, *51*(6), 675–683. doi:10.1002/mnfr.200700002 PMID:17533652

Zakaria, Z., Balan, T., Mamat, S., Mohtarrudin, N., Kek, T., & Salleh, M. (2015). Mechanisms of gastroprotection of methanol extract of *Melastoma malabathricum* leaves. *Complementary and Alternative Medicine.*, *15*(1), 135–150. doi:10.1186/s12906-015-0638-z PMID:25927982

Zanella, A. (1987). Desferrioxamine Loading of Red Cells for Transfusion. *Advanced Biosciences, 67,* 17–27.

Zeng, J. (2000). Mini-Review: Computational Structure-Based Design of Inhibitors that Target Protein Surfaces. *Combinatorial Chemistry & High Throughput Screening*, *3*(5), 355–362. doi:10.2174/1386207003331490 PMID:11032953

Zhang, A. H., Skupsky, J., & Scott, D. W. (2009). Factor VIII inhibitors: Risk factors and methods for prevention and immune modulation. *Clinical Reviews in Allergy & Immunology*, *37*(2), 114–124. doi:10.1007/s12016-009-8122-5 PMID:19199081

Zhang, B., Salituro, G., Szalkowski, D., Li, Z., Zhang, Y., Royo, I., & Moller, D. E. et al. (1999). Discovery of small molecule insulin mimetic with antidiabetic activity in mice. *Science*, *284*(5416), 974–977. doi:10.1126/science.284.5416.974 PMID:10320380

Zhang, C., Tan, C., Ding, H., Xin, T., & Jiang, Y. (2012). Selective VEGFR inhibitors for anticancer therapeutics in clinical use and clinical trials. *Current Pharmaceutical Design*, *18*(20), 2921–2935. doi:10.2174/138161212800672732 PMID:22571661

Zhang, F., Huang, X., Zhu, L., Guo, N., Niu, G., Swierczewska, M., & Chen, X. et al. (2012). Noninvasive monitoring of orthotopic glioblastoma therapy response using RGD-conjugated iron oxide nanoparticles. *Biomaterials*, *33*(21), 5414–5422. doi:10.1016/j.biomaterials.2012.04.032 PMID:22560667

Zhang, H., Saha, J., Byun, J., Schin, M., Lorenz, M., Kennedy, R. T., & Brosius, F. C. et al. (2008). …Brosius, F.C. Rosiglitazone reduces renal and plasma markers of oxidative injury and reverses urinary metabolite abnormalities in the amelioration of diabetic nephropathy. *American Journal of Physiology. Renal Physiology*, *295*(4), F1071–F1081. doi:10.1152/ajprenal.90208.2008 PMID:18667486

Zhang, L. J., Guerrero-Juarez, C. F., Hata, T., Bapat, S. P., Ramos, R., Plikus, M. V., & Gallo, R. L. (2015). Innate immunity. Dermal adipocytes protect against invasive Staphylococcus aureus skin infection. *Science*, *347*(6217), 67–71. doi:10.1126/science.1260972 PMID:25554785

Zhang, L., Xu, X., Yang, R., Chen, J., Wang, S., Yang, J., & Zhang, D. (2015). Paclitaxel attenuates renal interstitial fibroblast activation and interstitial fibrosis by inhibiting STAT3 signaling. *Drug Design. Development & Therapy*, *9*, 2139–2148. doi:10.2147/DDDT.S81390 PMID:25931810

Zhang, M., Chen, M., Zhang, H. Q., Sun, S., Xia, B., & Wu, F. H. (2009). In vivo hypoglycemic effects of phenolics from the root bark of *Morus alba. Fitoterapia*, *80*(8), 475–477. doi:10.1016/j.fitote.2009.06.009 PMID:19545615

Zhang, M., Feng, L., Gu, J., Ma, L., Qin, D., Wu, C., & Jia, X. (2014). The attenuation of Moutan Cortex on oxidative stress for renal injury in AGEs-induced mesangial cell dysfunction and streptozotocin-induced diabetic nephropathy rats. *Oxidative Medicine and Cellular Longevity*. PMID:24876912

Zhang, P., Luo, S., Li, M., & Tan, S. (2015). Artesunate inhibits the growth and induces apoptosis of human gastric cancer cells by downregulating COX-2. *Onco Targets & Therapy*, *8*, 845–854. doi:10.2147/OTT.S81041 PMID:25945055

Zhang, S. M., Cook, N. R., Albert, C. M., Gaziano, J. M., Buring, J. E., & Manson, J. E. (2008). Effect of combined folic acid, vitamin B6, and vitamin B12 on cancer risk in women: A randomized trial. *Journal of the American Medical Association*, *300*(17), 2012–2021. doi:10.1001/jama.2008.555 PMID:18984888

Zhang, S., Wang, J., Xue, H., Deng, Q., Xing, F., & Ando, M. (2002). Three new guaianolides fromSiyekucai (*Ixeris chinensis*). *Journal of Natural Products*, *65*(12), 1927–1929. doi:10.1021/np0202632 PMID:12502342

Zhang, Y., Ma, H., Zhang, J., Liu, S., Liu, Y., & Zheng, D. (2008). AAV-mediated TRAIL gene expression driven by hTERT promoter suppressed human hepatocellular carcinoma growth in mice. *Life Sciences*, *82*, 1154–1161. PMID:18485417

Zhao, Y., Sun, X., Zhang, G., Trewyn, B. G., Slowing, I. I., & Lin, V. S. (2011). Interaction of mesoporous silica nanoparticles with human red blood cell membranes: Size and surface effects. *ACS Nano*, *5*(2), 1366–1375. doi:10.1021/nn103077k PMID:21294526

Zheng, N., Lin, X., Wen, Q., Kintoko, , Zhang, S., Huang, J., & Huang, R. et al. (2013). Effect of 2-dodecyl-6-methoxycyclohexa-2,5-diene-1,4-dione, isolated from Averrhoa carambola L. (Oxalidaceae) roots, on advanced glycation end-product-mediated renal injury in type 2 diabetic KK Ay mice. *Toxicology Letters*, *10*(1), 77–84. doi:10.1016/j.toxlet.2013.03.001 PMID:23500658

Zheng, S. G., Wang, J. H., Koss, M. N., Quismorio, F. Jr, Gray, J. D., & Horwitz, D. A. (2004). CD4+ and CD8+ regulatory T cells generated ex vivo with IL-2 and TGF-beta suppress a stimulatory graft-versus-host disease with a lupus-like syndrome. *Journal of Immunology (Baltimore, MD.: 1950)*, *172*(3), 1531–1539. doi:10.4049/jimmunol.172.3.1531 PMID:14734731

Zhong, H., & Bowen, J. P. (2011). Recent advances in small molecule inhibitors of VEGFR and EGFR signaling pathways. *Current Topics in Medicinal Chemistry*, *11*(12), 1571–1590. doi:10.2174/156802611795860924 PMID:21510831

Zhou, C., Wu, Y. L., Chen, G., Feng, J., Liu, X. Q., Wang, C., & You, C. et al. (2011). Erlotinib versus chemotherapy as first-line treatment for patients with advanced EGFR mutation-positive non-small-cell lung cancer (OPTIMAL, CTONG-0802): A multicentre, open-label, randomised, phase 3 study. *The Lancet Oncology*, *12*(8), 735–742. doi:10.1016/S1470-2045(11)70184-X PMID:21783417

Zhou, T., Commodore, L., Huang, W. S., Wang, Y., Thomas, M., Keats, J., & Zhu, X. et al. (2011). Structural mechanism of the Pan-BCR-ABL inhibitor ponatinib (AP24534): Lessons for overcoming kinase inhibitor resistance. *Chemical Biology & Drug Design*, *77*(1), 1–11. doi:10.1111/j.1747-0285.2010.01054.x PMID:21118377

Ziemssen, T., & Schrempf, W. (2007). Glatiramer acetate: Mechanisms of action in multiple sclerosis. *International Review of Neurobiology*, *79*, 537–570. doi:10.1016/S0074-7742(07)79024-4 PMID:17531858

Zimmermann, U. (1973). *Jahresbericht der Kernforschungsanlage Julich GmbH*. Julich: Nuclear Research Center.

Zimmermann, U. (1983). Cellular Drug-Carrier Systems and Their Possible Targeting. In *Targeted Drugs* (pp. 153–200). New York, NY: John Wiley & Sons.

Zimmermann, U., Pilwat, G., & Riemann, F. (1975). Preparation of Erythrocyte Ghosts by Dielectric Breakdown of the Cell Membrane. *Biochimica et Biophysica Acta*, *375*(2), 209–219. doi:10.1016/0005-2736(75)90189-3 PMID:1168495

Zimmermann, U., Riemann, F., & Pilwat, G. (1976). Enzyme Loading of Electrically Homogenous Human Red Blood Cell Ghosts Prepared by Dielectric Breakdown. *Biochimica et Biophysica Acta*, *436*(2), 460–474. doi:10.1016/0005-2736(76)90208-X PMID:1276224

Zobayed, S. A., Afreen, F., & Kozai, T. (2005). Necessity and production of medicinal plants under controlled environments. *Environment Control in Biology*, *43*(4), 243–252. doi:10.2525/ecb.43.243

Zocchi, E., Tonetti, M., Polvani, C., Guida, L., Benatti, U., & De Flora, A. (1988). *In-Vivo* Liver and Lung Targeting of Adriamycin Encapsulated in Glutaraldehyde-Treated Murine Erythrocytes. *Biotechnology and Applied Biochemistry*, *10*, 555–562. PMID:3148305

Zoetendal, E. G., Raes, J., van den Bogert, B., Arumugam, M., Booijink, C. C., Troost, F. J., & Kleerebezem, M. et al. (2012). The human small intestinal microbiota is driven by rapid uptake and conversion of simplecarbohydrates. *The ISME Journal*, *6*(7), 1415–1426. doi:10.1038/ismej.2011.212 PMID:22258098

Zonana-Nacach, A., Barr, S. G., Magder, L. S., & Petri, M. (2000). Damage in systemic lupus erythematosus and its association with corticosteroids. *Arthritis and Rheumatism*, *43*(8), 1801–1808. doi:10.1002/1529-0131(200008)43:8<1801::AID-ANR16>3.0.CO;2-O PMID:10943870

Zou, J., Yu, X., Qu, S., Li, X., Jin, Y., & Sui, D. (2014). Protective effect of total flavonoids extracted from the leaves of *Murraya paniculata* (L.) Jack on diabetic nephropathy in rats. *Food and Chemical Toxicology*, *64*, 231–237. doi:10.1016/j.fct.2013.11.043 PMID:24309143

About the Contributors

Raj K. Keservani has more than 7 years of academic (Teaching) experience in various institutes of India imparting Pharmaceutical education. Mr. Keservani did his graduation (B. Pharmacy) from Department of Pharmacy, Kumaun University, Nainital (U.A.), India in 2005. Afterwards he qualified GATE in same year conducted by IIT Mumbai. He received Master of Pharmacy (M. Pharmacy) from School of Pharmaceutical Sciences, Rajiv Gandhi Proudyogiki Vishwavidyalaya, Bhopal (M.P.), India in 2008 with specialization in Pharmaceutics. Further, he has published 25 peer reviewed papers in the field of Pharmaceutical Sciences in national and international reputed journals, 10 book chapters, 2 co-authored books.He is also active as a reviewer in several scientific international journals. His research interest encompasses Nutraceutical and Functional Foods, Novel Drug Delivery Systems (NDDS), Transdermal Drug Delivery/ Drug Delivery, Health Science/Life Science, Biology/Cancer Biology/Neurobiology.

Anil K. Sharma has more than 6 years of academic experience in Pharmaceutical sciences. He did his graduation (B. Pharmacy) from University of Rajasthan, Jaipur, India in 2005. Afterwards he qualified GATE in same year conducted by IIT Mumbai. He received Master of Pharmacy (M. Pharmacy) from School of Pharmaceutical Sciences, Rajiv Gandhi Proudyogiki Vishwavidyalaya, Bhopal (M.P.), India in 2007 with specialization in Pharmaceutics. Further, he has published 25 peer reviewed papers in the field of Pharmaceutical Sciences in national and international reputed journals, 10 book chapters. His research interest encompasses Nutraceutical and Functional Foods, Novel Drug Delivery Systems (NDDS), Drug Delivery, Nanotechnology, Health Science/Life Science, Biology/Cancer Biology/Neurobiology. Currently he is working as lecturer at Delhi Institute of Pharmaceutical Sciences & Research, University of Delhi, India.

Rajesh K. Kesharwani has more than 7 years of research and 2 years of teaching experience in various institutes of India imparting bioinformatics and biotechnology education. Dr. Kesharwani did his graduation (B.Sc. Biology) from Ewing Christian College, Allahabad, an autonomous college of University of Allahabad and post-graduation (M.Sc. Biochemistry) from Awadesh Pratap Singh University, Rewa, Madhya Pradesh, India. He has qualified GATE 2005 and 2006, received Ministry of Human Resource Development, India fellowship to complete M.Tech-IT (specialization in Bioinformatics) degree from Indian Institute of Information Technology, Allahabad, India in 2008. He has completed doctorate (Ph.D.) from Indian Institute of Information Technology, Allahabad in 2014 and received Ministry of Human Resource Development, India fellowship and Senior Research Fellowship from Indian Council of Medical Research, India. Dr. Kesharwani has awarded Swarna Jayanti Puruskar by The National Academy of Sciences, India for best paper presentation. He has authored 29+ peer-reviewed articles, 5 book chapters and, one book as co-editor together with more than 10 book chapters has been accepted for publication with international publishers. He has been members of many scientific communities and reviewer of many international journals. His research fields of interest are Medical Informatics, Protein Structure and Function Prediction, Computer-Aided Drug Designing, Structural Biology, Drug Delivery, Cancer Biology and Next Generation Sequence Analysis.

* * *

Kamal Kumar Chaudhary has completed his M.Tech. and Ph.D. in Bioinformatics from IIIT-Allahabad.

Naihan Chen is a graduate student in the doctoral program in Pharmaceutical Sciences at The University of North Carolina at Chapel Hill. Her research focuses on the application of nanobiomaterials to enhance disease therapies through drug delivery. Ms. Chen received her Bachelor of Arts in Biochemistry from Smith College in 2014. She graduated with Summa Cum Laude and a high honor in Biochemistry.

Charu Gupta (Gold Medal; ICAR-NET, GATE qualified), Assistant Professor, Amity Institute of Herbal Research & Studies, Amity University Uttar Pradesh carries with over 8 years of experience in teaching and research at University level. She has published around 30 research and review papers in SCI journals, authored 4 books and 70 abstracts in both national and international conferences. During her tenure at Amity, she has filed several patents and related to the medicinal plants and microbiology. Her research interests are in probiotics & utilization of agro-industrial wastes for production of value added products.

Sarvesh Kumar Gupta has obtained M.Tech. in bioinformatics from IIIT- Allahabad.

Alejandra Hernández-Ceruelos is a professor researcher at the Medical School. Universidad Autónoma del Estado de Hidalgo. The areas of expertise are cytogenetics, natural products and pharmacology.

Urmila Jarouliya had 9 years teaching experience at graduate and postgraduate level. She qualified GATE (2013) and did her M.Sc and PhD in Biotechnology from Jiwaji University, Gwalior. She had published around 18 papers in national and international Journals and also contributed as author for various books. Her area of research is clinical Biochemistry, Industrial Microbiology and Immunology.

Rajesh K. Joshi was born in 1975 in Pamda (Barakot), District Champawat, Uttarakhand, India. He completed his PhD degree in Chemistry at Kumaoun University, Nainital, Uttarakhand in 2007. He was appointed as Senior Scientist in 2008 at Regional Medical Research Centre (Indian Council of Medical Research), Belagavi. He has established Phytochemistry Department with state-of-art facility laboratory at Regional Medical Research Centre-Belagavi. His main research interests are devoted to chemistry of natural products includes chemoprofiling of medicinal and aromatic plants of Western Ghats and anti-diabetic activity of phytoconstituents. He is also working on antimicrobial activity of lead phytoconstituents and endophytic fungi. Till 2015 he has authored more than 80 scientific publications in international journals and has supervised the research of a large number of Master students in various disciplines in addition to that mentor of one DHR fellow.

Tahir Mehmood Khan Is a lecture at school of pharmacy, Monash University. His research interest are in evidence based medicines in clinical aspect of drugs, and different pharmaceutical dosage forms. He is also Editor in Chief of Archives of Pharmacy Practice journal.

Long Chiau Ming is a senior lecturer in Division of Pharmacy, School of Medicine, University of Tasmania, Australia and a researcher at Unit for Medication Outcomes Research and Education . He obtained his BPharm (Hons) and Master (Clinical Pharmacy) degrees from Universiti Sains Malaysia. Then, he underwent PhD training on biopharmaceutics in University of Bath, UK. He teaches research methodology, pharmacoinformatics and clinical pharmacy subjects since 2007. He has a special interest in cosmeceutical science. Till Jan 2016 he has more than 50 journal publications; 30 conference abstracts and 2 book chapters. He had been awarded 9 research grants with a total amount of USD330k. He is actively supervising postgraduate students on research on cosmeceutical and pharmaceutical sciences.

Nidhi Mishra has obtained PhD from University of Delhi. She has worked at BITS Pilani and few UPTU colleges. Currently She is an assistant Professor at IIIT Allahabad.

Sergio Muñoz-Juarez is a professor researcher at the Medical School. Universidad Autónoma del Estado de Hidalgo.

Vivek Pandey is pursuing PhD in department of Medicinal Chemistry at Banaras Hindu University.

Jai N. Patel is employed as Chief, Pharmacology Research, Phase I Trials at the Carolinas HealthCare System's Levine Cancer Institute, where he currently leads the clinical pharmacology research program.

Kevin J. Peine is a Post-doctoral researcher in the UNC Eshelman School of Pharmacy at The University of North Carolina at Chapel Hill. His research uses microparticulate-based therapies for the treatment of Multiple Sclerosis and Type 1 Diabetes. Previously, as a graduate student at The Ohio State University, his dissertation work was on formulation of particulate-based immunomodulatory therapies for the treatment of diseases.

Dhan Prakash has 35 years of research experience in life sciences, worked as guest scientist at GSF-Munich, (GERMANY), Freiburg University, (GERMANY) and Ecole Normale Superieur, Lyon (FRANCE); guided more than 25 Ph. D. thesis, published 145 research papers in SCI journals, 28 book chapters, 173 abstracts in conferences, filed 35 patents and edited 5 books.

Boris V. Smirin is a postdoctoral researcher at A.I. Virtanen Institute, University of Eastern Finland. Dr. Smirin graduated from Moscow State University, and completed his PhD thesis in Institute of Pathology and Pathophysiology in Moscow, Russia.

Shivani Srivastava is pursuing PhD in Biochemistry from Department of Medicinal Chemistry, Institute of Medical Sciences, Banaras Hindu University, Studied B.Sc Botany (Hons.) and M.Sc Biochemistry from Banaras Hindu University. Also worked at the post of Senior Research Fellow (1.5 Years) in the Research scheme "Network Project on Transgenic Crops" in Indian Institute of Vegetable Research, ICAR, Varanasi, U.P., Qualified CSIR NET, GATE and UGC RGNFD Fellowship.

Premrutai Thitilertdecha, PhD, is a lecturer at Department of Research and Development, Faculty of Medicine Siriraj Hospital, Mahidol University, Bangkok, Thailand.

Patricia Vázquez-Alvarado is a professor researcher at the Dentistry School. Universidad Autónoma del Estado de Hidalgo.

Jeryl Villadolid is a Clinical Pharmacist Coordinator in Solid Tumor Oncology at the Carolinas HealthCare System's Levine Cancer Institute. She completed pharmacy school at University of Florida, trained in oncology pharmacy at Duke University Medical Center, and was a Clinical Pharmacy Specialist at University of Chicago Medicine. She has special interests in thoracic and head and neck cancers and has participated in research in pain and palliative care.

Maria A. Vlasova is currently working as a postdoctoral researcher at School of Pharmacy, University of Eastern Finland since 2007. Maria A. Vlasova graduated from Moscow State University with PhD in in 1999 specialsing in Cardiovascular physiology. Maria A. Vlasova has authored more than 20 publications in several high ranking peer reviewed journals.

Tin Wui Wong is an Associate Professor and Head of Non-Destructive Biomedical and Pharmaceutical Research Centre, iPROMISE, UiTM Malaysia.

Durgavati Yadav, MSc Biochemistry, is pursuing PhD in Biochemistry from BHU, Varanasi, India.

Quan Yang has obtained her PhD degree from the University of Bath. Her research focus was the assessment of skin barrier function using biophysics and bioengineering methods. She has also worked as a R&D research associate in Reckitt Benckiser, UK, with special interests in topical dermatological products.

Index

A

Adverse Effects 1, 8, 13, 17, 21, 54-55, 62, 229, 232, 235, 245, 291-293, 341, 353
Alpha Hydroxyl Acids 291, 308
Amino acids 130, 144, 162, 164, 168, 180, 182-183, 215, 235, 264-265, 278, 317, 342, 388
Anti-aging 263, 266, 287, 294, 296, 301, 314
Anticancer 7, 52-53, 74-75, 231, 233-234, 240-241, 243, 272-275, 278
Antimalarial 221, 240, 273
Antioxidants 166, 170, 180, 182-183, 206, 219, 264-265, 269-270, 272, 278, 294, 311, 316, 325, 328, 387, 405

B

Bioinformatics 115, 125-128, 130, 132-135, 143-145, 147-148, 152, 158, 244
Biomarker 4, 6-7, 52-54, 59, 62, 67, 75, 98-100, 104, 111, 114-115, 370, 382, 388-389
Biomedical 125-126, 147, 152, 158
Breast milk 309, 312, 320, 329, 331-332

C

Camel milk 309, 312-317, 320, 322-325, 328-331, 333, 335
Cancer 5, 12, 14, 23, 33-34, 52-53, 56-57, 59-65, 67-70, 72-73, 75, 98-99, 104-112, 114-115, 149, 161-163, 165-166, 168, 176, 218-219, 231, 233, 235, 240-244, 264, 266, 269-275, 278, 298, 310, 322, 327, 330, 332, 355
Carrier 35, 147, 294, 340-342, 345-347, 353-355, 357
Cheminformatics 126, 158
Chemo-preventive 263
Cosmeceutical 288-290, 293-295, 297-298, 300-302, 308, 310, 312, 314, 331, 334
Cosmeceuticals 287-291, 294, 298, 300-302, 308-310, 312-317, 319-322, 324, 328-333, 335
Cosmetic 208-209, 272, 287-290, 294, 297, 301, 311, 314-315, 317-318

D

Database 17, 125, 127-128, 130-132, 138, 145, 147, 158, 290
Depigmentation 291, 293
Diabetic Kidney Diseases (DKDs) 369, 404
Diseases 2, 9, 12-13, 23-24, 28-30, 34, 37-41, 97-100, 103, 111, 115, 134, 145, 147, 161, 163, 167, 175, 179-180, 183, 203, 212, 214, 218, 220-221, 229-230, 232-235, 240, 242-243, 248, 263-265, 267, 269-273, 275, 278, 310, 317, 320, 332, 342, 354, 368-371, 376-377, 379-380, 382, 385-386, 389-390, 404-405
Drug 1-7, 13, 15-16, 21, 23, 32-34, 40, 52-53, 55, 60, 62, 65-66, 68-75, 98, 100, 105, 108, 114, 129-130, 134-137, 139, 142, 144, 147-148, 151-152, 158, 164, 168, 181, 203-205, 207, 209, 212-214, 216, 229, 232-233, 235, 238-242, 244-248, 288-290, 293, 300, 309, 315, 330-331, 340-341, 346-354, 357, 392

E

Efficacy 2, 5, 7-8, 23-24, 26-30, 38, 40, 55, 61, 67, 70-72, 103, 107, 109, 180, 183, 202-203, 209, 212, 215-217, 220-221, 232-233, 235, 243, 247, 266, 277, 287-289, 292, 298, 302, 309, 320, 331, 348
Erythrocytes 31, 58, 66, 340-357

F

Fatty acids 161-162, 167, 180-181, 183, 212, 230, 265, 278, 301, 312, 333-334, 342, 390
Flavonoids 160-161, 171-172, 180, 182, 206, 209, 216, 219-220, 243, 246, 263, 266-271, 296, 300, 391
Functional foods 160-161, 163-165, 167-168, 170-171, 174, 177, 179-181, 184, 263-266, 277-278

G

Gene therapy 98-99, 101-102, 104-109, 113, 133, 147-148
Genomics 98, 105, 115, 126-128, 158, 244, 265
Germ-line 53, 64-65, 74-75
Glomerular Filtration Rate (GFR) 379, 388, 404

H

Hepatitis C 98-99, 112-115
HIV 135, 242
Homeostasis 218, 311, 376, 385, 387, 390
Hyperglycemia 57, 218, 368-369, 376, 378-379, 404

L

Liposomes 15-16, 32, 34, 37, 106-107

M

Mare milk 333-334
Medicinal plants 202-208, 230, 232-233, 244, 246, 248, 368, 394
Metabolic Syndrome 14, 368-369, 404
Microparticles 23, 32-37, 40, 213
Moisturizer 331-332
Multiple Sclerosis 23-25

N

Nano-bio Interactions 1, 8
Nanoparticles 5-10, 13, 17, 21, 32-33, 35-36, 38, 40, 106, 213
Nanotheranostics 1-2, 5-8, 14, 17, 21
Nanotoxicity 14
Nutraceutical 160-168, 170-171, 174, 177, 180-181, 183-184, 263-266, 273, 276, 278
Nutraceuticals 163, 171, 180-182, 184, 233, 244, 263-266, 272, 276-278
Nutrients 9, 160-162, 166, 174, 215, 244, 265, 310, 341-342, 344-345

O

Osmosis 346-348
Oxidative Stress 9, 114, 181-183, 221, 274, 297, 314, 342, 368-369, 371-372, 376, 385-386, 404

P

Personalization of Therapy 6
Personalized Protein Corona 2, 13
Personalized Therapy 21
Pharmaceutical 21, 75, 125-127, 129, 134-136, 138-141, 152, 158, 160, 163, 202-205, 208, 210, 212-213, 231, 233, 243-244, 246-247, 265-266, 273, 276, 287-288, 290, 301-302, 341, 380
Pharmaco informatics 126
Pharmacogenetic 53-54, 64-65, 68, 74-75
Pharmacoinformatics 158
Pharmacokinetics 15-16, 21, 32, 72
Phytochemicals 161, 171, 180, 205, 214, 232, 244, 246-247, 264, 266, 278, 368, 391
Phytopharmaceuticals 202-203, 205, 207, 216, 221, 229, 232, 235, 248, 263, 266, 278
Podocytes 373, 376-377, 379, 388-389, 405
Polymers 12, 15, 32, 34, 101, 105, 147, 265
Protein Corona 2, 10-13, 17, 21
Proteinuria 369, 371, 373-377, 379, 382, 388, 405
Proteomics 97-99, 104-105, 111-112, 114-115, 127-128, 130, 152, 158

Q

Quality 5, 23, 30, 39-40, 55, 133-134, 152, 183-184, 202-203, 205-211, 221, 247-248, 265, 271, 273, 288, 301, 317, 335

R

Repeated Administration 15-17
Resealed Erythrocytes 340-341, 345-348, 350, 352-355, 357
Retinoids 288, 294-296, 308
Rheumatoid Arthritis 23-24, 26, 98-100, 103-104, 115, 243, 385

S

Safety 2-5, 7-8, 14, 17, 25-27, 40, 62, 65, 103, 106, 161, 183, 202-203, 206, 211, 217, 232, 247, 287-290, 293, 297, 299-300, 302, 331
Somatic 53-54, 74-75, 246

T

Target 2, 6, 14-16, 23, 27, 32, 34, 54, 58, 62, 67, 70, 73, 98, 100-101, 106-107, 110-111, 113, 127, 129, 135-139, 141-142, 160, 214, 230-231, 244, 246, 297, 340-341, 347, 353-354
Therapeutic Window 2-4, 21, 32
Therapy 1-2, 6-7, 14-15, 21, 23-31, 35, 37-39, 52-53, 55-57, 59, 61-63, 65-67, 69-70, 75, 98-110, 112-114, 133, 145, 147-148, 150, 176, 181, 202-204, 231, 239, 242, 264-265, 271, 273, 287, 291, 293, 295, 302, 309, 323-324, 354-355, 389, 393
Traditional medicine 202-204, 215, 218, 229, 235
Type 1 Diabetes 23, 30, 368

V

Vitamins 160, 162, 168, 170, 180-181, 183, 204, 215, 244, 264-266, 278, 314, 317, 325, 333-334, 342, 353

W

Whitening 291, 308, 314

CPSIA information can be obtained
at www.ICGtesting.com
Printed in the USA
LVHW060156020721
691751LV00003B/3